Leadership and Management in Nursing

Anita W. Finkelman, MSN, RN

Senior Vice President for Nursing Operations
Orbis Education Services, Inc.

Adjunct Faculty
University of Oklahoma Health Sciences Center
College of Nursing

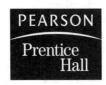

PEARSON
Prentice
Hall

Upper Saddle River, New Jersey 07458

Library of Congress Cataloging-in-Publication Data

Finkelman, Anita Ward.
    Leadership and management in nursing / Anita W. Finkelman.
        p. cm.
    Includes bibliographical references and index.
    ISBN 0-13-113869-3
    1. Nursing services—Administration. 2. Leadership. I. Title.
    RT89.F527 2006
    362.17'3'068—dc22

                                                    2005007483

Publisher: Julie Levin Alexander
Publisher's Assistant: Regina Bruno
Editor-in-Chief: Maura Connor
Acquisitions Editor: Pamela Fuller
Editorial Assistant: Aline Filippone
Director of Manufacturing and Production: Bruce Johnson
Managing Production Editor: Patrick Walsh
Production Liaison: Cathy O'Connell
Production Editor: Lynn Steines, Carlisle Publishing Services
Manufacturing Manager: Ilene Sanford
Manufacturing Buyer: Pat Brown
Design Director: Maria Guglielmo Walsh
Cover Designer: Amy Rosen
Interior Design: Carlisle Publishing Services
Director of Marketing: Karen Allman
Senior Marketing Manager: Frank Del Castillo
Marketing Coordinator: Michael Sirinides
Marketing Assistant: Patricia Linard
Associate Editor: Michael Giacobbe
Media Editor: John Jordan
Media Production Manager: Amy Peltier
Media Project Manager: Tina Rudowski
Composition: Carlisle Publishing Services
Printer/Binder: Banta/Harrisonburg
Cover Printer: Phoenix Color

Notice: Care has been taken to confirm the accuracy of information presented in this book. The authors, editors, and the publisher, however, cannot accept any responsibility for errors or omissions or for consequences from application of the information in this book and make no warranty, express or implied, with respect to its contents.

The authors and publisher have exerted every effort to ensure that drug selections and dosages set forth in this text are in accord with current recommendations and practice at time of publication. However, in view of ongoing research, changes in government regulations, and the constant flow of information relating to drug therapy and drug reactions, the reader is urged to check the package inserts of all drugs for any change in indications of dosage and for added warnings and precautions. This is particularly important when the recommended agent is a new and/or infrequently employed drug.

Pearson Prentice Hall™ is a trademark of Pearson Education, Inc.
Pearson® is a registered trademark of Pearson plc
Prentice Hall® is a registered trademark of Pearson Education, Inc.

Pearson Education Ltd.
Pearson Education Singapore, Pte. Ltd.
Pearson Education Canada, Ltd.
Pearson Education—Japan
Pearson Education Australia PTY, Limited

Pearson Education North Asia Ltd.
Pearson Educacíon de Mexico, S.A. de C.V.
Pearson Education Malaysia, Pte. Ltd.
Pearson Education, Upper Saddle River, New Jersey

10 9 8 7 6 5 4 3 2 1
ISBN: 0-13-113869-3

DEDICATION

To Fred, Shoshannah, and Deborah, my family. Nothing happens without their support and guidance.

CONTENTS

Nursing's Agenda for the Future (ANA, 2002) is an important document for the nursing profession. It describes the future vision of nursing in the following manner: "Nursing is *the* pivotal health care profession, highly valued for its specialized knowledge, skill and caring in improving the health status of the public and ensuring safe, effective, quality care. The profession mirrors the diverse population it serves and provides leadership to create positive changes in health policy and delivery systems. Individuals choose nursing as a career, and remain in the profession, because of the opportunities for personal and professional growth, supportive work environments and compensation commensurate with roles and responsibilities." This textbook uses the *Agenda for the Future* as its framework to address the critical issues that students will face during the transition to practicing nurse in a health care environment, an environment that increasingly expects nurses to be leaders.

Leadership and management are content areas included in all nursing programs; however, there is a great need to be current with the health care delivery system. This text provides opportunities for students to explore some of the current issues. New graduates usually do not serve in management positions immediately following graduation; however, they do need to demonstrate many leadership competencies, such as providing care, guiding others as team members and team leaders, communicating and collaborating with other health care professionals, and solving problems and making decisions to ensure that their patients receive quality, safe care. As new graduates become more involved in health care organizations they begin to participate in planning for the unit, on committees, and in other participatory opportunities, all of which require knowledge of the U.S. health care delivery system, health care organizations, nursing's roles in the delivery process, need to improve care, and what resources are needed to provide care effectively. Every nurse who strives to provide quality, safe care; continues to advocate for patients and their families; and strives to be recognized as a critical member of the health care team needs to demonstrate leadership.

Organization of This Textbook

This textbook is divided into eight sections, with each section focusing on one of the major domains described in *Nursing's Agenda for the Future*.

Section I Leadership and Planning focuses on introducing the student to the conceptual sis for leadership and management. Change, a critical issue today, and decision making are of un-Additional critical components of leadership are explored to allow the student an opportu ᶜ derstand the implications of collaboration, coordination, and conflict resolution᷉᷉er under- need to appreciate the need for effective communication and working relations᷉on the con-

Section II Delivery Systems/Nursing Models moves the student ᵗype of health standing of organizational structure that results in effective care deliv ᵃ understanding cepts introduced in Section I. More detailed information is provi ᶦᵒⁿ. Tools that are care organization, the acute care hospital, so that the new grad ᶜᵃˡ pathways, prac- of how this complex organization operates. Teams are emph ᵉˢues. Some nursing pro- used by many health care organizations to manage care d ᵗᵃⁿt for students to under- tice guidelines, and others, are discussed. ᵈ their practice. Health care

Section III Legislation/Regulation/Policy e ᵣˢtanding of their implications grams may have separate courses on these topic ᵐportant roles in policy making stand how these topics connect with leaders᷉ policy and legal and ethical issues are disc᷉ to practice. Consumers are included i᷉ and legal and ethical responses to᷉

Section IV Recruitment/Retention addresses the major concerns about the need to have qualified staff to provide care. Students need to understand this from the perspective of searching for their first nursing position and from the health care organization's perspective—how it needs to ensure that qualified staff are hired and maintained.

Section V Nursing/Professional Culture takes the focus of Section IV one step further and discusses two keys to professional success—career development and time management.

Section VI Economic Value approaches health care financial issues from the macrolevel or how health care is reimbursed, something that many students have little knowledge about but which still has a major impact on the nursing profession and nursing care, and the microlevel, which includes an introduction to some aspects of budgeting. It recognizes that new graduates do not typically get involved in this process but can benefit from understanding basic concepts and their effect on nursing care.

Section VII Work Environment focuses on two aspects of the health care work environment, technology and its impact and quality improvement and safety efforts from national, organizational, and professional perspectives.

Section VIII Diversity concludes the text. Diversity is explored from a variety of perspectives: patients, health care providers, healing environments, and the impact of the organization's culture. This domain from Nursing's Agenda for the Future recognizes that the health care organization of yesterday is a new organization today with complex needs. Nurses have major roles to play—each and every nurse needs to be a leader—to speak up for patients; to improve safe, quality care; and to provide input into responses to change that are present everyday in the health care delivery system and its multiple types of health care delivery organizations.

Features of the Textbook

This undergraduate textbook includes many teaching-learning features. It considers the needs of the student who now enters nursing with increased technology experience and who uses the computer daily. Each chapter includes the following features; some are found in the textbook, while others appear on the web. The text is available as a Flash e-Book, which is a new kind of textbook that combines the best elements of print and electronic media. Along with the print version of the text, students and faculty will have access to an online version of the text that is enhanced by a variety of multimedia elements, exercises, interactive quizzes, poll questions, and other activities to enhance learning.

Objectives—direct the reading and approach to the topic.

Exhibits and Figures—provide additional information or help to clarify content found in the chapter.

Test Your Understanding—allows the student to complete a short quiz to determine knowledge before beginning the chapter and highlights important themes. Feedback is provided to the student.

Benchmarks—allow the student to complete a short quiz at the end of each section within a chapter and provide a brief assessment of the student's knowledge of the material presented in the previous section. Feedback is provided to the student.

Current Issues—provide the student with examples from nursing literature, the Internet, and other sources that focus on current issues.

Your Opinion Counts—provides a poll question for students to respond to on the basis of material presented in the chapter. The focus is on opinion, and poll results from all students who may be currently using the text can be displayed.

Think Critically—provide interactive learning activities for students related to chapter content.

Summary and Applications—provide a variety of resources for the student: a chapter summary, ...ractice quiz with feedback, terms, additional learning activities, a case study, and Internet sites ...d to chapter content.

...ces and Additional Readings—provide references cited in the chapter and other refer-...may be of interest for further exploration of the topic.

...s Association. (2002). Nursing's agenda for the future. Washington, DC: American Nurses

ACKNOWLEDGMENTS

Projects like this one take time and certainly require support. My family deserves much of the credit for putting up with my endless writing projects. Carole Kenner, DNS, RNC, FAAN, Dean and Professor, University of Oklahoma Health Sciences Center, College of Nursing, continually provides professional support and friendship for which I will be forever grateful. Elizabeth Karle helped me design figures and found that piece of information I needed or lost and never found. To my colleagues who helped me formulate ideas when they did not even know they were helping, I offer my thanks. I thank members of the Prentice Hall team who have provided critical support for this project: Maura Connor, Pam Fuller and Lynn Steines.

Reviewers

Mary Louis Bost, DrPH, RN
Professor, Division of Nursing
Carlow College
Pittsburgh, PA

Darnell Cockram, EdD, RN, MSN, BSN
Educational Consultant
Danville Regional Medical Center
School of Nursing
Danville, VA

Janet Craig, RN, MSN, MBA, DHA
Assistant Professor
Clemson University
College of Health Education
Greenville, SC

Gloria Fowler, RN, MSN
Professor of Nursing
University of South Carolina
College of Nursing
Columbia, SC

Lucille Gambardella, PhD, RN, CS, APN-BC
Chair and Professor
Wesley College
Department of Nursing
Dover, DE

ABOUT THE AUTHOR

Anita W. Finkelman, MSN, RN, is Senior Vice President for Nursing Operations at Orbis Education Services, Inc. and Adjunct Faculty, University of Oklahoma Health Sciences Center, College of Nursing. She served as Director of Undergraduate Curriculum and Associate Professor/Clinical Nursing at the University of Cincinnati College of Nursing. She has a masters degree in psychiatric-mental health nursing from Yale University and post-masters graduate work in health care policy and administration from George Washington University. Additional work in the area of health policy was completed as a fellow of the Health Policy Institute, George Mason University. Ms. Finkelman's 35 years of nursing experience includes clinical, educational, and administrative positions. She has authored many books and journal articles and lectured on administration, health policy, continuing education, and psychiatric-mental health nursing, both nationally and internationally. She is a consultant to publishers and health care organizations and to a variety of educational institutions related to online course development. Other Prentice Hall publications include *Managed Care: A Nursing Perspective* (2001) and case studies in *Critical Thinking in Nursing: Case Studies Across the Continuum* (C. Green, Ed., 1999).

LEADERSHIP AND PLANNING

Leadership and planning are critical to the successful development and implementation of a strategic plan to achieve nursing's desired future state. Both are required to coordinate and monitor progress on the agenda, engage external stakeholders, and secure additional resources.

Desired Future Statement (Vision)

The nursing profession exhibits leadership through unified and systematic planning focused on the desired future state of the profession. This leadership behavior is driven by data/evidence and is implemented in a collaborative manner.

Four strategies are identified to achieve the vision and one of these is identified as the primary or driving strategy. They are:

Collaboration and accountability guide nursing in the development and implementation of its own plan: *Nursing's Agenda for the Future.* (Primary Strategy)

Unified commitment within nursing leads to success and a sense of shared accountability in accomplishing *Nursing's Agenda for the Future.*

Decision making and positive change are driven by reliable data.

Well-prepared nurse leaders assume positions of power and influence on key decision-making bodies throughout the profession and health care.

Objectives to Support the Primary Strategy

- Create a process that provides for ongoing communication, collaboration, support, and monitoring of the overall plan activities within the nursing community and among other health professions, the health care industry, and health care consumers.
- Influence public support and financial contributions to *Nursing's Agenda for the Future*, and direct those individuals and organizations working to support the plan to major funding sources.
- Maintain accountability for promoting and establishing a common focus within the nursing community and promote synergy of effort and resources, through utilization of a comprehensive plan to address staffing and shortage priorities: *Nursing's Agenda for the Future.*
- Develop clarity of purpose, roles, and process for the Call to the Nursing Profession Steering Committee.

SOURCE: American Nurses Association. (2002). *Nursing's agenda for the future. A call to the nation.* Washington, DC: Author. Reprinted with permission.

Conceptual Base for Leadership and Management

MediaLink
www.prenhall.com/finkelman

The Interactive Exercises for this chapter can be found in the OneKey course at www.prenhall.com/finkelman. Click on Chapter 1 to select from the following activities: Test Your Understanding, Benchmarks, Current Issues, Your Opinion Counts, Think Critically, and Summary and Applications.

What's Ahead

In the changing health care environment, nursing needs effective leaders who can understand change and take on opportunities as they arise. New graduates find that every nurse needs to be a leader—even nurses providing direct care. Sternweiler (1998) presents some interesting ideas about success in today's health care environment. Her motto is "be a willow tree." This unusual motto has relevance to many situations in which nurses find themselves today. Her comments focus on clinical specialists, but they also apply to all nurses. The first point she makes is that willow trees have many branches, and many branches are required to extend into all of the different areas in which nurses find themselves today. As new graduates begin to consider where they want to begin their practice of nursing, they are soon confronted with many wonderful choices. Many of these opportunities are clearly defined, while others are not. Willow trees also bend gracefully in the wind. This is a wonderful image of what nurses must do during change, which is a constant phenomenon today. Flexibility leads to more success than rigidity—the branch that refuses to bend often breaks. Willow trees have wide-reaching but shallow root systems. Uprooting deep, entrenched roots is much more painful than having an intricate, but shallow root system. Again, flexibility is the key to success during such a period. Each day brings a new piece of information, a new perspective, a new change, and a new challenge. All this requires nurses who are able to move thoughtfully with the changes. This image of nursing demonstrates that it is an exciting career, not a profession that does not change.

Nurse leaders, both formal and informal, need to set the stage for a positive approach to change and act as role models for staff; however, all nurses need to participate in making changes that improve care and the practice of nursing. Some of the key issues facing nurses today are:

1. The need to work together as a team, made all the more challenging as age differences and cultural diversity enrich the workforce and language and work ethics become more disparate.
2. Health care environments in which blame and punishment are practiced, even as those practices are disavowed on the surface.
3. Increasing pressure for results and less tolerance for mistakes. Burnout, anger, and other negative emotions still have a stronghold in many health care settings.
4. The need for greater creativity, collaboration, and learning, coupled with requirements for managers to do more with less.
5. The increasing press for successful recruitment and retention of current and future nursing personnel (Robinson-Walker, 2002, p. 148).

As leadership and management are explored in this chapter and throughout the text, many perspectives will be presented. Professional nurses need to open themselves up to a variety of ideas in order to arrive at a perspective of health care that enhances care delivery and the practice of nursing. This chapter discusses a variety of leadership and management theories and styles, nurse leadership, effectiveness, and managers. As nurses move through their careers some nurses will always provide direct care and yet still need to demonstrate leadership, some will decide to move into management positions and yet still need to demonstrate leadership, and then others may move back and forth between direct care and management positions. Being a nurse today requires leadership.

OBJECTIVES

Before you begin, take a moment to familiarize yourself with the key objectives of this chapter.

- Discuss the implications of change in the health care delivery system on nurse leadership.
- Describe key modern leadership theories.
- Compare and contrast leaders and managers.
- Discuss the importance of nurse leadership and its relationship to modern leadership theories.
- Explain the role of the clinical nurse as a leader and why it is important.

TEST YOUR UNDERSTANDING

Before we begin our exploration of this chapter, take a short "warm-up" test to see what you know about this topic.

Change in the Health Care Delivery System: Implications for Nurse Leadership

As new graduates enter the health care environment, they find an environment that seems to be constantly changing. It is easy to become frustrated with this as it is much easier to work when change is limited—one knows what to expect and when. However, the reality is not routine but instead requires health care organizations to cope with changes. Nurses must participate, too. What is meant by these changes that seem so important? Consider the examples of changes found in Box 1-1. Most students have observed most of these changing areas before they graduate.

This text includes content on all of these areas as they are important in understanding the nurse's role, as well as leadership and management. Chapter 2 specifically focuses on change and decision making. Porter-O'Grady closes his discussion on health care change by suggesting that, "Without engaging and embracing the issues around a new emerging foundation for nursing practice in the 21st century, it is quite possible that nurses will fail to find a meaningful place in the 21st century health service" (Porter-O'Grady, 2001, p. 186). This could be viewed as a pessimistic viewpoint, but it can also be viewed as a challenge to all nurses. Response will require leadership from all nurses.

To be successful in today's health care delivery system, a leader needs to actively pursue collaboration with peers and other health care professionals as well as reach outside of health care (for example, to consumers, local businesses, and local governmental agencies). Collaboration is "a dynamic transforming process of creating a power sharing partnership for pervasive application in health care practice, education, research, and organizational settings for the purposeful attention to needs and problems in order to achieve likely successful outcomes" (Sullivan, 1998,

BOX 1-1   A rapidly changing health care environment.

- New medical knowledge and technology
- Greater use of information technology
- Managed care and complex reimbursement system
- Greater use of a variety of settings where care is provided outside of acute care hospitals
- Increase in the uninsured and underinsured
- Greater diversity in patients and health care workforce
- Need to increase use of evidence-based practice
- Role changes (increasing use of unlicensed assistive personnel, and others) and implications for nursing roles and functions
- Use of advanced practice nurses, clinical nurse specialists, physician assistants, and hospitalists/intensivists
- Need for greater collaboration and interdisciplinary education and practice to prepare nurses and other health care professionals to work on interdisciplinary teams
- Greater importance of the consumer, the patient, and the patient's family
- Lack of health care policy or limited policy development in many areas, such as mental health, the uninsured, prescriptions for the elderly, chronic illness, and changing population demographics

p. 255). Collaboration requires that nurses work across professional boundaries, which has been difficult for them. Nurses need to work with physicians, social workers, pharmacists, physical therapists, admission staff, and many more. The meaning of collaboration implies the ability to be flexible, listen to others, include others, share information and ideas, and work toward the best solution to a problem. Nurses encounter many opportunities to collaborate every day. As theories of leadership and management are discussed and applied in this chapter's content, it is important to remember that collaboration is a key characteristic of effective leaders and managers. Collaboration is discussed in more detail in Chapter 3; however, collaboration is a critical component of effective leadership.

THINK CRITICALLY

Try this exercise to apply what you have learned about this topic.

Leadership and Management Theories and Styles

This section discusses modern leadership and management theories and styles. These theories and styles affect health care leaders and nurse leaders who work in all types of health care settings. One should not get the impression that only those who hold the highest nursing management position or other high management positions in health care organizations are necessarily nurse leaders. Nurse leaders do not even have to be in formal "management positions" with a management title. There are many more nurses who are in lower level "management positions," and if they demonstrate leadership competencies, they are considered nurse leaders (for example, nurse managers, charge nurses, team leaders, and others). All are important to the profession and to health care delivery. As leadership theories and styles are discussed in this chapter, it is noted that one can be a manager and yet not be a leader because to be a leader the manager must demonstrate leadership qualities and competencies, which include some competencies that are different from management competencies. Some staff are informal leaders and do not hold formal leadership positions. How this can occur will be discussed further in this chapter and in the remainder of the text. In the end, leadership competencies are something that every nurse should strive to reach. To do this, nurses need to have an understanding of relevant leadership and management theories and styles.

A historical perspective of leadership theories

There are many leadership theories and styles that have affected management and care delivery in health care organizations; however, it is important to understand some aspects of the history of leadership and the effects that some of the past theories and styles have had on modern theories. Typically, the theories of the past emphasized control, competition, and getting the job done. Creativity was not a critical part of past leadership theories. Leadership theories and styles have changed over time; some still apply and some do not, and some of them have been developed into modern theories. An historical review of the stages of leadership theory development indicates that there are four stages, which are highlighted in Box 1-2.

It is still possible to find leaders in health care organizations who use the theories that were developed in the first three stages; for example, there are still organizations that use the autocratic and bureaucratic approach to leadership and management as described in Box 1-3.

Modern or current leadership theories and styles

The modern or current leadership theories and styles have their base in earlier theories, but they have been developed as the needs of organizations have required different types of leaders and managers. Box 1-4 highlights the key theories and styles that are discussed in this section.

BOX 1-2   A review of the stages of leadership theory development.

Stage I *Leader Traits*

Emphasized up to the late 1940s. The theories tried to determine what personal qualities and characteristics were demonstrated by leaders. An important assumption with this approach was the belief that leaders were born rather than made. Many qualities and characteristics were examined during this time, and the conclusions served as the basis for other theories.

Stage II *Leadership Styles*

Began in the late 1940s and continued until the late 1960s. The emphasis was on training leaders, which was different from the earlier stage in which the emphasis was on the selection of leaders who innately had the required qualities. A critical concern was how to determine if someone was a leader prior to putting the person into a leadership position.

Stage II Focused on *Contingency Approach*

Began in the late 1960s and continued through the early 1980s. This approach examined all the situational factors surrounding leadership that might affect the effectiveness of different leadership approaches. What is happening in the environment and organization that might affect the leader?

Stage IV *New Leadership Approaches*

Began in the early 1980s and continues today. This stage is the focus in this text. Transformational Leadership, Charismatic Leadership, and Visionary Leadership, as well as others, have become more and more acceptable. There is increased interest in organizational culture and its effect on leadership as well as leadership's effect on organizational culture (Bryman, 2001).

BOX 1-3   What is autocratic, bureaucratic, and laissez-faire leadership?

What Is . . .

Autocratic (authoritarian, directive)

The leader makes decisions for the group and may do this by "simply issuing detailed orders and expecting them to be carried out automatically" (Curtin, 2001, p. 238). The leader assumes people are externally motivated and incapable of independent decision making. External motivators might be: salary and benefits or job security. Today, this style is most effective in emergencies (e.g., a fire on the unit or a cardiac arrest), when clear direction is required from one person. It is not as effective for long-term use.

Bureaucratic

The bureaucratic style is directly related to the autocratic style as the leader also presumes the group is externally motivated. The leader relies on organizational rules and policies, takes an inflexible approach, and gives directions, expecting them to be followed.

Laissez-faire (nondirective, permissive, ultraliberal)

The leader assumes the group is internally motivated by recognition, achievement, increased responsibility, and so on and needs autonomy and self-regulation. The leader uses a "hands-off" approach. This leadership style is directly opposite of autocratic and bureaucratic leadership as the leader allows staff to do as they please rather than telling them exactly what they must do. Sometimes this style can be too detached, resulting in no leadership and floundering staff. When staff on a patient care unit feel there is no real leadership or guidance, the nurse manager is probably using laissez-faire leadership, though the manager may not actually realize this is the approach.

BOX 1-4 Select modern leadership theories and styles.

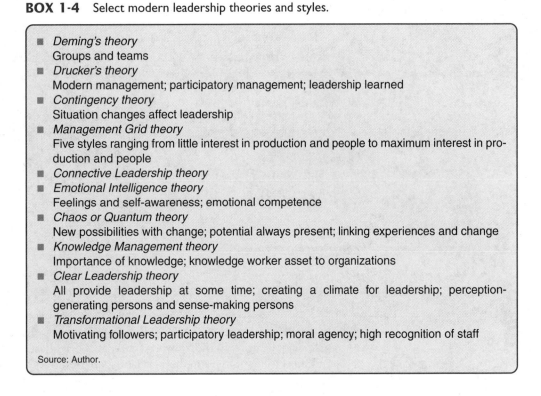

- *Deming's theory*
  Groups and teams
- *Drucker's theory*
  Modern management; participatory management; leadership learned
- *Contingency theory*
  Situation changes affect leadership
- *Management Grid theory*
  Five styles ranging from little interest in production and people to maximum interest in production and people
- *Connective Leadership theory*
- *Emotional Intelligence theory*
  Feelings and self-awareness; emotional competence
- *Chaos or Quantum theory*
  New possibilities with change; potential always present; linking experiences and change
- *Knowledge Management theory*
  Importance of knowledge; knowledge worker asset to organizations
- *Clear Leadership theory*
  All provide leadership at some time; creating a climate for leadership; perception-generating persons and sense-making persons
- *Transformational Leadership theory*
  Motivating followers; participatory leadership; moral agency; high recognition of staff

Source: Author.

Deming's theory

"The magic of Deming's management of leadership system is that it creates opportunities for management and staff to interact often. Personal interaction has the greatest potential for creating trust because it increases the likelihood of effective communication" (Crow, 2002, p. 10). Group or team work and team ownership of work are the focus in this theory. Despite the fact that Deming's approach was tried and successful in some U.S. businesses, it has had less of an immediate impact on health care organizations. Health care organizations still feature much centralized control, with upper management making many of the decisions rather than staff participation. There are, however, an increasing number of health care organizations that are slowly seeing the value of staff participation. Later leadership and management theories have included the need for greater staff participation.

Drucker's theory

Peter Drucker is considered to be the father of modern management (Porter-O'Grady & Finnegan, 1984). His view of management stimulated the shift toward the realization of the importance of participatory organizations, which is similar to Deming's approach. Drucker felt that staff should participate in as much of the planning and establishment of goals and decision making as possible. Individual autonomy is a critical part of this theory of management. Drucker believed that when staff participated in the core functions of management the organization would be more effective. For example, staff nurses should provide input into planning and changes that might be necessary on the unit, and nurse managers should seek out staff ideas and ask them to assist with planning. Drucker's theory includes the assumption that leadership can be learned. Leaders are not born, but rather staff can be nurtured to gain greater leadership competency. Clearly, this approach offers more opportunity to develop leaders and is important to nursing. Including leadership and management content in undergraduate education indicates that the nursing profession values leadership and recognizes the need to develop leadership and management competencies in students.

FIGURE 1-1 Contingency theory.

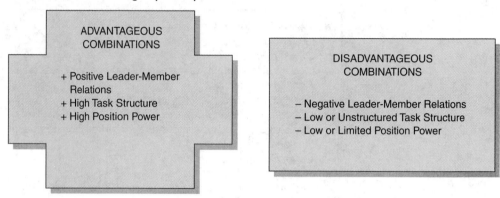

Contingency theory

In 1967, Fiedler developed the Contingency theory by focusing on the situational variables that affect the leader-member relationship, task structure, and position power (Fiedler, 1967; Huber, 2000).

1. The leader-member relationship variable describes the type and quality of the leader's personal relationships with the followers. This variable is affected by the amount of confidence and loyalty followers have in their leader (Grohar-Murray & DiCroce, 2003).
2. The task structure, the number of correct solutions to a given situational dilemma, focuses on the level of structure found in the group's task.
3. Position power, which addresses the power or amount of organizational support that the leader receives from the organization as a part of the position the leader holds, is critical to success.

Using these three major variables, Fiedler arrived at a number of combinations and identified which combinations were advantageous and which were disadvantageous to the organization and its leadership. These combinations are highlighted in Figure 1-1. He concluded that the best type of situation occurs when there are positive leader-member relations, high task structure, and high position power. Problematic situations are those in which the leader is disliked, "there is an unstructured task," and there is limited position power (Huber, 2000). Groups do change, which then changes the situational variables. Leadership, which is contingent on these variables, then must also change.

Management Grid theory

Another approach to understanding leadership is the Managerial Grid model (Porter-O'Grady & Finnegan, 1984). This model identifies five styles of leadership.

1. **Impoverished leadership.** In this style the leader has limited interest in production or people. Work requirements are established at a minimum level.
2. **Country club leadership.** This type of leader has an interest in people, and staff describe the leader as friendly and outgoing. Productivity, however, is not a major concern.
3. **Task leadership.** This type focuses on efficiency and getting the job done. This includes providing a work environment in which staff can be productive, but the leader has less concern for staff members as people.
4. **Team leadership.** This type of leader is very concerned about productivity and about the staff, morale, and satisfaction.
5. **Middle-of-the-road.** Using this style, the leader has a balanced approach with concern about productivity and efficiency as well as staff morale.

Another approach that is related to the Management Grid is the Leadership Grid, which was first described in 1964 to explore the relationship between leadership styles and how leaders respond to production and people. This theory was further developed in 1991 (Blake & McCanse, 1991; Milgram, Spector, & Treger, 1999). The Leadership Grid's two axes are concern for people and concern for production. Leaders are rated based on the level of concern that they have for each of these factors: people (staff, patients, families, co-workers) and products. The product in health care typically is referred to as the patient care that is provided to reach patient outcomes. The grid identifies a variety of leadership styles.

- The "cream puff" manager is a person who does not push for anything within the organization.
- The "do-gooder" manager is the manager who goes around taking care of staff in such a manner that it interferes with work.
- The "middle-of-the-road" manager approaches management so that just enough is done to balance staff needs and work needs, and performance is maintained at an adequate level.
- The "professional manager" is the manager who strives to develop the work team and is committed to the staff and the organization's need for production.
- The "paternalist manager" is the parent manager, rewarding and punishing staff as needed to improve production.
- The "opportunistic manager" changes management styles in order to get the most out of a situation and is particularly focused on self.

New graduates soon encounter managers who use a variety of leadership styles, some of which may have a major impact on how a new graduate adapts to the work environment and the nurse's roles.

Connective Leadership theory

Connective Leadership theory focuses on caring. Interconnectedness is a key element in health care today with the increasing emphasis on the continuum of services to meet the needs of patients and communities across the age span and different delivery settings. In this particular approach to leadership, the leader needs to promote collaboration and teamwork within the medical organization and among other organizations in the community. It recognizes that many groups exist within an organization and outside an organization that can affect leadership style. Connecting to others—individuals, groups, and organizations—leads to greater success. This viewpoint of leadership is incorporated in many of the current modern theories.

Emotional Intelligence theory

As leadership theory has moved toward considering the leader-follower relationship, theories have focused more and more on feelings and self-awareness, such as Goleman's theory of Emotional Intelligence (EI). Emotional competence is "a learning capability based on emotional intelligence that results in outstanding performance at work" (Goleman, 1998, p. 24). Emotional competencies are learning abilities or job skills that can be learned. A person has the potential to develop the necessary skills or required competencies (Goleman, 2001). This relates back to other theories that have been discussed that assume people can learn to be more effective leaders. Goleman identifies domains or dimensions that are important to Emotional Intelligence, which he calls clusters. Within each cluster there are identified competencies, which are highlighted in Box 1-5.

It might seem that all of these competencies stand alone; however, Goleman notes that they occur in groups, which is why they are described in clusters. Each competency is on a continuum in that an individual may perform the competency at different levels. As new graduates learn more about leadership and develop leadership competencies they can be found anywhere on the continuum. It takes time and support to learn about leadership. At some point an individual competency may reach what is called a "tipping point," which is when the individual excels in the competency (Goleman, 2001). For example, a team leader seems to have it all together—the team is functioning well; feedback is routinely given to team members by the team leader; team members are very active in planning and are able to speak up when they have concerns; team members support one another and feel the team leader will support the team; communication is clear—the work seems to flow.

BOX 1-5   EI: Clusters of competencies.

The Self-awareness Cluster

Understanding feelings and accurate self-assessment. Leaders recognize their own feelings and how they affect others and their performance. Self-assessment is important so that the leader can identify strengths and limitations. Leaders with these competencies try to find ways to improve, seek feedback, and actively learn from past experience. Self-confidence is a critical element in this cluster. It is easy to see how understanding oneself and using this information to improve oneself can lead to greater self-confidence.

The Self-management Cluster

Managing internal emotions, impulses, and resources. This cluster includes six competencies:

1. *Emotional self-control.* Most people have probably encountered persons who were in positions of authority and yet not able to handle their own emotions. Usually these leaders are described as ineffective leaders. Emotional self-control does not mean that the leader never expresses emotions but rather that the leader often expresses emotions appropriately.
2. *Trustworthiness.* "This competence translates into letting others know one's values and principles, intentions and feelings, and acting in ways that are consistent with them. Trustworthy individuals are forthright about their own mistakes and confront others about their lapses" (Goleman, 1998, p. 34).
3. Conscientiousness. This competency is demonstrated when the leader is careful, self-disciplined, and ensures that responsibilities are met.
4. *Adaptability.* This is a competence that really makes a difference in leaders today. Leaders with this competence are open to new ideas, search out challenges and opportunities, and use them to move forward. This is the leader who "thinks outside the box" and for whom a risk is not a barrier to moving forward.
5. *Achievement drive.* This is "an optimistic striving to continually improve performance" (Goleman, 1998, p. 35).
6. *Initiative.* People who take initiative act before they are found in situations where they may be forced to act. They are a step ahead at all times and seem to seek out opportunities before others are aware of them.

More nurse leaders who have these competencies are needed—leaders who can analyze a situation and create opportunities for nurses to expand their roles, improve staff roles, and develop leadership competencies, which will also improve patient care.

The Social Awareness Cluster

The focus is on reading people and groups accurately and includes three competencies.

1. *Empathy* or being aware of others' feelings, needs, and concerns. Self-awareness is required for successful empathy. Understanding oneself comes before understanding of others.
2. *Service orientation.* This is "the ability to identify a client's or a customer's often unstated needs and concerns and then match them to products or services" (Goleman, 2001, p. 36).
3. *Organizational awareness.* The leader is able to identify group feelings and organizational needs. This competence helps the leader to develop coalitions and to network. If a leader does not understand the feelings of others or their needs, it is difficult to get staff to work for the leader and the organization.

Relationship Management Cluster

This cluster focuses on inducing desirable responses and includes eight competencies.

1. *Developing others.* The leader knows when staff are ready for further development.
2. *Influence.* This is the ability of a leader to persuade others.
3. *Communication.* For leaders to be effective they need to have communication competence, the ability to communicate emotions and facts, listen, share information, and encourage sharing of information. In today's world information is a driving force in many work activities.
4. *Conflict management.* It is not easy to learn how to manage conflict, but leaders with emotional intelligence must develop this competence to be successful. Conflict management requires negotiation and the ability to see outside the box.
5. *Visionary leadership.* This is the leader who can develop a vision and includes staff in the vision for success.
6. *Change catalyst.* Leaders with Emotional Intelligence must see change as an opportunity, recognize barriers to change and remove them whenever possible, challenge the status quo, and involve as many of the staff as possible in the change process.
7. *Building bonds.* This competence assists the leader in finding ways to make connections with others, build trust, and recognize the importance of relationships.
8. *Collaboration and teamwork.* This competence depends on many of the earlier competencies that have been identified.

How does Emotional Intelligence leadership affect the organization's performance? This is an important question as there is no reason to continue with a leadership approach if it is not having a positive effect on the organization's staff and work. "The evidence suggests that emotionally intelligent leadership is key to creating a working climate that nurtures its employees and encourages them to do their best with enthusiasm, in turn this pays off in improved business performance" (Goleman, 2001, p. 40). Applying EI to leadership style requires that the leader demonstrate the EI competencies of self-confidence, empathy, change catalyst, and visionary leadership. "For jobs of all kinds, emotional intelligence is twice as important as a person's intelligence quotient and technical skills combined" (Strickland, 2000, p. 112). How smart a nurse is will not be as important as whether or not the nurse has, or is able to develop, critical EI competencies.

Much has been discussed about the positive aspects of EI leadership theory; however, caution needs to be exercised in connecting or applying Emotional Intelligence theory to workplace success even though it is very popular today (Vitello-Cicciu, 2002). New nurses typically need to develop at least some of the social and emotional competencies needed for effective performance in today's health care environment, and some new nurses demonstrate some of these competencies at the time of graduation. It still has not been proven that EI or the presence of emotional intelligence in leadership is a strong predictor of success. Tests to measure Emotional Intelligence have been developed, but many of these tests have been found to be less effective than had been hoped (Vitello-Cicciu, 2002). Many of the tests are self-assessment measures, which sometimes leads those who use them to respond in ways to impress others or what would be expected responses.

There is no doubt that nursing, as a "people-oriented" profession, is a profession in which emotional issues and responses are critical. It is also important for nurses to understand and manage their own emotions in an effective way. Nurse leadership is challenged to "create the climate for satisfied staff, patients, and their loved ones and diminish the degree of emotional labor which may cause burnout of nursing staff" (Vitello-Cicciu, 2002, p. 208). "Effective leadership is one of the most elusive keys to organizational success and yet it is the key ingredient to making any organization work. Leadership is also changing in nature" (Snow, 2001, p. 440). Those who support EI recognize that Emotionally Intelligent nurse leaders will bring the following to health care organizations.

1. Improved performance of nursing personnel
2. Improved retention of top talent
3. Improved teamwork among nurses
4. Increased motivation by team members
5. Enhanced innovation in the nursing group
6. Enhanced use of time and resources
7. Restored trust between nurses and their leaders (Snow, 2001, p. 443)

The outcome should be more satisfied patients, nurses, physicians, and families and a work environment that provides the best for all concerned—quality care, safe care, effective work environment, retention of staff, and an environment of improvement.

Chaos or quantum theory

Porter-O'Grady (1999) suggested that health care organizations have focused their organization and leadership approaches on Newtonian thinking, but what is needed is a change to a quantum thinking approach. "Classical Newtonian thinking reduces all complex things to a few simple rules that are absolute, unchanging, and stable. Quantum thinking sees that kinds of new possibilities emerge as a result of a combination of things. Everything has the potential to become more and different from that which it might be at any given time.... Everything is inextricably linked" (Porter-O'Grady, 1999, p. 37). Health care organizations in the past were able to rely on orderliness, following policies without considering options, viewing problems as having limited solutions, and creating clear lines of who reports to whom. This describes Newtonian thinking, which is no longer the reality. Problems and their solutions are not always clear, risk taking may be required, and mistakes will be made. Many factors affect how work is done and whether or not work processes need to be altered unexpectedly. Policies may not always be easily applied. Because of past experiences, health care managers have become quite good in using control, and many managers use it in such a way that staff do not complain about it. Neither of these approaches will result in positive outcomes in today's complex, changing environment where rigid approaches are not successful in the long run.

The relationship between people and management has also changed in the Quantum Age. As systems have become much more important, it is recognized that new forms of leadership are required. Creativity and health care worker knowledge are critical to the organization's success. Teams and partnerships continue to have a major impact on the organizational work. "The knowledge and authority essential to do great work needs to be located both where the work is done and within the roles of those who do it" (Porter-O'Grady, 1999, p. 38). **Accountability** needs to be in the hands of those doing the work, where there is more expertise. This is supported further by participative leadership, which is an important part of current leadership theories. All of these factors are integral parts of the Quantum Age.

To accomplish many of the needed changes in a health care organization's "chaos," a major role of the leader is to help staff adjust to new roles and strategies. What are some guidelines that leaders might use to address these new roles and strategies?

1. Leaders should not predict the future as no one really knows what the future may be.
2. Leaders need to be very sensitive to indicators of change and must respond when required.
3. The manager or leader should translate information so that it can be used to produce outcomes. With the increasing amount of information today, there is a critical need for analysis of information, which is related to the next theory, Knowledge Management (Porter-O'Grady, 1999, p. 39).

Knowledge Management theory

Sorrells-Jones (1999) noted that the emphasis on the knowledge worker, knowledge-intense organizations, interdisciplinary collaboration, and accountability found in the Information Age provides nurses with opportunities to improve and expand their practice.

Knowledge work is a combination of routine and non-routine knowledge-based work. Routine work (e.g., providing immunizations or other routine interventions or procedures) may require specialized knowledge that includes some level of predictability with anticipated probable outcomes. Non-routine knowledge work is full of exceptions, lacks predictability, requires interpretation and judgment, and may not be fully understood (e.g., altering care based on assessment data). Learning is an important component of knowledge work (Sorrells-Jones, 1999). Drucker (1993, 1994) first used the term *knowledge worker* when he described a person who works with both his or her hands and with theoretical knowledge. A knowledge-intense business organization is one in which 40% or more of the workers are knowledge workers (Sorrell-Jones, 1999). In this type of organization staff are the organization's knowledge assets or intellectual capital. Health care organizations meet the criteria for this type of organization.

This new age of knowledge requires workers who use information to produce knowledge, solve problems, and meet organizational goals (Weaver, 2001). Nurses should be viewed as knowledge workers, not laborers (Drucker, 1993). Today, a person's title is *not* the most important element; rather, it is the person's expertise in knowledge that is the critical element. As noted in EI theory however, some staff have "too much college, too little kindergarten" (Weaver, 2001, p. 82). This means that these staff may have expertise and knowledge, but they lack the insight that allows them to appreciate the impact of their behavior on other individuals. The latter represents a lack of kindergarten skills (for example, a sense of fair play, commitment to collaboration, willingness to share the limelight, and a growing sense of self that considers one's strengths and weaknesses). In addition, these skills are critical for the development of team effectiveness. It may not always be easy to clearly predict what may be the result when problem solving, which means that a person or team must be willing to take risks (Weaver, 2001). It is important to remember that when staff take a risk when making a decision there is some probability of loss. Therefore, the risk taker must work to decrease this probability (Milstead, 2004). It is, however, not always possible to have time to assess a situation to its fullest nor is it always possible to recognize all possible solutions to a problem. These factors can make risk taking difficult but should not eliminate the need for taking risks in some situations.

What does the manager in a knowledge-work environment do when the manager is no longer expected to tell staff what to do? This new manager brings people together with different knowledge bases in order to reach the most effective performance. The focus is on developing the most effective teams, leading change initiatives, coaching teams, providing performance expectations, helping knowledge workers (e.g., RNs) and knowledge work teams (e.g., care team) self-regulate themselves, teaching the team to use systematic decision making, and encouraging an attitude of continuous improvement (Mohrman & Mohrman, 1997). Knowledge-based managers must be leaders who are facilitators and integrators. They support diverse team members who work toward reaching a common goal. No single staff member can know everything that is required for practice today, and so the interdisciplinary team becomes the focus.

An important goal today is the development of staff so that they become the health care organization (Weaver & Sorrells-Jones, 1999). Team members should be viewed as assets; they are valuable to the team and the organization. A major goal is to maximize team member efficiency. It is important to decrease the time that team members spend doing functions and tasks that are not as important or, if they are professionals, functions that are not critical professional tasks. Examples of these are: (a) RNs transporting patients, (b) RNs completing paperwork that does not require professional competencies, and (c) RNs searching for equipment or needed supplies. RNs are team members who are knowledge assets due to their special knowledge and skills (Bahrami, 1992; Hammer, 1997; Weaver & Sorrells-Jones, 1999).

Clear Leadership theory

In Bushe's theory of Clear Leadership (2001) everyone provides leadership at some time. Staff switch back and forth between being leaders and followers. The history of organizations indicates that everyone can be a leader, though it usually takes time to develop leadership competencies. Clear Leadership occurs when "leaders create a climate in which people are willing to express their own truth and listen to other people's truth, where working together is based on accurate understanding, not assumptions" (Bushe, 2001, p. 2). When a manager and staff really listen to one another and consider what is being said, then active listening is present. This is critical for Clear Leadership.

In this approach to leadership, a critical factor is "Interpersonal Mush," which "occurs when people's understanding of each other is based on fantasies and stories they have made up about one another" (Bushe, 2001, p. 5). How does this "Interpersonal Mush" get in the way of work and productivity? For example, a team leader may think that the team members really do not like him or her based on negative feedback that was overheard. The team leader did not hear the entire conversation and then filled in what the leader thought might have been going on when in reality this negative viewpoint was not correct. If this "Interpersonal Mush" then affects how the leader approaches team members and he or she never openly discusses the issue with the members to discover the truth, this will interfere with effective leading. This is "Interpersonal Mush." Willingness to tell the truth about experiences and learn from them is critical for success in the newer approaches to management. Leaders need to be clear about themselves—who they are, their strengths and weaknesses—and know what should be taken on and when to pull back. Clear Leadership is a theory that also is closely related to EI theory with its concern about feelings, how people relate to one another, collaboration, and partnership.

Clear Leadership is based on two critical principles (Bushe, 2001):

1. Perception-generation is a process that is used constantly. Another term for this is the person's experience, which is made up of the percepts that a person generates and the person's reaction to these percepts. However, to be "interpersonally skillful you must give up the idea that what you believe you saw or heard is always the truth . . . treat your perceptions as hypotheses that always require further investigation and updating" (Bushe, 2001, p. 7). Each person's experience is not what happens to that person but rather the person's reaction to the experience.
2. Sense-making is also a key human process. "When we make sense we explain our perceptions within the framework that provides consistency and meaning to what we are perceiving" (Bushe, 2001, p. 8). It is like making up a story about the experience. Other aspects of Clear Leadership are highlighted in Box 1-6.

BOX 1-6   Clear leadership.

Self-awareness

The person as an Aware Self knows what she/he is thinking, feeling, observing, and wanting. This leader is aware of facts and what is sense-making. Some organizations have used the Myers-Briggs Type Indicator assessment (MBTI) to help staff gain a better understanding of their preferred styles of interaction and temperament, learning styles, and problem solving. It functions as a tool to help individuals in organizations: (a) understand themselves and their behaviors, (b) recognize differences in others so as to make constructive use of their contributions, and (c) value different ways in approaching problems, recognizing that the organization will be healthier and more productive over time.

Descriptiveness

The Descriptive Self focuses on the ability to help other people empathize with oneself. When someone uses descriptiveness as a leader the person is able to describe experiences clearly, including difficult, confrontational experiences, in a manner that is not defensive but causes others to listen and understand.

Curiosity

A leader who is using the Curious Self is able to get other people to be descriptive. Others feel comfortable telling this leader the truth about an experience, and the leader is able to use observations and questions to get to the truth.

Appreciation

The Appreciative Self uses imagination and conversation to recognize the best in people and processes/relationships.

CURRENT ISSUES

Learn about events around the globe that relate to the chapter content.

Clear Leadership focuses on humility. This means that leaders accept that it is not about them, but rather "A person provides leadership when they do something that helps a group or organization achieve its goals or increase its effectiveness" (Bushe, 2001, p. 11). If this is the case, who is a leader? The leader may very well be an informal leader. It is important to recognize that not everyone in a formal leadership/management position is a leader. Most people have experienced working for someone who was not a leader—"Leaders" who are never seen; appear in a crisis and fade into the woodwork; isolate themselves; send down dictums with little staff input; ask for staff input and then ignore it; hire people as their implementers who also have limited leadership skills or qualities; and so on. There seems to be a lot of this type of leadership in health care. Bushe (2001) suggests that the approach of Clear Leadership attempts to eliminate "Interpersonal Mush" and creates a climate in which people can feel free to:

■ Say what they really mean
■ Truly agree on goals and plans
■ Genuinely pull together as teams
■ Learn effectively

Applying Clear Leadership approaches assists teams in solving problems, making decisions, dealing with conflict, assessing performance, serving consumers, and managing change.

Transformational Leadership theory

Burns' theory of leadership incorporates central aspects found in EI, Chaos theory, Knowledge Management, Clear Leadership, and Contingency theory (1985). There are two major types of leaders, the Transactional Leader and the Transformational Leader (Curtin, 2001). The first, the Transactional Leader, is the most common type of leader found in health care organizations today, though this is changing in many health care organizations to Transformational Leadership, which is much more applicable in today's dynamic health care system. Some leaders may use both types of leadership depending on their needs. "The transforming leader looks for potential motives in followers, seeks to satisfy the needs and engages the full person of the followers. The result of transforming leadership is a relationship of mutual stimulation and elevation that converts followers into leaders and leaders into moral agents" (Curtin, 2001, p. 239). In addition, Burns emphasizes the importance of morals and ethics, which is particularly relevant to leaders who are also members of a profession that must meet professional ethical codes (Curtin & Falherty, 1993 p. 64).

1. What is Transformational Leadership?

Transformational Leadership is a theory that focuses on the need for leaders who are willing to embrace change, reward staff, guide staff in understanding their role within the organization and the importance of the organization or a positive work environment, and work toward developing a self-aware staff who are able to take risks to improve. This does not mean that the Transformational Leader is not concerned with the critical organizational functions that are required to get the work done that are emphasized in Transactional Leadership; however, the Transformational Leader begins with a vision. What is meant by a vision? A vision is a view of the organization in the future. What could the organization be? A mission statement, supporting the vision, describes the organization's purpose and the current position of the organization. Why is it so important to have a vision? The vision allows the organization, its leaders or managers and staff, to look into the future, based on reasonable facts and experience, and to use this vision to become involved in opportunities to improve.

2. Why did Transformational Leadership develop?

The key reason for the development of Transformational Leadership is change (Sullivan, 1998). "Transformational leadership has been suggested in the literature as a leadership model that best fits with the changing health care environment" (Bass & Avolio, 1997; as cited in Ohman, 1999, p. 16; Medley & Larochelle, 1985). As the health care system began to experience extreme and frequent change, it found that its leadership styles were not working in the chaotic change atmosphere. To cope, organizations needed the skills and knowledge of a greater number of the staff. The leader also needed to be ahead of the change as much as possible. This required vision, creativity, and new leadership styles that empower staff. These leaders typically exhibit both Transformational and Transactional Leadership; however, transformational is usually more predominant (Bass, 1998; Dunham-Taylor, 2000). As has been discussed, the characteristics described as part of Transformational Leadership are also focused in the theories of Clear Leadership, EI, Chaos theory, and Knowledge Management.

3. What are the qualities of a Transformational Leader?

Qualities that have been identified in Transformation Leaders are self-confidence, self-direction, honesty, energy, loyalty, commitment, and the ability to develop and implement a vision. Empowerment is an important component of Transformational Leadership. The more power the leader gives to staff, the more power the leader will gain (Fullan, Lando, Johansen, Reyes, & Szaloczy, 1998). The Transformational Leader who has these qualities is a "leader who motivates followers to perform to their full potential over time by influencing a change in perceptions and by providing a sense of direction. Transformational Leaders use charisma, individualized consideration, and intellectual stimulation to produce greater effort, effectiveness, and satisfaction and followers" (Huber, 2000, p. 65). This is different from a Transactional Leader who is "a leader or manager who functions in a caretaker role and is focused on day-to-day operations. Such leaders survey their followers' needs and set goals for them based on what can be expected from the followers" (Huber, 2000, p. 65). This leader is essential to any organization and works to produce the expected outcomes (Huber, 2000).

BOX 1-7 Transformational leadership errors.

- Lack of a sense of urgency
- Lack of a guiding coalition
- Lack of a vision
- Lack of communication about the vision
- Lack of removals of barriers to the vision
- Lack of systematic planning
- Declaring a victory too soon
- Lack of recognition of organization culture

4. Is Transformational Leadership always successful in all organizations?
It is not always successful, and when it fails, it is usually related to one of the errors that are highlighted in Box 1-7 (Kotter, 1995).

THINK CRITICALLY

Try this exercise to apply what you have learned about this topic.

A conclusion: Effective leadership

It is not easy to describe effective leadership. There is certainly no magic formula that will guarantee effective leadership. As noted in the previous discussion of leadership theories and styles, effective leaders have vision, influence, and power. The vision of the future guides the leader in making day-to-day decisions. Leaders use influence, which is the informal strategy of cooperation combined with formal authority of a position to develop trust. The leader needs to be persuasive and use productive communication. Power enables the leader to influence others, and by doing this, the leader can change staff attitudes and behavior, hopefully moving toward meeting expected outcomes.

Values, the importance that is attached to something that guides action, are more important today in understanding effective leadership. An example of the impact of values is found in health care organizations that focus on the bottom line, cutting costs with little concern about the effect this has on the quality of care. This communicates a particular value to their staff, patients, and community. Health care organizations, however, that communicate the importance of a caring environment where the highest quality care is provided to individual patients are communicating a different value. Leaders of these two types of organizations are actively involved in communicating critical values, though very different ones. The leader in the first type of organization focuses more on financial issues and is less willing to listen to staff concerns about the quality of care unless it has a major impact on costs. The leader in the second type of organization is more willing to look at the total care picture, listen to staff, and look for opportunities to improve care, but does not forget the need to monitor costs. Understanding a leader's values is critical to understanding how that leader might function in an organization and how the organization's values might mesh or collide with the leader's values, which has an impact on the effectiveness of leadership.

BENCHMARKS

Now let's take a moment to test your knowledge of the concepts you have studied in this section.

Leaders and Managers: A Comparison

Leadership and management are not the same. It is important to understand how these compare and recognize that the goal is really to have managers who are also leaders. The key functions of management are

- Planning
- Organizing
- Leading
- Controlling

There is no doubt, however, that leadership plays a critical role in management. In fact, a successful manager exhibits leadership qualities. The key difference between managers and leaders is that managers typically focus on managing or maintaining equilibrium, whereas leaders are focused more on change. Most people think of management as a particular position, and this is true. Leadership, however, does not require a specific position. Nursing requires management, but nursing also needs leadership. What are some examples of the differences between a leader and a manager? What does it mean for a person to inspire others as a leader? The leader communicates to staff the importance of staff contributions and recognizes staff members' successes. In doing so, the staff member is motivated to continue to improve and to be effective. Leaders are also persuasive in that they are able to convince others to make changes and to improve. Through the leader's influence care can be improved, and the work situation can become more productive. Leaders ask questions, take risks, and are challenged by change. In contrast, managers are typically less able to handle unstable or non-routine situations. Managers who develop leadership competencies are more effective and handle non-routine situations better.

With a greater understanding of leadership, it is important to consider how leaders and managers are compared and contrasted. "There is a profound difference—a chasm—between leaders and managers. A good manager does things right. A leader does the right thing" (Bennis & Goldsmith, 1997). The following descriptions provide examples of some of the differences.

- Leaders conquer the context always going on around them while managers surrender to it.
- Leaders assess reality, identify critical factors, and use analysis while managers accept the truth from others with few questions.
- Leaders focus on effectiveness; managers focus on efficiency.
- Leaders focus on what and why; managers focus on how.
- Leaders innovate and initiate; managers copy and keep the status quo.
- Leaders empower, compel others with their creative vision, and translate that vision into action; managers are less concerned with empowerment and vision.
- The manager administers; the leader innovates.
- The manager is a copy; the leader is an original.
- The manager maintains; the leader develops.
- The manager accepts reality; the leader investigates it.
- The manager focuses on systems and structure; the leader focuses on people.
- The manager relies on control; the leader inspires trust.
- The manager has a short-range view; the leader has a long-range perspective.
- The manager asks how and when; the leader asks what and why.
- The manager has his or her eye always on the bottom line; the leader has his or her eye on the horizon.
- The manager imitates; the leader originates.
- The manager accepts the status quo; the leader challenges it.
- The manager is a classic good soldier; the leader is his or her own person (Bennis & Goldsmith, 1997, pp. 4, 9–10).

Leaders gain their authority from their ability to influence others to get the work done; because of this, anyone has the potential to be a leader. A manager's authority comes from the manager's position in the organization, such as a team leader, nurse manager, assistant director of nursing, or vice president of nursing. There is no doubt that managers are different in not only what they do but also in how they do their work, staff roles, and authority.

Since the main goal of leadership is to have staff achieve their best, leaders cannot ignore quality and practice improvement (Heller, 1999). To be successful as a leader, leaders commit to lifelong learning and improvement. They also encourage staff to pursue lifelong learning goals and serve as coaches and mentors. This should help to reach the goal of improving care. Flexibility is a key factor in leadership. This is demonstrated when leaders must plan and respond to problems as well as work with others to achieve goals. This requires knowledge.

What are the key leadership roles?

1. **Expert.** An expert has an in-depth understanding of a particular topic or function. An expert will strive toward the best performance.
2. **Administrator.** The leader makes sure that the organization, unit, or service operates effectively. In this role, the leader looks for ways to improve efficiency and provides the framework for practice, such as policies and procedures, guidelines, values, systems, and other necessary rules, to get the job done.
3. **People person.** In this role the leader ensures that staff have the training and education to meet the performance requirements. In addition, the leader strives to provide a work environment in which staff feel comfortable to share information and their opinions and are willing to work as a group.
4. **Strategist or planning for the future.** The leader also takes on the role of change agent. In this role the leader strives to make the most of change to improve the organization, even taking risks to accomplish effective change.

If one rereads these descriptions of the roles, "manager" could be substituted for "leader" *if* the manager demonstrated leadership qualities.

In comparison, the focus of management is "the coordination and integration of resources through planning, organizing, coordinating, directing, and controlling to accomplish specific institutional goals and objectives" (Huber, 2000, p. 52). An overlap of management and leadership is found in the need for broad-perspective decision making, communication, and motivation of followers. Even management is changing, as managers today need management skills that:

- Change focus from process to outcomes
- Align role to information infrastructure rather than functional performance
- Focus on team results rather than individual performance
- Manage data complexes rather than individual events
- Facilitate resources that then direct work
- Transfer skill-sets rather than make decisions for staff
- Develop staff self-direction rather than giving direction
- Focus on obtaining value rather than simply finding costs
- Focus on consumer-driven structure rather than provider-based system
- Construct horizontal relationships rather than maintain vertical control mechanisms
- Facilitate equity-based partnerships rather than control individual behaviors (Porter-O'Grady, 1999, p. 40)

It is easy to assume that leaders can do it all. This is a myth. There are other myths about leadership, some of which are described in Box 1-8.

What are some differences between the nurse manager and the nurse leader (Laurent, 2000)? Registered nurses are clearly trained to manage patient care. The term *management* is used frequently in nursing. "Nursing managers are successful because of one word, control. Managers control their environment, things can be controlled, and patient care is manipulated or managed. In this process nurses learn about crisis management or how to re-establish control" (Laurent, 2000, p. 84). This has worked to nursing's benefit; however, the first step in moving from a

BOX 1-8 Myths about leadership.

There are many popular myths about leadership. Goffee and Jones (2000) identified some of these myths.

- *Everyone can be a leader.* This is not true. Everyone may have the potential to be a leader; however, the person needs to develop certain leadership competencies such as self-knowledge or authenticity to be a leader.
- *Leaders deliver business results.* They do not always deliver the desired outcomes.
- *People who get to the top are leaders.* This is not true as many people in management are not leaders and have limited leadership qualities. A manager may or may not also demonstrate leadership qualities and competencies.
- *Leaders are great coaches.* They are not always great coaches, as leaders cannot always share important technical skills while at the same time inspire staff.

nurse manager to a nurse manager who is also a leader is to give up this control. This is not always easy for new nurse managers to do, and many experienced nurse managers also have problems giving up control and allowing staff to participate more in decision making and planning.

THINK CRITICALLY

Try this exercise to apply what you have learned about this topic.

Who is a nurse leader?

To develop a fuller understanding of nurse leadership and the need to "step outside the box," it is important to have an appreciation of the following:

1. Where nursing leadership came from
2. Where nursing leadership is today
3. How nursing might be affected by leadership and management theories and styles

The manager's job is to accomplish the work of the organization. This is true regardless of the type of organization such as acute care hospital, home care agency, long-term care organization, clinic or a hospital unit, and so on. Manager roles and functions vary with the type of organization and the level of management. Typically, management is viewed from three levels: first-level, middle-level, and upper-level managers. First-level managers focus on managing the work of non-managerial staff or on the day-to-day activities of a specific work group. Examples of first-level managers are nurse managers and charge nurses. Middle-level managers focus on supervising several first-level managers. Examples of middle-level managers are a director of surgical services or women's health and a night supervisor. These managers also serve as liaisons between first-level managers and upper-level managers. The upper-level managers are responsible for establishing goals and strategic plans for the organization. They are the organization's executives and top administrators. Examples of upper-level managers are a nurse executive, vice president of patient services, chief executive officer, and medical director. Not all organizations have all three levels.

What is the historical development of the "nurse leader" in health care organizations (Ulrich, 2001)? The nurse leader in acute care settings was first called the director of nursing (DON). The DON focused on nursing care in hospitals and had limited interaction with hospital administration about planning. The DON had little idea about the budget and did not seem particularly interested in it. These positions were held for many years with very low turnover rates. Early on few of these nurses had advanced degrees. In the late 1970s and early 1980s, as the DON's power began to increase, some hospitals began to change the DON title to vice president of nursing, but the focus was still on nursing. In these cases, more of these nurses had advanced degrees.

Slowly, this nurse leader began to interact more with hospital administration and to assume more responsibility for the nursing department's planning and budget. The next step in title changes was the move to vice president of patient services. This was a significant change as it recognized that the nurse leader had the ability to have an impact on broader patient care issues, not just nursing. The nurse leader is responsible for nursing care, other clinical delivery services, and sometimes covers support services such as medical records. Health care organizations continue to vary in their views of the nurse leader. The last example of a vice president for patient services is not found in every acute care setting, but it is increasing.

In addition, more nurses are now moving into overall administration positions in health care settings such as acute care hospitals, home care, long-term care, and ambulatory care. When nurses hold the positions of chief executive officer (CEO) or chief operating officer (COO), they have reached the point where they oversee the entire health care organization. How did this happen? Some nurse leaders have clearly demonstrated to health care organizations that they can handle these responsibilities. In addition, many of the values that are important to nursing have become more important in health care in general (e.g., caring, respect for the patient, and identification and evaluation of outcomes). When nurses move into these higher positions they bring these values with them; however, to be successful these nurses also need to be competent in all of the administrative tasks that are involved in these high-level positions. Twenty-one key competencies for health care professionals in the 21st century have been identified. These competencies, which indicate that leadership is a key competency needed in health care professionals today, are identified in Box 1-9.

Preparation and development of nurse managers

The nurse manager role

Nurse managers are directly responsible for maintaining standards of care, managing fiscal resources, and developing staff. Some of the titles for this middle management position include "nurse manager," "head nurse," "nursing unit manager," and "nursing or nurse coordinator."

BOX 1-9   Health care professional competencies for the 21st century.

- Embrace a personal ethic of social responsibility and service.
- Exhibit ethical behavior in all professional activities.
- Provide evidence-based, clinically competent care.
- Incorporate the multiple determinants of health in clinical care.
- Apply knowledge of the new sciences.
- Demonstrate critical thinking, reflection, and problem-solving skills.
- Understand the role of primary care.
- Rigorously practice preventive health care.
- Integrate population-based care and services into practice.
- Improve access to health care for those with unmet health needs.
- Practice relationship-centered care with individuals and families.
- Provide culturally sensitive care to a diverse society.
- Partner with communities in health care decisions.
- Use communication and information technology effectively and appropriately.
- Work in interdisciplinary teams.
- Ensure care that balances individual, professional, system, and societal needs.
- Practice leadership.
- Take responsibility for quality care and health outcomes at all levels.
- Contribute to continuous improvement of the health care system.
- Advocate for public policy that promotes and protects the health of the public.
- Continue to learn and help others learn.

Nurse manager responsibilities vary from organization to organization. Some positions focus more on management and others more on clinical care. "Nurse managers are internal stakeholders who play essential roles in managing change, cultural integration, retention, and direction of staff attitudes toward changing health care structures" (Mathena, 2002, p. 136). Many nurse managers are not prepared to deal with staff stress, low morale, staff uncertainty, and turnover, all of which are common problems today (Singleton & Nail-Hall, 1995). Nurse managers who are also leaders will be involved in visioning, interdisciplinary team building, workload and work process analysis, stakeholder analysis, and interactive planning (Mathena, 2002). Critical competencies to accomplish these activities include:

- Directing others
- Group management
- Interpersonal sensitivity
- Self-confidence
- Use of influence strategies
- Analytical thinking
- Initiative
- Achievement orientation
- Direct persuasion

The Peter Principle

The **Peter Principle** (Peter & Hull, 1969) describes a major leadership and management problem in bureaucratic organizations (Milgram, Spector, & Treger, 1999). The problem occurs when staff are promoted for doing a good job with their assigned tasks; however, as they climb up the hierarchical ladder, they eventually are promoted to a position for which they are not competent. An example is the staff nurse who provides quality care and is considered to be an expert clinician who is then promoted to a management position. It is assumed that because the nurse is an expert clinician that he or she will be an effective manager. This is not necessarily the case, and even if the nurse has the potential to be an effective manager he or she would still need to develop additional leadership and management competencies. The danger of this type of promotion is that demotion is not something that is done very easily. Typically, the staff member stays in the position though the staff member may be incompetent as a manager and a leader. The reward system in nursing has typically been to reward good clinical staff with a management position, which has led to problems and is an example of the Peter Principle.

Nurse management development

Hill (1993) conducted long-term surveys of new managers in businesses and was able to identify many needs and concerns of the new managers that can also be applied to nursing. The most difficult task for these new managers was developing interpersonal skills. Many of the current theories that have been discussed, such as EI, Clear Leadership, and Transformational Leadership, emphasize the importance of interpersonal skills. Development of self-awareness and personal growth are clearly the most challenging experience for staff nurses who move into a manager role. How do managers change? Typically, they learn slowly over time, and they are not always aware of what they are learning. Most managers seem to learn on the job with limited formal training or education in management; however, formal training and education in management makes the transition to the position much easier. This is just as true in health care organizations as it is in other types of businesses.

In one study of nurse managers (Mathena, 2002) the managers felt that they needed further education to develop financial management competency and technical skills such as data analysis. Even though nurse managers recognized the importance of communication skills they did not rank it as high. The health care environment with its increased interest in reducing health care costs is probably a major reason for identifying the need for more financial information by managers, who are typically responsible for their unit's budget. There is no doubt that nurse managers who have an understanding of budgets and costs will be more effective.

Management development is a long-term self-learning process, as was noted in Hill's study of business managers. As the manager learns, it is important for the manager to receive feedback and guidance. "Adopting attitudes and a psychological perspective consistent with their new role can be even more demanding" (Hill, 1993, p. 155). A manager needs to actively use introspection, which requires much adaptation. New managers often have many misconceptions about management and about themselves. The most important guideline for leadership success is the importance of using self-learning. Having access to peers for discussion and feedback assists the manager when new tasks and responsibilities are learned.

New managers need mentors and coaches. Ideally, the new manager's supervisor should form a relationship with the new manager that encourages feedback and open discussion. The supervisor may need to reach out first to the new manager, as it may be difficult for the new manager to ask for help. When managers gain interpersonal judgment this increases self-confidence and self-assurance. They are then more able to delegate and give up some control. To do this, new managers need to learn how to listen before making rapid decisions and consider factors that affect decisions and delegation. New managers often first adopt a hands-on **autocratic** approach to management because they want to influence results. When they do this, they appear to be very directive. However, despite the fact that they really are directive, when new managers are asked to describe their management style, they typically describe it as consultative rather than authoritative. Over time new managers discover the limits of their formal authority. They may give staff directions, but that does not mean staff will follow them. It is at this point that the manager learns about the need for persuasion. When managers finally learn that staff are more motivated when they can offer their own reactions and input into decisions, managers experience greater success.

Hill also identified concerns that new managers have about the process of administration. Managers often define "administration as routine communication activities such as paperwork and exchange of information. . . . Their administrative responsibilities seemed to be constraints that interfered with their autonomy and stole precious time for more important responsibilities" (Hill, 1993, p. 24). Nurse managers also often experience this concern when they try to do their jobs and examine quality of care and requests from higher management (administration) that demand certain responses. They must work with multiple disruptions, which is probably different from the managers that Hill followed. Interdisciplinary issues also make the management process more complex.

Nurse managers work in complex health care environments just as the managers in Hill's study worked in complex organizations. Working in complex environments, whether health care or business, implies that the following are part of the leadership/management process.

1. Leaders manage not simply by directive, but by persuasion, motivation, and empowerment; they identify and gain commitment to an exciting or challenging vision.
2. Leaders manage not only individual performance, but also group performance; as a way of exercising authority, they create the appropriate organizational context (Hill, 1993, p. 111).

To accomplish this, managers need to remember that actions speak louder than words. Managers need to establish a culture of high standards and openness, and empower or share power with their staff.

Nurse manager competencies

As has been discussed, the best managers are also leaders. Key skills and competencies that assist managers are:

- Critical thinking—Verbs that can be used to describe the critical thinking skills required for managers are: evaluate, select, analyze, utilize, consider, align, proactive, plan, think, recognize, and predict. All of these are active verbs. Critical thinking requires an active stance rather than a passive one (Child, Lingle, & Watson, 2001).
- Communication skills
- Networking
- Managing resources (e.g., budgeting, staffing)
- Enhancing employee performance (e.g., mentoring)

- Team-building
- Evaluating effectiveness and efficiency
- Delegating
- Clinical and organizational expertise
- Flexibility
- Collaboration (multidisciplinary)
- Coordination
- Outcome oriented
- Problem solving
- Evaluation and analysis

In fact, these skills are important for every RN, and this is one reason why this content is important for all nursing students. It is easy to say, "I am not going to be a manager," but many management skills as well as leadership skills are required in the daily practice of every RN.

A key job of a manager is to make sure that the staff understand instructions and that these instructions are carried out effectively. In doing this, the manager is exercising authority. The manager establishes an environment in which the staff understand that it is acceptable to identify problems and to speak out when their performance has not been as effective as possible. Staff should not fear that they will be reprimanded and should feel that they can trust their manager rather than be concerned about negative outcomes.

Caring and trust

Managers who are leaders need to care for their staff. What does this mean? This means that the manager listens to staff, recognizes when staff need special support and guidance, and takes time to respond to the staff. There are times when staff lack confidence, and it is then the role of the manager to help increase staff confidence. To accomplish this, the manager may provide positive feedback and guidance or provide additional educational opportunities to develop new competencies. Giving staff recognition for positive performance develops staff confidence. It may be simply recognizing a staff member with a kind word and comment. When errors occur, and they do, a manager who is also a leader does not punish staff but uses the mistake as an opportunity for improvement. Managers also need to be able to admit failure themselves, and in doing so, act as role models for staff by demonstrating that managers also need to improve. The effective manager will be seen as a leader, inspire excellence, and motivate others to excellence.

There are four critical qualities that are important in developing trust: competence, congruity, constancy, and caring. In today's health care environment, the complex work environment may be tense; staff may be tired; morale may be low; and work requirements may have increased. Leaders must constantly foster trust by demonstrating loyalty and supporting staff. Staff need to feel that they can share their feedback, whether positive or negative, and not feel threatened when they disagree with the manager or for their creative ideas.

How does a manager develop trust? First, the manager needs to have competence, hopefully leadership competencies. How do staff recognize when a person is a leader? Usually, staff will say that they have a feeling that the manager is able to accomplish what is supposed to be accomplished. They describe a manager as a person of integrity. Staff want their manager to be on their side and do not want to be left alone when things get difficult at work. This is particularly important when there is conflict. Managers who make promises to staff need to keep them. In addition, managers need to demonstrate to their staff that they trust that staff performance will be effective. Most people have likely experienced relationships in which trust was not present. Typically, these relationships involve situations where the person's actions and words did not mesh. If this becomes a pattern, then trust never develops or is destroyed. It is then very difficult to regain trust. Managers must be honest and play fair with their staff.

Consistency is critical in any leadership position and is also related to caring and trust. When authority is exercised it must be consistent in order to develop staff respect for the manager. If staff feel that some staff are given extra credit, rarely receive criticism when it is deserved, or are assigned less work, staff will feel uncomfortable with the manager and resentment will build (Heller, 1999). Distrust will develop. In these situations staff will not respect the manager, and this will affect work outcomes and patient care.

Leadership in community health

Is leadership in the community different from leadership in other health care settings? As the level of health care delivered in the community increases, nurse leadership will need to become more effective in this setting (Koerner, 2000). Today, more nurses are needed to assist in developing leadership within the community. Nurses who function in the community should not take over the leadership and direct the community but rather should facilitate the building of community leadership by providing their expertise and guidance. To do this nurses need the following skills: "capacity to create negotiated partnerships and shared responsibility and accountability as they work with other professions and members of the community; capacity to create new order by seeing relationships between unrelated parts and can anticipate and plan for the future . . . to approach the situation with an open mind and improvise inadequate reaction requires a different set of skills. It is based on the knowledge that there are multiple ways to address the situation and that the best solution resides within the problem itself" (Koerner, 2000, pp. 16–17). Community health nursing has become more important in nursing. Community leadership should not be ignored in this setting; however, nurses may need to consider new and different competencies for this environment.

There is also no doubt that, despite the many exciting new opportunities, the U.S. health care delivery system has major problems, and this text discusses many of them. Wolf (2000) seems to think that a major reason for these problems or the chaotic health care delivery system is that health care delivery has lost its focus on what is truly important to the people it serves, the patients. She believes that to transform health care organizations, staff who are responsible for providing care need to take a serious look at their roles and their practice. In addition, the future health care system will require active participation of health care consumers. "It will require those who deliver care to focus on developing innovative ways of providing this care. An organization approach to learning and development, with a focus on innovation and creativity will become essential" (Wolf, 2000, p. 46). Wolf also describes a key transformational model of care that has four components that can be applied to any type of health care organization. The components of this model are highlighted in Box 1-10. This model can be helpful in integrating the

BOX 1-10   Transformational model of care.

1. The *first component of the model is a professional practice component,* which focuses on deliberate critical thinking, negotiation, and decision making. In this process, individual needs of patients, professional recommendations, and effective resource management are considered. It is important that each health care discipline consider its practice and what elements of its practice are critical for patient outcomes. Wolf identifies four concepts that are important to this component: Transformational Leadership, care delivery systems, professional growth, and collaborative practice.

2. The *second component focuses on process,* which includes the processes that each health care professional group uses in its practice (for example, the nursing process). However, it is important that nurses as well as other health care professionals continually evaluate routines of care to determine if they continue to be necessary. As is done in nursing, it is important for other health care professionals to consider the patient as a partner in the care development process.

3. The *third component is the primary outcome,* and here the emphasis is on the relationship of patients to the process and outcome of care delivery.

4. The *fourth component focuses on identifying strategic outcomes related to the organization,* such as the ability to adapt to change, compete financially, and so on. Wolf also identifies strategic outcomes related to the profession which are professional organization, education, research, and professional publications.

health care system as well as developing and maintaining an organization's cultural identity and its leaders and staff.

The image of nursing

The image of nursing is an important aspect of nursing leadership. How nurses are viewed affects if they may be seen as possible leaders and whether or not nurses can be more effective. A *New York Times* article (Villarosa, 2001, May 22) on the image of nursing noted that national polls consistently confirm that nursing is viewed as one of the most trusted professions; however, the image of the profession is not that positive. A survey of schoolchildren indicated that they saw nursing as a "scary, stressful, low-status job, terrible hours, and an ugly uniform" (Villarosa, 2001, May 22, p. D7). Nursing's image has suffered over the past few years (Vestal, 2002). One reason for this is that consumers do not really have a complete or accurate view of the roles that nurses play throughout the health care system. "However, the side of nursing that involves human caring and making a difference in people's lives was not part of the story. If the image of nursing continues to be one that detracts from our ability to recruit new professionals, then we have to work on our stories that go out to the public" (Vestal, 2002, p. 4). Nursing still must contend with the fact that it is primarily a women's profession. There have been many media stories about how difficult the job is and how the work environment is stressful with staff shortages. As people who might consider the profession are listening to these messages, they do have an effect on the recruitment of potential students. More needs to be done to ensure that there is a more consistent message. Johnson and Johnson partnered with nursing to develop some excellent television ads that demonstrate positive qualities of nursing as a career choice. This is an important goal—to make sure that nurses see their choice of nursing as a lifetime commitment to a career and that nurses have a sense of pride in their profession, and then communicate this to the public, especially to groups who might consider it as a possible profession to enter. Leadership can play an important role here. Nursing needs to emphasize how nurses can be, and in many cases are, leaders in the health care environment. Leadership is a critical component of the profession. The ANA's *Nursing's Agenda for Change* (2002), which is discussed later in this chapter and provides the framework for this text, identifies a major goal related to public relations/communications and nursing: "Nursing's pivotal role in health care will be demonstrated on a regular basis to various publics outside of the profession" (p. 14). This will not be easy to accomplish, but it is a critical goal.

Making a difference: Increasing nurse leaders

How do nurses become leaders? "Nurse leaders do not just appear. It is a professional responsibility for all of us to become leaders and to mentor future leaders" (Anderson, 2000, p. 47). Nursing education should take advantage of leadership opportunities. The first step is to make a commitment to lifelong learning. As students enter clinical practice and then their careers, they will be confronted with change. Leaders use change as opportunities for learning. Becoming involved in professional organizations is also an important part of developing leadership. This may begin with participation in the National Student Nurses Association, Sigma Theta Tau, the nursing honor society, or other campus organizations. Mentoring is also part of leadership. Some nursing programs have mentoring programs so that students can help one another. Networking, which can be helpful, can begin as a student. It is important to remember that faculty, peers, and nurses in the clinical settings, as well as nurses who might be met outside of school or clinical practice, may at some point be important individuals in a nurse's career. Through networking, connections are made to assist a nurse throughout the nurse's career.

There are not enough nurses to fill all the nurse leadership positions that are available today. Some nurses will eventually move into formal management positions, and others will apply leadership skills in non-management positions. Nursing must find a way to increase the pool of potential nurse leaders. Some solutions to this problem include: (a) develop clinical/career ladders for nursing managers, (b) define goals and competency-based outcomes to direct manager growth and development within organizations and within the profession, (c) provide mentorship, and (d) develop a system for identifying novice to expert among nurse leaders (Coughlin, 2002). Clinical ladders are used in many health care organizations to recognize performance and competencies. Typically, a new nurse enters the organization at the lowest level and then must meet specific criteria and competencies to move "up the ladder" to different clinical levels. Leadership is included in the criteria and competencies, (e.g., membership on committees, chair of committees, development of unit-based materials such as patient education or a change in a policy or procedure, mentoring new nurses, preceptor for nursing students, implementing evidence-based practice, or developing research). "The American Organization of Nurse Executives (AONE), professional association for nurse executives and nurse leaders, is committed to identifying and adopting evidence-based management practices. AONE believes that nursing leadership plays an extremely important role in creating the work environments that attract and keep nurses and that current management practices are not uniformly successful" (Watson, 2004, p. 207).

As organizations and the nursing profession consider the best methods for leadership development, there are guidelines that should not be forgotten. Leaders need to "exemplify leadership, not formulas; demonstrate empowerment by developing, not ruling followers; learn to provide leadership opportunities for others, all the while learning to coach. Leaders need nurses to expand their own definitions of themselves and their role" (Ferguson & Brindle, 2000, p. 5).

CURRENT ISSUES

Learn about events around the globe that relate to the chapter content.

New graduates do not usually graduate and step into management positions, and in fact, the majority will never be in a formal management position. So why all this interest in leadership and management? "Is there a magic formula to resuscitate today's management? Perhaps, but formula or not, the antidote for today's management dilemma is leadership" (Stahl, 1998, p. 7). It is important to recognize that leadership skills are not only required for those in high positions in nursing. "In today's increasingly less hierarchical and more lateral organizational structures, leadership is not about position of authority, as much as it is a role of influence. Staff nurses can and must lead through teamwork, the development of better practices, through the development of centrality in communication networks, and in contributing to the strategic management of the units and departments. The leadership role and task is pivotal, not peripheral to the success of health care facilities" (Ferguson & Brindle, 2000, p. 5). Ferguson's comments about leadership are very important and timely. In May of 2003, the American Association of Colleges of Nursing (AACN) published a White Paper, *The Role of the Clinical Nurse Leader* (2003). The position of the AACN is that leadership is very important in nursing. This position is supported in recent Institute of Medicine reports related to the quality and safety of health care in which nurses are described as leaders and important in making a difference in the quality and safety of health care. There needs, however, to be greater recognition that leadership is required for all nursing positions. To meet this need for nursing leaders, the AACN recognizes the need to incorporate more leadership development in undergraduate and graduate programs. This decision is based on 10 assumptions about the health care delivery system and nursing.

1. Practice is at the systems level. Nurses must practice in all types of settings and are accountable for care outcomes of clinical populations (e.g., mothers in labor population, patients in a clinic, children in a community).
2. Population-level care outcomes are the measure of quality practice. Performance will be measured by clinical and cost outcomes.
3. Practice guidelines are based on evidence.

4. Client-centered practice is intra- and interdisciplinary.
5. Information will maximize self-care and client decision making.
6. Nursing assessment is the basis for theory and knowledge development.
7. Good fiscal stewardship is a condition of quality care.
8. Social justice is an essential nursing value.
9. Communication technology will facilitate the continuity and comprehensiveness of care.
10. The CNL must assume guardianship for the nursing profession (American Association of Colleges of Nursing, 2003, pp. 5–9).

These assumptions are clearly related to current leadership and management theories and styles that have been discussed in this chapter and will be emphasized throughout the text. The role of nurse leader is critical for patients, their families, and the delivery system as a whole. Nurses have really been in this role for a very long time. Some were more prepared than others for it, and now it is important to recognize that every nurse needs to develop leadership qualities and competencies, whether or not they are in a formal management position.

BENCHMARKS

Now let's take a moment to test your knowledge of the concepts you have studied in this section.

Chapter Wrap-Up

Now that you've reached the end of the chapter, you may wish to explore the concepts you've been reading about in greater detail or test yourself to see how well you've comprehended the material.

SUMMARY AND APPLICATIONS

- Summary
- Practice Quiz
- Key Terms
- Tying It All Together

- Experiential Exercises
- Case 1
- Links

REFERENCES

American Association of Colleges of Nursing. (2003, May). *White paper on the role of the clinical nurse leader*. Retrieved on June 16, 2003, from http://www.aacn.nche.edu.

American Nurses Association et al. (2002). *Nursing's agenda for change*. Retrieved on May 16, 2002, from http://www.nursingworld.org/naf.

Anderson, C. (2000). The critical path to leadership development: A student perspective. *Imprint, 47*(4), 47–48.

Bahrami, H. (1992). The emerging flexible organization: Perspectives from Silicon Valley. *California Management Review, 34*(4), 33–52.

Bass, B. (1998). *Leadership and performance beyond expectations*. New York: Free Press.

Bass, B., & Avolio, B. (1997). *Transformational leadership development: Manual for multifactor leadership questionnaire*. Palo Alto, CA: Consulting Psychologists Press.

Bennis, W., & Goldsmith, J. (1997). *Learning to lead: A workbook on becoming a leader*. Reading, MA: Perseus Books.

Blake, R., & McCanse, A. (1991). *Leadership dilemmas—Grid solutions*. San Francisco: Jossey-Bass.

Bryman, A. (2001). *Leadership in organizations*. In A. Bryman (Ed.), *Organizational studies* (pp. 276–292). Thousand Oaks, CA: Sage Publishers.

Burns, J. (1985). *Leadership*. New York: Harper Collins.

Bushe, G. (2001). *Clear Leadership*. Palo Alto, CA: Davies-Black Publishing.

Child, R., Lingle, G., & Watson, P. (2001). Managing diversity in the environment of care. *Seminars for Nurse Managers, 9*(2), 102–110.

Coughlin, C. (2002). Saving nursing management. *Journal of Nursing Administration, 32*(4), 178–179.

Crow, G. (2002). The relationship between trust, social capital, and organizational success. *Nursing Administration Quarterly, 26*(3), 1–11.

Curtin, L. (2001). Guest editorial: EQ is more important now than ever before. *Seminars for Nurse Managers, 9*(4), 203–205.

Curtin, L., & Falherty, M. (1993). *Nursing ethics: Theories and pragmatics*. Upper Saddle River, NJ: Prentice Hall.

Drucker, P. (1994). The age of social transformation. *Atlantic Monthly, 274*(5) 53–80.

Drucker, P. (1993). *Post-capitalistic society*. NY: Harper Business Publications.

Dunham-Taylor, J. (2000). Nurse executive transformational leadership found in participative organizations. *Journal of Nursing Administration, 30*(5), 241–250.

Ferguson, S., & Brindle, M. (2000). Nursing leadership: Vision and the reality. *Nursing Spectrum, 10*(21DC), 5.

Fiedler, F. (1967). *A theory of leadership effectiveness*. New York: McGraw-Hill.

Fullan, C., Lando, A., Johansen, M., Reyes, A., & Szaloczy, D. (1988). The triad of empowerment: Leadership, environment, and professional traits. *Nursing Economics, 16*(5), 254–257.

Goffee, R., & Jones, G. (2000). Why should anyone be led by you. *Harvard Business Review*, Sept.–Oct., 63–71.

Goleman, D. (1998). *Working with emotional intelligence*. New York: Bantam Books.

Goleman, D. (2001). An EI theory of performance. In C. Cherniss & D. Goleman (Eds.), *The emotionally intelligent workplace* (pp. 27–44). San Francisco: Jossey-Bass.

Grohar-Murray, M., & DiCroce, H. (2003). *Leadership and management in nursing* (3rd ed.). Upper Saddle River, NJ: Pearson Education.

Hammer, M. (1997). The soul of the new organization. In F. Hesselbein, M. Goldsmith, & R. Beckhard (Eds.), *The organization of the future* (pp. 27–31). San Francisco: Jossey-Bass.

Heller, R. (1999). *Learning to lead*. New York: DK Publishing, Inc.

Hill, L. (1993). *Becoming a manager: How new managers master the challenges of leadership*. New York: Penguin Books.

Huber, D. (2000). *Leadership and nursing care management*. Philadelphia: W.B. Saunders Company.

Koerner, J. (2000). Nightingale II: Nursing leaders remembering community. *Nursing Administration Quarterly, 24*(2), 13–18.

Kotter, J. (1995). Leading change: Why transformation efforts fail. *Harvard Business Review, 73*(3), 59–67.

Laurent, C. (2000). A nursing theory for nursing leadership. *Journal of Nursing Management, 8*(2), 83.

Mathena, K. (2002). Nursing manager leadership skills. *Journal of Nursing Administration, 32*(3), 136–142.

Medley, F., & Larochelle, D. (1995). Transformational Leadership and job satisfaction. *Nursing Management, 26*, 64JJ–64LL, 64NN.

Milgram, L., Spector, A., & Treger, M. (1999). *Managing smart*. Houston, TX: Cashman Dudley.

Milstead, J. (2004). Challenging five traditional leadership principles. *Policy, Politics, & Nursing Pratice, 5*(1), 5–9.

Mohrman, S., & Mohrman, A. (1997). *Designing and leading team-based organizations*. San Francisco: Jossey-Bass.

Ohman, K. (1999). Nurse manager leadership. *Journal of Nursing Administration, 29*(12), 16, 21.

Peter, L., & Hull, R. (1969). *The Peter Principle: Why things go wrong*. New York: William Morrow.

Porter-O'Grady, T. (1999). Quantum leadership: New roles for a new age. *Journal of Nursing Administration, 29*(10), 37–42.

Porter-O'Grady, T. (2001). Profound change: 21st century nursing. *Nursing Outlook, 49*(4), 182–186.

Porter-O'Grady, T., & Finnegan, S. (1984). *Shared governance for nursing: A creative approach to professional accountability*. Gaithersburg, MD: Aspen Publishers Inc.

Robinson-Walker, C. (2002). Guest editorial: Coaching culture. *Seminars for Nurse Managers, 10*(3), 148–149.

Singleton, E., & Nail-Hall, F. (1995). Charting the course for merger: Key concepts for nurse executive. *Journal of Nursing Administration, 25*(5), 47–54.

Snow, J. (2001). Looking beyond nursing for clues to effective leadership. *Journal of Nursing Administration, 31*(9), 440–443.

Sorrells-Jones, J. (1999). The role of the chief nurse executive in the knowledge-intense organization of the future. *Nursing Administration Quarterly, 23*(3), 17–25.

Stahl, D. (1998). Leadership in these changing times. *Nursing Management, 29*(4), 16–18.

Sternweiler, V. (1998). Career journeys: How to be a successful conical nurse specialist—be a willow tree. *Advanced Practice Nursing, 3*(4), 31–33.

Strickland, D. (2000). Emotional Intelligence: The most potent factor in the success equation. *Journal of Nursing Administration, 30*(3), 112–117.

Sullivan, T. (1998). Transformational leadership. In T. Sullivan (Ed.), *Collaboration: A health care imperative* (pp. 467–497). New York: McGraw-Hill.

Ulrich, B. (2001). Successfully managing multigenerational workforces. *Seminars for Nurse Managers, 9*(3), 147–153.

Villarosa, L. (2001, May 21). Working to burnish nursing's image. *New York Times*, D7.

Vestal, K. (2002, July). The big picture. *Newsweek*, p. 4.

Vitello-Cicciu, J. (2002). Exploring Emotional Intelligence: Implications for nursing leaders. *Journal of Nursing Administration, 32*(4), 203–210.

Watson, C. (2004). Evidence-based management practices. *Journal of Nursing Administration, 34*(5), 207–209.

Weaver, D. (2001). Transdisciplinary teams: Very important leadership stuff. *Seminars for Nurse Managers, 9*(2), 79–84.

Weaver, D., & Sorrells-Jones, J. (1999). Knowledge workers and knowledge-intense organizations, Part 2: Designing and managing for productivity. *Journal of Nursing Administration, 29*(9), 19–25.

Wolf, G. (2000). Vision 2000: The transformation of professional practice. *Nursing Administration Quarterly, 24*(2), 45–51.

ADDITIONAL READINGS

Allen, D. (1998). How nurses become leaders: Perception and beliefs about leadership development. *Journal of Nursing Administration, 28*(9), 15–20.

American Nurses Association. (2001). *Code of ethics for nurses with interpretive statements*. Washington, DC: Author.

Bennis, W., & Thomas, R. (2002). Crucibles of leadership. *Harvard Business Review, 80*(9), 39–45.

Bertholf, L., & Loveless, S. (2001). Baby boomers and generation X: Strategies to bridge the gap. *Seminars for Nurse Managers, 9*(3), 169–172.

Bower, F. (Ed.). (2000). *Nurses taking the lead: Personal qualities of effective leadership*. Philadelphia: W. B. Saunders.

Brooks, A., Thomas, S., & Dropplemann, P. (1996). From frustration to red fury: A description of work-related anger by male registered nurses. *Nursing Forum, 31*(3), 4–15.

Byers, J. (2000). Knowledge, skills, and attributes needed for nurse and non-nurse executives. *Journal of Nursing Administration, 30*(7/8), 354–356.

Cherniss, C., & Goleman, D. (Eds.). (2001). *The Emotionally Intelligent workplace*. San Francisco: Jossey-Bass.

Cook, M. (2001). The renaissance of clinical leadership. *International Nursing Review, 48*(1), 38.

Curtin, L. (2001a). Leadership—The gold standard. *Seminars for Nurse Managers, 9*(4), 238–240.

Curtin, L. (2001b). To get there together. *Curtin Calls, 3*(4), 1–2.

Davis, S. (2001). Diversity and generation X. *Seminars for Nurse Managers, 9*(3), 161–163.

De Ruiter, H., & Saphiere, D. (2001). Nurse leaders as cultural bridges. *Journal of Nursing Administration, 31*(9), 418–423.

Dixon, D. (1999). Achieving results through transformational leadership. *Journal of Nursing Administration, 29*(12), 17–21.

Dochterman, J., & Grace, H. (2001). *Current issues in nursing* (6th ed.). St. Louis, MO: Mosby, Inc.

Doty, E. (2002). Organizing to learn: Recognizing and cultivating learning communities. *Seminars for Nurse Managers, 10*(3), 196–211.

Farrell, M. (2002). Setting the vision: The CEO's perspective. *Seminars for Nurse Managers, 10*(1), 38–42.

Felgen, J., & Kinnaird, L. (2001). Dynamic dialogue: Application to generational diversity. *Seminars for Nurse Managers, 9*(3), 164–168.

Finkelman, A. (2001). *Managed care: A nursing perspective*. Upper Saddle River, NJ: Prentice Hall.

Forman, H. (2002). Is shared governance still relevant? *Journal of Nursing Administration, 32*(2), 97.

Freshwater, D. (2004). Tool for developing clinical leadership. *Reflections on Nursing LEADERSHIP*, second quarter, 20, 22, 26.

Freshwater, D., & Stickley, T. (2004). The heart of the art: Emotional Intelligence in nurse education. *Inquiry, 11*(2), 91–98.

Fullam, C., et al. (1998). The triad of empowerment: Leadership environment and professional traits. *Nursing Economics, 16*(5), 254–257.

George, V. (2003). Women as leaders: Changing the workplace. *Nurse Leader, 1*(1), 44–45.

Gerke, M. (2001). Understanding and leading the quad matrix: Four generations in the workplace: The traditional generation, boomers, gen-X, nexters. *Seminars for Nurse Managers, 9*(3), 173–181.

Giannelli, P., Morrison, M., & Spivak, L. (2001). Nurse manager exemplar: A journey out of the glass house. *Seminars for Nurse Managers, 9*(2), 126–131.

Haigh, C. (2002). Using Chaos theory: The implications for nursing. *Journal of Advanced Nursing, 37*(5), 462–469.

Hepner, L., & Hopkins, L. (2000). Partnership 2000: A journey to the 21st century. *Nursing Administration Quarterly, 24*(2), 34–44.

Herrin, D. (2004). Shared governance: A nurse executive response. *Journal of Issues in Nursing, 9*(1). Available at http://www.nursingworld.org/ojin/topic23/tpc23_1.htm.

Herzberg, F. (1987). One more time: How do you motivate your employees? *Harvard Business Review, 65,* 109–120.

Hess, R. (2004). From bedside to boardroom—Nursing shared governance. *Journal of Issues in Nursing, 9*(1). Available at http://www.nursingworld.org/ojin/topic23/tpc23_1.htm.

Hunt, P. (1999). How to lead departments outside your clinical competence. *Nursing Management,* December, 28–31.

Johns, C. (2004). Becoming a transformational leader through reflection. *Reflections on nursing LEADERSHIP, second quarter,* 24–26.

Kerfoot, K. (1996). The emotional side of leadership: The nurse manager's challenge. *Nursing Economics, 14*(1), 59–62.

Kerfoot, K. (2002). The leader as chief knowledge officer. *Nursing Economics, 20*(1), 40–41, 43.

Kerfoot, K., & Simpson, R. (2002). Knowledge-driven care: Powerful medicine. *Reflections on Nursing LEADERSHIP,* third quarter, 22–24.

Kondrat, B. (2001). Operating room nurse managers competence and beyond. *AORN Journal, 73*(6), 1116–1130.

Laschinger, H., & Wong, C. (1999). Staff nurse empowerment and collective accountability: Effect on perceived productivity and self-rated work effectiveness. *Nursing Economics, 17*(6), 308–316, 351.

Marquis, B., & Huston, C. (2000). *Leadership roles and management functions in nursing.* Philadelphia: J. B. Lippincott.

McGuire, E. (1999). Chaos theory: Learning a new science. *Journal of Nursing Administration, 29*(2), 8–9.

Mintzberg, H. (1996). Musing on management. *Harvard Business Review, 74,* 61–67.

Morgan, B. (2000). Testing leadership and management concepts. *Nurse Educator, 25*(4), 181–185.

Morrison, R., Jones, L., & Fuller, B. (1997). The relation between leadership style and empowerment on job satisfaction of nurses. *Journal of Nursing Administration, 27*(5), 27–34.

Neault, G. (2001). Developing nursing leadership in an ambulatory surgical center through shared responsibility. *Insight, 26*(1), 10–12.

Neuman, B., Newman, D., & Holder, P. (2000). Leadership-scholarship integration: Using the Neuman Systems Model for 21st century professional nursing practice. *Nursing Science Quarterly, 13*(1), 60–63.

O'Neil, E., & Pew Health Commission. (1995). *Critical challenges: Revitalizing the health professions for the 21st century.* San Francisco: Center for Health Professions.

Perra, B. (2000). Leadership: The key to quality outcomes. *Nursing Administration Quarterly, 24*(2), 56–61.

Porter-O'Grady, T. (2001). Into the new age: The call for a new construct for nursing. *Geriatric Nursing, 22*(1), 12–15.

Purnell, L. (1999). Health care managers' and administrators' roles, functions, and responsibilities. *Nursing Administration Quarterly, 23*(3), 26–37.

Ray, M., Turkel, M., & Marino, F. (2002). The transformative process for nursing in workforce redevelopment. *Nursing Administrative Quarterly, 26*(2), 1–14.

Reese, S. (1999). The new wave of gen X workers. *Business and Health, 17*(6), 19–23.

Russell, G., & Scoble, K. (2003). Vision 2020, Part II: Educational preparation for the future nurse manager. *Journal of Nursing Administration, 33*(7/8), 404–409.

Schmieding, N. (2000). Minority nurses in leadership positions: A call for action. *Nursing Outlook, 48*(3), 120–127.

Scoble, K., & Russell, G. (2003). Vision 2020, Part I: Profile of the future nurse leader. *Journal of Nursing Administration, 33*(6), 324–330.

Scott, J., Sochalski, J., & Aiken, L. (1999). Review of magnet hospital research: Findings and implications for professional nursing practice. *Journal of Nursing Administration, 29*(1), 9–19.

Snow, J. (2001). Looking beyond nursing for clues to effective leadership. *Journal of Nursing Administration, 31,* 440–443.

Sorrells-Jones, J., & Weaver, D. (1999a). Knowledge workers and knowledge-intense organizations, Part 1: A promising framework for nursing and healthcare. *Journal of Nursing Administration, 29*(7/8), 12–18.

Sorrells-Jones, J., & Weaver, D. (1999b). Knowledge workers and knowledge-intense organizations, Part 3: Implications for preparing healthcare professionals. *Journal of Nursing Administration, 29*(10), 14–21.

Spellerberg, D. (2001). What does it mean to lead? *Nursing Spectrum Metro* (August), 18MW.

Stordeur, S., Vandenberghe, C., & D'hoore, W. (2000). Leadership styles across hierarchical levels in nursing departments. *Nursing Research, 49*(1), 27–43.

Sullivan, E. (2002). In a woman's world. *Reflections on Nursing LEADERSHIP,* third quarter, 10–11, 17.

Sullivan, T. (1998). *Collaboration: A health care imperative.* New York: McGraw-Hill.

Swanson, J. (2000). Zen leadership: Balancing energy for mind, body, and spirit harmony. *Nursing Administration Quarterly, 24*(2), 29–33.

Tichy, N., & Devanna, M. (1990). *The transformational leader.* New York: John Wiley and Sons.

Trofino, A. (2000). Transformational Leadership: Moving total quality management to world-class organizations. *International Nursing Review, 47,* 232–242.

Trossman, S. (2002). Envisioning a brighter future. *American Journal of Nursing, 102*(7), 65–66.

Verdejo, T. (2001). Leading into the 21st century: Changing the vision and leading toward success. *Seminars for Nurse Managers, 9*(2), 115–118.

Vitello-Cicciu, J. (2002). Exploring Emotional Intelligence. *Journal of Nursing Administration, 32*(4), 203–210.

Vitello-Cicciu, J. (2003). Innovative leadership through Emotional Intelligence. *Nursing Management, 34*(10), 28–32.

Weaver, C. (2002). Nurses in corporate America: Embracing power through influence. *Seminars for Nurse Managers, 10*(2), 117–119.

Wenger, E., & Snyder, W. (2000). Communities of practice: The new organizational frontier. *Harvard Business Review, 78*(1), 139–145.

Wieck, K., Prydum, M., & Walsh, T. (2002). What the emerging workforce wants in its leaders. *Journal of Nursing Scholarship,* third quarter, 283–288.

Change and Decision Making

CHAPTER OUTLINE

MediaLink
www.prenhall.com/finkelman

The Interactive Exercises for this chapter can be found in the OneKey course at www.prenhall.com/finkelman. Click on Chapter 2 to select from the following activities: Test Your Understanding, Benchmarks, Current Issues, Your Opinion Counts, Think Critically, and Summary and Applications.

What's Ahead

"In the 21st century, the demand of change and innovation is challenging and enormous. . . . Effective leaders need to do far more than simply manage change; they need to passionately champion both change and innovation" (Gebelein et al., 2000, p. 24). Staff tend to think that leaders and managers will save the day by helping them cope with the ever-changing health care environment. The truth is that most managers will not be able to do this, as many are not prepared to cope with this rate of change (Bennis & Goldsmith, 1997). What does this mean? Nurses at all levels must make a commitment to the change process and take active roles in the process. Change that comes from and is totally managed by a manager will not be successful today. Staff who pull back and wait for the manager to make the difference will also find that changes will occur but without their input. "Understanding change and its potential landmines are important to be successful today, but we must also recognize the benefits of change, though we often complain about it. Change can invigorate us. If we had no change, there would be no need for critical thinking. After a time we would know all of the answers or approaches to expected problems. I am sure after a time we would also find this to be a rather boring environment in which to work, though for most of us it would be comfortable initially. Complacency and isolationism can be very destructive landmines" (Finkelman, 2001, p. 195). This chapter focuses on change and decision making in organizations—what are the critical change and decision-making processes and the impact of change on staff, health care organizations, and their decisions? It is difficult to separate change from decisions as responding to change requires that decisions are made; some minor, some more important and complex. Nurses participate in the change process and make decisions wherever they practice.

OBJECTIVES

Before you begin, take a moment to familiarize yourself with the key objectives of this chapter.

- Discuss critical nursing issues related to reengineering, redesigning, re-regulating, rightsizing, and restructuring.
- Discuss why the concept of change is important in the health care environment and to nursing leadership and management.
- Discuss external trends and factors that impact nursing practice and health care organizations.
- Define two key change theories.
- Describe eight key steps in the change process.
- Discuss resistance to change and how it can be handled.
- Identify strategies to improve responses to change.
- Apply the decision-making process.
- Describe the keys to successful planning.
- Distinguish between strategic and project planning.

TEST YOUR UNDERSTANDING

Before we begin our exploration of this chapter, take a short "warm-up" test to assess what you know about this topic.

The Five "Rs": Change and Decision Making in Action

The health care delivery system has been adjusting to managed care, staff shortages, budget cuts, technology, role changes, and much more, all of which have had a major impact on nursing. Change has driven the need for the five "Rs," which particularly affect health care organizations, nursing education, and nursing practice. The five "Rs" are:

1. Reengineering the health care organization
2. Redesigning the workforce
3. Re-regulating professional practice
4. Rightsizing the workforce
5. Restructuring nursing education.

Each one of the five Rs is about change and requires decision making on the part of the organization and its staff. Understanding their impact provides an introduction to the importance of change and decision making for nurses.

Reengineering the health care organization

Reengineering has been occurring in many health care organizations for a number of years. This management trend, borrowed from business, has been defined as "the fundamental rethinking and radical redesign of business processes to achieve dramatic improvements in critical, contemporary measures of performance, such as cost, quality, service and speed" (Hammer & Champy, 1993; as cited in Beyers, 1999, p. 163). This is more than a minor organizational change—it is a reinvention or recreation of processes, work, and systems. Often reengineering is not easy for nurses to accept as they may radically change how nursing is practiced, and thus nurses may be reluctant to participate. To actively participate in reengineering, nurses need to understand their own work and be willing to explore improving their practice. This requires flexibility, creativity, and the ability to use resources differently (Beyers, 1999).

What really is reengineering? The core features of reengineering include:

- **Discontinuous thinking.** Breaking away from the past requires reinvention. This is not easy for every organization to do and can be very frightening to staff. In order to survive in a competitive health care environment, it is necessary to reassess all aspects of the organization as some may need to be changed or eliminated.
- **Cross-functional approach.** Processes and systems do not work in isolation. This approach is critical in health care and greatly affects nurses, nursing education, regulation, rightsizing, and work redesign. Nurses may be trained to work in different specialties so that they can be shifted from one area to another when staffing requires adjustment.
- **Major, radical change.** The focus is not on fixing. Organizations that undergo reengineering should appear very different when final outcomes are reached.
- **Futuristic imperative.** The beginning point for reengineering is the future. The organization then looks backward to determine where changes need to be made to get ready for future needs. This requires a vision of what the organization should look like as well as support from top-level management. *Reengineering* is a term that is used frequently today, but many organizations are not really applying reengineering to their organizations; rather, they are just chipping away with minor changes (Hammer & Champy, 1993, p. 107).

The following do not represent reengineering, though they are often identified as reengineering.

- Accomplishing incremental or small-scale change
- Reducing full-time equivalents (FTEs), staff who have full-time positions, to control costs
- Switching vendors or changing products
- Offering contests, slogans, or gimmicks to get staff involved
- Providing quality improvement initiatives
- Remodeling the physical plant
- Restructuring the organization
- Improving processes
- Developing new services
- Automating existing processes
- Improving systems
- Decreasing health care services (Flarey & Smith, 1999, pp. 21–22)

Many of these techniques or outcomes *may* be a part of reengineering, but they do not represent the essential features of reengineering, which must affect the entire organization.

Nurses have experienced what has been described as reengineering when the major focus actually was only on reducing full-time equivalents (FTEs), primarily nursing, developing or reducing services, or decreasing length-of-stay. This has usually been done with limited nursing input.

Varied reengineering strategies are used. An important strategy for nursing is that of patient-focused care, a combination of reengineering and work redesign. The goals are to improve patient and customer satisfaction, quality of care, and cost reduction (Turner, 1999). This idea of arranging work around the patient rather than specialized departments has great potential for providing an opportunity to deliver nursing care that meets patient needs; however, this has not been easy to accomplish. It takes time and commitment and requires significant change in the organization. Over many years, patient care has been delivered in hospitals with the number of departments increasing and more and more staff interacting with the patient. Specialization has led to problems of poor communication, complex processes, increased paperwork, poor collaboration, and error. "A primary goal of the patient-focused design is to provide at least 70% of all services on the patient unit" (Truscott & Churchill, 1995, p. 5). What would this mean in most hospitals? How would a hospital go about doing this? What role would nurses play? These are critical examples of decisions that must be made as planning is done to make major changes in health care organizations. Reengineering is considered to be the approach that will solve many of today's health care organization problems. The result, however, will not be known for several years, until retrospective evaluation can occur to assess the outcomes.

Redesigning the workforce

Demands that managed care have placed on clinical settings to increase productivity and patient and customer satisfaction, and at the same time provide lower cost quality care, have pressured nurse executives and managers to institute work redesign. With the nursing shortage, the need for work redesign is even more important. Improved efficiency that results in more effective practice with less staff is critical. This has led to the development of, and changes in, inpatient care delivery models, such as the use of patient-focused care and changing staff mix such as decreasing the number of RNs, increasing the number of unlicensed assistive personnel (UAPs), increasing licensed practical nurses (LPNs/LVN), and cross training.

If nurses do not take active roles in **redesigning** work, it will be done *for* nurses rather than *by* nurses (Hoover, 1998). Traditional nursing roles and activities need to be assessed, and then often rejected, to allow for more innovative approaches. Nurses need to provide supportive data to demonstrate the impact that their own roles and activities have on efficiency, improved care, and patient outcomes. The problem, however, is that there are many perspectives on nursing work redesign. Research in this area has been inadequate, and duplication of studies to demonstrate that previous results were accurate is lacking. Patient outcomes also have not played a major role in redesign evaluation. Determining the best way to design how staff work together to provide quality, safe care that includes patients is the key issue.

When health care organizations confront the need to make changes in responsibilities, functions, and tasks in the delivery system, the most common reasons have been due to (a) the supply of nurses, (b) the cost of nursing salaries, (c) rethinking the role of nursing, and (d) changes in other professions within the health care system that impact nursing (Kerfoot, 1997). Work redesign is used to address these concerns; however, there are other factors that need to be considered. Nurses are responsible for ensuring a baseline level of performance. If UAPs are used, nurses need to ensure that training and supervision are provided to the UAPs to ensure patient safety and quality care. The nursing profession must also be careful about new delivery models or how staff are organized to provide care (for example, the use of teams). There needs to be more research to validate the outcomes of these models. The bottom line is nursing needs data to support these delivery changes.

- Are they effective?
- If not, why?

■ What can be done to make them more effective?

■ Should the model be used?

■ Under what circumstances is the model effective or ineffective?

Nurses should be asking these questions and not waiting for others to do so. They should also be directly responsible for finding the answers, analyzing the results, and making decisions about changes that need to be made.

Professional nursing organizations need to look at methods of examining best practices such as the Magnet Recognition Program (Kerfoot, 1997). This program, which is discussed in more detail in Chapter 6, identifies health care organizations that are providing excellent nursing care and have work environments that support professional nursing.

Re-regulating professional practice

Why is **re-regulating professional practice** an important change issue today? Nurses have discovered that many of the changes that are taking place in health care, such as the use of tele-health, workforce mobility, and mergers (or several health care organizations forming one organization, which may then have parts of the organization in different states), are affecting licensure. It is predicted that many nurses will be involved in providing care across state lines and in situations in which the patient is in a different state from the one in which the nurse is licensed and located (Hutcherson & Williamson, 1999). The use of telenursing is also growing, which allows for greater opportunities to provide nursing care over distances using telecommunication technology and other technology. This type of care is considered to be within the practice of nursing, even if it is not "hands-on care" or direct care. In addition, restructuring of health care has led to an increase in multistate health care systems, and this has affected how nurses are employed and where they work.

In order to understand the recent proposed changes in regulation, it is important to understand how regulation is applied. The purpose of practice regulation is to ensure public safety. Boards of nursing, which regulate nursing practice, began in the early 1900s (Hutcherson & Williamson, 1999). The right of states to regulate practice is based on the Tenth Amendment of the U.S. Constitution, the states' rights amendment. This amendment provides each state with the right to regulate nursing practice within its own state but not within other states. This is why nurses who move from one state to another to work must obtain licensure in the new state. Reciprocity or the right to practice is primarily based on national board scores; however, the nurse must still apply for an RN licensure in the state, meet individual state requirements such as continuing education, and pay state fees. Due to changes in health care, boards of nursing and nursing organizations have been discussing changes that need to be made in the regulation of nursing practice nationally. The dilemma is that licensure remains state-based and yet state lines may no longer bind nursing practice. Various options were considered by the National Council of State Boards of Nursing (NCSBN) to resolve this dilemma, but the option selected to address this licensure problem is mutual recognition. The implementation of this type of licensure requires an interstate compact, which is an agreement between two or more states, entered into for the purpose of addressing a problem that transcends state lines. Compacts are created when two or more states enact identical statutes establishing and defining the compact and its role. The result is the creation of both state law and an enforceable contract with other states that adopt the compact (Hutcherson & Williamson, 1999). Not all states have made decisions to make this change and collaborate with adjacent states about RN licensure, but there is a trend to move in this direction.

THINK CRITICALLY

Try this exercise to apply what you have learned about this topic.

Rightsizing the workforce

Rightsizing and *downsizing* are terms that cause nurses to shudder, as they suggest that the health care organization might reduce staff. In 1996, the *American Journal of Nursing* published a patient care survey of 7,560 nurses (Shindul-Rothschild, Berry, & Long-Middleton, 1996). The results identified problems that nurses saw in clinical settings and their reactions to downsizing. This survey is several years old; however, it does indicate areas that need to be watched carefully as more changes occur in health care delivery. In fact, many of the issues that were identified continue to be major problems today. After many hospitals decreased their staff and beds, they had to reverse these decisions or have tried to do so. More beds have been needed in many areas of the country; therefore, the hospitals want the nurses back. This has not been easy to accomplish. Some nurses simply did not want to come back, but along with this response is the fact that there are fewer nurses available to fill the need. The nursing shortage continues, and hospital acuity remains high. Concerns identified by the nurses in this survey are highlighted in Box 2-1 (Shindul-Rothschild, Berry, & Long-Middleton, 1996).

In the 1990s, 675 acute care hospitals closed. These changes directly affected health care in general, nursing care, and the nursing profession. Sovie and Jawad (2001) examined the impact of hospital restructuring on 29 university teaching hospitals. At these hospitals RN staff and management staff were reduced, UAPs were increased, and the UAP role was expanded. The goal was to reduce costs; however, this study indicated that costs actually increased per patient discharge. In addition, these hospitals experienced higher rates of patient falls and lower rates of patient satisfaction with their pain management.

Rightsizing focuses on how many staff are required to do the job, and this has never been easy to predict. Since education for health care professionals takes time, it is important to try to predict future needs. The goal is to determine how many health care professionals need to be educated to meet the needs and ensure that there will be jobs for them when they complete their education and training. It is clear that there are not enough nurses now, and the predictions for the future are also bleak. Many more nurses will be needed to fill future empty positions. Approaching the problem only from the point-of-view of getting the "right" number of nurses is not a helpful approach. Since it will probably not be possible to get the number of nurses desired, other strategies will be needed to change how nursing care is provided to reduce the number of nurses required.

BOX 2-1   1996 survey of nurses.

- Decrease in continuity of care
- Increase in unexpected readmissions
- Variability in perception of quality care
- Increase in number of part-time or temporary nurses
- Increase in substitution of unlicensed assistive personnel for registered nurses
- Increase in work-related injuries (particularly in the specialty services of psychiatric/mental health, orthopedic, neurology, operating room/post-anesthesia care, primary care, and emergency department)
- Increase in workplace violence (particularly in the specialty services of psychiatric/mental health, primary care, and emergency department)
- 25% said they would not remain in nursing
- Two out of five nurses would not have their family members in their hospitals
- Increase in number of patients assigned
- Increase in cross-training
- Organizational changes: closing beds or units, construction or renovation, establishing/acquiring community services, loss of managed care contracts
- Less time to provide required care

Source: Author created and summarized results from Shindul-Rothschild, J., Berry, D., & Long-Middleton, E. (1996). Where have all the nurses gone? Final results of our patient care survey. *American Journal of Nursing*, 96(11), 25–39.

The American Organization of Nurse Executives (AONE), in collaboration with ANA and the Division of Nursing, surveyed hospital managers from 388 acute care hospitals (AONE, 1999). AONE, a subsidiary of the American Hospital Association, is the professional organization for nurses in leadership positions. This survey addressed the concern about an impending nurse shortage, which is now a reality and predicted to increase. The results indicated that this nursing shortage was different from others in the past in that there was also an increased demand for nurses in specialty areas. The following are specific findings from this survey.

- Hospitals are experiencing competition for nurses from managed care, pharmaceutical, and non–health-related companies.
- There is regional variation in the ability of hospitals to recruit nurses.
- It is taking longer to recruit nurses.
- Urban hospitals are having more problems in filling positions.
- Small hospitals are having more problems filling positions for obstetrical nurses.
- Larger and urban hospitals are using more agency and contract nurses.
- Recruitment and retention are problems. Incentives that are used include flexible hours, bonuses, and child care.

The report on this survey concluded that there are three nursing staff priorities.

1. The first is to find nurses with appropriate skills, competency, and experience, and this is as true today as it was in 1999 when the survey was reported. This is a problem because a lack of educational resources exists to keep nurses up-to-date, and many educational programs are not providing content and experience related to practice in the clinical settings—the "real world."
2. The second priority is managing flexible staffing to accommodate the fluctuating patient census and the use of temporary staffing.
3. The third priority relates to organizational issues that affect staff and retention, such as the amount of paperwork and decreased financial support for nursing management support systems. Retention of nurses requires the creation of work environments when professional practice and leadership are recognized, and there is educational support for ongoing professional development and career opportunities. There is no doubt that wages in other types of settings in which nurses are now finding new employment opportunities will continue to entice nurses away from the more traditional work settings; however, strategies need to be developed and implemented to retain nurses.

CURRENT ISSUES

Learn about events around the globe that relate to the chapter content.

Restructuring nursing education

When restructuring nursing education is discussed there are two critical focus areas. The first is academic education, and the second is continuing education for nurses who are practicing.

Nursing education must make curriculum changes in order to prepare nurses who meet today's and tomorrow's health care needs. The importance of the consumer as a significant player in the health care environment must be part of this preparation; however, this is not new to nursing education as nursing has always emphasized the importance of the patient's role. Understanding the interplay of values, motivations, and incentives of the major players or stakeholders in health care including insurers, providers, purchasers of health care, and consumers, helps nurses understand the health care culture in which they practice. Stakeholders sometimes have competing interests that affect decisions. Health care markets continue to change, which means nurses at all levels need to be aware of these changes and also know how to react positively to change, and in many cases to even anticipate it. Understanding the reasons health care delivery has become more business oriented and knowing its effect on nursing practice is also important. Today, there is a greater emphasis on service, innovation, cost-effectiveness, and customer service. To be successful in the more business-oriented health care environment, nurses need to be flexible. Nurses do need to have some understanding of the impact of costs on care and recognize that nurses have a fiscal responsibility or should be active in trying to reduce costs whenever it is possible. Lack of understanding about this responsibility is no longer an acceptable reason for not participating in reducing costs. All nurses need to be prepared to be leaders as well as team members, and restructuring education needs to provide content and learning experiences that assist students in developing leadership competencies.

The second area of concern about nursing education is the need for continuing education. All nurses need to be lifelong learners. Practice should be based on current knowledge. Not only is current information needed, but there also needs to be opportunities to understand and apply the knowledge.

The education needs of both groups, practicing nurses and nursing students, must be met to ensure that nurses are able to practice and participate actively in the change process within the health care delivery system, as well as make decisions.

CURRENT ISSUES

Learn about events around the globe that relate to the chapter content.

Several important factors in gaining a better understanding of the changing health care environment are particularly related to nursing.

1. Demographic trends are a very important issue related to workforce needs. Racial distribution and gender disparity in the nursing profession are problems. Another fact related to the future of health care delivery is the aging of the nursing workforce. Who will replace nurses as large numbers retire?

2. Another issue is the changing demand for nursing services, something that continues to be very difficult to determine. The present nursing shortage is the number one topic in nursing today. The shortage has had a major impact on the effectiveness of the entire health care delivery system.

3. The shifting nursing employment settings is a critical topic in both education and practice. Patients are sicker in the hospital, requiring complex care, and more and more care is provided outside the hospital and in the community. How are nurses prepared to meet both the needs of the acute care patient and the patient in the community?

4. The separation of nursing education and practice has provided many advantages for developing university-based nursing education, but it has caused problems for employers who want a more clearly articulated continuum of education and practice. Employers have become more involved in identifying minimum competencies for employment.

5. The changing nursing workforce competencies require that nurses possess **critical thinking** skills, independent clinical judgment, management and organizational skills, leadership abilities, technological understanding, and the ability to practice in a variety of settings. Nurses, not just nurse managers, need to be able to manage and coordinate personnel, services, data, and resources. They also need to demonstrate leadership.

6. There is a need for greater integration of research and nursing practice. Isolating education and research from the clinical setting is not helpful to nursing practice. Evidence-based practice is having an important impact on the application of research findings in practice as well as the use of standards, clinical guidelines, and clinical pathways.

Every nurse has a daily opportunity to be a nurse leader. Nurses use leadership skills when caring for individual patients and groups of patients and also when working with other health care workers.

The Concept of Change

Change is the "process of making something different from what it is" (Sullivan & Decker, 2001, p. 249). There is no doubt that change has become the normal state for all health care providers, but what is being changed? In general, everything; however, the important examples of change are related to an organization's structure, roles and responsibilities, communication methods and systems, policies and standards, culture, leadership and management approaches, and competencies and attitudes. In fact, before one change is completed there seems to be another one waiting in the wings to come on center stage. Some changes even come together, forcing staff and management to juggle multiple changes at one time. Change can be viewed from three interrelated perspectives as described in Figure 2-1 (Fisher, 1996).

Change disturbs the equilibrium, and so there also needs to be an effort to learn how to work in an environment whose equilibrium is frequently out of balance. Every staff member and nurse manager needs to understand their own personal response to change, both effective and ineffective responses. One concern is there are organizations or units in organizations that feel stability and security are more important than looking forward to the opportunities that are offered by the change process. In these organizations, staff feel frustration as they struggle with change that will inevitably occur and yet experience a leadership that says, "We want things to stay the same."

So why bother with change if it causes so much stress and problems? External factors outside the health care organization are a key driver in the need for change. Some changes are actually made so that the organization can survive. Many health care organizations today function from day-to-day, and in the long term they may close or merge with other health care organiza-

FIGURE 2-1   Interrelated perspectives.

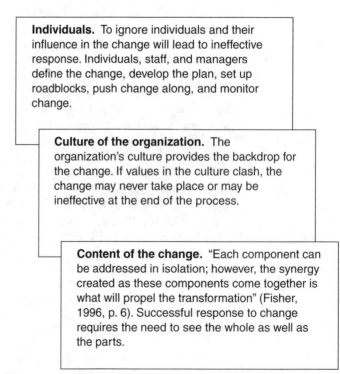

Individuals. To ignore individuals and their influence in the change will lead to ineffective response. Individuals, staff, and managers define the change, develop the plan, set up roadblocks, push change along, and monitor change.

Culture of the organization. The organization's culture provides the backdrop for the change. If values in the culture clash, the change may never take place or may be ineffective at the end of the process.

Content of the change. "Each component can be addressed in isolation; however, the synergy created as these components come together is what will propel the transformation" (Fisher, 1996, p. 6). Successful response to change requires the need to see the whole as well as the parts.

Source: Author.

tions. Nurses work daily in environments where external factors have an impact on what they do and on their ability to influence the health care delivery system. Each nurse has opportunities to be a change agent, but these opportunities are driven by and affected by many critical external factors. Box 2-2 identifies examples of these external factors that may affect change in health care delivery.

BOX 2-2 External factors that affect change.

- Local, state, and federal government: policy, laws, and regulations
- Technology
- Economics
- Reimbursement
- Competition
- Providers
- Managed care
- Providers of all types
- Medicare and Medicaid
- Demographics
- Nurse Practice Acts
- Health care professional organizations
- Health care professional standards
- Accreditation of health care organizations
- Malpractice issues
- Community culture
- Nurse recruitment and retention
- Community support of health care organizations
- Labor unions
- Research
- Local businesses
- Transportation services
- Marketing
- The uninsured and underinsured
- Pharmaceutical industry
- Consumers and consumer organizations
- Information technology
- Social service agencies
- Health status of the community
- Media and image
- Patient rights, privacy, and confidentiality
- Disasters and response

Source: Author.

THINK CRITICALLY

Try this exercise to apply what you have learned about this topic.

Examples of change theory

There are many theories about change, but only two theories are discussed in this chapter: Lewin's theory, which is frequently referred to, and Quinn's theory, which is a newer theory.

Lewin's force-field model of change

Lewin proposed a change theory that he called a force-field model of change, which includes three stages (Dessler, 2002; Lewin, 1947).

1. **Unfreezing stage.** This stage focuses on developing problem awareness and decreasing forces that maintain the status quo. This includes the recognition of a problem and whether or not there is a feeling that the problem can be improved. Methods that might be used to promote unfreezing are interview results, surveys, or meetings in which there is an open discussion of relevant issues. The result should be a better understanding of the issue or problem.
2. **Moving stage.** In this stage the issue or problem is clearly identified, and goals and objectives are developed. Strategies are developed and implemented. This is the working stage of the process where new values, attitudes, and behaviors are promoted.
3. **Refreezing stage.** This stage occurs when the change becomes a part of the work environment and its processes. This stage may take some time as it is easy to slip back to the way things were, so during this phase, the goal is to prevent a return to the past. In today's health care environment an organization is typically experiencing refreezing for one change while beginning another change. This is something that was not as critical when Lewin developed his theory.

Force-field analysis is used to improve the change process. In this analysis the manager (change agent) and staff identify the driving forces or factors that will help to move the situation in the direction of the anticipated change or the desired outcome. To be effective this should be a collaborative process between the manager and staff. If the manager identifies these forces and analyzes them without staff input, the analysis may not be as effective. Frequently staff are able to identify factors that might make a strategy more effective. Examples of driving forces are increasing staff, increasing staff time to provide direct care, decreasing costs, or increased availability of expertise. The focus should be on increasing acceptance of the change.

Restraining forces or forces that may keep the change from occurring should not, however, be ignored. What might be a restraining force? Examples are staffing concerns, increased safety risks, or decreasing quality. After the driving and restraining forces are identified, there are three possible approaches that might be used to cope with driving and restraining forces, which are described in Figure 2-2:

1. Increase the number or strength of the driving forces
2. Decrease the number or strength of the restraining forces
3. A combination of both

It is easy to apply these approaches in health care, but it does require information about the organization, staff, processes, and the change issue or problem. It is also important to include the informal processes such as the grapevine and informal leaders who may or may not be supportive. This information must be carefully analyzed using each of the approaches described in Lewin's theory.

Quinn's theory of change

When an organization experiences change it usually faces a major dilemma of a "slow death" or "deep change" (Quinn, 1996, 2000). When does "slow death" occur? If an organization finds it is more comfortable accepting the status quo and not changing, "slow death" occurs. This is demonstrated when staff experience burnout, lack energy, or feel hopeless or trapped. Staff are seen as pulling back and running around doing insignificant things. " 'Slow death' exists when self-interests triumph over collective responsibilities" (Pesut, 2001, p. 118). There is no vision or clear description of the future for the organization.

How do organizations and their leaders typically cope with "slow death"? The first method is probably obvious: they resign themselves to the situation. The second method is to try to find

FIGURE 2-2 Force-field analysis.

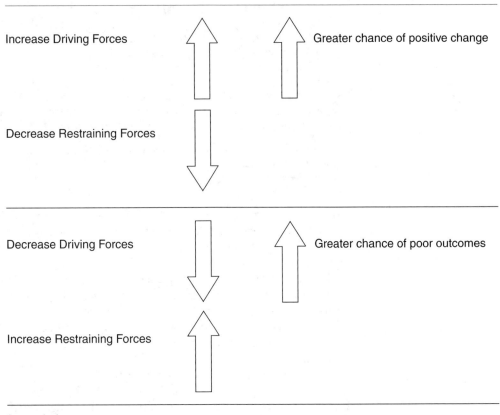

Source: Author.

a way around the problem or a way out, hoping that the "slow death" will not cause a major problem. These two methods are not positive responses and usually make the situation worse as the organization will not adapt when it is needed. The last coping method is the positive approach of engaging in "deep change," which is the method that a Transformational Leader would take. This requires that the need for change is understood and accepted and that adjustments are made in the organization to respond to the need. **Quinn's theory of change** is an approach that is easily applied with current leadership theories discussed in Chapter 1 such as Transformational Leadership, Clear Leadership, and Emotional Intelligence.

The process of change

The literature discusses many approaches to change. Dessler (2002) describes one of these in his eight-step process for leading organizational change that is helpful in understanding the key elements of the change process. When the eight steps of the change process are experienced, change can occur at all levels of the organization (for example, within a unit or division, at one location such as a community clinic, or throughout the entire organization). Regardless of where or how much of the organization is affected, **resistance** and acceptance will be experienced. The following steps, which are highlighted in Box 2-3, provide some description about what happens during the process and also apply Lewin's theory of change.

1. **Create a sense of urgency.** Applying unfreezing means that staff need to be motivated to make the changes. "Urgency does more than overcome employees' traditional reasons for resisting change: It can also jar them out of their complacency" (Dessler, 2002, p. 302). Staff need to feel that change is required. If, however, change occurs too fast, the organization and its staff may not be able to respond effectively, and this may affect other organizational functions.

2. **Create a guiding coalition and mobilize commitment.** Clearly, the change agent is important during change. The change agent (e.g., a nurse manager, team leader, staff nurse, or any

BOX 2-3   The change process.

> 1. Create a sense of urgency
> 2. Create a guiding coalition and mobilize commitment
> 3. Develop and communicate a shared vision
> 4. Empower employees to make the change
> 5. Generate short-term wins
> 6. Consolidate and produce more change
> 7. Anchor the new ways of doing things in the organizational culture
> 8. Monitor progress and adjust the vision as required
>
> Source: Author created summarization of content from Dessler, G. (2002). *Management*, pp. 302–306. Upper Saddle River, NJ: Prentice Hall.

member of the management team) is the person(s) who works to bring about the change. Focusing just on the change agent, however, is not enough. It is important to also have coalitions or groups of staff that can help push the change forward. This means the change agent seeks political support for the change—gaining staff support and agreement. Task forces often play this role and provide a place to develop a shared understanding. Many ideas will be discussed, and this is exciting. If, however, the discussion never gets to planning, it can sometimes act as a barrier. It is thus important to "Distinguish between and respect the two phases of your creative process: voicing creative ideas, where the quantity of suggestions prevails (diverging process), and sorting out the answers, where the quality of the suggestions prevails (converging process)" (Gebelein et al., 2000, p. 25).

3. **Develop and communicate a shared vision.** The **vision** provides direction for the change. Staff need to know what that vision is and how it relates to them. After they agree on what the outcome should be—a view of the future—then specific objectives need to be identified to reach the outcome. Change agents need to keep the vision simple and real, and it needs to mean something to the staff. Sharing the vision with staff so that they can understand and participate actively requires multiple methods, forums, and repetition to ensure that all staff gain an understanding.

4. **Empower employees to make the change.** Major changes in an organization require empowerment of staff so that they can actively participate in all phases. Empowerment is the "sense that one is not only capable of acting but expected and encouraged to act" (Tappen, 1995, p. 50). When staff feel empowered then they are more committed to the change and buy into it. It is at this time that barriers, such as resistances, are dealt with in order to move the change process along.

5. **Generate short-term wins.** If a change process only focuses on the long-term results, management and staff will lose steam somewhere along the way. Change takes time, but people need to feel that they are moving along. Identifying short-term goals and then evaluating when they are met will help management and staff feel that they can make it to the end point and they can see that some progress has been made. These short-term wins do much to build morale and a sense of success. They act as benchmarks that keep the change process on target.

6. **Consolidate and produce more change.** It is at this point that complacency can return. Staff may feel that things really are fine and nothing more needs to be done. When short-term goals are met and recognized, this helps staff to recognize that there is movement, hopefully positive movement, toward the goal. Staff may need to be reminded that some changes take time. A typical problem that is encountered with change is how to keep it going. Many managers and staff seem to be able to recognize a need for change, plan for change, and even implement change with greater ease than maintaining the change. There is a greater risk of slowing down the change process at this point, almost as if all involved say, "Okay we did it. What's next?" If this occurs, then the final goal(s) will not be met. Stopping too soon often is the reason staff feel that the organization never seems to make changes effectively—it never completes anything.

7. **Anchor the new ways of doing things in the organizational culture.** Shared values are important in every organization. As change occurs, there may need to be changes in these val-

ues so that there is a match between the change and the organizational culture. One example of values are recognition of the importance of staff involvement in decisions, diversity, and management that respects the employee. Changing values must be done carefully and only when absolutely necessary. This can cause stress as management and staff may feel insecure when values are challenged, but this can be worked through with recognition of new shared values. For example, if an organization wants more staff input and will use this feedback, but this approach has not been valued in the past, staff may be unsure about this change in values. Some may wonder why managers are now interested in what they have to say. Some may doubt that the change will actually happen. Management will need to take time to explain why they now value staff input, and then managers at all levels will have to demonstrate that they mean it. It is important, however, to recognize that not all changes require changes in values.

   8. Monitor progress and adjust the vision as required. Evaluation should never be ignored. Changes that organizations and their staff undergo are not written in stone. As has been noted in this chapter, change is constant now, so getting too settled is not a good idea. Organizations not only have to be concerned with future change, but they also need to monitor each change process. Adjustment may be needed, and if so, it needs to take place as soon as possible. Staff will become very discouraged if this does not occur. The inability to adjust can do considerable damage to morale, recruitment and retention, productivity, and quality of care. It also affects future changes as staff will not be as willing to go through "this process" again (Dessler, 2002, pp. 302–306).

Readiness for change

Readiness for change means that staff and management are willing to take on the challenge of change and to invest in the effort. At this time they are ready to begin the work of change. Not all staff will be ready at the same time, and some will never be ready. Readiness is affected by trust, the relationship between staff and management, fear and concern about what might be lost, staff experience, seriousness of the change, past history with both personal and work related change, effectiveness of communication, staff and management commitment to the organization, and the planning process or lack of a process.

   Many barriers and facilitators that affect the change process can be found in any organization. Some of the typical barriers are:

- Staff are too focused on their specialty and not able to see beyond it—they are focusing on parts and unable to see the whole, which often results in isolationism and territoriality.
- When managers overdirect, overobserve, or overreport, staff will not be innovative—staff feel they will be taken care of by the manager.
- When staff or managers say, "This is the way things have always been done," "They'll never accept it," or "We can't"—they see no need to respond positively to change.
- Policies and procedures can be barriers if they prevent staff from approaching change in a creative way.

Clearly, some policies and procedures must be followed; however, if they interfere with the consideration of alternative options and the change process then they act as barriers.

- Staff or managers with hidden agendas or motives are barriers.
- Criticizing staff when they make suggestions and identifying them as troublemakers act as barriers when the appropriate response should be rewarding staff who challenge and question ideas, thereby contributing new ideas.
- Organizational inertia or organizations that just do not seem to be changing or keeping up with current trends act as a barrier to effective organizations.
- Budgetary constraints can act as a barrier—if there is not enough money to make changes. This can be deadly for the organization.
- Bureaucratic organizations set up too much "red tape" and thus limit creativity—there are too many steps and staff to consult to get something accomplished.
- **Sensory overload** that occurs when staff have just experienced too much change in a short period of time acts as a barrier—staff need a break to recoup.

■ Fear of failure will always act as a barrier if one cannot get over it and move on. This prevents risk taking, which is necessary for successful responses to change.

■ The complexity of a needed change may make it difficult to initiate change that requires major planning—initiating a response to change may require funding, excessive staff time, additional staff, and so on.

■ Change means there needs to be a willingness to alter direction. When a change decision is viewed as written in stone, this then acts as a barrier (Fisher, 1996; Gebelein et al., 2000).

Facilitators are situations, factors, and behaviors that can reduce or eliminate barriers to change (Fisher, 1996). They make it possible to make a change. Managers who use self-reflection to understand behavior and how behaviors affect the organization's response to change are more effective facilitators of change. They are visible and accessible, and thus better able to lead the staff. The staff can easily communicate with their manager to express their reactions and ideas. Getting teams or groups involved in the change process facilitates change. Staff who feel that they can participate and have some freedom to act will improve the change process to reach a more effective outcome. Few situations are so clear that there is only one approach. Recognizing this acts as a facilitator. "When organizations are rigid and job descriptions are defined too precisely, little room for flexibility and shifting of responsibility is possible" (Fisher, 1996, p. 56). Wiggle room that allows for flexibility helps organizations to develop creative approaches to change.

Empathy is a critical key to readiness for change, and when it is present there is a greater chance of reaching a successful outcome (Kirkpatrick, 2001). It is related to effective communication and participation, which are always important. What is empathy? Empathy occurs when one is able to put oneself in the shoes of another person. It is empathy that helps in the understanding of acceptance, resistance, or a mixed reaction to change. With this information, concerns can be better addressed, and hopefully, the change process will go more smoothly. If managers and staff take time to get to know one another, this will improve empathy. Then there will be some ability to anticipate how one another might respond. "Communication means to create understanding" (Kirkpatrick, 2001, p. 58). This is more than just sending and receiving information. Staff need to understand the "why," "what," and "how" about the change. Change cannot be really successful without some empathy and effective communication.

Participation from all staff involved also improves communication and the final outcomes. Participatory management/leadership sometimes is viewed as the miracle that will solve all problems. Just get the staff involved, and the task is accomplished. It does not work this way. Participation must be managed and used carefully. Timing and clear direction must be part of the process. An important factor is how much management really believes that staff participation is critical to success. Lip-service acceptance of the need for staff participation will only be more destructive. Staff will know when management is asking for participation because it is "the thing to do" rather than from a deep-seated belief that this is the best approach. Empathy clearly affects readiness for change since understanding, which is improved with empathy, is required for readiness.

Resistance to change

Most staff and managers have experienced forced change, change that appeared to be useless, as well as times when it would just be better to have things stay the way they were, protecting the status quo. Staff resistance to change places major roadblocks to success and progress. Why might staff or even managers be resistant to a change? Typically, change means someone has to give up something or make some adaptation, and this is stressful. Along with the stress, the person may not be able to see the benefits and no one points the way to the positive aspects of the change. The person is concerned about

1. his/her *fears and biases* due to lack of understanding;
2. *perceptual issues* when the person cannot appreciate the situation around the change;
3. *economic threat*, which may lead to job change, job loss, decreased salary, and lack of promotion; and
4. *social threat* when the social structure of the organization changes.

Resistance to change is inevitable, and it can be experienced by managers, staff, the organization as a whole or parts of it, or the community outside the organization, and by consumers. Most people do not like disequilibrium as it makes them feel uncomfortable. Resistance to change is often the first response to disequilibrium. With the need for change occurring rapidly today, there is less time for adjustment though staff do need time to do this. When there is little time for adjustment, resistance can be greater. What are some of the typical reasons for manager and staff resistance that need to be considered before a change is instituted?

- Staff or managers see no need for a change and feel that the way things are done is fine—the effect of habit and inertia.
- Staff or managers see the need for change as a personal criticism.
- Staff or managers feel that the organization is constantly changing and do not feel a sense of stability anywhere in the organization.
- Staff and a new nurse manager or new team leader may not have had enough time to develop the relationship that is critical to successful response to change.
- Staff or manager may have developed a negative attitude toward their manager/supervisor, the nursing department, or the organization and view all changes negatively.
- Staff do not respect their nurse manager, or the nurse manager does not respect the staff and is unable to be objective.
- Staff do not hear about a change directly from their manager but rather as secondhand information.
- When staff or managers have a negative attitude toward the organization, this results in a negative attitude toward change.
- The change will add to work, and thus it is viewed as a burden.
- Staff or manager may feel that the change may cause more problems than it solves.
- Staff or manager may fear the unknown and the loss of predictability.
- Administration or management may not have admitted that some past decisions related to change were inadequate.
- Change that is directed rather than participatory tends to experience more resistance (Finkelman, 1996; Kirkpatrick, 2001).

Though all of these are possible reasons for resistance, the most common reason for resistance is lack of staff input and participation. Sometimes it is difficult to identify the reasons for resistance; however, it is important to try and identify these reasons. If this can be done, strategies can then be taken to prevent them or make an attempt to decrease their impact, such as by applying Lewin's theory to decrease the barriers and increase the facilitators.

Loss plays a role in resistance to change and should be included in the assessment of resistance. Loss is a natural experience with change. What is loss? Examples of loss that staff may experience are old ways of doing things, old job responsibilities, a manager or staff person who may leave his or her job, or old structure. Staff need to grieve these losses and then move on. Some staff do this with greater ease than others. Grieving requires (a) recognition of the loss, (b) letting go, and (c) moving on. Some of the common losses that those who resist change are concerned about when change is introduced include:

- **Security.** Staff may lose their jobs.
- **Money.** Staff may experience a decrease in salary, overtime, benefits, travel expenses, education expenses, or budget level.
- **Pride and satisfaction.** Job redesign may mean that the job is less prestigious or less interesting.
- **Friends and important contacts.** Change may bring an alteration in staff interactions on the job.
- **Freedom.** Freedom may lead to changes in the ability to function independently or the assignment of a new manager who does not allow as much freedom.
- **Responsibility.** The level of responsibility may decrease or it could increase, leading to a loss of competency in the job.

- **Authority.** Power and authority over others may change or be lost with reorganization.
- **Good working conditions.** Staff may experience a change in space, location, sharing more with others, work hours, and so on.
- **Status.** Staff may fear reduction to a low level or less recognized position (Kirkpatrick, 2001, pp. 20–21).

Management and staff can experience any of these losses. These possible losses will be on their minds as change occurs. It is natural for staff to want to protect what is valuable to them, and this can then become a resistance to change.

Is there value to this resistance to change? Yes, there can be value to resistance as it can force management or the change agent to clarify the need for change and then develop a plan with a clearer statement of purpose. Those who question may be providing valuable information of flaws that can be solved before more serious errors are made. Resistance may indicate that the communication process has not worked in getting a clear message across, and this should not be ignored. Sometimes resistance is used against those who are resistant. Staff who are resistant may be identified as non-team players. This approach can be very destructive, as it sets a tone of clamping down on those who offer a different point of view. Resistance should be viewed as a motivator to make the message clearer and to use input from others. Further assessment is then required to improve the plan and clearly state the outcomes.

A critical factor in coping with resistance to change is the long-term relationship that exists between management and staff. If this relationship has been good, with trust and open communication, then resistance can usually be handled effectively. If this relationship does not exist, then coping with resistance will be more difficult. As has been discussed in Chapter 1, managers must spend time on building and maintaining staff relationships as this will be the key to success. Managers who demonstrate leadership competence will understand the need to respond in the following way: "I need to stop and listen."

Since some resistance should be expected, planning for resistance needs to be included whenever change is occurring. First, staff need to understand why change is needed—the vision for change, advantages and disadvantages, how it might adversely affect staff, how change relates to competitive needs, and the financial benefits. Losses may occur, and this potential requires open discussion. Alliances need to be formed to gain political support for the change. What is political support? This is when one person supports another because that person feels a personal allegiance and will support the person's ideas. When leaders allow staff to openly discuss concerns without fear or punitive actions, resistance can be dealt with openly. Clearly, data that can be provided to support the need and direction for change are very important. It may be necessary to stop doing what is being done and take a step back. Resistance needs to be viewed as an honest friend or a cue. Allowing others to tell their story or express their concerns will help make resistance a positive experience rather than a barrier to success. When children cross the street, they are taught to, "Stop, look, and listen." This is what needs to be done when resistance occurs.

YOUR OPINION COUNTS

Find out what others think about this topic. Post your response and check out other opinions.

Acceptance of change

After this discussion of resistance to change, it is easy to assume that all staff resist change, but this is not true. What is different about situations that are accepted and in some cases welcomed (Kirkpatrick, 2001)? There is no doubt that when a situation is very bad staff tend to welcome change, hoping it will improve a dysfunctional situation. What about the situations that are not so extreme? The key issue in acceptance is not what might be lost, but rather what will be gained. This is where the focus should be, though concerns about what might be lost should not be ignored. These gains are related to the loss factors, but they focus on the positive. Staff feel they will be more secure in their jobs and more of their skills will be used. There may be an increase in money through salary, benefits, and other incentive changes. There may be an improved over-all budget. Someone may receive a promotion or a new manager may be assigned who may give staff more authority. Status and prestige may improve with more space, special responsibilities, or a new location. Job responsibilities may change and improve. Better working conditions may be gained with new equipment, work schedule, or better workspace. Self-satisfaction in the job or the work environment may occur. Staff may find themselves in work situations that provide them with better personal contacts or social relationships. The change may require less time and effort to get the job done because work will be more efficient. In conclusion, there may also be some staff who have mixed reactions to change—some resistance with some acceptance. How an individual identifies or predicts what will be gained and what will be lost are critical factors in directing the individual's response to change—whether it be resistance, acceptance, or some-where in-between.

Where to begin when confronted with change

There are internal and external key factors that influence how an organization responds to change (for example, a change in policy, regulations and accreditation, organization, and finan-cial issues). Each of these factors need to be considered.

1. **Internal and external policies.** It is important to understand how change affects and is affected by **internal** and **external policies** before actions are taken. Are there health policies such as state or federal laws that would affect a decision about the need for a decision? External poli-cies may seem to be disconnected but really provide required direction (for example, a state's nurse practice act describes what RNs may do). Internal policies are those that exist within an organization. Clearly, internal policies might be changed and may again be changed to adapt to a situation; however, what is the policy's present status? An example is the increased use of UAPs, which has caused much concern in nursing. If a hospital wanted to increase the use of UAPs in the organization, what does the hospital policy say about the UAP's present role, and how does this role relate to the change the hospital wants to make? What does the board of nurs-ing say about the UAP role (for example, can the UAP administer medications)? If a hospital then decided that UAPs could administer oral medications, this would probably be in conflict with the board of nursing and the nurse practice act. This is an example of the relevancy of in-ternal and external policies. Changes in external policy require political advocacy.

2. **Regulations and accreditation.** Regulations are very important. They describe how laws are to be implemented, and they are developed by governmental agencies after legislative bod-ies pass laws, as in the previous example regarding boards of nursing that develop regulations re-lating to nurse practice acts. Another example is the Department of Health and Human Services in Washington, DC, which develops regulations for specific laws passed by Congress (for exam-ple, when laws about Medicare are passed there still needs to be rules set up to address imple-mentation of the law that are much more detailed than the law). Standards and accreditation also have an impact on change (for example, nursing standards of care and the standards devel-oped by the Joint Commission on Accreditation of Healthcare Organizations (JCAHO) that are used when health care organizations are evaluated for accreditation).

3. **Organization.** Organizational issues, such as the organization's vision statement of how it views itself in the future; structure (departments, who reports to whom); size, roles, and func-tions of staff and administration; communication; morale and culture; willingness to change; fi-nancial status; quality improvement; and the organization's position and relationship with the community, are all key to understanding the organization, how it will respond to change, and what needs to change. For example, if a health care organization is experiencing low staff morale as well as having financial problems, it will have problems responding to a need to change its documentation system. Staff will probably not be eager to make changes, and there may be lim-ited funds to develop a new system.

4. **Financial issues.** Costs can never be ignored, and during change responses may be costly. Change may actually be driven by increased cost. For example, a hospital may decide to eliminate

its obstetrical service as it is not getting enough admissions and is in competition with another hospital that has a large obstetrical service. In an uncertain health care industry, two things are facts. First, regardless of the decision maker (government, managed care organizations/insurers, businesses, health care organizations), cost constraints will continue to tighten. Second, as data become more available and more reliable, data will increasingly be used in decision making. Data will drive how care is delivered by driving improvement opportunities and how the organization competes with other health care organizations.

Along with the consideration of influences on the organization, an organization needs to include total quality improvement in the change process. In doing this, the organization's leaders create a plan for excellence and better ensure implementation of the plan.

Strategies to respond to change are very important throughout the change process. To adjust to change, nurses need to develop their mental flexibility, which is the ability to consider new information and a broad range of alternatives (Gebelein et al., 2000). When a nurse uses mental flexibility, the nurse listens to others and avoids snap judgments. This is an attitude of "yes and . . ." rather than "yes, but. . . ." This nurse will ask others who are trusted for honest feedback, develop personal creativity, and will improve coping with change through these acts. How can coping with change be improved? Examples of guidelines are found in Box 2-4 (Gebelein et al., 2000; Marrelli, 1997).

The change agent

During the change process, the change agent, who may be a nurse executive, nurse manager, nurse team leader, staff nurse, and so on, has four major leadership functions: charismatic, enabling, instrumental, and missionary (Dessler, 2002). There is no doubt that leadership is one of the most critical factors affecting change, particularly major changes, in a health care organization.

1. The charismatic change agent is an envisioning leader who can describe the vision, set high expectations, and is a role model for staff. In this process the change agent needs to energize others and be excited and stimulated about the potential opportunity.

BOX 2-4   Guidelines for coping with change.

- During the creatively stage, give up critical judgment; avoid using, "It won't work."
- Instead of asking, "Why?"; ask, "Why not?"
- Use a multidisciplinary group to develop responses to change needs.
- Expect that resistance to change is a fact, but approach it as a problem, not a character flaw.
- Talk, talk, talk to get the ideas flowing. Be challenged by opposite points-of-view. Try taking the opposite point-of-view and defend it.
- Generate as many options as possible. This will lead to finding the best method of coping with change.
- Do not throw out ideas too quickly. These may be important ideas.
- Join together with the change champions in the organization, those who seem to do well with change.
- View change as a challenge or opportunity for innovation.
- Control is very important as it means that the staff feel that they can make a difference.
- Commitment is part of a successful response to change.
- Working together and using social support can give staff extra energy and resources.
- Use stress management when stress increases, as it often does during the change process.

Source: Author content and summary of content from Dessler, G. (2002). *Management.* Upper Saddle River, NJ: Prentice Hall; Robbins, S., & Decenzo, D. (2001). *Fundamentals of management.* Upper Saddle River, NJ: Prentice Hall.

2. As an enabling change agent, the change agent expresses personal views, empathizes, and lets others know that they can do it.
3. Change agents need to also demonstrate instrumental leadership, which is the management component of leadership referred to as Transactional Leadership, by providing staff with resources they need to do their jobs (funds, appropriate staff levels, supplies and equipment, and so on).
4. As a missionary change agent, the change agent shares and clearly communicates the vision that is required to meet the goals (Dessler, 2002, p. 307).

Like their staff, managers must cope with frequent changes. It is important for staff to understand the manager's response to change as it affects staff involvement. The major role of the manager is to implement change as directed from administration or management about the manager. Some managers will feel that they must respond positively to all requests even if they disagree with the need or the specific change. Why do they do this? They may be afraid about what might happen to them if they do not agree. They may want to be seen as a loyal manager. If the manager does disagree, the manager may decide to ask why this change is required. The manager may then need to explain why he or she disagrees with the change and to make recommendations for other approaches. There are certainly managers who have come to the point where they cannot agree with higher management directives for change, and if they cannot influence the change process, they may then leave their positions. During these times, stress will be very high, and undoubtedly this will spill over onto the staff.

There are other roles that managers need to take. Change agents do not wait for change—they look for it and embrace it as an opportunity. In addition, a manager may implement some change independently from the total organization, without involvement from those above the manager. These changes usually pertain to the manager's unit or department and do not affect others outside that area. There are fewer and fewer situations that can meet this criterion as collaboration across areas is becoming more important in successful organizations. If the budget is involved, then the manager must carefully consider how to respond and how to involve upper management. It takes courage to initiate change as it involves risk taking, a higher risk than just implementing change that may be directed from above. Staff need to be involved and understand that the risk taking includes them. The manager may risk altering staff morale, loss of staff, loss of quality care, loss of money from the budget, poor image, and so on. Participation from staff means they become direct participants, adding their input to the plan. Changes that are implemented when there is a crisis carry with them an even higher risk for success. At this time careful planning may be put aside; the result is then often a haphazard response.

Change agents need to be very effective in initiating adaptive work (figuring out the best way to adapt how work is done and still meet the work demands). Certainly change is stressful for everyone, and yet this cannot be used as a barrier to improvement. Six principles for leading adaptive work include the following.

1. **"Get on the balcony."** See the context, the environment, or situation for change or create it. This requires seeing the larger picture.
2. **Identify the adaptive challenge.** How can improvement occur? It is important to clearly identify the issue or problem, or the plan for change will not be effective.
3. **Regulate the distress caused by adaptive challenge.** Managers or change agents need to recognize that work and change need to be paced. This requires asking tough questions without getting anxious. Staff need to have confidence in the change agent; therefore, the change agent needs to remain calm during stress.
4. **Maintain disciplined attention.** Watch for signs of work avoidance; expose conflict, do not hide it—all these can lead to a source of creativity and learning. It is easy to get distracted so it is important for the change agent to recognize distractions and intervene to prevent them.
5. **Give the work back to the people.** Distress can lead to passivity and dependency on management—move to getting staff to assume responsibility. Many staff expect the change agent to take on most of the responsibility. Some of this is from habit when staff expect the manager to carry the responsibility, and some is because it is easier to say it is someone else's responsibility.
6. **Protect voices of leadership from below.** Listen to those who identify contradictions, though they seem to upset the status quo. Leadership can come from all levels of the staff,

and it needs to be encouraged. Initially, leadership from the staff may not be perfect, but it should be nurtured and encouraged to grow (Heifetz & Laurie, 2001, p. 131).

During the change process, it is also important to consider the impact of the organizational culture (Dessler, 2002). How does the change agent create and sustain the right culture? Change agents demonstrate through their words and actions the critical values. As managers who are change agents manage the environment and work, they also provide a vision for the staff. This is a time when words and actions need to match. It is not a time for conflict or inconsistency. For some changes, the culture also needs to change. This is not easy to do and requires a planned approach. During the change process, staff empowerment becomes important. "Empowering employees means giving employees the authority, tools, and information they need to do their jobs with greater autonomy, as well as the self-confidence required to perform the jobs effectively" (Dessler, 2002, p. 246). This helps to increase motivation. When staff are empowered they need to know their responsibilities and be given the authority that they need to get the job done. If training or further education is required, then staff need assistance in getting it. In order to move forward with change, staff need information, and standards need to be clear. There are several critical factors that can make a change more effective:

1. Exhibit a high level of commitment to change and are fully involved.
2. Motivated to ensure a successful change.
3. Use professional judgment in the change process.
4. Understand the need for change and the change process.
5. Exercise high levels of communications throughout the change.
6. Recognize that a high quality of outcome from the change will result in enhanced patient care (Carney, 2002, p. 297).

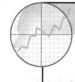

THINK CRITICALLY

Try this exercise to apply what you have learned about this topic.

BENCHMARKS

Now let's take a moment to test your knowledge of the concepts you have studied in this section.

A Decision: A Response to Change

"You may notice that the planning process parallels the decision-making process; this makes sense, since developing plans involves deciding today what you'll do tomorrow. Both involve establishing objectives or criteria, developing and analyzing alternatives based on information you obtain, evaluating the alternatives, and then making a choice" (Dessler, 2002, p. 93). This section of the chapter focuses on decision making and planning, which are functions that every nurse uses in the practice of nursing. Any response to change requires decisions, and many of these decisions require careful **planning**.

"Decision making is a process that begins with the identification of a problem and ends with the evaluation of the choices and taking a course of action" (Bernard & Walsh, 1990, as cited in Krairiksh & Anthony, 2001, p. 16). Decisions are a means rather than ends. They are used to achieve a goal. When decisions are made, the goal is usually related to both tasks and relationships. Some decisions may focus more on one than the other (Gebelein et al., 2000). Those who make decisions must learn to cope with being right some of the time and also learn to live with imperfect solutions. To make sound decisions, which is what people desire to do, the most important consideration is the criteria that are used to make the decision. Some examples of the criteria that might be used are: "(1) Minimally impacts current operations, (2) Helps achieve important priorities, (3) Is consistent with values, (4) Is acceptable to those involved in the decision, (5) Can be implemented with the constraints (time, resources, other priorities), and (6) Considers pros, cons, and risks" (Gebelein et al., 2000, p. 114).

How is decision making related to planning? Nurses actively use decision making in a variety of situations, particularly during planning—patient care planning, planning the work day, and more involved planning for specific projects such as changing documentation or how the unit is organized. "Planning is setting goals and deciding on courses of action, developing rules and procedures, developing plans (both for the organization and for those who work for it), and forecasting (predicting or projecting what the future holds for the organization)" (Dessler, 2002, p. 3). During all phases of the planning process, decisions are made. Each day a nurse makes multiple decisions that affect the nurse, the patient, other staff, patient's family, and many others as nursing practice is made up of a series of decisions.

"A problem is a discrepancy between a desirable and an actual situation" (Dessler, 2002, p. 68). Decisions are required to resolve this discrepancy. Typically, decision making and problem solving are used interchangeably though decisions do not always focus on problems. Decisions, however, are made when problems are solved. Figure 2-3 describes some of the key reasons for planning.

Decision styles

Why is creativity important in the decision-making process? Stepping "outside the box" is mentioned frequently today in all types of organizations. Decision making that routinely results in similar outcomes and does not consider innovative outcomes will not be as effective in the long run. Styles of decision making are affected by creativity or innovation. The common types of styles are unilateral, individual, and authoritarian decision making, all of which focus on one person making a decision with limited or no input from others. The opposite of this style is participative and consensus decision making. Here the emphasis is on including others in the decision

FIGURE 2-3   Reasons for planning.

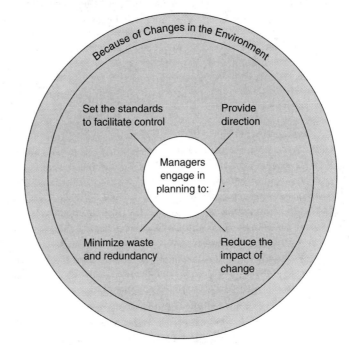

Source: Robbins, S., & Decenzo, D. (2001). *Fundamentals of management*, p. 81. Upper Saddle River, NJ: Prentice Hall. Reprinted with permission.

making, even if an individual must make the final decision. The individual, however, who uses this style would pay close attention to feedback from others before making the final decision.

Other **decision-making** styles that have been described are: **decisive**, **integrative**, **hierarchic**, and **flexible** (Milgram, Spector, & Treger, 1999). These styles apply to managers and to staff. The difference in these four styles is in the amount of data that is used to make a decision and the options that are considered.

- The decisive style depends on less data to arrive at one decision.
- The integrative style uses all available data and identifies multiple alternatives.
- The hierarchic style focuses on a large amount of information but arrives at one alternative or solution.
- The flexible style uses a small amount of data while generating multiple alternatives and may change as information is reinterpreted.

It is typical for managers to primarily use one style, though some managers use mixed styles or may switch styles depending upon the situation. For example, as was discussed in Chapter 1 about Contingency Leadership theory, when a situation changes different factors become more important, and the manager may change styles to adjust. A nurse manager may encourage staff participation in decisions and allow time for this, but if the unit is suddenly short staffed then the manager may need to step in and make decisions quickly.

Systematic versus intuitive decision styles are two other approaches to decision making (Dessler, 2002). **Systematic decision makers** form their decisions more logically and use a structured approach. **Intuitive decision makers** are at the other end of the spectrum; here the focus is on a trial-and-error approach. They may ignore information and change their alternatives if it does not feel right. This is the "gut" approach. A staff member will say, "I just had a feeling about it." Again, the situation can make a difference. When a nurse has expertise in an area, decisions may appear to be more intuitive because the nurse may feel more confident and can rely more on a "gut feeling," though the decision is probably supported by expertise.

Group decision making is another style that is used more today. It focuses on synergy, which is the combination of people's efforts that results in an output which is greater than the sum of the parts. Multiple ideas and experiences come together to form a decision. There are advantages and disadvantages to using group decision making. Advantages clearly focus on the fact that ideas from more than one person tend to improve other ideas and the final decision. As group members discuss an issue, ideas tend to bounce off of each other, which stimulates further ideas. The major disadvantage is it takes longer to make a decision. Some issues or problems are made worse by group decision making (for example, during an emergency when decisions must be made quickly and clearly so that all can follow them). The need during a crisis is for someone to make a decision and move the process along. Staff need to know that their ideas are important though they cannot always be used. These ideas or suggestions can be considered after the potential crisis has passed and then be used to improve future decisions. When feedback is not recognized, those giving the feedback will feel left out and wonder why they wasted their time. Managers sometimes think that they use staff feedback and this should be obvious, but often it is not so obvious to staff. Recognition goes a long way to improve morale, encourage staff to increase participation, and improve group decision making.

Dessler (2002) identifies additional advantages and disadvantages for using group decision making. The generally accepted advantage is "two heads are better than one." This allows for more points of view and develops more acceptance and commitment from those who participate. The result usually is greater effort to make the decision work during implementation. Why would there be disadvantages to group decision making? The process may actually shorten or interfere with the decision-making process, which affects the quality of the outcome. There may be greater pressure for consensus when members may not actually agree. Some groups experience dominance by one individual, diluting the effect of group input. Group members can believe so much in their own ideas that they are unable to openly consider other ideas. Group decisions can also take longer, which for some situations may be a disadvantage.

Groups can, of course, be quite successful in making decisions, but decision making does not just happen. There usually must be some guidance or facilitation. Brainstorming requires that all members are clear about what the issue is about and what it is not about. Setting a reasonable time limit pushes staff to move toward a result. Ground rules should make clear that the following are not helpful: (a) digression into details, (b) focusing on reasons about why it will not work or the constraints, and (c) criticism of ideas or evaluation of alternatives (Gebelein et al., 2000). While the group develops ideas, recording them is important so that they are not lost.

There are methods other than brainstorming that also facilitate group decision making, such as idea-generating questions (for example, "If we had enough staff, what would we do?" and "If we had the funding, how would we solve the problem?"). It is helpful to stimulate the group so that the group considers how similar problems were solved in the past, and then the group compares and contrasts the past with the present problem. Taking a different point of view than what would normally be taken may help the group understand the problem or issue from another perspective, which may lead to different alternatives, moving the decision making "out-of-the-box."

Types of decisions

Are there any major differences in the types of decisions? There are two major types that most staff encounter. The first is the need for **programmed decisions**. These decisions are more repetitive and routine. They take less time and typically are related to a policy or procedure. For example, if a patient leaves the hospital against medical advice (AMA), there is a procedure for an AMA discharge, or if a nurse misses an order for a medication, there is a procedure to follow such as whom to notify, what to document, and so on. Most decisions are of this type, which is a good thing as these take less time. The second type, **non-programmed decisions**, are not so routine, and some may be crises. Situations that require this type of decision require more time, collection of data, critical thinking and analysis, and may require consultation with others. These decisions may be completely new experiences. They require more judgment, or the "cognitive or thinking aspects of the decision-making process" (Dessler, 2002, p. 68).

Another view of the types of decisions considers the focus of the decision (Anthony, 1997, 1999; Blegen et al., 1993; Krairiksh & Anthony, 2001). One type is patient care decisions that nurses make in their practice that affect direct patient care. The second type is decisions about the condition of work. This type affects the work environment, groups of patients, and how work is conducted. Most nurses tend to participate more in the first type of decision, those with direct care implications (Krairiksh & Anthony, 2001). This, however, is changing as nurses become more involved as leaders in the health care delivery system.

The decision-making process

The decision-making process is a dynamic process. The most effective decisions are made in collaboration with others in the organization. Collaboration between nurses and physicians also affects nurses' participation as it provides greater opportunities for nurses to participate. When collaboration is present nurses and physicians share responsibility and hopefully respect one another more. Knowledge, ideas, and skills are shared. This type of relationship can only improve decision making. The key steps in the decision-making process are identified in Figure 2-4.

FIGURE 2-4   The decision-making process.

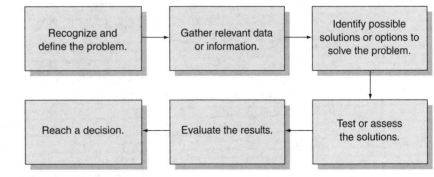

Source: Author.

Nursing and critical thinking

Nursing has become very complex with change occurring almost daily in nursing management and clinical practice. This complex, changing environment often leads to stress for all levels of staff. Managers and team leaders need to be particularly skilled in coping with stress and embrace opportunities to make change a positive experience for themselves, all staff, and the organization and to actively use critical thinking. "A more progressive, holistic way to define critical thinking is a commitment to look for the best way, based on the most current research and practice findings; for example, the best strategy to manage pain in a specific person or situation. Critical thinking in nursing means constantly striving to find a better way by focusing on two key questions: What are the outcomes? And how can we do better?" (Alfaro-LeFevre, 2001, p. 26). Another definition is "Critical thinking is reasoning in a manner that generates and examines questions and problems. Intuition and feelings are considered as an individual weighs, clarifies, and evaluates evidence, arguments, and conclusions" (Stark, 1996, p. 168). Those who use critical thinking incorporate the following in their thinking process:

- Reasoning
- Generates and examines questions and problems
- Intuition and feelings
- Weighs, clarifies, and evaluates evidence

Box 2-5 identifies some critical thinking skills. Nurses use critical thinking as they provide direct care, but they also use it as they coordinate care; advocate for the patient; work with other staff to resolve issues on the unit; ensure that quality, safe care is provided on the unit; and collaborate with others. Nurses who serve on committees and task forces use critical thinking in the work that must be done.

As decision making is experienced, it is easy to slip into **dichotomous thinking**. This should be avoided because when it is used, problems and situations are viewed in a polarized manner—things are seen as either "good" or "bad." This approach can lead to ineffective decision making as it limits choices for patients and for other types of decisions that need to be made. Some strategies that can prevent dichotomous thinking and improve critical thinking include the following.

- Replace "I don't know" and "I'm not sure" with "I'll find out."
- Turn errors into opportunities.
- Anticipate questions others might ask.
- Ask, "What if?"
- Look for flaws in one's own thinking, and ask others to identify flaws (Alfaro-LeFevre, 2001, p. 27).

Critical thinking should be part of problem solving and decision making in response to change. It is important, however, to note that critical thinking is not the same as problem solving or decision making. Nurses who develop critical thinking skills will relieve their own stress, solve

BOX 2-5   Critical thinking skills.

- Knowledge, experience, judgment, and evaluation
- Interpretation
- Affective listening
- Application of moral reasoning and values
- Comprehension, application, analysis, and synthesis
- Awareness of self
- Mistakes happen and we learn from them

Source: Author.

TABLE 2-1 Comparison of critical thinking, decision making, and problem solving.

CRITICAL THINKING	DECISION MAKING	PROBLEM SOLVING
Definition: "A process of examining underlying assumptions, interpreting and evaluating arguments, imagining and exploring alternatives, and developing relative criticism for the purpose of reaching a reasoned, justifiable conclusion" (Sullivan & Decker, 2001, p. 151). • Seeks no single solution. • Focuses on creativity and innovation. • Purposeful and constantly re-evaluating. • May be used in both decision making and problem solving. • Allows the person to "think outside the box" and consider many ideas without prejudice.	Definition: "A process whereby appropriate alternatives are weighed and one is ultimately selected" (Sullivan & Decker, 2001, p. 153). • Decisions are made daily by nurses: care decisions, management decisions, professional decisions. • Decisions may not involve a problem. • Ideally, critical thinking is used when decisions are made. • Decisions require a choice between alternatives.	Definition: "A process whereby a dilemma is identified and corrected" (Sullivan & Decker, 2001, p. 153). • A problem is a gap in how things are and how they might be. • Problem solving requires that the problem is identified or diagnosed. • There may not be the need to select a correct solution—for example, there may be no response to the problem. This in itself is a form of a decision. • Resolving a problem may include critical thinking—and the best resolutions include critical thinking. • Resolving a problem includes many decisions, typically some minor and some major. • Problem-solving process: define the problem, gather information, analyze the information, develop solutions, make a decision or choose the solution, implement the decision (solution), and evaluate the decision (solution). • The problem-solving process corresponds to the nursing process.

Source: Author. Adapted from Sullivan E., & Decker P. (2001). *Effective leadership and management in nursing.* Upper Saddle River, NJ: Prentice Hall.

problems, and make more effective decisions. Table 2-1 compares critical thinking, decision making, and problem solving.

How does one describe a critical thinker? Some authorities have identified key traits. Paul (1995) identifies the following four traits.

1. **Intellectual humility.** The person is willing to admit what is not known.
2. **Intellectual integrity.** The person continually evaluates his or her own thinking and is willing to admit when wrong.
3. **Intellectual courage.** The person is aware of the need to confront ideas fairly, even when negative reactions toward the ideas may be present.
4. **Intellectual empathy.** The person makes a conscious effort to understand others.

CURRENT ISSUES

Learn about events around the globe that relate to the chapter content.

Identify the need for decision making: What is the problem?

After a review of related issues, the need to make a decision should be carefully defined. A solution cannot be found for something that is truly unknown or poorly understood. Clarifying the problem is not always easy. Staff may have different perspectives on the issue. For example, one

BOX 2-6   Identifying the need for decision making: Questions to ask.

- What is the issue or problem? State the issue or problem in terms of need rather than a solution, using terms that are understood.

- What important, critical facts are known? Describe these as clearly as possible.

- What is unknown? How important is the unknown? Who might know the information or how can it be obtained? Be willing to identify factors that might be negative or different.

- When does the problem occur? When is it absent? Consider days of week, time of day, and factors that might affect timing.

- What is the consequence of the problem or issue? This step should include negative and positive consequences.

- What has been tried in the past to deal with the situation? This may be an action that occurred within the organization or externally considered (literature review, network with others, and so on). What happened as a result of these actions?

- How do people feel about the situation and changes to it?

- What related problems are present? If something changes, what else will likely change as a result of the initial change?

- What assumptions—about people, technology, systems, funding—have been made that might need to be challenged?

Source: Author content and some summarized content from Gebellin, S., et al. (2000). *Successful manager's handbook*. Minneapolis, MN: Personnel Decisions International Corporation; Marrelli, T. (1997). *The nurse manager's guide*. St. Louis, MO: Mosby-Year Book, Inc.

staff member may think a problem about quality care might be due to low staffing and another may attribute it to lack of appropriate training of unlicensed assistive personnel. The questions found in Box 2-6 should be considered in this step of the process.

After the analysis of the answers to the questions found in Box 2-6, goals need to be established so that all staff know the direction that is to be taken. Identifying goals is the only way to know if results are met. Who sets the goals? This can vary. The typical situation is the manager of change agents sets the goals, or this is done by higher levels of managers. As discussed throughout this text, however, the more staff are involved the better the decision-making process. Setting goals is part of this process. Team leaders also set goals, and individual staff may also set goals as they do their work. In the end, who sets the goals depends on the issue or problem that is being addressed.

What are some guidelines for setting goals (Milgram, Spector, & Treger, 1999)? Goals need to be reasonable. By evaluating strengths and weaknesses, additional information can be identified to assist in setting realistic goals. Setting goals should not be done in a vacuum. If consideration is not given to external factors that might affect the goals, the goals may not be what should be achieved, may be unreasonable, or may not receive critical support. Throughout the decision-making process, perception is a critical factor. "Perception is the selection and interpretation of information we receive through our senses and the meaning we give to the information" (Dessler, 2002, p. 75). Many factors influence how stimuli are perceived, such as level of participation, past history with decision making, how and what information is shared, who is involved, commitment to the issue or problem, morale and stress level, level of staffing, and so on.

Proactive planning helps to improve decision making and decrease stress about decisions that need to be made. This means there must be some anticipation of problems. Those who understand trends, past history, risks, and how problems are connected to one another, as well as identify signs that might indicate a need for a response, will be more able to anticipate and begin decision making early rather than later when the problem may be more complicated.

Decision-making conditions

When discussing decision-making conditions the first major issue is who is responsible for making the decision. Managers and staff can get themselves into further problems when they take on decisions that are not theirs to make or they do not make decisions they are responsible for making. How does one find out about who is responsible for a decision? Position descriptions should clarify some of this. The immediate supervisor is also an important resource to help clarify this responsibility. During the hiring process and orientation, staff need clear direction about their responsibilities. If they are confused or unclear about their decision-making responsibilities, they are responsible for asking about them to gain greater clarification. A staff member's comfort level with making decisions is also very important. Staff who feel uncomfortable may avoid decisions, let others make the decision, execute the decision-making process poorly, or arrive at poor decisions, which only makes them more uncomfortable. Those who work with this staff member will also feel uncomfortable about the decisions that are made, which affects morale, productivity, safety and quality, and the overall working environment.

What are the key reasons for staff discomfort with decision making (Gebelein et al., 2000)? When a person feels that there is a lack of knowledge about the true risk of the alternatives, then discomfort increases. Further data collection and analysis are important at this time. Some staff are uncomfortable with the possible consequences of risk taking. When this occurs, the staff member might ask what is the worst thing that could happen. It is important to consider impact and strategies to reduce risks. Maybe the person is focusing too much on the negative aspects? Others feel uncomfortable when the risk factors are unknown. Again, there needs to be more data collection, analysis, and talking to others who may help clarify the issue. Others find they are uncomfortable when certain types of decisions must be made such as those dealing with budget, staffing, or termination of personnel. If this is the case, it is important to learn more about these areas and gain some expertise and confidence. Improving decision-making competency is important for all staff and managers. Increasing knowledge, researching to gain more information, and getting additional experience helps to improve decision making. Discussing concerns with colleagues is an important strategy for every nurse to use.

Barriers to decision making

Barriers to decision making may focus on a variety of factors, and they are similar to barriers to change. Whenever barriers are considered, it is critical to be clear about the barriers that exist within the organization. Examples of typical barriers are dysfunction, poor communication, lack of staff participation, changing organization ownership or administration, inadequate staff, poorly prepared managers, inadequate budget, inadequate staffing levels, policies and procedures, and poor relationships with the community and consumers. There are other barriers that focus more on the individuals who make the decisions (Dessler, 2002). Taking decision-making shortcuts can be an advantage, but this can also be a barrier to success when the shortcut limits data collection, analysis, and the quantity and quality of alternatives that are considered. If description of an issue or problem is really off track, this can act as a barrier. A frequent error in describing an issue or problem occurs when the person unconsciously considers some information to be more important when it is not (Dessler, 2002, p. 76). An individual's psychological set, which is a rigid strategy or point-of-view, is another major barrier. When a staff member enters the decision-making process with a rigid idea about possible cause(es) or strategies, there is an immediate block to success. Because barriers change they need to be considered throughout the decision-making process.

Data collection

Data that are collected are determined by the need and the objectives. It is important first to complete the analysis of the issue or problem. What is the issue or problem? This will then direct data collection. It is easy to get carried away with data collection, which can lead to a situation of just collecting data for the sake of collecting it. The first consideration must be existing data. What data are already available that were collected for another reason but could be used for this new purpose? When existing data are used, it is important to determine if the data meets the specific need. Four common data collection methods used in nursing are described in Box 2-7.

BOX 2-7   Common data collection methods.

Interview

Interviews can be unstructured or structured. The unstructured interview provides opportunity to gain more detailed information with limited boundaries. Structured interviews, which use a standard form and/or format, are less flexible and collect standardized data. For both types of interviews, after the interviews are conducted, data must be summarized and analyzed, and this can take time.

Observation

Observation is often used when complex data are required. It might be used if a clinic needed data about the flow of work in the clinic. Observation may be used to document what staff were doing, time factors, and impact of the physical layout. This type of observation would require a standard checklist or documentation form for the observers and clear guidelines as to what is to be observed and recorded.

Questionnaire/survey

This perhaps is the simplest method, and it is used frequently. It can be less expensive to administer. The questionnarie or survey may be used to collect information about facts such as how many staff are working at a particular time or how many patients were assigned particular staff members. Another type of data is procedure performance data. Evaluative data can also be obtained; for example, how does the staff feel about a change in the admission procedure or a change in documentation. Questions can be asked as to whether or not the procedure was followed or does staff feel prepared for the change.

Source: Author.

Data are then analyzed to determine the cause, which requires objectivity. It is easy to assume something is the cause and then unconsciously insert this assumption into the analysis of the data collected. Getting different perspectives of the data is also important rather than relying on just one individual or a few. Figure 2-5 provides a number of examples of tools that can be used in collecting and analyzing data.

Selecting alternatives

For most problems there are multiple alternative solutions that could be used to solve the problem, or prevent one if that is the goal. It is best to have a number of alternatives from which to select. When the final alternative is selected, it needs to meet the critical criteria that were identified as important for success such as time limitation and resources including staff, space, expertise, and educational level of staff. Alternatives are usually evaluated according to three conditions.

1. Certainty indicates that there is considerable information about the issue or problem indicating a very high probability of the outcome.
2. A second condition is uncertainty, which indicates there is no knowledge of the probability of success.
3. The third condition is risk, which indicates that some information is known but not a high level.

To select the third type of alternative is risky, but this is how most alternatives are selected. Most staff can provide many examples of situations when problems were confronted, and there was thought to be a high probability that the alternative selected was going to achieve the goal desired, and yet this did not occur.

Selecting alternatives also requires a reflection on past experience, which provides data about the probability of success as mistakes can teach staff what not to do or which directions usually do not lead to success. In this selection, trading off or compromise often is required. Decision making is a dynamic process, so give and take is part of the process. Organizational and individual values will affect the alternatives selected, and thus it is difficult to avoid ethics

FIGURE 2-5 Making sense of data: Methods.

Cause-and-effect diagram. This is a diagram that describes a specific process with its causal factors and their consequences. The focus is on improving understanding of possible causes. Another term for this diagram is a *fishbone diagram.*

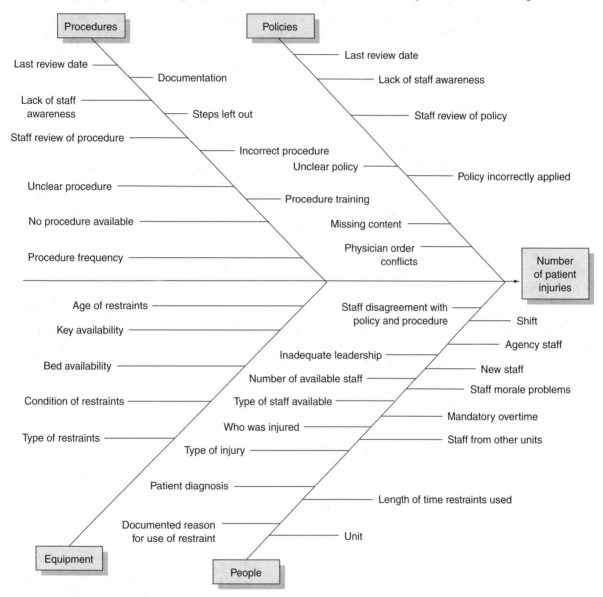

Pareto chart. This method may be used after a cause-and-effect diagram is developed in order to identify the causes of primary importance. Data are described according to the frequency of each cause and displayed according to the most frequent and least frequent. This will help to narrow the data so that the data can be used to determine the best action to take.

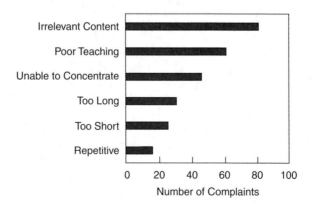

Staff Evaluation of Staff Education

(continued)

FIGURE 2-5   Making sense of data: Methods. *(continued)*

Graph. A graph is used to describe performance over a period of time in an attempt to identify trends. The line graph, used in this example, can describe one or more sets of data. This example describes two sets of data: the number of procedures and the clinical units. Then the data can be compared.

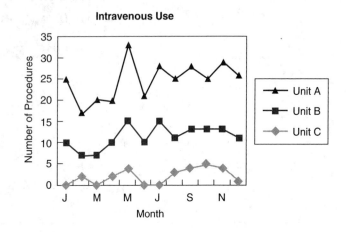

Flowchart. This is a type of chart that is helpful when there is a need to describe a decision-making process. The chart should be developed by a group or team who are involved in the process. The flowchart helps all focus on the process rather than just seeing one part or a part that relates to them as individuals. Typically these charts use common symbols, for example, (A) box represents a function, task, or department; (B) a diamond represents a decision; and (C) arrows indicate the flow of information. After the flowchart is developed, it is then easier to identify repetitive steps, unnecessary steps, or other steps that just do not make sense in the process.

Histogram. This is a bar graph, which illustrates the frequency distribution of a variable or variables in continuous data.

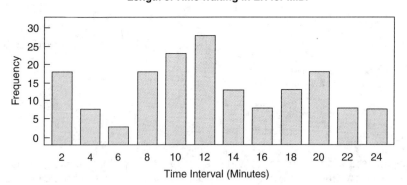

FIGURE 2-5 Making sense of data: Methods. *(continued)*

Pie chart. This is another type of graph that provides a description of percentages of the whole. This is a common graph that most have seen.

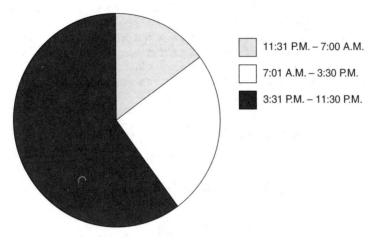

11:31 P.M. – 7:00 A.M.

7:01 A.M. – 3:30 P.M.

3:31 P.M. – 11:30 P.M.

Cost-benefit analysis. This is a method that is used to analyze two or more alternatives in order to determine which alternative will bring the greatest rewards or benefits compared with the costs. Cost-effectiveness is the focus. Both tangible and intangible benefits and costs are considered. Tangible costs might include funds, supplies, space, equipment, staff salaries and benefits, loss of staff, orientation costs, recruitment costs, and so on. Intangible costs might include downtime, staff resistance, decrease in morale, increase in errors, and changes in quality. Intangible benefits might include improved morale, improved level of staffing, increase in communication, and so on. Tangible benefits might include an increased number of patients seen or admitted, decrease in length-of-stay or complications, money saved, decrease in incidents, and so on. The cost benefit ratio can then be determined, which is represented by benefits divided by costs.

COST-BENEFIT ANALYSIS

Solution:

Tangible Costs	Dollar Amounts	Intangible Costs
✓	$	✓
✓	$	✓
✓	$	✓
✓	$	✓
		✓
Total Costs	$	

Tangible Benefits	Dollar Amounts	Intangible Benefits
✓	$	✓
✓	$	✓
✓	$	✓
✓	$	✓
		✓
Total Costs	$	

$$\text{Cost Benefit Ratio} = \frac{\text{Benefits} (\quad)}{\text{Costs} (\quad)} = \underline{\quad}$$

(continued)

FIGURE 2-5   Making sense of data: Methods. *(continued)*

WOTS-up. This is a method that is used to analyze the weaknesses, opportunities, threats, and strengths of a particular situation. Weaknesses focus on internal factors such as lack of management development, qualifications of staff, level of staffing, staff expertise, financial status, marketing efforts, location, quality of services, and so on. Opportunities are the factors that are viewed as positive and have the potential to move the organization forward. Examples are nurse and physician recruitment levels, new programs or services, new markets, population growth, improved technology, new drugs, and new facilities. Threats are serious factors that might hold the organization back such as staff shortage, decreased patient satisfaction, decrease in insured patients, decrease in demand for services, accreditation problems, malpractice litigation, and legislative changes. The fourth category includes the organization's strengths, which might include management style, qualifications and expertise of staff, financial status, increased demand for services, location, and quality of services.

Weaknesses	Opportunities	Threats	Strengths

Solution analysis grid. This method first identifies the problem and the objective. Then each suggested alternative to resolve the problem is analyzed as to how it might contribute to meeting the objective by ranking whether it would have a high, medium, or low contribution; cost in dollars; timeframe or the amount of time it will take to implement (for example, short range, long range, or immediate); and feasibility. The latter is simply a "yes" or "no" response.

SOLUTION ANALYSIS FIELD

Alternative Solution	Cost Solution to Objectives	Cost $	Time	Feasibility

Source: Author.

when some decisions are made. For example, organ transplants involve a decision-making process, one that is highly structured, and this is certainly a decision process that involves ethical issues.

When alternatives are selected, it is critical to ask if an alternative is practical. Some alternatives are not practical and pursuing them will only increase frustration and cause more problems. Collaborating with others by asking them if they think it is practical and what might be some of the "real" concerns about the selection of the alternative usually improves decisions. There needs to be realistic estimates of resource requirements (staff, supplies and equipment, and so on) during the planning. At this point planning also includes an assessment of staff capabilities (not just staff numbers), and how they relate to the plan and its implementation. If additional capabilities are required, then this needs to be included in the plan (for example, a consultant or an expert to teach staff new computer skills so that a new computerized physician order system can be implemented that will affect how nurses review orders). Timelines are identified for all of the activities in the plan so specific steps and accountabilities for staff can be identified. Throughout the process it is important to be a step ahead. This can be done by frequently asking "what if" to identify those situations that might arise to block the solution or make strategies or interventions ineffective.

Implementing and selling the decision

Selling the decision focuses on decision acceptance. How committed to the decision are those who will be affected by the decision? This is a key question. Earlier in this chapter resistance to change was discussed. This information applies to commitment to decisions. Decisions that meet strong resistance will fail. Those who are needed to move the decision forward need to understand what is behind the decision.

Some decisions require a detailed action plan, but most do not. The key to implementation is timing. When to make the decision and when to implement it are frequently difficult to determine. Procrastination is common in decision making. If a decision is delayed, the typical reasons for this are (a) lack of information, (b) unclear course of action, (c) lack of time for thought, and (d) fear of negative consequences (Gebelein et al., 2000). Each of these reasons have very clear solutions. All relate to getting more information, planning, and developing a clear viewpoint of the issue at hand. Another problem is making impulsive decisions. These decisions lead to more problems. If pressure is felt to make a decision now, then it is best to stop and consider why and what could be done to improve the decision making. It is rarely helpful to make decisions when emotions such as anger are strong. Those who want to jump in too soon should step back and take time to collaborate with others to work through the decision and to write plans down. Time taken to do this will decrease impulsiveness. The plan needs to include specific information as to actions and responsibilities.

Evaluating results

Evaluating results of decisions is never easy. By the time one thinks this should be done, another change, decision, and plan are in process. However, neglecting evaluation has long-term consequences. The quality of a decision depends heavily on the goals selected and the strategies used to achieve them. Evaluation is thus intricately tied to the beginning, the middle, and the end of the decision-making process. In addition, evaluation itself does not just happen at the end of the process, but rather needs to be incorporated in all of the steps. This provides valuable data about when approaches need adjustment to prevent the situation from becoming too complex.

Those who were involved in decision making should be involved in the evaluation. This does require objectivity. Staff who buy into a plan may be reluctant to say it needs adjusting or has failed. For one reason, it probably means more change and stress; however, if this is not done, greater stress can also be expected.

The following are some keys for improving decision making and planning that can be used in a variety of situations.

- Take time whenever possible to think through the process, avoiding impulsive decision making
- When appropriate, include others
- Use creative techniques

- Listen and consider ideas from others
- Stay open to ideas and perspectives, even those that are very different
- Challenge self and develop new thinking skills: critical thinking, conceptual thinking, creative thinking, and intuitive thinking
- Recognize the broad implications of issues
- Identify relationships
- Balance short-term and long-term priorities (Gebelein et al., 2000, p. 213)

Planning

Why is it important to plan? If organizations or staff go off without a plan or map, will they get to their goals or their destination? An analogy would be traveling to an unknown place without a map. Getting lost increases stress, takes time, may increase expenses, and may interfere with reaching the destination, which is the goal. Most nurses have worked in situations where there were no goals, or the goals were unclear or kept a secret. This is not a great way to work. What if patients were cared for without a plan? How would staff know if outcomes were met? How organized would the care be? How would staff know their responsibilities? Crisis management seems to be more the norm in health care organizations. It is certainly important to learn how to deal with crises, but a better approach, whenever possible, is to plan, both long range and short range. Leaders do not have the luxury of saying, "I don't have time to plan." Organizations cannot afford not to.

When there is recognition that change is needed, particularly one that is fairly major, the planning process goes into action. A plan is a picture of a future vision, ideally painted by a group or team. Planning includes multiple decisions and is directly affected by change. Planning is the pivotal step in the process of getting there. There are three types of planning:

1. **Policy planning.** This planning focuses on changing the value system or laws and regulations. It is health planning in its broadest concept (see Chapter 10).
2. **Strategic planning.** This is the planning that an organization does when it considers longer range issues and goals, which is discussed in more detail in Chapter 6. It includes planning that is done by the organization's components, such as its departments or services. The organization looks at its vision and its organizational assessment data, and then asks where are the gaps? What would it take to get there? A typical result is the organization's plan for the next 5 years.

CURRENT ISSUES

Learn about events around the globe that relate to the chapter content.

3. **Project planning.** This planning focuses on operational matters in the organization. Examples include a plan to change documentation, introduce a new admission procedure or new service, or change staff roles. Project planning must take into account strategic plans so that there is no conflict, and project plans should help the organization reach strategic goals. For example, if one of an organization's strategic goals is to develop the use of interdisciplinary teams in all departments and units, a project plan that focuses on training staff would need to be developed by staff education.

CURRENT ISSUES

Learn about events around the globe that relate to the chapter content.

BENCHMARKS

Now let's take a moment to test your knowledge of the concepts you have studied in this section.

Chapter Wrap-Up

Now that you've reached the end of the chapter, you may wish to explore the concepts you've been reading about in greater detail, or test yourself to see how well you've comprehended the material.

SUMMARY AND APPLICATIONS

- Practice Quiz
- Key Terms
- Tying It All Together
- Experiential Exercises

- Companion Web Site
- Case 1
- Links

REFERENCES

Alfaro-LeFevre, R. (2001). Improving your ability to think critically. *Nursing Spectrum Metro Edition*, (March), 25–30.

American Organization of Nurse Executives. (1999). *Nurse staffing survey*. Chicago, IL: American Hospital Association.

Anthony, M. (1999). The relationship of authority to decision-making behavior, implications for redesign. *Research Nursing Health, 22*, 388–398.

Bennis, W., & Goldsmith, G. (1997). *Learning to lead*. Reading. MA: Perseus Books.

Bernhard, L. & Walsh, M. (1990). Leadership: The key to the profession of nursing (2nd Ed.). St. Louis, MO: C. V. Mosby.

Beyers, M. (1999). Reengineering patient care in multi-institutional systems. In S. Smith & D. Flarey (Eds.), *Process-centered health care organizations* (pp. 161–176). Gaithersburg, MD: Aspen Publishers, Inc.

Blegen, M., et al. (1993). Preferences for decision-making autonomy. *Image Journal of Nursing Scholarship, 25*, 339–344.

Carney, M. (2002). The management of change: Using a model to evaluate the change process. *Seminars for Nurse Managers, 10*(3), 206–211.

Dessler, G. (2002). *Management*. Upper Saddle River, NJ: Prentice Hall.

Finkelman, A. (1996). *Psychiatric nursing administration manual*. Gaithersburg, MD: Aspen Publishers, Inc.

Finkelman, A. (2001). *Managed care: A nursing perspective*. Upper Saddle River, NJ: Prentice Hall.

Fisher, M. (1996). *Redesigning the nursing organization*. Albany, NY: Delmar Publishers.

Flarey, D., & Smith. S. (1999). Reengineering: The journey to a process-centered organization. In S. Smith & D. Flarey (Eds.), *Process-centered healthcare organizations* (pp. 17–44). Gaithersburg, MD: Aspen Publishers, Inc.

Gebelein, S., et al. (2000). *Successful manager's handbook*. Minneapolis, MN: Personnel Decisions International Corporation.

Hammer, M., & Champy, J. (1993). *Reengineering the corporation: A manifesto for business revolution*. New York: Harper Business.

Heifetz, R., & Laurie, D. (2001). The work of leadership. *Harvard Business Review, 79*(12), 9–18.

Hoover, K. (1998). Nursing work redesign in response to managed care. *Journal of Nursing Administration, 28*(11), 9–18.

Hutcherson, C., & Williamson, S. (May 31, 1999). Nursing regulation for the new millennium: The mutual recognition model. *Online Journal of Issues in Nursing*. Retrieved on July 16, 1999, from http://www.nursingworld.org/ojin/topic9/topic9_2.htm.

Kerfoot, K. (December 22, 1997). Role redesign. What has it accomplished? *Online Journal of Issues in Nursing*. Retrieved on July 16, 1999, from http://www.nursingworld.org/ojin/topic5/topic5_3.htm.

Kirkpatrick, D. (2001). *Managing change effectively*. Boston: Butterworth-Heinemann.

Krairiksh, M., & Anthony, M. (2001). Benefits and outcomes of staff nurses' participation in decision-making. *Journal of Nursing Administration, 31*(1), 16–23.

Lewin, K. (1947). Group and social change. In T. Newcomb and E. Hartely (Eds.), *Readings in social psychology*. New York: Holt, Rinehart & Winston.

Marrelli, T. (1997). *The nurse manager's guide*. St. Louis, MO: Mosby-Year Book, Inc.

Milgram, L., Spector, A., & Treger, M. (1999). *Managing smart*. Houston, TX: Cashman Dudley.

Paul, R. (1995). *Critical thinking: How to prepare students for a rapidly changing world*. Santa Rosa, CA: Foundation for Critical Thinking.

Pesut, D. (2001). Deep change. *Nursing Outlook, 49*(3), 118.

Quinn, R. (1996). *Deep change: Discovering the leader within*. San Francisco: Jossey-Bass.

Quinn, R. (2000). *Change the world: How ordinary people can accomplish extraordinary results*. San Francisco: Jossey-Bass.

Shindul-Rothschild, J., Berry, D., & Long-Middleton, E. (1996). Where have all the nurses gone? Final results of our patient care survey. *American Journal of Nursing, 96*(11), 25–39.

Sovie, M., & Jawad, A. (2001). Hospital restructuring and its impact on outcomes: Nursing staff regulations are premature. *Journal of Nursing Administration, 31*(12), 588–600.

Stark, J. (1996). Critical thinking for outcomes-based practice. *Seminars for Nurse Managers, 4*(3), 168.

Sullivan, E., & Decker, P. (2001). *Effective leadership and management in nursing*. Upper Saddle River, NJ: Prentice Hall.

Tappen, R. (1995). *Nursing leadership and management*. Philadelphia: F. A. Davis.

Truscott, J., & Churchill, G. (1995). Patient-focused care. *Nursing Policy Forum, 1*(4), 5–12.

Turner, S. (1999). *The nurse's guide to managed care*. Gaithersburg, MD: Aspen Publishers, Inc.

ADDITIONAL READINGS

Aiken, L., Clarke, S., & Sloane, D. (2000). Hospital restructuring. Does it adversely affect care and outcomes? *Journal of Nursing Administration, 30*(10), 457–465.

Anthony, M. (1997). The participation in decision questionnaire: Development and testing of nurse decision-making behavior. *Journal of Shared Governance, 4*(2), 15–23.

Blythe, J., Baumann, A., & Giovannetti, P. (2001). Nurses' experiences of restructuring in three Ontario hospitals. *Image: Journal of Nursing Scholarship*, first quarter, 61–68.

Branowicki, P., Shermont, H., Rogers, J., & Melchiono, M. (2001). Improving systems related to clinical practice: An interdisciplinary team approach. *Seminars for nurse managers, 9*(2), 110–114.

Capuano, T., Bokovoy, J., Halkins, D., & Hitchings, K. (2004). Work flow analysis. *Journal of Nursing Administration, 34*(5), 246–256.

Child, R., Lingle, G., & Watson, P. (2001). Managing diversity in the environment of care. *Seminars for Nurse Managers, 9*(2), 102–110.

Clancy, T. (2003). The art of decision-making. *The Journal of Nursing Administration, 33*(6), 343–349.

Coe, S. (2001). Healthcare delivery in the future. In C. McCullough, (Ed.), *Creating responsive solutions to healthcare change* (pp. 235–262). Indianapolis, IN: Center Nursing Press.

Docimo, A., et al. (2000). Using the online and offline change model to improve efficiency for fast-track patients in an emergency department. *Journal of Quality Improvement* (September), 503–514.

Drenkard, K. (2001). Creating a future worth experiencing. *Journal of Nursing Administration, 31*(7/8), 364–376.

Duck, J. (1993). Managing change: The art of balancing. *Harvard Business Review, 71*(6), 109–118.

Dumpe, M., Herman, J., & Young, S. (1998). Forecasting the nursing workforce in a dynamic healthcare market. *Nursing Economics, 16*(4), 170–188.

Farson, R., & Keyes, R. (2002). The failure-tolerant leader. *Harvard Business Review, 80*(8), 64–72.

Ficaro, C., & Elberth, W. (2001). Reengineering patient care: A multidisciplinary approach—an interview. *Seminars for Nurse Manager, 9*(2), 121–125.

Flarey, D. (Ed.). (1995). *Redesigning nursing care delivery*. Philadelphia: J.B. Lippincott Company.

Foglia, D., Davis, J., & Black-Wieber, D. (2001). Nothing for granted. *Reflections on Nursing LEADERSHIP, 27*(3), 17–20.

Hanneman, E. Nurse-physician collaboration: A post-structionalist view. *Journal of Advanced Nursing, 22*, 359–363.

Hansten, R., & Washburn, M. (2000). Intuition in professional practice: Executive and staff perceptions. *Journal of Nursing Administration, 30*(4), 185–189.

Harrison, J. (1999). Influence of managed care on professional nursing practice. *Image: Journal of Nursing Scholarship, 31*(2), 161–166.

Havens, D. (2002). Measuring staff nurse decisional involvement: The decisional involvement scale. *The Journal of Nursing Administration, 33*(6), 331–336.

Huber, D. (2000). *Leadership and nursing care management*. Philadelphia: WB Saunders Company.

Huntington, J. (1997). Healthcare in chaos. Will we ever see real managed care? *Online Journal of Issues in Nursing*. Retrieved on May 4, 1999, from http://www.nursingworld/ojin/tpc2/tpc2_7.htm.

Ingersoll, G., et al. (2000). Relationship of organizational culture and readiness for change to employee commitment to the organization. *Journal of Nursing Administration, 30*(1), 11–20.

Ingersoll, G., et al. (2002). Patient-focused redesign and employee perception of work environment. *Nursing Economics, 20*(4), 163–170, 187.

Johnson, S. (1998). *Who moved my cheese?* New York: G. P. Putnam's Sons.

Jones, K., & Redman, R. (2000). Organizational culture and work redesign: Experiences in three organizations. *Journal of Nursing Administration, 30*(12), 604–610.

Knox, S., & Gharrity, J. (2002). Transitions in American hospitals: The necessary reshaping is taking place. *JONA's Healthcare Law, Ethics, and Regulation, 4*(1), 13–17.

Laschinger, H., Finegan, J., Shamian, J., & Almost, J. (2001). Testing Karasek's demands-control model in restructured healthcare settings. *Journal of Nursing Administration, 31*(5), 233–243.

Lassen, A., Fosbinder, D., Minton, S., & Robins, M. (1997). Nurse/physician collaborative practice: Improving healthcare quality while decreasing cost. *Nursing Economics, 15*(2), 87–91.

Manthey, M. (2003). Guest editorial aka primary nursing. *The Journal of Nursing Administration, 33*(7/8), 369–370.

National Council of State Boards of Nursing. (1998). *Revised approved interstate compact language*. Retrieved July 7, 1999, http://www.ncsbn.org/files/msrtf/compact9811.pdf.

Newhouse, R., & Dan, D. (2001). Measuring changes for nurses. *Journal of Nursing Administration, 31*(4), 173–175.

O'Connor, M. (2002). Nurse, leader: Heal thyself. *Nursing Administration Quarterly, 26*(2), 69–79.

O'Neil, E., & Coffman, J. (1998). *Strategies for the future of nursing*. San Francisco, CA: Jossey-Bass.

O'Neil, E., & the Pew Health Professions Commission. (1998). *Recreating health professions practice for a new century*. San Francisco, CA: Pew Health Professions Commission.

Pew Health Professions Commission. (1995). *Reforming the health care workforce regulation: Policy considerations for the 21st century*. San Francisco, CA: Pew Health Professions Commission.

Pike, A., et al. (1993). A new architecture for quality assurance nurse-physician collaboration. *Journal of Nursing Care Quality, 7*(3), 1–8.

Porter-O'Grady, T. (2000). Visions for the 21st century: New horizons, new healthcare. *Nursing Administration Quarterly, 25*(1), 30–38.

Purdum, T. (1999). California to set level of staffing for nursing care. *New York Times*, A1, A21.

Sanders, T. (1998). *Strategic thinking and the new science: Planning in the midst of chaos, complexity, and change*. New York: The Free Press.

Sternweiler, V. (1998). Career journeys: How to be a successful clinical nurse specialist—be a willow tree. *Advanced Practice Nursing Quarterly*, (3), 31–33.

Tonges, M. (1989). Redesigning hospital nursing practice: The professionally advanced care team (ProACT) model: Part 1. *Journal of Nursing Administration, 19*(7), 31–38.

Tracey, D. (1990). *Steps to empowerment*. New York: William Morrow.

Urden, L., & Walston, S. (2001). Outcomes of hospital restructuring and reengineering. *Journal of Nursing Administration, 31*(4), 203–209.

Verdejo, T. (2001). Leading into the 21st century: Changing the vision and leading toward success. *Seminars for Nurse Managers, 9*(2), 115–118.

Keys to Working with Others: Collaboration, Coordination, and Conflict Resolution

CHAPTER OUTLINE

MediaLink
www.prenhall.com/finkelman

The Interactive Exercises for this chapter can be found in the OneKey course at www.prenhall.com/finkelman. Click on Chapter 3 to select from the following activities: Test Your Understanding, Benchmarks, Current Issues, Your Opinion Counts, Think Critically, and Summary and Applications.

What's Ahead

Collaboration, coordination, and conflict resolution are skills needed by every nurse regardless of the specialty or type of setting where the nurse works. These skills are directly related to effective leadership and management. Health care organizations in which staff collaborate with one another, work together to coordinate care delivery, and strive to resolve conflicts that inevitably will occur will be successful in meeting their goals—to provide quality, safe care. This chapter discusses these three critical skills that are needed by each nurse.

OBJECTIVES

Before you begin, take a moment to familiarize yourself with the key objectives of this chapter.

- Describe key aspects related to collaboration.
- Identify barriers to achieving effective collaboration.
- Discuss the skills that are needed to improve collaboration.
- Discuss the impact collaboration has on nursing staff and interdisciplinary interactions.
- Describe key aspects related to coordination.
- Identify barriers to achieving effective coordination.
- Discuss the skills that are needed to improve coordination.
- Discuss the impact coordination has on nursing staff and interdisciplinary interactions.
- Describe key aspects related to conflict.
- Identify methods to prevent conflict.
- Discuss how individuals respond to conflict.
- Discuss the skills that are needed to respond to conflict.
- Explain conflict management and strategies that might be used.
- Discuss the impact conflict has on nursing staff and interdisciplinary interactions.

TEST YOUR UNDERSTANDING

Before we begin our exploration of this chapter, take a short "warm-up" test to see what you know about this topic.

Collaboration

Definitions

Collaboration is a cooperative effort that focuses on a win-win strategy. To collaborate each individual needs to recognize the perspective of others who are involved and eventually reach a **consensus** of a common goal(s).

> The benefits of collaboration are well supported in the literature. These include, but are not limited to, reduced mortality, morbidity, nosocomial infection rates, shorter lengths of hospital stays, more satisfied consumers, and happier staff/health care providers. Collaborative practice teams foster collegial relationships, cooperation, and more effective conflict resolution practices; build mutual trust, respect and caring attitude among team members; encourage appreciation and understanding of each team member's role, knowledge, skills, and contributions to the overall care; and ensure a better work environment. Members of collaborative practice teams complement one another's expertise, which, in turn, improves outcomes and enhances savings as well as fosters an environment conducive to peer-to-peer mentoring and ongoing learning. (Tahan, 2001, p. 71).

This statement demonstrates the broad impact that collaboration can have on care and the work environment. The American Nurses Association's *Standards of Professional Performance* also identifies the need for collaboration, emphasizing that all nurses are expected to collaborate. Box 3-1 provides information about this standard. Clearly, collaboration is important, but how does one develop this skill and use it effectively?

Key concepts related to collaboration are: (a) partnership, (b) interdependence, and (c) collective ownership and responsibility. Considering these concepts and those identified by Tahan helps us understand the impact of collaboration. Sullivan (1998a) defines collaboration as "a dynamic, transforming process of creating a power sharing partnership for pervasive application in health care practice, education, research, and organizational settings for the purposeful attention

BOX 3-1   Standards of professional performance.

> **Standard VI. Collaboration**
> The nurse collaborates with the patient, family, and other health care providers in providing patient care.
>
> **Measurement Criteria**
>   1. The nurse communicates with the patient, family, and other health care providers.
>   2. The nurse collaborates with the patient, family, and other health care providers in the formulation of overall goals and the plan of care, and in decisions related to care and the delivery of services.
>   3. The nurse consults with other health care providers for patient care, as needed.
>   4. The nurse makes referrals, including provisions for continuity of care, as needed.
>
> Source: American Nurses Association. (1998). *Standards of Professional Performance.* Washington, DC: American Publishing Inc., p. 14. Reprinted with permission.

to needs and problems in order to achieve likely successful outcomes" (p. 6). Another definition is proposed by Disch, who says collaboration is "the process of joint decision-making among interdependent parties, involving joint ownership of decisions and collective responsibility for outcomes" (2001, p. 275). Both of these definitions and perspectives indicate that staff must work with others to be effective. Collaboration is also a process. It is not stagnant but rather changes, which requires staff to make adjustments as situations change in order to collaborate with others. Most people can remember experiences when working with others where the work just seemed to flow with less stress and good communication. This probably means that the people working together were collaborating.

Collaboration should be a positive experience, but this is not always the case. If it is not positive, it will not be effective. If a group of nurses was surveyed, it would be surprising to get a consensus that collaboration was always a positive experience. Often attempts at collaboration mean struggle, conflict, and sometimes ineffective results. Some research has been conducted to assess the effectiveness of collaboration. A review of 100 studies, however, indicates that studies of collaboration have not been scientifically rigorous enough to prove that collaboration improves care (Dechairo-Marino, Jordan-Marsh, Traiger, & Saulo, 2001; Hammick, 2000; Zwarenstein, Bryant, Bailie, & Sidthorpe, 1997). Others have noted that collaborative studies have focused more on the relations between nurses and physicians (Aiken, Smith, & Lake, 1994). Collaboration is an area that requires further research, as a need exists to determine the best methods for improving collaboration.

Barriers to effective collaboration

"One of the paradoxes of being a nursing leader today is the need to passionately promote nursing and concurrently work to create strong interdisciplinary teams through collaboration" (Disch, 2001, p. 275). How does the profession arrive at the right balance, one that focuses on nursing and its professional role and needs, while simultaneously developing nurses who can work collaboratively with others to meet patient outcomes? Collaboration requires an interactive process. If staff are not willing to interact or have any other barrier to interaction, collaboration cannot take place. Lack of understanding about the roles and responsibilities of others and lack of respect for what others contribute interferes with effective collaboration. How much do nurses know about what physicians do and vice versa, or social workers and nurses, or physical therapists and nurses, and so on? If there is distrust, collaboration is hindered because distrust affects willingness to share information, which is an integral component in the collaborative relationship. Disch (2001) suggests an analogy to support her recommendation for greater interdisciplinary collaboration, "A violinist needs to develop expertise and be the best violinist possible. But when working in a group, the violinist must weave his or her melodies into making the string quartet the most impressive it can be" (p. 275). This analogy demonstrates how collaboration can result in an effective or ineffective team. If each violinist continued to play as if he or she was the only one present, ignoring the others, the music would not come together. Although each nurse must develop individual expertise, this expertise must come together with others' expertise. Few nurses really can work effectively in isolation. Nursing is a profession that requires contact with others—patients, other nursing staff, other health care professionals, families, community members, and so on.

Some staff will "not play fairly," and this will be a major barrier to effective collaboration (Marriner-Tomey, 1992). In these situations, staff may attack one another by asserting their position, or by attacking ideas. In some cases, they attack one another personally. The first response typically is to attack back, which acts as an additional barrier to effective collaboration. Steps, however, can be taken to respond positively.

1. Try to understand what is behind the other party's idea.
2. Avoid defending your idea but rather ask the other party for advice and comments.
3. "Reframe the attack on you as an attack on the problem," making it less personal (Marriner-Tomey, 1992, p. 300).

The goal is to break down the barrier by avoiding counterattacking and focusing on common interests and resolutions.

Collaboration often is used to reach an agreement during a conflict. This is often true with nurse-physician collaboration, though ideally collaboration should be part of all of their interactions. Nurse-physician relationships are complex. There is overlapping of focus in that both are concerned about the patient though maybe from different points-of-view, and this is not always understood or appreciated. There is also some confusion about roles, which can lead to problems. In some cases there is a certain amount of competition, which really is a sad statement as the goal should be focused on what is best for the patient.

Nurse-physician relationships

Nurses have long worked on teams, mostly with other nursing staff. However, the nurse-physician relationships have become more important in the changing health care environment with the greater emphasis on interdisciplinary teams. Others suggest that because nurses and physicians use different methods to resolve conflict this affects the ability to develop collaboration. Nurses use more avoidance, accommodation, or competition while physicians use bargaining or negotiation (Saulo, 1987; Weisbord & Goodstein, 1978). This demonstrates two different approaches to conflict resolution, which will be discussed later in this chapter.

Nurse-physician interactions and communication have been discussed for a long time in health care literature. Ladden (2001) notes that most of this discussion is found in nursing literature, not medical literature. Of the 300 articles reviewed by Ladden, 62% were published in nursing journals, 27% in medical journals, 9% in journals of other health professionals, and 2% in non-health professions journals. This probably indicates that nursing is more interested in this issue, or at least interested in discussing it in their professional literature. The focus of these articles can be categorized into three areas: (a) review articles that describe the collaboration, (b) proposals for a theoretical basis about the reasons for the barriers to collaboration, and (c) research reports on interventions that have been used to measure or improve collaboration.

A study that explored the impact of nurse-physician relationships on nurse satisfaction and retention, conducted by a physician, was reported in 2002 (Rosenstein, 2002). The results of the survey of 1,200 nurses, physicians, and hospital executives "suggests that daily interactions between nurses and physicians strongly influence nurses' morale (Rosenstein, 2002, p. 26). Overall, 96% of the nurses had witnessed or experienced disruptive physician behavior, including yelling or raising the voice, disrespect, condescension, berating colleagues, berating patients, and use of abusive language. The survey found 344 nurses who knew of other nurses who had left the hospital due to disruptive behavior. These nurses did not feel that the administration supported the resolution of conflict between nurses and physicians. This study recommended the following improvement strategies, which could apply to most health care organizations.

■ Create more opportunities for collaboration and communication through open forums, group discussions, and collaborative relationships.

■ Increase availability of training and educational programs for nurses and physicians that focus on improving teamwork and working relationships (for example, sensitivity training, assertiveness training, conflict management, time management, and phone etiquette, with emphasis on courtesy, respect, promptness, and preparation).

■ Improve organizational processes by requiring administrators to take a more proactive approach to avoiding potential confrontations related to staffing, scheduling, and equipment.

■ Establish a zero-tolerance policy for disruptive behavior, holding nurses and physicians more accountable for their actions.

■ Disseminate code-of-conduct policies and reporting guidelines to both nurses and physicians, and apply policies consistently and quickly, providing feedback to all involved.

■ Ensure appropriate nurse competencies.

■ Have physicians sign a code-of-conduct policy when they are credentialed or re-credentialed.

■ Appoint a physician leader who will take charge of training and education programs.

■ Provide an ongoing forum to increase physician awareness of the issues addressed in this survey and raise awareness of other factors that increase nurses' stress levels.

■ Place physicians on nurse recruitment teams, enabling them to gain a better understanding and appreciation of the factors that are important to nurses as they consider employment opportunities.

■ Provide a case study or conduct role-play exercises that allow physicians a firsthand understanding of nurses' responsibilities and work flow (Rosenstein, 2002, pp. 32–33).

THINK CRITICALLY

Try this exercise to apply what you have learned about this topic.

Physicians, however, are not the only health care providers that nurses must work with while they provide care (for example, nurses work with other nursing staff, social workers, support staff, laboratory technicians, physical therapists, pharmacists, and many others). There are also new members joining the health care team such as alternative therapists (massage therapists, herbal therapists, acupuncturists, etc.), case managers, more actively involved insurers, and so forth. The future will probably bring other new members into the health care delivery system. Nurses need to develop the skills necessary to participate effectively on the team, which requires collaboration, communication, coordination, delegation, and negotiation. Communication and delegation are discussed in other chapters.

It is difficult to practice today in any health care setting without experiencing interdisciplinary interactions such as nurse-physician. As teams work together, effective teams:

■ Work together (collaborate)
■ Recognize strengths and limitations
■ Respect individual responsibilities
■ Maintain open communication

If every nurse was committed to improving collaboration, this would have a major impact on the practice of nursing and the leadership role that nurses need to reach.

Skills to achieve effective collaboration

Collaboration is a critical skill required to practice in any health care setting. The increased emphasis on interdisciplinary teams to meet the patient's needs across the continuum of care requires the skill of collaboration. The very nature of a team implies that there is more than one idea or approach and not all can usually be accomplished. Decisions need to be made; this is where collaboration comes into play. "Collaboration is the vehicle for bringing disparate disciplines and organizations together to act in ways that they could not act on their own to resolve needs and concerns that they are not able to address on their own" (Sullivan, 1998b, p. 56). It is important to remember that collaboration is also a critical factor in the nurse-patient relationship. Nurses need to actively pursue patient collaboration to ensure that patients are involved in their own care. The nursing profession has long emphasized patient participation in planning care and in patient education. Collaboration is also important in the development of effective management.

To be effective in collaboration, staff require a number of skills.

■ Communication skills are critical, which are discussed more in Chapter 4. Verbal skills are the focus; however, in some instances written communication is also important as information and process are described in written format.

■ Staff also need to be aware of their own feelings, as was discussed in some of the leadership theories such as Emotional Intelligence.

■ Staff need to be able to make decisions to solve problems effectively.

■ As is discussed in this chapter, coordination is also important when collaborating with others.

■ Conflicts will arise, which may interfere with collaboration. Staff need to develop negotiation skills to be used in resolving difficult conflicts.

■ Assessment skills are also required as information needs to be collected and analyzed as relationships move toward greater collaboration. Box 3-2 highlights these skills.

Collaborative care is central to the success of efficient, outcome-driven care. With the complex health care system, specialization of many health care professionals, variety of health care settings, complex reimbursement systems, technology, and new drugs, collaboration is the only way that patients will receive quality, cost-effective care. Today, the health care system is an interdependent system with multiple settings and a variety of health care professionals, who are dependent on one another. The increased use of case management can be very supportive in developing collaborative care. Care requires flexibility to adjust to the changing needs of the complex health care environment. The process of collaboration includes shared planning, goal setting, decision making, interventions, and problem solving (Sullivan, 1998b). All of these activities are integral to successful case management as the case manager works with many different health care providers, within many different health care settings, and with the patient and family to ensure quality, cost-effective care for the patient.

Collaborative planning, or joining together to form alliances or partnerships (coalitions), is an important method used to address the following (Puetz & Shinn, 2002).

1. Maximize resources such as funding, equipment and supplies, space, and staff.
2. Minimize duplication of work.
3. Improve relationships.

This type of planning also recognizes that collaboration has a positive effect on achieving patient outcomes (Disch, 2001). Collaborative planning requires that all parties agree on the mission and goals of the partnership so that they have common expectations. All members of the effort

BOX 3-2   Collaboration: Skills needed.

■ Communication
■ Awareness of personal feelings
■ Problem solving
■ Negotiation
■ Assessment

Source: Author.

need to commit to open and honest communication, which is essential to sharing. This can be difficult in some organizations, components of an organization such as specific units or departments, and for some individuals. Those who fear competition and are concerned about power will struggle with the need to share.

Regular evaluation needs to be built into collaborative planning. This evaluation should not only focus on the content of the planning but also on the process—how is the collaborative relationship working? This is something that is often neglected. Power, which is discussed later in this chapter, plays an important role in collaboration. Usually some of the partners in a relationship have more power than others. "Any imbalance in capacity and capability can be smoothed out by the establishment of mutually agreed-upon goals and expectations. Clarity about outcomes and inputs can help build trust and buy-in from the outset" (Puetz & Shinn, 2002, p. 183). When partners work through the collaborative planning process, some issues may interfere with the process. These may include:

- Preconditions
- Lack of commitment
- Changing players in midstream
- Saboteurs and rumors
- Diversions from the timeline (Puetz & Shinn, 2002)

Recognizing these potential issues should be a priority to prevent barriers to success. What can be done to prevent them? Clear communication about purpose, particularly identifying issues from the past that may affect the collaborative planning, can help to clear up misconceptions. Team members need to accept the importance of effort and commit to it. All efforts should be made to keep team membership committed. Evaluation data about the collaborative effort can help to improve team functioning.

CURRENT ISSUES

Learn about events around the globe that relate to the chapter content.

Application of collaboration

What is gained from collaboration? "The essence of collaborating involves working across professional boundaries" (Liedtka & Whitten, 1998, p. 186). The complex health care delivery system requires many skills, and no one health care profession has all of the necessary skills to provide all the care that is required. Interdisciplinary teams and effective collaboration are critical.

CURRENT ISSUES

Learn about events around the globe that relate to the chapter content.

The Magnet Hospital Recognition Program has also considered the impact of collaborative relationships on care and the work environment for nurses by assessing the presence of collaboration when determining if a hospital meets criteria for excellence in nursing. (See Chapter 6 for more information on Magnet hospitals.) By including collaboration, this recognition program establishes that collaboration is a critical component in the delivery of care.

How do health care professionals develop the skills necessary for collaboration? There is a great need to incorporate more interdisciplinary educational experiences into all health care professional education, including nursing. Students from the various health care professions need to have some experiences learning together in the same classroom and participating in clinical experiences together. Learning separately makes it very difficult to expect that at the time of graduation new health care professionals will easily collaborate when they have had limited collaborative experience with other health care professional students or health care professionals. They do not understand or respect the knowledge and learning experiences of other students, or their roles and typical communication methods and processes. They may not even value or respect what other health care professionals offer to the team and to the patient. This causes serious problems as new health care professionals begin to work and are then confronted with working with one another. In addition, nurses need to have a positive understanding of their own roles and responsibilities—what they have to offer is valuable—so that they can approach collaboration while understanding that they have important knowledge and competencies to add to the collaboration. This, however, must be accomplished *not* from the perspective of "I am better than you" but rather "How can we bring our respective skills and knowledge together to provide comprehensive, consistent care?"

YOUR OPINION COUNTS

Find out what others think about this topic. Post your response and check out other opinions.

Interdisciplinary relationships and activities can result in positive, collaborative outcomes; however, it is not easy to establish these relationships and maintain them over time. The goal is to combine "the complementary skills, knowledge, and approaches of the various disciplines" (Long, 2001, p. 279). Long also notes that those who have been successful with interdisciplinary work indicate that it requires an incremental approach and committed leadership (Long, 2001). It takes time. Other recommendations are to set realistic goals with commitment from all involved disciplines to these goals; negotiate the means to meet the goals; avoid battles that only serve as barriers such as turf battles; and measure the success based on the established goals. All along it is important to remember that "Deep-seated professional traditions result in a desire to protect the identity and stature of one's own profession. Underlying feelings of distrust or even dislike for the other profession are often manifested in heated disagreements about mundane issues" (Stumpf & Clark, 1999; as cited in Long, 2001, p. 281). This response is clearly a danger, and it can be seen in most health care organizations, including nursing education.

If the idea is to improve interdisciplinary and collaborative relationships, what might be the results? Cody summarizes possible desired outcomes that can result from collaborative interdisciplinary relationships and activities described in the literature. These outcomes include:

- Professionals will be more familiar with one another's activities and roles, thereby improving interprofessional communication.
- Professionals will be better able to work collaboratively, thereby improving care.
- Professionals will have broader repertoires of knowledge and skills, thereby in effect increasing access to care for the people.
- Professionals will have more career mobility as health care systems change.
- With larger, more diverse research teams, research productivity on issues of importance in health care will increase.
- Cross-disciplinary peer review and critique of practice and research will be more available and more intellectually sound.
- Cross-fertilization with creative ideas from many sectors will enhance and accelerate innovations in health care (Cody, 2001, p. 276; Finch, 2000; Gueldner & Stroud, 1996; Hammick, 2000).

If these results or outcomes can be reached the working environment will be improved.

Coordination

Definitions

"Coordination is the process of achieving unity of action among interdependent activities. Coordination is required whenever two or more interdependent individuals, groups, or departments
must work together to achieve a common goal" (Dessler, 2002, pp. 143–144). **Coordination** is
related to collaboration, and in fact, it is very difficult to do one without the other. When considering patient care, however, there is a critical difference between the two. Collaboration with
a patient requires a direct interaction with the patient. Coordination of care usually takes place
before or after patient care is provided or interwoven in the care. In the latter situation a nurse
may ensure that all the plans for the patient's discharge are complete or that the various treatment and exam procedures are scheduled appropriately for the patient's needs. Coordination
does not mean that the patient is not involved because patient input is critical, but the nurse
may do the coordination such as calling for supplies or making sure a treatment is scheduled
when not in the presence of the patient or while providing direct care. Both coordination and
collaboration are also found daily in staff-staff interactions. Collaboration focuses on solving a
problem with two or more people working toward this goal. Coordination is done to ensure that
something happens such as the provision of services.

Barriers to effective coordination

As health care organizations and services become more complex and they use more interdisciplinary teams, team members may not always have the same view of the patient, problems, or priorities, and yet it is critical that the team find a way to work collaboratively to provide coordinated
patient care and prevent errors, disorganized care, and care that does not reach effective outcomes.
Team members need to have a better understanding of individual responsibilities and their own
stress in order to appreciate each other and develop more realistic working relationships. Coordination is also more effective when those involved have a better understanding of their respective
roles and work stresses. Recognizing this will make coordination less frustrating. If resources are
not available when and in the manner required, this will act as a barrier to coordination. Staff who
are not willing to listen and include others will find that coordination may not be as successful as
planned. Other barriers are a lack of interdisciplinary understanding, lack of resources, and inadequate communication. Ineffective problem solving is also a critical barrier.

Skills to achieve effective coordination

For staff to provide effective coordination, they need to make decisions to solve problems, plan,
use the abilities of other staff, identify resources required, communicate, and be willing to collaborate. Delegation often is required, so delegation skills are important. (See Chapter 8 for more
discussion on delegation.) The nurse also needs to develop evaluation skills to determine if outcomes are met as well as when to change course or make adjustments. The skills required for coordination are the same ones required for collaboration with the primary goal of working together
to reach agreed upon goals. Box 3-3 highlights the skills needed for effective coordination.

BOX 3-3   Coordination: Skills needed.

- Problem solving
- Plan
- Use abilities of others
- Identify needed resources
- Communication
- Collaboration
- Delegation
- Evaluation

Source: Author.

Application of coordination

Coordination is integral to daily operations, short- and long-range planning, and the daily care process. All of these activities require coordination of clinical and administrative resources. The following strategies are helpful in improving coordination.

- All staff should have a clear understanding of goals.
- All staff should use voluntary coordination in horizontal relationships with an understanding of one another's needs.
- All staff should have knowledge of policies and procedures with an understanding of what has to be done, by whom, and how it will help to facilitate coordination.
- Improved organizational performance will depend on coordination at all levels in the organization.
- Orientation and staff development programs should emphasize the importance of coordination and how to use it.
- Coordination requires effective communication.
- Coordination through supervision occurs as staff are taught how to work together, how to communicate with each other, and how to respond to each other's needs.
- All staff need to accept that different expertise is required to meet complex patient needs (Finkelman, 1996, p. 1–1:17).

Health care uses many tools that focus on coordination of care. Some of these are case management, clinical pathways, practice guidelines, and disease management. (See Chapters 9 and 15.) To be successful and meet expected outcomes, these tools also require collaboration with the patient, patient's families and significant others, and other health care staff, and they are very useful when coordination is required. With managed care's emphasis on effective and efficient care, coordination plays a major role in reaching this goal. Coordination requires that the nurse understand patient needs and the resources that are available to meet these needs. An awareness of the association of costs and services is part of coordinating patient care. In addition, coordination is a very important part of management within the health care delivery system. This system has become more complex, which has made communication and coordination more complex. Coordination is required to get resources, schedule staff, plan work activities, implement quality improvement, and perform all types of management functions.

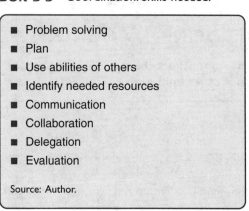

BENCHMARKS

Now let's take a moment to test your knowledge of the concepts you have studied in this section.

Negotiation and Conflict Resolution

Definitions

Conflict can never be eliminated in organizations; however, conflict can be managed. Typically, conflict arises when people feel strongly about something. Conflicts can take place between individual staff, within a unit, or within a department. They can be inter-unit and interdepartmental, affect the entire organization, or even occur between multiple organizations, between or within teams or units, or between an organization and the community. Conflict is the "tension arising from compatible needs, in which the actions of one frustrate the ability of the other to achieve a goal" (Boggs, 2003, p. 366).

There are three types of conflict: individual, interpersonal, and intergroup/organizational (Dessler, 2002).

■ The most common type of individual conflict in the workplace is role conflict, which occurs when there is incompatibility between one or more role expectations. When staff do not understand the roles of other staff this can be very stressful for the individual and does affect work. Staff may be critical of each other for not doing some work activity when in reality it is not part of the role and responsibilities of that staff member, or staff may feel that another staff member is doing some activity that really is not his or her responsibility.

■ Interpersonal conflict occurs between people. Sometimes this is due to differences and/or personalities, competition, or concern about territory, control, or loss.

■ Conflict also occurs between groups (e.g., units, services, teams, health care professional groups, agencies, community and a health care provider organization, and so on).

"Conflict is merely individuals or groups experiencing differences in views, goals, or facts that place them at opposite poles. It usually involves areas of differing expertise, practice, or authority" (Cesta, Tahan, & Fink, 1998, p. 68). Something is out of sync, usually due to a lack of clear understanding of one another's roles and responsibilities.

Conflict can be overt or covert, and both can lead to problems as well as opportunities.

> However, covert conflict processes, obviously, tend to be fluid and difficult to describe. It is in behaviors between individuals and groups, as well as individual behaviors that are observable. These behaviors can be categorized as reactive, repressive, or avoidant. Reactive behaviors include high levels of competition, inefficiency, 'yesing' people with no real attempt to understand, whining, complaining, destructive behavior, counter organization moves, and passive-aggressive behaviors such as escapist drinking, irregular output, or frequent expression of low job satisfaction. In workplaces that are ripe with unacknowledged conflict, rumor mills flourish. Repressive behaviors include absenteeism, whereas avoidant behaviors can include withholding information, avoidance of contact with managers or other team members, or 'hiding out' on the job. (Clement, 2001, p. 212)

Everyone has experienced covert conflict. It never feels good and increases stress quickly. Distrust and confusion about the best response are also experienced. Acknowledging covert conflict is not easy, and staff will have different perceptions of the conflict since it is not clear and below the surface. Overt conflict is obvious, at least to most people, and thus coping with it is usually easier. It is easier to arrive at an agreement that conflict is present and easier to arrive at a description of the conflict.

The common assumption about conflict is that it is destructive, and it certainly can be. There is, however, another view of conflict. "Despite its adverse effects, conflict is viewed by most experts today as potentially useful because it can, if properly channeled, be an engine of innovation and change. This view explicitly encourages a certain amount of controlled conflict in organizations because lack of active debate can permit the status quo or mediocre ideas to prevail" (Dessler, 2002, p. 315). In reality, staff really cannot avoid conflict because some conflict is inevitable. The following quote speaks to the need to recognize most conflict as opportunity.

> When I speak of celebrating conflict, others often look at me as if I have just stepped over the credibility line. As nurses, we have been socialized to avoid conflict. Our modis operandi has been to smooth over at all costs, particularly if the dynamic involves individuals representing roles that have significant power differences in the organization. Be advised that well-functioning transdisciplinary teams will encounter conflict-laden situations. It is inevitable. The role of the leader is to use conflicting perspectives to highlight and hone the rich diversity that is present within the team. Conflict also provides opportunities for individuals to present divergent yet equally valid views that allow all team members to gain an understanding of their contributions to the process. Respect for each team member's standpoint comes only after the team has explored fully and learned to appreciate the diversity of its membership. (Weaver, 2001, p. 83)

This is a very positive view of conflict, which on the surface may appear negative. If one asked nurses if they wanted to experience conflict, they would say "no." Probably behind their response is the fact that they do not know how to handle conflict and feel uncomfortable with it. Avoidance of conflict, however, usually means that it will catch up with the person again, and then it may be more difficult to resolve. There may then be more emotions attached to it, making it more difficult to resolve.

Causes of conflict

Effective resolution of conflict requires an understanding of the cause of the conflict; however, some conflicts may have more than one cause. It is easy to jump to conclusions without doing a thorough assessment. Some of the typical causes of conflict between individuals and between groups include:

- Inadequate communication
- Incorrect facts
- Lack of trust
- Unclear position descriptions
- Misunderstanding of roles and responsibilities
- Unclear or conflicted goals and objectives
- Inadequate action plans
- Directions
- Unstable leadership
- Receiving direction from two or more "bosses"
- Inability to accept change
- Lack of leadership
- Lack of or limited staff participation in decision making
- Power issues (Finkelman, 1996, p. 1–1:17)

Dessler (2002) discusses three additional major causes of inter-group conflict found in management literature that are also relevant to health care settings.

- The first view is that groups that must work interdependently and compete for scarce resources will experience more conflict (Walton & Dutton, 1969). For example, if units or services are competing for staff, a scarce resource, conflict may arise as they try to "prove" to administration that they need the staff more than another unit or service.
- The second cause focuses on differences in goals. This can be more than just the content of the goals; it may also include issues of flexibility, measurement of performance, and differences between the goals and societal needs (Dutton & Walton, 1966). This can certainly be seen in individuals, but groups who need to work together will find tension rising if they do not agree on the goals.

BOX 3-4   Possible causes of inter-group conflict.

Interdependence and competition

Differences in goals

Differentiation of co-workers

Inconsistency with actual authority and prestige

Source: Author.

■ The third cause is related to the amount of differentiation between co-workers (Lawrence & Lorsch, 1961). A common example in nursing is conflict between professional nursing staff and non-professional nursing staff such as UAPs or LPNs. When there is inconsistency with a group's actual authority and its prestige there can be inter-group conflict (Seiler, 1963).

These causes are highlighted in Box 3-4.

Two predictors of conflict are the existence of competition for resources or inadequate communication. It is rare that a major change on a unit or in a health care organization does not result in competition for resources (staff, financial, space, supplies) so conflicts will arise between units or between those who may or may not receive the resources or may lose resources. As has been demonstrated in some of the examples, causes of conflict can be varied. An understanding of a conflict requires as thorough an assessment as possible. Along with the assessment, it is important to understand the stages of conflict.

Stages of conflict

There are four stages of conflict that help describe the process of conflict development.

1. **Latent conflict.** This stage involves the anticipation of conflict. Competition for resources or inadequate communication can be predictors of conflict. Anticipating conflict can increase tension. This is when staff may verbalize, "We know we are going to have a hassle with this" or may feel this internally. The anticipation of conflict can occur between units who accept one another's patients when one unit does not think that the staff on the other unit is very competent and yet they must accept orders and patient plans from them.

2. **Perceived conflict.** This stage requires recognition or awareness that conflict exists at a particular time. It may not be discussed but only felt. Perception is very important as it can affect whether or not there really is a conflict, what is known about the conflict, and how it might be resolved.

3. **Felt conflict.** This occurs when individuals begin to have feelings about the conflict such as anxiety or anger. Staff feel stress at this time. If avoidance is used at this time, it may prevent the conflict from moving to the next stage. Avoidance may be appropriate in some circumstances, but sometimes it just covers over the conflict and does not resolve it. In this case, the conflict may come up again and be more complicated. Trust plays a role here. How much do staff trust that the situation will be resolved effectively? How comfortable do staff feel in being open with their feelings and opinions?

4. **Manifest conflict.** This is overt conflict. At this time the conflict can be constructive or destructive. Examples of destructive behavior related to the conflict are: (a) ignoring a policy, (b) denying a problem, (c) avoiding a staff member, or (d) discussing staff in public with negative terms. Examples of constructive responses to the conflict are: (a) encouraging the group to identify and solve the problem, (b) expressing appropriate feelings, or (c) offering to help out a staff member (Finkelman, 1996; Marriner-Tomey, 1992).

Figure 3-1 highlights the stages of conflict.

FIGURE 3-1 Stages of conflict.

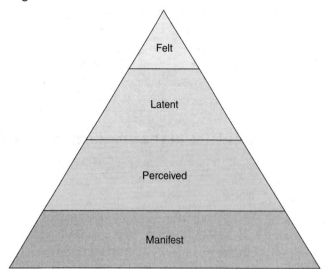

Source: Author.

THINK CRITICALLY

Try this exercise to apply what you have learned about this topic.

Prevention of conflict

Some conflict can be prevented so it is important to take preventive steps whenever possible to correct a problem before it develops into a conflict. Prevention of conflict should focus on the typical causes of conflict that have been identified in this chapter. Clear communication and delineation of roles and responsibilities will go a long way toward preventing conflict. If the goal is to eliminate all conflict this will not be successful, because it cannot be done. A staff group or organization that says it has no conflicts is either not aware of conflict or prefers not to acknowledge it. The following are important in the prevention of conflict.

- Allocate resources fairly
- Clearly state expectations (at all levels)
- Avoid sudden unexplained changes in processes
- Address staff fears (Milgram, Spector, & Treger, 1999, p. 297)

Since not all conflict can be prevented, staff and managers need to know how to manage conflict and resolve conflict when it exists. It is important to identify potential barriers that can make it more likely that a situation will turn into a conflict or will act as barriers to conflict resolution. First and foremost, if all staff make an effort to decrease their tension or stress level, this will go a long way in preventing or resolving conflict. In addition to this strategy, the following are important.

- Deal with difficult issues when they occur. Do not put off interventions as this will only make the tension rise.
- Avoid behavior that might lead to defensiveness or counteractions. Examples of this behavior are threats, limited patience, and use of hot-button or demoralizing words (for example, "never").

- Observe nonverbal communication that might indicate staff are upset (for example, sarcasm, body posture, raising voice or tone of voice, hand movements).
- Treat others with respect, which will decrease defensiveness.
- Avoid arguments. Sometimes people do need to vent, and as long as it is done appropriately and in a private place, it may be helpful in decreasing tension.
- Listen to each other.
- Consider the phases of conflict resolution (Milgram, Spector, & Treger, 1999, p. 296).

Conflict management: Issues and strategies

Conflict management is critical in any organization. When conflicts arise then managers and staff need to understand conflict management issues and strategies. The major goals of conflict management are:

1. To eliminate or decrease the conflict
2. To meet the needs of the patient, family/significant others, and the organization
3. To ensure that all parties feel positive about the resolution so that future work together can be productive.

When staff experience conflict, powerlessness and empowerment, as well as aggressiveness and passive-aggressiveness, become important.

Powerlessness and empowerment

1. **Power and powerlessness**

    When staff feel that they are not recognized, appreciated, or paid attention to, then they feel **powerlessness**. What happens in a work environment when staff feel powerlessness? First, staff do not feel that they can make an impact—they are unable to change situations that they feel need to be changed. Staff will not be as creative in approaching problems. They may feel that they are responsible for tasks and yet have no control or power to affect change with these tasks. The team community will be affected negatively, and eventually the team may feel it cannot make change happen. Staff may make any of the following comments: "Don't bother trying to make a difference," "I can't make a difference here," and "Who listens to us?" Morale deteriorates as staff feel more and more powerless. New staff will soon pick up on the feeling of powerlessness. In some respects, the powerlessness really does diminish any effort for change. As was discussed in Chapter 2, responding to change effectively is very important today.

    Power is about influencing decisions, controlling resources, and affecting behavior. It is the ability to get things done—access resources and information, and use it to make decisions. Power can be used constructively or destructively. The power a person has originates from the person's personal qualities and characteristics, as well as the person's position. Some people have qualities that make others turn to them—people trust them, consider their advice helpful, and so on. A person's position, such as a team leader or nurse manager, has associated power.

    Power is not stagnant. It changes as it is affected by the situation. Fisher (1996) describes power and influence as parts of a continuum. In this viewpoint, power is seen as control over others to reach a goal or outcome; whereas, "influence is a dynamic process; it seeks not to control but to set in place an interdependence that fosters cooperation" (Carr, 1992; Fisher, 1996, p. 114). The concept of influence is a much more positive viewpoint and indicates support of the importance of collaboration and recognition of staff. In this situation, it is more likely that communication, decision making, cooperation, conflict resolution, and collaboration will improve.

    There are a number of sources of power. Each one can be useful depending on the circumstances and the goal. An individual may have several sources of power; for example, a team leader may have legitimate power due to the position held, expert power due to team members' recognition of the team leader's expertise in care of oncology patients, and persuasive power as the team leader is able to convince team members the best steps to take to solve a problem. The common sources of power include the following.

    - **Legitimate power.** This power is what one typically thinks of in relation to power. It is power that comes from having a formal position in an organization such as a nurse manager, team leader, or vice president of patient services. These positions give the person who holds one of them the right to influence staff and expect staff to follow requests. Staff recognize that they have tasks to accomplish and job requirements.

■ **Reward power.** A person's power comes from the ability to reward others when they comply. Examples of reward power include money (such as an increase in salary level), desired schedule or assignment, providing a space to work, or recognition of accomplishment.

■ **Coercive power.** This type of power is based on punishment when a person does not do as expected or directed. Examples of this type include denial of a pay raise, termination, and poor schedule or assignment. This type of power leads to an unpleasant work situation. It is important to remember that "the stronger the power used, the greater the resistance that can be anticipated" (Carr, 1992). Staff will not respond positively to coercive power, and this type of power has a strong negative effect on staff morale.

■ **Referent power.** This informal power comes from others recognizing that an individual has special qualities and is admired. This person then has influence over others because they want to follow the person due to the person's charisma. Staff feel valued and accepted.

■ **Expert power.** When a person has an expertise the person can have power over others who respect that expertise. When this type of power is present, the expert is able to provide sound advice and direction.

■ **Informational power.** This type of power arises from the ability to access and share information, which is critical in the Information Age.

■ **Persuasive power.** This type of power influences others by providing an effective point-of-view or argument (Bennis & Goldsmith, 1997; Dessler, 2002; Finkelman, 1996; Marriner-Tomey, 1992).

Box 3-5 highlights the types of power.

It is important to note that a leader must have legitimate power. "A mugger on the street may have a gun and power to threaten your life, but not qualify as a leader, because leading means influencing people to work *willingly* toward achieving your objectives. That is not to say that a little fear can't be a good thing, at least occasionally" (Dessler, 2002, p. 212). This is a critical concept to understand about leadership and power. However, it takes more than power to be an effective leader and manager. "If you have the traits and you have the power, then you have the *potential* to be a leader" (Dessler, 2002, p. 212).

All organizations experience their own brand of "politics." Some staff and managers find themselves maneuvering to acquire power within the organization. This is directly influenced by the goals that people feel are important to them. These goals may come in conflict with the goals of others, and when this happens, holding greater power may make a difference in who "wins." Political power maneuvering can become unpleasant for staff and managers and can also damage the organization's culture. Trust may decrease, along with effective communication, coordination, collaboration, and resolution of conflicts. This is not to say that all political power in the organization is negative, but it is a slippery slope and needs to be carefully observed. Part

BOX 3-5   Types of power.

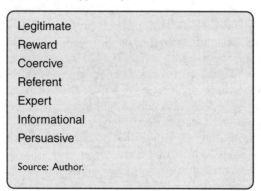

Legitimate
Reward
Coercive
Referent
Expert
Informational
Persuasive

Source: Author.

of this process is the need to identify where the power is coming from and to learn how to access the power to meet goals (Marrelli, 1997). As has been said, power can be used negatively, and this can also lead to the unethical use of power or not doing the right thing with the power. Chapter 10 discusses examples of ethical issues. There is no doubt that there are managers who use their power to control staff, as well as staff who use power to control other staff, but this is not a healthy use of power. Rather, it is a misuse of power and does not demonstrate nursing leadership.

How do people see themselves in relation to power? This issue is not always openly discussed, but it is present in all situations. There are several stages that a person may experience.

- ▓ Powerless. Many nurses see themselves as victims. "It doesn't make any difference, so I'm not going to do it."

- ▓ Power-seeking. With this view, nurses seek those who have power and build relationships with them for the purpose of gaining power. "It's who I know."

- ▓ Power symbols. This view identifies symbols that should indicate power such as degrees, new office, better home, and so on.

- ▓ Power by reflection. This is when the nurse is concerned with congruence. "I really want congruency between who I am and what I'm doing."

- ▓ Power by purpose. This is the final stage when the nurse knows the direction and purpose that is important. "I know who I am. I know what I'll do, and I can play ball regardless of external circumstances" (Hagenow, 1999, pp. 31–32).

A self-appraisal of a person's personal view of power allows the individual to better understand how power is used and how it then affects the person's decisions and relationships. This can lead to more effective responses to change during planning and decision making, coping with conflict, and the ability to collaborate and coordinate.

2. Empowerment

Empowerment is often viewed as the sharing of power; however, it is more than this. "To empower is to enable to act" (Finkelman, 1996, pp. 1–1.6). Power must be more than words, but rather it must be demonstrated. "Empowered leaders can educate and encourage trusting relationships by practicing and modeling sharing, listening, accepting, learning, consideration, consistency, and purposeful activity. . . . We must throw away the victim mentality and move the business of providing health care into the 21st century" (Smith, 2000, pp. 2–3). Participative decision making empowers staff, but only if staff really do have the opportunity to participate and influence decisions. Recognizing that one's participation is accepted makes a difference. True empowerment gives the staff the right to choose how to address issues with the manager.

Should all staff be empowered? A critical issue to answer this question is whether or not staff can handle decision making. This implies that staff need leadership qualities and skills to make sound decisions and participate together collaboratively. They need to be able to use communication effectively. When staff are selected, all these factors become important. Empowerment is not gained just by being a member of the staff, but rather staff gain empowerment because they are able to handle it. Management that wants to empower staff must transfer power over the staff, but they must first feel confident that staff can handle empowerment.

When staff are empowered some limits or boundaries need to be set or conflict may develop. Some of these boundaries are established by the organization's policies, procedures, and position descriptions, education and experience, and by laws and regulations (for example, nurse practice acts). The manager must be aware of these boundaries and establish any others that may be required (for example, direct involvement of staff in the selection process for new equipment). If staff are involved in the decision making, then they should first be given a list of several possible equipment choices that meet the budgetary requirements from which to choose. It is critical that the manager make clear the boundaries, or staff will feel like their efforts are useless if their suggestions are rejected because they were not given the boundaries. What does this mean? "Boundaries are key constraints such as costs, schedules, and consumer or customer requirements. Staff who are told that they are free to develop plans of care for patients as long as specific requirements are met will feel more in control" (Finkelman, 1996, p. 1–1:7). At the same time the nurse manager or the team leader must not control, dominer, or overpower staff. This type of response is usually seen in new nurse managers or team leaders who feel insecure. Ineffective use of empowerment can be just as problematic as a lack of empowerment.

Organizations that actively use empowerment demonstrate some important qualities (Bennis & Goldsmith, 1997).

- Staff feel significant as they make a difference in the organization and in its success.
- The organization emphasizes that learning and competence are critical. Failure is not an issue as mistakes are seen as opportunities for improvement.
- Staff feel that they are part of a team or community, which implies trust and commitment.
- Staff who are empowered usually feel that their work is exciting. "An essential ingredient in organizational leadership is that the leader pulls rather than pushes people along. A pull style of influence works by attracting and energizing people to enroll in their vision of the future. It motivates through identification rather than through rewards and punishments" (Bennis & Goldsmith, 1997, p. 165).

What type of power would be less common in this type of organization? Coercive power would not be effective as it is not supportive of empowerment.

"Empowerment is an interrelationship between authority, resources, timely and accurate information, and accountability. A nurse manager who is providing staff an environment in which empowerment is valued works to see that all four of these elements are present for the staff in their daily work environment" (Finkelman, 1996, p. 1–1:6). It requires a focus on established goals and communication that encourages feedback. When nurses stay focused on quality care, they cannot allow the hierarchy in the organization to interfere with required care (Cesta, Tahan, & Fink, 1998). Nurse leaders need to do the following to empower staff.

- Teach and provide staff development opportunities—growth opportunities
- Remove barriers
- Set meaningful goals that are communicated to staff
- Provide access to resources such as staff, money, technology, equipment, and supplies
- Foster independence by encouraging decision making and delegation
- Offer opportunities to network and gain others' acknowledgment, support, and cooperation
- Provide access to information
- Develop trust and express confidence in staff
- Ask for staff feedback and respond to the feedback
- Support staff
- Decentralize decision making (Finkelman, 1996; Laschinger, Finegan, Shamian, & Casier, 2000; Lee, 2000)

Although empowering one's self may seem like an unusual concept, it is an important one. Situational anger may be the force that moves nurses to empower themselves (Lyon, 2000). The amount of power a person has in a relationship is determined by the degree to which someone else needs what the other person has. Anger is related to expectations that are not met, and when these expectations are not met, the person may act out to gain empowerment. It is the responsibility of the nursing profession to communicate what nurses have to offer to patient care and to the health care delivery system, but individual nurses also need to understand what they have to offer as nurses. To have an impact this communication and development must be ongoing. Empowerment can be positive if the strategies that are used to gain empowerment are constructive (for example, gaining new skills, speaking out constructively, networking, using political advocacy, increasing involvement in planning and decision making, getting more nurses on key organization committees, improving image through a positive image campaign, and developing and implementing assertiveness skills. There are many other strategies that can result in empowerment that improves the workplace and the nurse's self-perception.

Aggressive and passive-aggressive behavior

Aggressive and passive-aggressive behavior can interfere with successful conflict resolution and might even be the cause of conflict. When staff are hostile to one another, the team leader, or the nurse manager, anxiety rises. Hostile behavior can be a response to conflict. It is important to recognize personal feelings. The first response should be to get under control and communicate control to the hostile staff member. The nurse manager or team leader may be the one who is hostile, which makes it even more complex and requires assistance from higher level management. Hopefully, someone will recognize the need to bring the situation under control and try to move to a private place. Demonstrations of open conflict with hostility should not take place in patient or public areas. If the suggestion to move to a private area does not work and the situation continues to escalate, simply walking away may help set some boundaries. Cool down time is definitely needed.

There are many times when more information is really required before a response can be given. If this is the case, everyone concerned needs to be told that when information is gathered the issue or problem will then be discussed. No one should be pressured to respond with inadequate information as this will lead to ineffective decision making and may lead to further hostility. It is critical that after further assessment is completed that there be additional discussion and a conclusion. "Unless the behavior of a difficult person is physically threatening, try ignoring it. Deal only with the heart of the matter. Focus your attention on the issue and work at refocusing your 'opponent's' attention. Repeatedly use his or her name. State and restate the problem. Try to defuse emotion—yours first, because ultimately the only person you really control is yourself" (Forman, 2001, p. 13). These are methods that can help move a negative situation into a positive one.

When there are problems with patients and families, what is the best way to cope? Many of the same strategies can be used. Safety is the first issue, as it must be maintained. It is never appropriate to allow patients or families to demonstrate anger inappropriately. When this occurs, someone needs to set reasonable limits that are based on an assessment of the situation. There may be many reasons for anger and inappropriate behavior, such as pain, medications, fear and anxiety, psychosis, dysfunctional communication, and so on. Staff need to avoid taking things personally, as this will interfere with thoughtful problem solving. When one gets defensive or emotional, interventions taken to resolve a conflict may not be effective. Active listening is critical to cope with emotions. If a different culture is involved, then this factor needs to be considered (for example, some cultures consider it appropriate to be very emotional and others do not). In the long term, clear communication is critical during the entire process.

How do individual staff members cope with conflict?

Not everyone responds to conflict in the same way, and individuals may vary in how they respond dependent upon the circumstances. Four typical responses to conflict are avoidance, accommodation, competition, and collaboration (Boggs, 2003).

■ Avoidance occurs when a person is very uncomfortable and cannot cope with the anxiety effectively. This person will withdraw from the situation to avoid it. There are times when this may be the most effective response, particularly when the situation may lead to negative results, but in many situations this will not be effective in the long term. This response might occur when a staff member is in conflict with a manager and disagrees with the manager. The staff member must consider whether it is worth it to disagree publicly. Typically, avoidance occurs when one side is perceived as more powerful than the other. It is a helpful approach when more information is needed or when the issue just is not worth what might be lost.

■ A second response is accommodation. How does this occur? The person tries to make the situation better by cooperating. The critical issue may not be resolved, or not be resolved to the fullest satisfaction. The goal is just to eliminate the conflict as quickly as possible. Accommodation works best when one person or group is less interested in the issue than the other. It can be advantageous as it does develop harmony, and it can provide power in future conflict since one party was more willing to let the conflict deflate.

BOX 3-6   Examples of conflict management styles.

Confrontation

"In recent meetings we have had a thrashing around about our needs. At first we did not have much agreement, but we kept thrashing around and finally agreed on what was the best we could do."

Smoothing

"I thought I went to great lengths in our group to confront conflict. I said what I thought in the meeting, but it did not bother anybody. I guess I should have been harsher. I could have said I won't do it unless you do it my way. If I had done this, they couldn't have backed away, but I guess I didn't have the guts to do it. I guess I didn't pound the bushes hard enough."

Forcing

"If I want something very badly and I am confronted by a roadblock, I go to top management to get the decision made. If the research managers are willing to go ahead [my way], there is no problem. If there is a conflict, then I take the decision to somebody higher up."

Avoidance

"I'm not going to discuss that with you."

Competitive

"You don't know what you're doing." "You need to get to work; if you can't get your job done, get out." "This is your doing, not mine."

Compromise and collaboration

"I'm sure we can figure out a way to solve this together." "We're all in the same boat in this matter." "Let's see how we can work this out."

Accommodating

"Calm down so we can work this out." "Let's see how we can work this out."

Source: Author created and summarized from Thomas, K. (1976). Conflict and conflict management. In M. Dunnettte (Ed.), *Handbook of Industrial and Organizational Psychology*. Chicago: Rand McNally, pp. 900–902; Carrell, M., Jennings, D., & Heavrin, C. (1997). *Fundamentals of organizational behavior.* Upper Saddle River, NJ: Prentice Hall, pp. 505–509.

■ A third response is competition. How does this work? Power is used to stop the conflict. A manager might say, "This is the way it will be." This closes further efforts from others who may be in conflict with the manager.

■ Collaboration is the fourth response, which has been discussed in this chapter. This is a positive approach, with all parties attempting to reach an acceptable solution, and in the end both sides feel that they won something. Collaboration often involves some compromise, which is a method used to respond to conflict.

Using the best conflict resolution style can make a difference in success. There are many ways that a conflict can be resolved. Box 3-6 provides a review of other examples of conflict management styles and statements. Some of these are less effective, but their effectiveness depends on the situation.

When conflict occurs each person involved has a personal perspective of the issue and conflict. Today there is more conflict in the health care delivery environment with increased workplace stress that may lead to misunderstandings, ineffective communication, and reduced productivity (Iacono, 2000). The following strategies were developed by a specific health care organization, the St. Joseph Hospital Health Center in Syracuse, New York, to assist staff with conflict resolution. This demonstrates how serious this organization considers the problem of conflict in the workplace.

1. Identify the problem behaviors. It is important to focus on behaviors, not personalities.
2. Collect facts about the problem behaviors. Clear and specific description of the problem behaviors is critical. Problems should be kept separate so that the focus is clear.
3. Document the facts and their sources.
4. Ensure privacy when the behaviors and related issues are discussed.
5. Explore the different perspectives. In this discussion make sure that understanding of the issue and expectations is present.
6. Use counseling sessions as a learning opportunity for growth, which requires objective feedback and encourages active participation.
7. Document both the manager's and employee's personal reactions to the counseling and the results.
8. Document employee's response to counseling and the corrective action.
9. Clarify with the employee who has access to the documentation, who will be told about the counseling session and action plan, and the timeline for change.
10. Report the results to the appropriate supervisor, if required (Iacono, 2000, p. 261).

Gender issues

Are there differences in the way that women and men negotiate? Wyatt (2000) discusses factors related to these differences. Men tend to negotiate to win while women focus more on what is fair. It is believed that this is related to the way children play through sports and activities. Women will make an effort to reach win-win solutions. Men will test the limits that have been set more overtly than women, so it is important for women to ensure that limits are set and maintained. "Managerial women, however, demonstrate less confidence than men when anticipating negotiation and feel less satisfaction with their performance when the process is completed" (Robbins, 1998; as cited in Wyatt, 2000, p. 43). It is important, despite the differences described, to avoid stereotyping.

How can women participate more positively in negotiations? The key is in planning. "Negotiation is 80% planning, and 20% action" (Wyatt, 2000, p. 45). How do the differences in women and men affect this process?

■ During the first step of preparation and planning, women tend to take things more personally. At this time women can use their skills to positively engage in personal relationships. Power bases are evaluated during this step. Appearance can make a difference in how a person's power might be perceived.

■ During the second step, defining the ground rules, the boundaries are set and issues such as the time and place for meeting or whose turf will be used becomes important. Body language is important as well as a display of confidence.

■ Clarifying and justifying is the third step in the process. This is when both sides educate one another about the issue. "Sex differences become readily apparent during this step because once a women states her proposal, she often characterizes her explanation using adjectives, adverbs, and expletives less powerful than those commonly used by males. This manner of speech conveys triviality by male standards. When women use these patterns of communication, they are perceived as incompetent, whereas if men use them, they are perceived as polite" (Lenz, 1990, as cited in Wyatt, 2000, p. 44). Using assertiveness skills is important.

■ During the fourth step, the focus is on bargaining and problem solving. Both parties will have to compromise and make concessions. Communication skills will be critical. When men and women have similar expertise, men tend to talk longer than women and thus are viewed as being more dominant. Men also interrupt more when they want to demonstrate their dominance. Women need to be assertive and not give up their time to express their views or allow the interruptions to occur (Lenz, 1990). This is when emotions increase, and all parties, women and men, must control themselves.

■ The final step is closure and implementation. Afterwards, an agreement is formalized.

Nurse-physician relationships

Though the nurse-physician relationship should be the strongest relationship that nurses have in order to meet the needs of the patient, it frequently is not. Both sides of the relationship play a role in the inadequacies of this relationship. Conflict does occur, and this conflict can act as a barrier to effective patient care. Literature about Magnet hospitals distinguishes between collegial and collaborative relationships and between nurses and physicians (Kramer & Schmalenberg, 2002). Collegial relationships are those where there is equality of power. This power is different but equal power and knowledge. In contrast, collaborative relationships between nurses and physicians focus on mutual power, but the physician's power is greater. The nurse's power is based on the nurse's extended time with patients, experience, and knowledge. In addition to power, this relationship requires respect and trust between the nurse and physician. Due to these factors, it is a complex relationship.

Positive professional communication is critical. Both sides should initiate positive dialogue rather than adversarial positions. Cooperation and collaboration are also integral to the success of this relationship. A frequent question discussed in the literature is, "Why is there conflict between nurses and physicians?" One approach that has been taken to this question is to suggest that the conflict exists because the two professions structure their work differently (Finkelman, 1996; Sheard, 1980). This perspective identifies the key elements that are important in the work structure, which are sense of time, sense of resources, unit of analysis, sense of mastery, and type of rewards.

- The nurse is focused on shorter periods of time, and time is usually short, with frequent interruptions. The physician's sense of time focuses on the course of illness.
- If a physician gives a stat order, the physician has problems understanding what might interfere with the nurse making this a priority. There is a lack of understanding of the nurse's work structure.
- Physicians often are not concerned with resources, though this is certainly changing as physicians do recognize that there is a shortage of staff as well as issues about costs and reimbursement for care. They, however, may not be willing to accept these factors as relevant when their patients need something. There are, of course, other resources such as equipment availability, supplies, and funds that can cause problems and conflicts. Nurses are typically more aware of the effect that these factors have on daily care.
- Unit of analysis is another factor; for example, nurses are caring for groups of patients even though care is supposed to be individualized. Physicians may not have an understanding of this if they have only a few patients in the hospital.
- Physicians also do not have an understanding of nursing delivery models such as team nursing or primary nursing, and often nurses themselves are not clear about them. This affects nurses' ability to explain how they work.
- Clearly, the sense of reward is different. Nurses work in a task-oriented environment and typically get paid an hourly rate. Most physicians are not salaried and are independent practitioners though some are employees of the organization (hospital, clinic, and so on).

Conflict and verbal abuse are related. Verbal abuse occurs in health care settings between patients and staff, nurses and other nurses, physicians and nurses, and all other staff relationships. This abuse can consist of statements made directly to a staff member or about a staff member to others. A common complaint from nurses regards verbal abuse from physicians. "Some nurses, particularly new ones, allow physicians to verbally abuse them because they are insecure about their knowledge base" (Parks, 2001, p. 20MW). Verbal abuse affects turnover rates and contributes to the nursing shortage so it is has serious consequences (Stringer, 2001). "Poor physician-nurse interaction also compromises patient care" (Stringer, 2001, p. 7).

How can this problem be improved? A critical step is to gain better understanding of each profession's viewpoint and demonstrate less automatic acceptance of inappropriate behavior. This requires that management become proactive in eliminating negative communication and behavior. Some hospitals have tried a number of strategies to deal with verbal abuse. Some of these are: (a) encouraging staff to report abuse by allowing anonymity, (b) using physician-nurse counseling teams to act as liaisons with employees, (c) encouraging staff to speak firmly and address abuse, and (d) introducing staff to new physicians and encouraging them to come for assistance (Stringer, 2001).

What can nurses do about this? One suggestion is to improve their own knowledge base and thus develop more self-confidence. "Remind yourself that you have many valuable skills, and you don't deserve to be verbally abused. These efforts will help decrease the feelings of intimidation" (Parks, 2001, p. 20MW). Another problem is that nurses think they must resolve all problems and "make things" work correctly when this may not be realistic. The nurses then become scapegoats. Verbal abuse, no matter who is doing it, physician or nurse, should not be tolerated. Those involved need to be approached in private to identify the need for a change in behavior. All staff need to be respected.

CURRENT ISSUES

Learn about events around the globe that relate to the chapter content.

Application of negotiation to conflict resolution

Negotiation is the critical element in making conflict a nightmare or an opportunity. Negotiation can be used to resolve a conflict, and some types of negotiation, such as mediation, can be very structured. When two or more people or organizations disagree or have opposing views about a problem or solution, a conflict exists. To resolve the conflict, the involved people need to discuss resolution in a manner that is acceptable to all of those involved. Although it does not have to take long, in some cases it may be very long, such as what might occur in a union–employer negotiation for a contract.

Principled negotiation can be helpful in resolving problems and conflict. It focuses on four basic points: "(1) separate the people from the problem, (2) focus on interests instead of positions, (3) generate a variety of options before deciding what to do, and (4) insist that the result be based on an objective standard" (Marriner-Tomey, 1992, p. 299). This approach may be more successful than others because it is a mixture of hard and soft negotiating. Hard approaches focus on winning and assuming that if one waits long enough the other side will give in. The soft approach focuses on prevention of conflict and concessions. In this case, the soft negotiator does not feel positive at the end but rather is bitter (Marriner-Tomey, 1992).

Conflict resolution includes the use of a variety of skills and strategies. Four key needs are clarification, performance, questioning, and expectations (Marrelli, 1997). As the process begins it is important to *clarify* all of the issues and parties who are involved in the conflict. *Performance* or potential outcomes should be established early in the process. *Questioning* is important throughout resolution. For example, it is important to ask about behaviors that started the conflict and how to avoid them in the future. Management needs to be clear about *expectations* and provide these in writing, which helps to decrease conflict over critical issues.

What strategies might be used to resolve specific conflicts?

- Help involved parties settle their differences themselves whenever possible rather than stepping in and taking over.
- Maintain an objective approach.
- Communicate trust to the staff and communicate that it is believed that they can resolve problems.
- Avoid criticizing or denying feelings.
- Use a problem-solving approach.
- Provide privacy for sensitive discussions.
- Identify staff who chronically complain and work with them to adapt their behavior as this behavior can increase the risk of conflict and interfere with resolving it when it does occur.

- Listen with understanding rather than judgment. This is important throughout the resolution process and can also assist with prevention of conflict.
- Provide opportunities for all staff to improve their problem-solving and communication skills (Marrelli, 1997, pp. 101–102).

Since conflict is inevitable, all staff nurses will encounter it. Knowing how to manage conflict will be of great benefit to the individual nurse as well as improve the working environment and ability to better reach patient outcomes. There are several conditions that are important to consider in negotiation (Tappen, 1995).

1. The first condition is a recognized conflict of interest or incompatibility between those involved. If a conflict is not identified though it is present, it can damage patient care and staff relationships.
2. Negotiation involves offers and counteroffers, and this inevitably leads to emotions, which are also present before negotiation even begins.
3. The relationship between the parties in the negotiation must be voluntary, which means all must recognize that anyone may remove him- or herself from the negotiation process at any time. If one is forced to negotiate, success in reaching effective conflict resolution is not likely.
4. There may be superficial resolution, but beneath the surface there may be many negative emotions that will act as barriers to further success when the resolution is implemented.
5. The conclusion or solution should be a win-win situation. This is not easy to accomplish because often people go into negotiation with the attitude of obtaining a win-lose result. Strategies to improve the negotiating process include establishing a cooperative climate, supplying information that supports a viewpoint or proposal, appealing to fair play, and rewarding work rather than making threats.

Why is negotiation identified as a critical skill for nurses in the health care environment? Patients should not become part of staff or organizational conflicts, and there is risk that this may occur. These conflicts need to be resolved or patient care may suffer negative consequences. Consider these examples.

- The interdisciplinary team cannot agree on a treatment approach and must do this by the end of the team meeting.
- A patient's managed care organization or health plan refuses to allow the patient to stay two more days in the hospital. As the hospital's nurse case manager you must work with the managed care representative to reach a compromise.
- Staffing in a hospital is being reduced, and the nurses are convinced that the new staffing level will be unsafe for patients. Something must be done to resolve this issue.
- A home care agency has learned that the Medicare contract has decided that specific patients will receive fewer visits.

How can these examples be resolved satisfactorily so that the quality of care does not suffer? Finding a mentor to discuss the process as well as vent feelings may be very helpful. Developing negotiation skills makes conflicts easier to handle and less stressful. Nurses who become involved in unions will find that negotiation skills are also very important. If negotiation is not used effectively, all of these conflict examples can lead to major problems for the patient and/or staff.

When approaching conflict resolution, it is important to recognize that both sides contributed to the conflict. One side cannot have a conflict by itself as it takes at least two. Consider how each side has contributed to the conflict. Another critical issue is to carefully consider if this is the time and place to address the conflict. "Define the conflict in terms of needs, not solutions. People may disagree about the right solution, but they can agree on needs and thus focus on creative problem solving and looking at alternatives" (Gebelein, 2000, p. 469). When the environment is too emotional, conflict resolution will be difficult. Stepping back or taking a break may be the best position to take. The following are strategies that can be used to effectively negotiate.

- Negotiate for agreements—not winning or losing. Clearly state that your desire is to find a solution and to work together.

- Separate people from positions.
- Establish mutual trust and respect.
- Avoid one-sided or personal gains.
- Allow time for expressing the interests of each side/party.
- Listen actively during the process, and acknowledge what is being said; avoid defending or explaining yourself.
- Use data/evidence to strengthen your position.
- Focus on patient care interests.
- Always remember that the process is a problem-solving one, and the benefit is for the patient and family.
- Clearly identify the priority and arrive at common goal(s).
- Avoid using pressure.
- Identify and understand the real reasons underlying the problem.
- Be knowledgeable about organizational policies, procedures, systems, standards, and the law, applying this knowledge as needed.
- Try to understand the other side, and ask questions and seek clarification when unsure or uncertain; understanding the other side first before explaining yours increases effectiveness.
- Avoid emotional outbursts and overreacting if the other party exhibits such behavior; depersonalize the conflict.
- Avoid premature judgments, blame, and inflammatory comments.
- Be concrete and flexible when presenting your position.
- Be reasonable and fair (Cesta, Tahan, & Fink, 1998; Gebelein et al., 2000).

Mediation

There are some conflicts that will require a third-party negotiator to reach a more effective resolution. This is needed when there is no opportunity for cooperative problem solving and objectivity is required. "Mediation is a form of dispute resolution that has been used in many cultures throughout history. . . . Mediation is a problem-solving process in which a neutral third party (who has no stake in the outcome of the process) helps people who have a disagreement or dispute reach a mutually satisfactory resolution. Mediators are facilitators, not decision makers (as in the case of arbitrators). In mediation, the people with the dispute have an opportunity to tell their story and to be understood, as well as to listen to and understand the story of the other party. The process itself generates an atmosphere of mutual respect and valuing of opinions and abilities" (Clement, 2001, p. 216). A key factor in mediation is the need for all parties to willingly participate in the process. The mediator guides the process and discussion. Certain guidelines are established for the discussion that all parties must follow throughout the process (for example, allowing each party time to speak and complete a statement without interruption, calling for a break when needed, enforcing time limited meetings, substantiating comments with facts, and so on). With these guidelines and the presence of a mediator, this type of negotiation can result in positive outcomes. It provides protection for both sides.

BENCHMARKS

Now let's take a moment to test your knowledge of the concepts you have studied in this section.

Chapter Wrap-Up

Now that you've reached the end of the chapter, you may wish to explore the concepts you've been reading about in greater detail or test yourself to see how well you've comprehended the material.

SUMMARY AND APPLICATIONS

- Summary
- Practice Quiz
- Key Terms
- Tying It All Together

- Experiential Exercises
- Case 1
- Links

REFERENCES

Aiken, L., Smith, H., & Lake, E. (1994). Lower Medicare mortality among a set of hospitals known for good nursing care. *MedCare, 32,* 771–789.

American Psychiatric Nurses Association. (1999). *Position statement: Collaboration.* Washington, DC: Author.

Bennis, W., & Goldsmith, J. (1997). *Learning to lead.* Reading, MA: Perseus Books.

Boggs, K. (2003). Resolving conflict between nurse and client. In E. Arnold & K. Boggs (Eds.), *Interpersonal relationships: Professional communication skills for nurses* (4th ed., pp. 368–388). Philadelphia: W.B. Saunders Company.

Carr, C. (1992). *Team power.* Upper Saddle River, NJ: Prentice-Hall.

Cesta, T., Tahan, H., & Fink, L. (1998). *The case manager's survival guide: Winning strategies for clinical practice.* St. Louis: Mosby-Year Book, Inc.

Clement, J. (2001). The leadership imperative: Managing conflict and resolving disputes creatively. *Seminars for Nurse Managers, 9*(4), 211–217.

Cody, W. (2001). Interdisciplinarity and nursing: "Everything is everything," or is it? *Nursing Science Quarterly, 14*(4), 274–280.

Dechairo-Marino, A., Jordan-Marsh, M., Traiger, G., & Saulo, M. (2001). Nurse/physician collaboration. *Journal of Nursing Administration, 31*(5), 223–232.

Dessler, G. (2002). *Management: Leading people and organizations in the 21st century.* Upper Saddle River, NJ: Prentice Hall.

Disch, J. (2001). Strengthening nursing and interdisciplinary collaboration. *Journal of Professional Nursing, 17*(6), 275.

Dutton, J., & Walton, R. (1966). Interdepartmental conflict and cooperation: Two contrasting studies. *Human Organization, 25,* 207–220.

Finch, J. (2000). Interprofessional education and teamworking: A view from the education providers. *British Medical Journal, 321,* 1138.

Finkelman, A. (1996). *Psychiatric nursing administration manual.* Gaithersburg, MD: Aspen Publishers, Inc.

Fisher, M. (1996). Dynamics of implementation. In M. Fisher (Ed.), *Redesigning the nursing organization* (pp. 114–130). Albany, NY: Delmar Publishers.

Forman, H. (2001). Difficult people? What's the problem. *Nursing Spectrum Metro Edition,* August, 12–13.

Gebelein, S., et al. (2000). *Successful manager's handbook.* Minneapolis, MN: Personnel Decisions International Corporation.

Gueldner, S., & Stroud, S. (1996). Sharing the quest for knowledge through interdisciplinary research. *Holistic Nursing Practice, 103*(3), 54–62.

Hagenow, N. (1999). Become architects of your future. *Nursing Management February, 30*(2), 31–35.

Hammick, M. (2000). Interprofessional education: Evidence from the past to guide the future. *Medical Teacher, 22,* 461–467.

Iacono, M. (2000). Managing conflict/employee counseling. *Journal of Perianesthesia Nursing, 15*(4), 260–263.

Kramer, M., & Schmalenberg, C. (2002). Staff nurses identify essentials of magnetism. In M. McClure & A. Hinshaw (Eds.), *Magnet hospitals revisited. Attraction and retention of professional nurses* (pp. 25–59). Washington, D.C.: American Nurses Publishing, Inc.

Ladden, M. (2001). Physician-nurse collaboration: The view from PubMed. Retrieved on May 15, 2003, from http://www.mceconnection.org/mce/topic/topic.asp?tpcId=0.

Laschinger, H., Finegan, J., Shamian, J., & Casier, S. (2000). Organizational trust and empowerment in restructured healthcare settings. *Journal of Nursing Administration, 30*(9), 413–425.

Lawrence, P., & Lorsch, J. (1961). The horizontal dimensions in a bureaucracy. *Administrative Science Quarterly, 6,* 298–333.

Lenz, E. (1990). The influence of gender on communication for nurse leaders. *Nursing Administrative Quarterly, 15*(1), 49–55.

Liedtka, J., & Whitten, E. (1998). Enhancing care delivery through cross-disciplinary collaboration: A case study. *Journal of Healthcare Management, 43,* 186.

Long, K. (2001). A reality-oriented approach to interdisciplinary work. *Journal of Professional Nursing, 17*(6), 278–282.

Lyon, B. (2000). Situational anger and self-empowerment. *Reflections on Nursing LEADERSHIP, 26*(3), 26–27.

Marrelli, T. (1997). *The nurse manager's survival guide.* St. Louis, MO: Mosby-Year Book, Inc.

Marriner-Tomey, A. (1992). *Guide to nursing management.* St. Louis, MO: Mosby-Year Book, Inc.

Milgram, L., Spector, A., & Treger, M. (1999). *Managing smart.* Houston, TX: Cashman Dudley.

Parks, S. (2001, August). Silence verbal abuse. *Nursing Spectrum Metro Edition,* 20MW–21MW.

Puetz, B., & Shinn, L. (2002). Strategic partnerships. *Journal of Nursing Administration, 32*(4), 182–184.

Robbin, S. (1998). Organizational behavior. Englewood Cliffs, NJ: Prentice-Hall, Inc.

Rosenstein, A. (2002). Nurse-physician relationships: Impact on nurse satisfaction and retention. *American Journal of Nursing, 102*(6), 26–34.

Saulo, M. (1987). Teaching conflict resolution. *Nurse Education, 12*(4), 14–17.

Seiler, J. (1963). Diagnosing interdepartmental conflict. *Harvard Business Review,* Sept.–Oct., 121–132.

Sheard, T. (1980). The structure of conflict in nurse physician relationships. *Supervisor Nurse, 11*(9), 14.

Smith, S. (2000). Modeling interpersonal competencies enhances patient care and organization. *INSIGHT, 25*(1), 2–3.

Stringer, H. (2001). Raging bullies. *Nursing Week, 1*(2), 6–7.

Stumpf, S. & Clark, J. (1999). The promise and pragmatism of interdisciplinary education. Journal of Allied Health, 28(1), 30–32.

Sullivan, T. (1998a). Concept analysis: Part I. In T. Sullivan (Ed.), *Collaboration: A health care imperative* (pp. 3–42). New York: McGraw-Hill.

Sullivan, T. (1998b). Concept analysis: Part II. In T. Sullivan (Ed.), *Collaboration: A health care imperative* (pp. 43–64). New York: McGraw-Hill.

Tahan, J. (2001). A story from the bedside: The primary nurse as an integral health care team member. *Seminars for Nurse Managers, 9*(2), 68–72.

Tappen, R. (1995). *Nursing Leadership and Management.* Philadelphia: F.A. Davis.

Walton, R., & Dutton, J. (1969). The management of interdepartment conflict: A model and review. *Administrative Science Quarterly,* March, 73–84.

Weaver, D. (2001). Transdisciplinary teams: Very important leadership stuff. *Seminars for Nurse Managers, 9*(2), 79–84.

Weisbord, M., & Goodstein, L. (1978). Towards healthier medical systems: Can we learn from experiences? Introduction. *Journal of Applied Behavioral Science, 14*(3), 263–264.

Wyatt, D. (2000). Negotiation savvy: Level the playing field by understanding sex differences. *Dimensions of Critical Care Nursing, 19*(1), 43–45.

Zwarenstein, M., Bryant, W., Bailie, R., & Sidthorpe, B. (1997). Interventions to promote collaboration between nurses and doctors. *The Cochrane Library,* 2.

ADDITIONAL READINGS

American Association of Colleges of Nursing. (1995). *Interdisciplinary education and practice. Position statement.* Washington, DC: Author.

American Hospital Association. (2002). *In our hands: How hospital leaders can build a thriving workforce.* Chicago: Author.

American Nurses Association. (1998). *Standards of clinical nursing practice.* Washington, DC: American Nurses Publishing.

Baker, C., et al. (2000). Transforming negative work cultures. *Journal of Nursing Administration, 30*(7/8), 357–363.

Cox, K. (2001). The effects of unit morale and interpersonal relations on conflict in the nursing unit. *Journal of Advanced Nursing, 35*(1), 17–25.

DeMarco, R., & Roberts, S. (2003). Negative behaviors in nursing. *American Journal of Nursing, 103*(3), 113, 115–116.

Edwards, J., & Lenz, C. (1990). The influence of gender on communication for nurse leaders. *Nursing Administrative Quarterly, 15*(1), 49–55.

Knox, S., & Irving, J. (1997). An interactive quality of work life model applied to organizational transition. *Journal of Nursing Administration, 27*(1), 39–47.

Lake, M., Keeling, P., Weber, G., & Olade, R. (1999). Collaborative care: A professional practice model. *Journal of Nursing Administration, 29*(9), 51–56.

Lee, L. (2000, October). Buzzwords with a basis. Motivation, mentoring, and empowerment aren't just management jargon—they're resources you use every day. *Nursing Management, 31*(10), 25–27.

Malloch, K., Sluyter, D., & Moore, N. (2000). Relationship-centered care. Achieving true value in healthcare. *Journal of Nursing Administration, 30*(7/8), 379–385.

Mason, D. (2002). MD-RN: A tired old dance. *American Journal of Nursing, 102*(6), 7.

Parker, M., & Gadbois, S. (2000). The fragmentation of community: Part 1, the loss of belonging and commitment at work. *Journal of Nursing Administration, 30*(7/8), 386–390.

Rosenstein, A. (2002). Nurse-physician relationships: Impact on nurse satisfaction and retention. *American Journal of Nursing, 102*(6), 26–34.

Tracy, M., & Ceronsky, C. (2001). Creating a collaborative environment to care for complex patients and families. *AACN Clinical Issues, 12*(3), 383–400.

Woods, D. (2002). Realizing your marketing influence, Part 1: Meeting patients' needs through collaboration. *Journal of Nursing Administration, 32*(4), 189–195.

CHAPTER 4

Effective Staff Communication and Working Relationships

CHAPTER OUTLINE

What's Ahead
Objectives
Test Your Understanding
Communication: What Is It?
  Communication systems and lines of
    communication
  The communication process
  Communication component systems:
    Verbal, nonverbal, and
    metacommunication
  Assessment of communication
    effectiveness
Think Critically
Your Opinion Counts
Think Critically
Benchmarks

Communication Methods
  Written communication
  Face-to-face communication
  Storytelling
  Information technology and
    communication
  Resolving communication problems and
    improving communication
Current Issues
Current Issues
Think Critically
Benchmarks
Chapter Wrap-Up
Summary and Applications
References
Additional Readings

MediaLink
www.prenhall.com/finkelman

The Interactive Exercises for this chapter can be found in the OneKey course at www.prenhall.com/finkelman. Click on Chapter 4 to select from the following activities: Test Your Understanding, Benchmarks, Current Issues, Your Opinion Counts, Think Critically, and Summary and Applications.

What's Ahead

Communication is part of everything that is done within the health care system. It can appear as staff-to-staff communication and patient-to-staff communication. Communication includes verbal, nonverbal, written, and electronic communication. The major goal of staff communication is the effective exchange of information that assists staff in meeting outcomes. The survival of each organization is dependent upon the transfer of information and actions taken based on information or communication; therefore, this process serves to integrate the organization's activities. Critical to effective communication is respect for another's values, feelings, opinions, and trust. Typically, when groups or teams work together one of the first signs that productivity

98

is down will be an increase in communication problems. Decreasing communication has a direct negative effect on decision making, collaboration, coordination, and prevention of conflict. Communication is expensive as it consumes staff time and affects the organization and patient outcomes. When outcomes are not met, this affects costs. New information technology, such as computer hardware, software, information specialists, maintenance, repair and upgrade of hardware and software, and staff training in use of information technology, is very costly. This chapter discusses many of these issues concerning communication, and how communication affects the work environment and outcomes.

OBJECTIVES

Before you begin, take a moment to familiarize yourself with the key objectives of this chapter.

- Describe the critical elements of communication.
- Distinguish between the four lines of communication.
- Describe the communication process.
- Identify several examples for each of the communication component systems.
- Describe what might be included in an assessment of a work group's communication.
- Identify three barriers to communication and how to resolve them.
- Describe four communication methods, including the most effective use of the method.
- Identify two strategies for resolving communication problems.
- Assess your own communication style.

TEST YOUR UNDERSTANDING

Before we begin our exploration of this chapter, take a short "warm-up" test to see what you know about this topic.

Communication: What Is It?

Communication, a key to successful teamwork, is a complex process that should never be ignored. Nurses need this skill daily in their work as they communicate with patients, families, co-workers, physicians and other health care providers, administrators and managers, support staff, case managers, utilization management staff, community agencies, and so on. Although communication cannot be avoided, nurses can provide inadequate or ineffective communication. Communication is a two-way process that is used to convey a message or an idea between two or more people. "The way in which people connect with each other, through conversation, discussion, and even body language, has a significant effect on the nature of the work relationships" (Comack, Paech, & Porter-O'Grady, 1999, p. 61). This process is used to share thoughts, attitudes, information, and feelings. Effective care, which should be the goal, requires a focused exchange of ideas, feelings, and attitudes. Communication is best described as a complementary process with sender and receiver roles and, as such, is a process that happens between people and within people. Organizations must exert considerable effort in ensuring that effective communication occurs within the organization, with other external organizations, and with people who are important to the organization. Key issues are: (a) who says what, (b) to whom, (c) in what way, and (d) with what effect.

Nurses need to understand the **communication process** and use it to benefit patient care and the work that needs to be done to reach identified outcomes. As staff communicate, they become involved in discussions and in dialogue. "Discussion is characterized by a sustained emphasis on winning or having one's views accepted by the group. Dialogue is a process in which all individuals gain insights that could not be achieved individually. Complex issues are explored from many points of view through the practice of concrete skills: advocacy, inquiry, listening, and silence. People participate in developing a pool of common meaning by suspending assumptions and exploring experience and thought, a process that enables individuals to move beyond their original viewpoint" (Comack, Paech, & Porter-O'Grady, 1999, p. 61). Effective communication broadens an individual's and a group's view of issues and how best to work with one another. The result should be better outcomes for patients and the organization.

Four fundamentals of communication theory are helpful in expanding our understanding of the definition of communication and the process of communication.

1. **Communication is perception.** Who is doing the perceiving in the communication process? The receiver uses perception to receive the message. The sender only sends the message. Due to this factor, effective communication requires that the receiver must be capable of perceiving. Perception is experience, not logic.

2. **Communication is expectation.** Typically, people perceive what they expect to perceive. The unexpected may be ignored, not heard or seen, or misunderstood. It is this frame of expectations that makes change difficult. Communication, too, confronts expectations. The sender may not, and often does not, know the receiver's expectations. To be effective the sender should try to understand the receiver's expectations as much as possible.

3. **Communication makes demands.** It demands that the receiver think about something, do something, believe something, and so on.

4. **Communication and information are different and indeed largely opposite—yet interdependent.** What is information? "Where communication is perception, information is logic. As such, information is purely formal and has no meaning. It is impersonal rather than interpersonal. The more it can be freed of the human component, that is, of such things as emotions and values, expectations and perceptions, the more valid and reliable does it become. Indeed it becomes increasingly informative" (Drucker, 1974, p. 487). How are effective communication and information different? Effective information is always specific, but too much information is seen as overload or less effective. Information presupposes communication as the information comes through the communication. Information needs to be encoded or understood by the receiver. However, communication "may not be dependent on information. Indeed, the most perfect communications may be purely 'shared experiences' without any logic whatever. Perception has primacy rather than information" (Drucker, 1974, p. 489).

Communication systems and lines of communication

Typically, communication is thought of as taking place in a straight line, from the sender to receiver; however, in most situations communication is much more complex. Its direction can be downward, upward, lateral, or diagonal. "Downward communications go from superior to subordinate, and consist of messages regarding things like corporate vision, what a job entails, procedures and practices to be followed, and performance appraisals. Lateral, or horizontal, communications go between departments or between people in the same department. Upward communication (from subordinates to superiors) provides management with insights into the company and its employees and competitors" (Dessler, 2002, p. 260). What do these descriptors really mean to nurses?

Downward communication

Communication is downward when a team leader tells a team member that a specific task must be done. Lines of communication typically relate to the organizational structure. The organizational chart provides the best illustration of these lines of communication. Those at the top levels communicate to those below that level and so on. **Downward communication** is the most typical and is found in the traditional bureaucratic organization, although it is used in many types of structures at some time or another. In line with this type of organization, this communication is directive and used primarily to coordinate activities to ensure that outcomes are reached. Examples of when downward communication might be used are: (a) the organization's policies and procedures, (b) position descriptions, (c) any employee rules and regulations, (d) written communication from administration, and (e) other forms of organizational communication that come from above. Performance evaluations traditionally have been primarily downward; however, this type of performance evaluation is less effective, as will be discussed in Chapter 12. Many organizations now require that staff participate in their own performance evaluation, thereby changing this communication line.

Organizations' changing organizational structures and leadership approaches have required changes in their communication. Consider what was discussed about Transformational Leadership in Chapter 1. Dictates from above or downward communication are not a communication approach that supports this type of leadership. As a consequence of leadership change, downward communication is becoming less common as more staff are encouraged to participate in organizational decisions and be innovative and initiate changes, which would encourage more upward communication and other communication forms in which staff interact in a participatory environment.

Drucker (1974) felt that downward communication did not work. Why is this so? Communication really is the act of the message's receiver. Does communication really occur if there is no active receiver? Downward communication can only send commands or directions. "One cannot communicate downward anything connected with understanding, let alone motivation. This requires upward communication, from those who perceive to those who want to reach their perception" (Drucker, 1974, p. 490). Communication needs to begin with the intended receiver rather than the sender. Downward communication comes after upward communications have been successful. It is a reaction rather than an action, or response rather than an initiative.

Upward communication

Communication is upward when a staff nurse tells a nurse manager that the schedule for the month does not meet the staff nurse's needs or when staff are involved in decision making at the unit level. Examples of upward communication, which are increasing in most health care organizations, include staff meetings, staff-to-staff or staff-to-manager communication, and communication that occurs on a daily basis in the work setting. Other examples are a manager's use of an "open door" policy so that staff can feel free to come to the manager with issues or concerns, shift reports, team or project communication and their written reports, the grievance procedures, staff development evaluation feedback, exit interviews, use of a suggestion box, staff satisfaction surveys, union communication, and the grapevine. Shared governance, a form of organizational process and structure, requires that staff participate actively in organizational decision making, which is upward communication; however, if there is limited lateral and diagonal communication, this still limits active staff participation in communication and decision making. Both downward and upward communication are similar in that communication goes from one level to another, but only in a different direction from bottom to top or the reverse. Those who receive the message last may not receive the exact message that was sent. This can be a disadvantage as it is critical that the message be received as sent. This can be an advantage if the message's content has been improved with the creative process of the ideas of more than one staff member, but this still means that not all staff received the same message. The issues of perception and expectations will always be a factor in limiting consistent communication.

Lateral communication

Lateral or horizontal communication is typically used to coordinate activities. This type of communication takes place between staff who are in the same or similar hierarchical level or departmental level in that one does not have formal power over the other (for example, between a staff nurse and another staff nurse or between two nurse managers, one from the cardiac care unit and the other from a medical unit). Typically, this communication is informal and might involve sharing information about patients, committee communication, and communication among team members and workgroup project members. As organizations begin to incorporate more teamwork and emphasize the value of working in teams, this type of communication develops and becomes critical for success.

Diagonal communication

Diagonal communication, another form of communication, is informal. This communication typically occurs when staff who are from different hierarchical levels are working on projects together, but when they work on a project they are equal. This, too, is a growing form of communication because more staff from different departments or units are working together. It also applies to the relationship between a nurse and a physician or a nurse and a patient. For example, if a health care organization is developing a new admission procedure, the project's team *may* include a physician, several nurse managers, several staff nurses, a patient transportation supervisor, the director of medical records, the director of information system management, a patient representative, an ombudsman or patient advocate, an admission department representative, an administrator, and the chief financial officer. This team has representatives from different departments, units within departments, management, administration, and an insurer representative; different hierarchical levels; consumers; and external representatives. The goal of diagonal communication is to improve communication so that all can work together to meet the team's goal.

Four basic principles of communication

There are four basic principles of communication theory that are important to remember as communication is discussed.

1. One cannot avoid communication. It is impossible not to communicate as there is a message in everything that is done. Communication, however, can be effective or ineffective. A critical element of communication is that once a message is sent it cannot be taken back. Everyone has experienced regret at times once the words are out. E-mail provides a common example: The send button is clicked, and once the message flies through the Internet Highway, the sender experiences regret in sending the message. This is why thinking before communicating is so important.
2. Every communication has a content and a relationship aspect, which is called **metacommunication**. The content is the message itself, and this is what most people think is the communication. There is much more to it, though. The relationship between the sender and receiver cannot be ignored as it has an effect on how the message is both sent and received. This relationship actually becomes a message in itself due to the impact it has on the message and the communication process. Consider the example of two nurses who frequently disagree. If one of the nurses tells the other what needs to be done at the end of a shift, how might past experiences in their relationship affect the communication? The content ("You need to check all IVs immediately.") is clear, but if one of the nurses feels that the other is always dictatorial and also panics easily, the nurse may not respond as quickly to the content of the message to check the IVs.
3. A series of communications can be viewed as an uninterrupted series of interchanges. Messages are not sent or received in a vacuum. All have a history behind them, and a future ahead, which can affect accuracy in reception.
4. All communication relationships are either symmetrical or complementary, depending on whether they are based on equality or inequality. A **symmetrical relationship** is one in which both persons are of equal status and position and neither is considered to be superior to the other. A **complementary relationship** is a relationship that is affected by the power and status of each person (for example, nurse-physician relationships). Understanding symmetrical and complementary relationships becomes very important as nurses take new positions (Power, 1999; Watzlawick, Beavin, & Jackson, 1967).

Figure 4-1 highlights these principles.

There is also increasing evidence suggesting that clinical errors are often related to ineffective communication patterns between members of the health care team. The Institute of

FIGURE 4-1   Basic principles of communication.

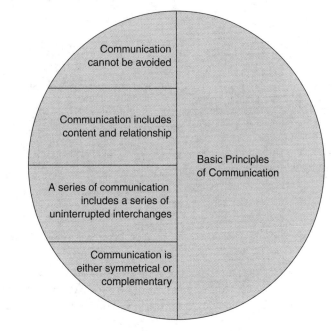

Source: Author.

Medicine report, *To Err Is Human,* discusses the problem of increasing errors in health care (Institute of Medicine, 1999). (See Chapter 17.) The report defines an error as "the failure of a planned action to be completed as intended or the use of a wrong plan to achieve an aim" (Institute of Medicine, 1999, p. 3). Considering this definition, it is difficult to exclude communication as a major factor in errors. Ineffective communication, problems with communication flow, poor feedback, and difficulty in getting relevant patient information are all mentioned in the report.

The communication process

The transmission of information and understanding of that information in the message takes place on many different levels: individual-to-individual, in small groups, in large organizations, and between large organizations. Each level of the process requires:

1. **Encoding** or translation of the communicator's ideas into language
2. **Message** or the result of the encoding process
3. **Medium** or the carrier of the message (e.g., face-to-face, memo, medical record, group meeting, computer, policy statement); it can be an unintended message that is sent by silence or inaction
4. **Decoding** or the process the receiver goes through to receive and interpret the message
5. **Feedback**, an important component of two-way communication

Figure 4-2 describes this process.

   Why should one be concerned about this process? First, the process can be used to analyze communication. Where was communication effective or ineffective? Was there a problem when the message was developed by the communicator? For example, if a nurse is too tired to be clear when giving directions to an unlicensed assistive personnel (UAP), this then affects the message—instead of telling the UAP to take blood pressures on four patients, one patient is forgotten. Sometimes a less-effective medium is chosen; for example, a memo may be sent when it would have been better to call the person to get more immediate feedback. Taking apart a communication by using the process as a framework of analysis can help to identify where the communication process needs to be improved.

FIGURE 4-2   Communication process.

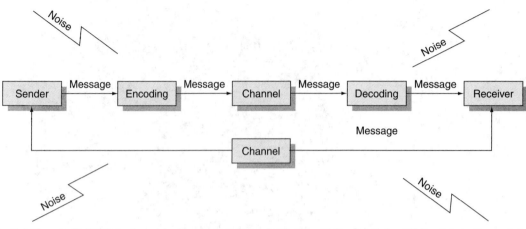

Source: Robbins, S., & Decenzo, D. (2001). *Fundamentals of management.* Upper Saddle River, NJ: Prentice Hall, p. 377. Reprinted with permission.

The communication process is affected by many factors that are external to the environment in which the communication may take place. Managed care is one of these factors as it has made communication in health care even more complex. Sometimes just trying to get approval for a patient procedure can strain a staff member's patience. There may need to be telephone calls, written documentation of needs, and in some cases, actual face-to-face contact, and the result may still be unsatisfying. Some external factors cannot be controlled. An example is state health departments that require all cases of child abuse to be reported. If there is a breakdown in this legally mandated communication, the child may suffer physically, and the health care organization may suffer severe consequences such as fines and discipline of specific health care providers. In this situation, the health care organization has no choice but to build in a communication process to ensure that this information is communicated.

The communication process is made up of five elements. It is important to recognize the use of the term *process,* which indicates that communication is a dynamic interaction. The following are the five elements.

1. The sender is the individual who initiates the message, which may be verbal and/or nonverbal. Communication may also be written. Verbal communication always includes nonverbal communication. There are many factors that affect the sender and the message (e.g., the sender's attitude toward self and toward the receiver, the situation in which the message is sent, timing, and purpose of the message). The sender uses encoding when decisions are made about what to include in the message and how to transmit the message. Then the message is sent.
2. The message includes both verbal and nonverbal information as well as the sender's attitude toward self, receiver, and the message.
3. The receiver is the person(s) to whom the message is sent. The receiver decodes the message so that it can be fully understood. This includes the actions necessary to understand the message (for example, listening, reading a memo or an e-mail message, or reviewing a chart of data).
4. The feedback is the message or response that the receiver may send back to the sender. Feedback may be verbal, nonverbal, or both. Clearly, the receiver's feelings, attitudes, experiences, relationship with the sender, the communication climate, cultural factors, and so on affect the decision to respond—the message and method chosen for the response. As discussed earlier, the receiver's perception and expectations are important. This is often referred to as "noise" or that which might interfere with communication. If response occurs, then the process turns around with the receiver becoming the sender and the original sender becoming the receiver. The receiver may also then communicate with other receivers. Two-way communication has then occurred.

5. The context is the situation or environment in which the communication takes place (for example, the nurse's station, patient's room, patient's home, the hallway, the clinic, the school nurse's office, staff meeting, or during shift report). This aspect of the process is very important and takes into consideration factors such as noise, number of people present, stress level, emergency or routine, presence of management or supervisors, privacy in the patient care area, organizational culture, morale, ethics and legal requirements, technology and information systems, and so on (Finkelman, 1996, p. 1–1:10).

Communication component systems: Verbal, nonverbal, and metacommunication

Typically, communication is identified as verbal, nonverbal, and metacommunication. These are the component systems of communication.

Verbal communication

Verbal communication is considered to be the most common type of communication. It is complex and can be described with many different characteristics, including written or oral, tone, language, volume, frequency, choice of words, rate, and accent. Verbal communication, like all other types of communication, is affected by a person's gender, age, culture, stereotypes and biases, education, and impairments such as hearing or sight loss. Individuals are highly dependent on verbal communication, and often are less aware of nonverbal communication and metacommunication.

Nonverbal communication

Nonverbal communication is frequently used in clinical situations when staff assess patients and their responses. Staff, however, are often not as aware of their own use of nonverbal communication with other staff, patients, and families. The major functions of nonverbal communication are expression of emotion; expression of interpersonal attitudes; maintenance of rituals; support of verbal communication; establishment, development, and maintenance of relationships; and self-presentation. Nonverbal communication is not something that is always in the awareness or control of the individual. To improve communication a person needs to increase awareness of the impact of nonverbal communication and increase assessment of nonverbal communication during the communication process. Nonverbal communication can consist of facial expressions, body movements or posture, gestures, volume of speech, tone of voice, gait, and physical appearance. Body language typically includes facial expression, eye movements, body movements, posture, gestures, and proxemics or distance between individuals. This assessment must not only include the nonverbal communication that the other party uses but also self-assessment of nonverbal communication. It is more difficult to be aware of how one is using nonverbal communication while one is using verbal communication. For example, when a nurse is discussing a procedure with a patient, is the nurse aware of personal facial expressions, body language, and tone of voice, or is the nurse just focused on the procedure and maybe the patient's nonverbal communication? Some nonverbal factors that are important to consider are:

- Maintain eye contact and a relaxed manner as this communicates sincerity.
- Smile if it is appropriate to the content, but do not smile constantly because this tends to make the receiver distrust the sender and the message.
- A neutral environment might be useful in circumstances in which meeting in one's office or on one's own territory might make the other person feel uncomfortable.
- If a person stands over or leans over another, it can make that person uncomfortable and feel a loss of power.
- Pulling away or appearing too casual may communicate superiority or disinterest.

Cultural issues are also important because there is great variation in nonverbal communication among different cultures and interpretation of nonverbals. Examples of questions to consider with different cultures are: (a) Do men look directly at women who are not their wives? (b) How do people greet one another? (c) Does the husband speak for the wife? Answers to these questions and many others are important to know if a nurse is trying to teach a woman and her husband is present.

Nonverbal communication frequently causes problems because it is often difficult to assess and interpret. This communication includes anything other than the spoken word. It can be deliberate or unintentional, and when it is unintentional, it is out of the control of the sender or the receiver. When there is doubt about the interpretation, the best approach is to ask for clarification about the meaning; however, this is not always easy to do. The receiver may be hesitant, feel incompetent, may be concerned that asking for information may be threatening, or may not know how or what to ask. Comparing the nonverbal with the verbal may assist in greater understanding, but this is not always the case as a person's nonverbal communication may be different from the verbal. Nurses tend to use comparison of verbal and nonverbal communication more during their communication with patients than with co-workers. Nonverbal communication, however, is very important in work-related communication and should not be ignored.

Metacommunication

"Metacommunication is a broad term used to describe all of the factors that influence how the message is perceived" (Boggs, 1999, p. 196). It includes the verbal communication and all of its factors, which include culture, native language, gender, vocal pitch, and so on, as well as the nonverbal communication and all of its factors, which include body language, culture, gender, appearance, and so on. Interpretation of meaning through verbal and nonverbal clues is very important when understanding metacommunication. It is at this time that the focus is on the whole rather than on the parts of the communication.

Assessment of communication effectiveness

Communicators want to have productive communication when the sender sends a message. The goal is that the message will be received and understood as sent. Productive communication can lead to many positive benefits for individual staff, teams, structural units within the organization, the organization, the community, and for the patient and family. Some of these benefits are:

- A group spirit with a common understanding and staff working toward common goals
- Participative management providing the staff with the opportunity to express different points of view and develop the best approach to problems
- Quick resolution of misunderstandings
- A comfortable environment that supports a motivational climate
- More creative thinking by nursing management and nursing staff
- Less staff turnover
- Less evidence of a rumor mill
- Clarification of responsibilities (Finkelman, 1996, pp. 1–1:13–14)

Team leaders, charge nurses, and nurse managers need to periodically evaluate the effectiveness of the communication—their own communication, individual staff members, and group communication, which could be a team, unit, department, or entire organization.

- What might be some indicators of staff communication problems?
- Do staff feel comfortable expressing their feelings and opinions?
- Are some staff trying to get on the good side of the nurse manager or leader?
- During meetings or in shift report, do staff ask questions?
- Do staff contribute their ideas to the discussion when there are problems? Silence may be positive as it can be used for thinking before responding; however, if staff are silent for long periods without contributing to the discussion, this can be an indicator of a communication problem.
- What about when messages do not seem to be understood or are misinterpreted?

These questions represent some of the many aspects that need to be considered when communication is evaluated.

THINK CRITICALLY

Try this exercise to apply what you have learned about this topic.

Staff-staff communication provides the critical framework in which care occurs. Imagine how a nurse might provide care without using communication. The care would have to occur on an isolated island, and even in that situation, the nurse would still have to communicate with the patient. Problems, however, do occur even in the best communication situations. The following are some examples.

■ Discussing patients and their care is part of staff responsibilities. This takes time and needs to be considered a critical aspect of each staff member's role. This is not to say that too much time can be spent talking about care rather than providing care. Undoubtedly, every nurse encounters staff members who seem to talk too much, neglect work, interrupt others' work, and cause tension. This may mean that the team leader or nurse manager will need to talk to the staff member and determine the reason for this type of communication problem, discuss how it interferes with the work and care of patients, and arrive at strategies to improve the staff member's communication and reduce the interruptions. Other staff may even discuss it with the staff member; however, this should be offered as positive criticism and in private.

■ Competition among staff can interfere with productive communication. It can lead to withholding of information, distortion of information, and poor morale. Why would staff be competitive? They might be seeking recognition for work, better assignments, better work schedules, or feel that some staff members are treated differently. Clearly, this indicates that there are major problems in the work environment that need to be addressed so that communication can improve.

■ Confidentiality is an ever present need in all clinical setting interactions. This has been reinforced by the new law related to privacy and confidentiality (see Chapter 10). Discussing staff and patient issues where others who should not hear about them might hear the conversation is very easy to do. Staff get involved and forget; however, the problems that can occur from this can be very serious. Staff are busy and so they "reach out" to other staff for these discussions when they can (for example, in the hallway, elevator, cafeteria, etc.). These are not private areas. Even the nursing station must be considered an open area unless it is enclosed. Telephone conversations can also be easily overheard. Many health care organizations now give staff cellular telephones to use in the clinical setting. These telephones are frequently used where conversations may be overheard. Nurses who work in the community must be particularly aware of this as they frequently use cellular telephones where the public can overhear confidential information or misinterpret what might be said by a health care professional (for example, taking calls while taking a lunch break in a public restaurant or telephoning a patient while in another patient's home making a home visit).

■ There needs to be greater consideration of staff feelings in the workplace. With heavy workloads it is easy to forget about the feelings of co-workers. Dashing around, communicating in short sentences, and moving on creates an environment in which staff forget to connect and to listen. A critical element of positive communication is the comfort level. Do staff feel comfortable saying "I need help?" "I am overwhelmed?" Or do staff feel that this will be seen only in a negative light? Staff communication may be sharp and caustic, leading to hurt feelings or anger, setting up barriers to future effective communication.

■ Medical records and documentation are very important parts of communication in the health care delivery system. This form of communication must be clear and provide critical information that is required. Requirements come from the nursing profession, state boards of nursing, standards, state and federal laws and regulations, managed care organizations/insurers, legal cases, and the organization's policies, procedures, and quality improvement program. Assessment of this type of communication must include these regulations. It is particularly important today to follow managed care or insurer requirements, particularly when describing patient problems, plan of care, and outcomes. This information affects decisions that are made and changes that are instituted, directs care evaluation, communicates responsibilities, identifies outcomes that should be met and (if they are met) determines reimbursement, and guides staff. The common response to medical malpractice issues, "If it is not documented, it did not happen," says much about the importance of this documentation. If a list was made of health care communication concerns, documentation would be a top priority.

YOUR OPINION COUNTS

Find out what others think about this topic. Post your response and check out other opinions.

- When a staff member does not understand something or what is to be done, it is important to ask to have the information or instruction repeated or explained. If it is something that makes the staff member feel uncomfortable, these feelings should be discussed. This is very important in delegation, as is discussed in Chapter 8.
- Mutual trust is something that is not easy to accomplish or assess today. Poor or inconsistent communication, inadequate staff input during the change process, and fears such as job loss or change can damage trust. This trust is a critical component of communication. Developing strategies to build mutual trust is important. Effective timing is something that should be considered for an important communication and assessment of the communication process. Box 4-1 identifies some techniques to promote trust.

BOX 4-1   Techniques designed to promote trust.

- Convey respect
- Consider the person's uniqueness
- Show warmth and caring
- Use active listening
- Give sufficient time to answer questions
- Maintain confidentiality
- Show congruence between verbal and nonverbal behaviors
- Use a warm friendly voice
- Use appropriate eye contact
- Smile appropriately
- Be flexible
- Be honest and open
- Give complete information
- Provide consistency
- Plan schedules
- Control distractions
- Set limits
- Follow through on commitments
- Use an attending posture: arms, legs, and body relaxed, leaning slightly forward
- Confirm responses

Source: Author.

- At times there seem to be several different "stories" or different versions of information from different staff. This causes major communication and morale problems. Getting facts from the source and discussing them openly helps to resolve this problem.

- Intuition during communication is used by many people, often unconsciously, and when it is used it may predict what will happen within the communication or within a situation. This may or may not be helpful as it may cause the sender or receiver to make the wrong assumption.

- Sometimes it is difficult to know when to use face-to-face communication and when to use the telephone or e-mail. Telephone and e-mail usually take less time, but if it is important to have a face-to-face conversation, then time needs to be taken for this. Telephone and e-mail offer more control: The sender selects the time when it is done; the time it takes is usually shorter; it is easier to take notes while in the middle of the communication; and e-mail provides more time to think about what will be said. Although physical nonverbal communication cannot be observed with these methods, tone and use of words communicated in an e-mail can communicate some aspects of nonverbal communication.

- Staff should not be left hanging. Feedback and follow-up are necessary for the development and maintenance of trust and to encourage two-way communication. It takes time to provide feedback, but it is time well spent.

- Interdepartmental/unit communication helps the nurse manager and staff see problems from the other department/unit's point-of-view. Without this communication, it is easy to be isolated and only see one viewpoint.

- There are times when communication in the nursing station, desk area, or the work area (such as in a clinic) is impossible or undesirable. If it is very busy, the message may be lost amid the confusion. If a sensitive topic is to be discussed, this location is too public. Never assume that this area is private.

- Selecting the appropriate time to discuss a sensitive issue or even to communicate daily work-related information can make a critical difference. If a staff member is busy with patient care or documentation, this is not the best time. There are times, such as immediately after a critical clinical incident, that staff are not able to discuss fully what has occurred due to emotions or fatigue. Often the first response is to discuss the situation; however, the best approach is to identify another time within a reasonable time frame to discuss the incident. Putting off a discussion is not always negative if it is done thoughtfully and follow-up action is actually taken (Finkelman, 1996, p. 1–1:14–15).

Barriers to communication

"Interpersonal communication occurs between two people; organizational communication is the exchange of information and transmission of meaning among several individuals or groups throughout the organization" (Dessler, 2002, p. 260). Communication, however, is not always successful. There are many barriers to communication that an organization, its management, and staff need to be aware of that affect short-term and long-term activities. The following list is far from complete, but it provides many critical examples of these barriers.

- **Failing to listen to others and not recognizing them:** This leads to negative feelings and responses. Active listening can improve this problem.

- **Using selective listening so that one hears only what one wants to hear:** This is often due to the inability to recognize the needs and problems of others. Active listening and gaining more understanding of others' expectations can also improve this problem.

- **Failing to probe or inquire further when encountering vague information, obtaining inadequate answers, reaching a confusing interpretation, or following procedures and standards so closely that the message is missed:** Using open questions will make a difference with this problem.

- **Making overly judgmental statements:** This often occurs when the receiver decides what is the overall value of the message (e.g., a staff member who always complains may not be heard when there is legitimate need for complaint). Active listening, trying to understand other viewpoints, and stopping before responding may decrease this barrier.

■ Expressing opinions while intentionally or unintentionally intimidating others: Asking for feedback can be helpful so that steps can be taken to improve. Being direct rather than aggressive avoids setting up barriers.

■ Overusing reassuring statements and rejecting statements: These types of statements cut off communication. More open communication that respects the other person can limit this barrier.

■ Using a defensive stance stops open communication: The communicator needs to be more open and recognize that there is more than one point-of-view.

■ Making a false inference: This often occurs when someone jumps to a conclusion without enough information. Getting more information before responding or communicating can limit this barrier.

■ Using personal criticism, profanity, and crudity: These act only as barriers to effective communication and also are very destructive to the communication climate. Respecting others is critical in communication and can help to limit this barrier.

■ Responding to spatial issues: Space can be a barrier—too close and people feel uncomfortable, particularly if a person crosses too far into the safe zone or people feel distant. Important spatial factors that can make a difference are: (a) How close are the receiver and sender? (b) Has one of them crossed into personal space that makes the other person uncomfortable? (c) What are the cultural issues related to space? (d) What is the space between the staff and the patient? (e) In a group meeting how are people sitting: at a table, in a circle, and so on? (f) What is the distance between them? and (g) Is it easy to have eye contact?

■ Keeping secrets: Secrecy is very destructive to communication and to organizations. It decreases staff trust, and this leads to ineffective communication. Communicating fully and openly will increase effective communication, and keeps the channels of communication open. "Open communication will increase confidence and trust in the staff, which can lead to increased risk-taking behavior and creativity" (Flarey & Smith, 1999, p. 142). It is not easy to develop and maintain a culture in which open communication is valued. Chapter 1 emphasizes the importance of this type of communication in leadership theories such as Emotional Intelligence and Clear Leadership. "Sometimes the very idea of open communication seems too utopian. Some people don't know what information to share, who would be interested in it, or how to communicate so others will pay attention to their message. Others don't want to get involved in the politics of communication. Still others hold onto what's always been done because it takes less time and is predictable" (Gebelein et al., 2000, p. 502).

In an open communication environment staff know that their ideas are respected and should be shared. Management will openly discuss communication and the need for greater communication with staff. Communication is considered when organizational goals are evaluated—assessment of the organization's communication is integrated into the process. Managers and leaders advocate that each staff member has a responsibility to contribute ideas and opinions, and they ask staff to contribute. Communication is part of performance evaluation for each staff member throughout the organization. In this open environment managers might use the following to support open communication.

■ Identifying all the methods available for soliciting and receiving input and experimenting with new ones: By understanding that different methods can be used, some of which are discussed in this chapter, staff will be more effective in selecting the best method because some may act as barriers if used inappropriately; for example, performance feedback should not be sent in an e-mail.

■ Giving staff time to respond when input is solicited: Time may be needed to develop an effective response. Cultural factors may also affect how quickly a staff member might respond.

■ Identifying and reinforcing behaviors that facilitate sharing of information: Behaviors that do not lead to sharing should not be encouraged.

■ Looking for opportunities to interact more with staff: It is easy to become isolated, and this will interfere with communication (Gebelein et al., 2000, p. 506).

Information overload

Today, in most organizations, it is very easy for staff to experience information overload. Information is coming from multiple sources at one time. It is difficult to decide what is important, and it seems that everyone feels that their needs are more important and require an immediate response. With the growth of information technology there is now an increased burden of too much communication, often with less real people contact. E-mails, faxes, the Internet, memos, letters, reports, and more are added to the pile. Medical record documentation also increases the amount of information that nurses have to cope with today. With the increase in quantity there is also increased speed—staff get information faster and then feel compelled to respond faster. This increasing speed of communication receipt has also spoiled staff to expect information quickly, and when it does not come quickly, staff experience stress.

What are the critical issues with information overload? Staff need to consider the following questions: What information is important, and what is extraneous? How quickly is a response expected, and what is a realistic response time? What is the purpose of the information? Does the information need to be saved? How should it be saved? Is this the end point of the information or should it be sent on to another? If so, to whom and why? What is the quality of the information? Who sent the information? What is the source of the information? It is very helpful when the sender indicates a time frame for response. This simple intervention can do much to decrease the stress of feeling compelled to respond quickly.

Importance of feedback: Giving and receiving feedback

Feedback is a part of all communication. To become an effective communicator nurses need to learn how to give and receive feedback. First and foremost, feedback should not be described as negative. Most staff immediately assume that feedback means "bad news." Positive feedback, what has been done well and so on, is critical. There are several types of feedback: oral, unspoken or nonverbal, substantiated, and perceptive (Milgram, Spector, & Treger, 1999).

- Oral feedback is also referred to as interactive feedback in that a person asks another or a group for clarification, and interpretation is shared.
- Unspoken or nonverbal feedback includes any form of nonverbal communication that indicates how one person is responding to the communication from another. A person might appear uninterested, taking steps out of the office, looking at his/her watch, smiling and moving forward in a move of acceptance, raising one's voice, and so on. Sometimes the unspoken feedback sends a message that is different from the verbal message and may be viewed as the most important part of the message. For example, a nurse is very upset about information that the nurse manager is giving in a meeting. The nurse says, "I agree with what you are saying." At the same time, the nurse appears anxious, taking steps toward the door, and the tone of voice is tight.
- Substantiated feedback is used to obtain accurate and specific data, and to ensure that the message is understood.
- Perceptive feedback concerns whether or not the message behind the words is understood. This gets to the "why" behind the message and "what" the sender or receiver really thinks. Empathy plays a role in the process; however, this type of feedback is difficult to discern. Feedback that is rarely used will soon send a negative message. Likely responses to this lack of interest will be decreased feedback. This may lead to decreased interaction, anger, decreased morale, and criticism, which may be given indirectly via gossip and the grapevine.

Feedback should flow in four directions in health care organizations: (a) from manager to staff, (b) from staff to managers, (c) from staff to staff, and (d) from staff to patients and families/significant others. The first type, between managers and staff, can be difficult, especially if staff feel uncomfortable and threatened in the work setting. How can organizations encourage staff to give feedback to managers so that it is not just manager to staff? Typical methods that are used to increase staff feedback are managers asking directly for feedback, allowing time in staff meetings for feedback, suggestion boxes, surveys, informal meetings such as at lunch or during break time, problem solving or project teams, an open door policy when the manager has open office hours, and walk-around management in which the manager is present on the clinical units and staff can approach the manager with comments and issues. When feedback can be given freely and received without undue stress, the work environment is a much more positive environment. In supervisory feedback the focus should: (a) be on the behavior, not on the person; (b) provide observations, not inferences; (c) avoid judgmental attitude and discuss specifics rather than generalizations; (d) share ideas and information rather than giving advice; and (e) consider the amount of information given at one time (Power, 1999).

How should staff respond to supervisory feedback? The most common response is to jump into a defensive response, but the better approach is to carefully consider what is shared. Listening is just as important in this type of communication as in other types. The tendency is to immediately try to explain actions or become defensive rather than to first listen. Sometimes a supervisor is only offering an alternative solution that needs to be thought about. If managers or supervisors do not offer feedback, staff need to ask for it. Staff sometimes think that supervisory feedback means that all of their co-workers think the same thing as the nurse manager. Supervisory feedback should represent the manager's opinion. If there are specific areas of concern that a nurse may have about work, the nurse should ask the nurse manager or, if appropriate, the team leader about this concern and not wait for the annual performance appraisal or for the manager to address the concern (Power, 1999).

Improving feedback communication can be done by using several techniques and considering some factors related to feedback (Milgram, Spector, & Treger, 1999).

- Definitions can make a difference in effective and ineffective communication. What do the words and phrases mean? Different people may use different definitions. Jargon and unfamiliar terms can confuse conversation requiring feedback for clarification.

- Simple and clear language is always better. It is easy to make assumptions about communication (for example, what the sender meant, what the feelings and attitudes are behind the message, or whether or not the sender really wanted to communicate).

- Feedback can be used to avoid the dangers of assumptions.

- Questions can also be used to clarify and to stimulate feedback.

- Observation plays an important role in the communication process, and nonverbal feedback is part of this process. What is the nonverbal feedback indicating? Is the message clear? Does the recipient appear involved, bored, angry, uncomfortable, and so on? Is more feedback required?

- A team leader or a nurse manager often must give team members or staff direct one-to-one feedback. This may be difficult, but the best approach is to focus on the behavior rather than making it personal. All feedback needs to be approached from a constructive perspective with a healthy positive attitude. Downgrading and making remarks that are hurtful are not effective feedback.

- Follow-up is also an important technique to improve communication. In the busy clinical setting it is easy to forget to follow-up. Nurses use various methods such as notebooks with lists to remind themselves. Even computer methods can be utilized as computers get smaller.

- Empathy is important. It means that the sender needs to be receiver oriented or have a greater understanding of the receiver, to be in the place of the receiver. This is closely related to the need for mutual trust between the sender and receiver. Those who use empathy recognize that it is important to understand another person. Questioning and active listening improve empathy. This process requires that the person focus on what is happening and avoid thinking of other things or allowing one's mind to wander.

- Sometimes the sender may find it helpful to repeat information in order to ensure that it was received as sent. Typical situations when information may need to be repeated are during delegation, orientation of new staff, training programs, and working with students (e.g., nursing, medical, and so on).

As team leaders, nurses must give feedback to team members. What is the best way to do this? If this type of communication is new to the team leader, the leader may be hesitant to give feedback, but team members nonetheless expect to receive feedback. In summary, the following guidelines about feedback can be helpful.

- Use specific examples and focus on behavior, not personal criticism.
- Provide feedback that is as immediate as possible to the situation.
- Give honest feedback in a simple and direct manner.
- If feedback is always positive, it probably means that the whole truth is not shared.
- Discuss the effects of positive and negative behavior on patient care, the unit, the clinic, the department, co-workers, nursing, the organization, and so on.
- Tell team members what is expected of them.
- Give positive and negative feedback as it is easy to forget to tell team members that they have done a great job or it was a tough day and they got through it.
- Reinforce positive behavior.
- Ask the team member for strategies to improve.
- Allow team members to give feedback to the team leader.
- Solicit feedback rather than waiting for it to come (Milgram, Spector, & Treger, 1999).

Box 4-2 provides some guidelines for giving and receiving criticism.

THINK CRITICALLY

Try this exercise to apply what you have learned about this topic.

Grapevine: Is it good or bad?

The grapevine is present in every organization, within its service areas, units, and departments. The grapevine can be positive or negative. Clearly, information can be distorted in the grapevine, individual feelings can be hurt, and information can be very difficult to control. The grapevine can affect staff morale when information that should not be communicated is shared; when communication is distorted and its meaning causes damage; or when staff feel left out. Efforts to eliminate the grapevine will undoubtedly fail as grapevines seem to be ingrained in all organizations and have a life of their own. Managers need to learn how to use the grapevine to their advantage. If the manager wants to get a message out quickly, the grapevine can be used if the leader knows how to access the grapevine. In addition, corrected information can be put into the grapevine.

> When information is not shared with employees, they perceive the existence of a gap. The presence of this gap is the basis for the creation of what is commonly referred to as the 'grapevine.' A grapevine can be extremely damaging. It can be fraught with fantasies, misconceptions, harmful rumors, and other problems. Grapevines are nothing more than a community's attempt to have some information. It is not necessary that the information be factual. Rather, it is more essential that there be some information. Even distorted, untruthful information is better than no information at all. The premise to remember is that communication is the most needed and the most effective strategy for any plan for change and transformation. (Beard, 1999, p. 109)

Given this information about the grapevine, what is the best way to decrease the damage that the grapevine can cause? The best approach is keeping staff informed. This is particularly important when there are critical issues (for example, budget, staffing, and plans for change). Staff need to also be careful with the grapevine, recognizing that factual information may not always be found in communication that is received via the grapevine.

BENCHMARKS

Now let's take a moment to test your knowledge of the concepts you have studied in this section.

BOX 4-2   Giving and receiving criticism.

Giving Constructive Criticism

When you offer criticism, use the following steps to communicate clearly and effectively:

Criticize the behavior rather than the person. In addition, make sure the behavior you intend to criticize is changeable. Chronic lateness can be changed; a physical inability to perform a task cannot.

Define specifically the behavior you want to change. Try not to drag any side issues into the conversation.

Balance criticism with positive words. Alternate critical comments with praise in other areas.

Stay calm and be brief. Avoid threats, ultimatums, or accusations. Use "I" messages; choose positive, non-threatening words, so the person knows that your intentions are positive.

Explain the effects caused by the behavior that warrants the criticism. Help the person understand why a change needs to happen, and talk about options in detail. Compare and contrast the effects of the current behavior with the effects of a potential change.

Offer help in changing the behavior. Lead by example.

Receiving Criticism

When you find yourself on the receiving end of criticism, use these coping techniques:

Listen to the criticism before you speak up. Resist the desire to defend yourself until you've heard all the details. Decide if the criticism is offered in a constructive or unconstructive manner.

Think the criticism through critically. Evaluate it carefully. While some criticism may come from a desire to help, other comments may have less honorable origins. People often criticize others out of jealousy, anger, frustration, or displaced feelings. In cases like those, it is best (though not always easy) to let the criticism wash right over you.

If it is unconstructive, you may not want to respond at that moment. Unconstructive criticism can inspire anger that might be destructive to express. Wait until you cool down and think about the criticism to see if there is anything important hiding under how it was presented. Then, tell the person that you see the value of the criticism, but also communicate to him or her how the delivery of the criticism made you feel. If he or she is willing to talk in a more constructive manner, continue with the following steps below. If not, your best bet may be to consider the case closed and move on.

If it is constructive, ask for suggestions of how to change the criticized behavior. You could ask, "How would you handle this if you were in my place?"

Before the conversation ends, summarize the criticism and your response to it. Repeat it back to the person who offered it. Make sure both of you understand the situation in the same way.

If you feel that the criticism is valid, plan a specific strategy for correcting the behavior.
Think over what you might learn from changing behavior. If you don't agree with the criticism even after the whole conversation, explain your behavior from your point-of-view.

Source: Katz, J. (2001). *Keys to nursing success* (pp. 272–273). Upper Saddle River, NJ: Prentice Hall. Reprinted with permission.

Communication Methods

Four communication methods will be described that are used by staff and management: written communication, face-to-face communication, storytelling, and information technology and communication. With each of these methods, timing needs to be considered. What is the best time to use a particular communication method? Sometimes it is better to talk to someone face-to-face while at other times an e-mail will be just as effective. The time it takes to complete the communication is another concern. How quickly does the communication need to occur? Today, with the technology that is available communication can be delivered quickly. This may or may not be a positive outcome. What is the best time to initiate communication? The situation, the sender, the receiver, stress, energy level, and support that might be needed are some of the factors to consider. "Many opportunities for successful communication have been lost because of timing" (Sullivan, 2004, p. 57). Each of the following communication methods are important for nurses in their daily practice.

Written communication

With so many communication options available today it is often difficult to know when to use each method. Written communication is most effective when the message needs to be documented, the message is complex, the message needs to be given to several people, and it is difficult or inconvenient to communicate face-to-face (Milgram, Spector, & Treger, 1999). It is particularly important to use this method when a record needs to be kept (e.g., document an important one-to-one meeting; minutes of a team, staff, or project meeting; disciplinary meeting; performance evaluation; reimbursements; and so on). It is important to remember that longer messages do not necessarily include more useful information. Time is important so messages need to get to the point and include required information.

When writing a message, the sender needs to consider what type of reaction is wanted from the message's receiver (Milgram, Spector, & Treger, 1999). There are two types of messages, direct and indirect. The latter is typically used when the sender expects the receiver to have a negative response to the message. This is the message that begins with general comments, and the bad news is buried near the end. An example might be the letter that comes after a job interview with an introduction describing the wonderful candidates who applied and how difficult the decision was to make, and is followed by the section that says someone else got the job. A direct message gets right to the point, and this type is used when the receiver is expected to respond positively to the information. This does not mean, however, that bad news should not be communicated with a more direct style. Often the sender's comfort level determines the method. Breaking bad news gently seems to make it less bad or less difficult for the sender. Written communication needs to be reviewed and edited before sending. A timely response is always appreciated. This communication method, as is true of all communication, needs to be adapted for the audience. Graphics and other visuals may be appropriate and added to written communication, but they should augment the message, not detract from it.

Written communication can be sent in several ways: hard copy via interdepartmental mail, e-mail, fax, U.S. postal service, non-U.S. postal service delivery companies, or hand delivered by the sender. The form that this type of communication takes can also vary: an informal note, memorandum (memo), formal letter, minutes, policy or procedure, surveys, data collecting tools, or performance evaluation. Most organizations have specific forms or formats that need to be used for memos, minutes, policies, procedures, and performance evaluation. Memos need to follow the organization's format with a clear identification of the subject or topic. Careful consideration needs to be given as to who should receive the memo. Content should be concise and relevant. A memo is not a lengthy report, but rather short and to the point. Clearly, all patient care documentation is a critical component of written communication.

Face-to-face communication

Face-to-face communication is the most frequently used communication method. There are times when it is the preferred method, particularly when personal sensitive information needs to be discussed. When a dialogue is needed with greater give and take, in-person communication is better. If in-person communication cannot be done and is needed, then the next choice is the telephone or, when possible, synchronous online conversation. Some health care organizations, especially large health care networks, have equipment for videoconferencing, which is discussed later in this chapter. This is another alternative to in-person communication. Box 4-3 shows examples of communication techniques.

Active listening, a technique that is critical for effective communication, means listening for the message's full meaning and ensuring that judgment of interpretations does not interfere

BOX 4-3   Communication techniques.

> Listening
>
> Silence
>
> Establish guidelines
>
> Giving broad openings
>
> Reducing distance
>
> Questions: closed, open, circular
>
> Acknowledgment
>
> Touch
>
> Restating
>
> Clarification
>
> Consensual validation
>
> Focusing
>
> Summarizing and planning
>
> Paraphrasing
>
> Reflection
>
> Source: Author.

with the understanding of the message. This takes concentration and involvement on the part of the listener. Listening also means that the person is willing to listen even when it means that what is heard may be negative or unpleasant. Seeking out information sometimes means taking risks. It is not uncommon for staff to tell nurse managers what they think the nurse manager wants to hear rather than providing a full disclosure. This does not demonstrate a staff who feel empowered, and it is not productive communication. Staff want to feel that managers and other staff are communicating *with* them, not *to* them, and the presence of listening increases the chance that communication will be a joint endeavor. Barriers to effective listening include: (a) preconceived beliefs, which are more prevalent when the communicators have known each other and assumptions are made without really listening; (b) lack of self-confidence, which interferes with any communication as the person is concerned about how he or she might appear, and so on; (c) decreasing energy limits listening which requires energy; (d) defensiveness; (e) and habit, which leads a person to think ahead, thereby interfering with listening to the now (Sullivan, 2004).

Questioning can help to resolve some communication problems to get more information and open up the communication. An open-ended question is a question that requires a more extensive answer that a simple "yes," "no," or "I agree." Why is this type of question more effective in most cases than the closed question? Mainly because it expands and facilitates the dialogue between the sender and the receiver, allowing for greater exchange of information.

Storytelling

Storytelling is a useful communication technique that can be used to clarify a confusing message, inspire others, and make communication more interesting. As Denning (2001) describes storytelling, he emphasizes that it is a way to get inside the minds of an organization's individuals and affect "how they think, worry, wonder, agonize, and dream about themselves and in the process create—and re-create—their organization" (p. xiv). Storytelling can be used in many situations, but it is particularly effective during times of change when innovation is needed. It supplements analytical thinking in organizations. Springboard stories are used to enable staff to move to the next level of understanding. As Denning notes, not all stories result in this type of effect. Typically, stories that have the perspective of a single protagonist who was in a predicament that was prototypical of the organization are the most successful. It needs to be familiar to the staff for it to be effective, and yet it must get their attention. When stories are told, they need to be brief and get to the point. Storytelling can be difficult, particularly if the audience is skeptical, but even under normal circumstances the story-teller, just like any sender of a message, must consider the situation, the receiver, and the nature of the message.

> Communicating a complex message to an audience with strong views of its own can be likened to row-ing a boat across a fast-moving river. If we aim the boat precisely toward the point to which we want to arrive, on the opposite shore, we can be sure that we will not arrive where we want to go, and instead, we will arrive somewhat further down river. If we want to arrive at a certain point, we need to ascertain in which direction the river is flowing and how fast, and then point the boat somewhat upstream, so that combination of our initial aim and the impact of the flow of the river will take us to our destina-tion. We might make many course corrections while making the crossing so that our estimates of the interaction between the speed of our rowing and the speed of the river can be calibrated in real time. If we are focusing solely on the message we are trying to send, we will see the speed and force of the in-tervening river—the inputs from the listeners—as regrettable interference or distortion, something un-fortunate that has to be minimized or eliminated, if at all possible . . . if we take advantage of a story, and its accompanying springboard effect, the inputs from the listeners enter the picture as energy-generating enhancements that help to get us to our intended destination (Denning, 2001, p. 83).

Denning's description highlights how important it is to understand the purpose of communi-cation, choose the right method and time while considering contextual factors, and above all adapt when cues are picked up indicating that the communication is not effective.

Storytelling is associated with Knowledge Management theory. With staff who are learning on the job; identification of knowledge gaps; staff research and analysis; and staff searching for knowledge from outside sources, there is a greater need for Knowledge Management, and then knowledge must be applied in the clinical setting. Storytelling can be used in the first phase of the creation of "cutting edge" knowledge, in the Knowledge Management system, and in the ap-plication of knowledge, which are all critical in today's health care environment.

Information technology and communication

"An information system (IS) consists of an organized combination of people, computer hardware, software, communications networks, and data resources that collect, transform, and spread infor-mation throughout an organization. Users of IT are the end users, the people who use the infor-mation, and the information system specialists, who are the staff who work with the IS and the technology behind it" (Milgram, Spector, & Treger, 1999, p. 72). With the increased development of communication technology, there has also been an increase in problems that are encountered with this type of communication (for example, hackers and viruses). The information highway grows, and those who want to interfere with communication and productivity increase. Hackers who interfere with computer transmission and can break into secure information are of major con-cern for health care providers due to the need of maintaining records and patient information con-fidentiality. In addition, viruses can also destroy software and crucial databases of patient and organization information. Health care providers, like all who use or interact with computers, have experienced times when the "system was down" or inaccessible. This is a major problem in health care organizations when clinical staff need this information and access to interactive communica-tion to provide care. Back-up plans are clearly critical for every health care organization. Staff need to be informed about these plans and when they should be used. (See Chapter 15 for more infor-mation on technology.)

Telephone

The telephone is certainly the most basic of the technology options available today, and yet it con-tinues to be a very important one. Use of cellular telephones, however, is relatively new and has been increasing. There are some simple reminders to improve the telephone communication method.

- Answer the phone with your name and title.
- When taking a message, repeat the information for the caller. Leave the message where the person addressed in the message will get it.
- With the increasing use of voice message systems, be prepared to leave a message.

- Keep emotions under control. Some callers may not be doing this and may say things that increase emotions. Stick to the point and get the information you need. If you do not have the answer, tell the caller you will return the call by a certain date/time or ask someone else to call.
- When you conclude a conversation that requires action, summarize the key issues and actions to be taken.
- Health care staff frequently receive calls that must be transferred. Check the number you are transferring to and tell the caller this number. The caller will then not have to call the wrong number again if the call fails to connect (Milgram, Spector, & Treger, 1999).

Voice mail has become so much a part of the workplace that it is easy to get frustrated when someone does not have voice mail or it is not working. This method can be used to send routine information and information that does not require a response. It can be used at any time and, in fact, is a method that is often used when the sender does not really want to talk to the receiver but rather just wants to get the message sent. When a message is left, clearly identify who is calling; from what location or organization, if relevant; date/time; purpose of call; and, if response is required, provide suggested times and method for a return communication. Callers need to speak slowly, repeating numbers and e-mail addresses. Some thought needs to be given to the message's content so that the caller does not appear confused and the message remains clear. Long messages should be avoided. If possible, identify good times to return the call. Confidentiality is important, so it is important to consider the message that is left and the nature of the message, which may be heard by others.

E-mail

Some organizations have e-mail policies and procedures, and these policies need to be communicated to staff when they receive their e-mail addresses. E-mail etiquette has been developing over the years. It is easy to forget in the world of rapid fire messaging that there are important legal and confidentiality issues that need to be considered. Use of patient names and other significant personal information or identifiers should not be used (see Chapter 10). Care needs to be taken when sending copyrighted material. As this requires permission, policies and procedures should be followed. Security within the organization's e-mail system is an important concern. Using passwords, not sharing passwords, and remembering that even when messages are deleted they may stay on the server and thus are accessible are factors that need to be reviewed with all staff. Organizations have policies about who may access sensitive information, and these policies must be followed. Some organizations have policies about using the organization's e-mail system for personal messages. Thought needs to be taken when writing messages, remembering that once they are sent they cannot be retrieved. E-mail is a good method for sending routine messages. The following are some e-mail etiquette guidelines.

- Remember that e-mail may not be read quickly so when the message is urgent a telephone call may be a better method. At a minimum, indicate the message is "urgent" or "priority."
- E-mail should be used thoughtfully. Sending too many messages that are unimportant may mean that important messages are ignored.
- Usually, this method should not be used for formal responses. It has become more acceptable to attach formal letters or resumes to an e-mail, but the sender should first inquire if this is acceptable.
- Acronyms and emoticons (symbols) should not be used in business e-mails.
- Break up content by using paragraphing. This makes it easier to read. Use bulleting or numbering to highlight information. Put the most important information at the beginning of the message to ensure that it is read.
- Color can also be used for emphasis, but it should be used carefully. Some colors do not show up well on the screen. When printed, the message probably will be printed in black and white. Complex graphics should be avoided as they take longer to download.

- When forwarding messages, include only relevant information from the original message to reduce the amount of reading required and length of time for receiving the message. The forwarded message should be clearly distinguished from the original message. When a message is forwarded consideration should be given as to who are the appropriate people to receive the message. The sender may not have intended for the message to be sent to others.
- When using reply, check to make sure that the reply message should go to all recipients automatically.
- There are times when a recipient may need more time to respond to a message; for example, to obtain more information. When this occurs, the recipient should acknowledge receipt of the message and indicate when a more detailed message will be sent.
- Not all messages sent via e-mail are received, and messages stating that there was a problem sending the message are not always sent. It is a good idea to ask the recipient to acknowledge receipt of important messages so that the sender can be sure the message was received.
- Use of virus protection is critical. Downloading messages, attachments, and information from the Internet is a good way for an entire system to get a virus, so it is important to make it a practice to check for viruses first.
- When an attachment is sent, double-check to see if the correct attachment is attached before hitting the send button. Another common problem is to say a document is attached and then forget to attach it. Extremely long attachments should be avoided unless the receiver has been consulted about the length.
- Do not use all caps, as this indicates shouting (Milgram, Spector, & Treger, 1999).

Videoconferencing

The advantage to **videoconferencing** is it is a live interaction with visual images while the communication takes place. It also can reduce costs and time as staff do not have to travel to another physical location. However, the initial cost of the equipment must be considered. Staff require some training in the use of the equipment, but it is not difficult. Videoconferencing is also used in telehealth. One example of its use is in providing medical consultations between rural health care providers and academic medical centers. More common uses are for meetings and educational programs.

Web pages

Web pages are very common today; most organizations have them or are developing them. They are used by organizations to communicate to a broad audience such as staff, patients, families, health care providers, consumers, the public, and so on. They need to be designed carefully with consideration given to ease of use, accuracy, timeliness and current information, level of information that might require secure entry, ethics of advertising on the page, and graphics and audio, which often take time to open. Nursing staff should be involved in the development of web pages and consider what should be included that would be helpful to the nursing staff and the care they provide. Pages can be useful in sharing patient and family health prevention education material, contact information for questions and further information, guidance for admission preparation, links to reliable websites that can provide additional information, and support information (for example, related to cancer, diabetes, arthritis, new mothers, breastfeeding, and many other health issues). It is critical that the web page is monitored and updated. Responsibility for the monitoring needs to be clearly defined. If information is not current, this acts as a barrier to effective communication.

Resolving communication problems and improving communication

The nurse manager plays a critical role in setting the tone for communication and maintaining open communication channels so that staff can do their work and patient care outcomes can be reached. The manager must continuously assess the communication climate to ensure that it supports effective communication. Marrelli (1997) identifies the manager's role in defining values and setting goals, including the following:

- Initiating and facilitating discussion to elicit clarification of values
- Recording written value statements, seeking staff feedback, and incorporating revisions into the organizational review process
- Initiating discussion of goals at the unit and individual levels with the staff that the manager directly supervises
- Bringing pertinent directives, regulations, accreditation standards, or other factors needing consideration to the discussion
- Recording written goals and action plans for achieving them
- Maintaining momentum of progress toward goals, giving positive and constructive feedback to promote progress toward meeting deadlines
- Communicating to staff the progress toward goals through the use of visual tools (p. 81)

When staff want to improve their communication, the first step is to assess current communication skills (Gebelein et al., 2000). Asking others for feedback is helpful and requires that this information is considered carefully. Include an assessment of nonverbal communication as it can make the difference between effective and non-effective communication. Specific methods that can be used to improve communication when it occurs are increased use of paraphrasing, reflection, and summarization. When paraphrasing is used, a person restates what has been said by another and asks for confirmation of what was said. The focus is on facts, and the statement should be short. Reflection focuses on the speaker's feelings, and the receiver of the message restates what the receiver thinks are the feelings expressed. Again, this is done for confirmation. Summarization combines content and feelings, by restating both of these elements for confirmation. Additional strategies that can be used to improve staff communication include the following.

- Communicate the "why" behind the "what."
- Realize that effective communication takes time.
- Accept negative news as information and do not take it personally.
- Respond non-defensively when people express differing or contradictory ideas and views.
- Report situations as accurately as possible and avoid downplaying negative factors.
- Send important organizational messages by at least two methods (for example, e-mail and a written memo or verbally and written).
- Do not rely so much on written communication as people often do not read it.
- Use active listening in all conversations.
- Select the location for discussing sensitive issues carefully.
- Say what you mean; avoid assumptions and ensure that the receiver has less need to turn to assumptions.
- Validate to ensure that what has been said has been heard and understood.
- Stress can interfere with communication, while managing stress can improve communication.
- Use appropriate eye contact.
- State information clearly backed up with research to get to the facts.
- Think before speaking.
- If you do not have the answer, state this and that you will look for the information and follow-up.
- How something is said can be as important as what is said.
- Summarize at the end of a lengthy conversation and ask for confirmation from the other party.
- "I" statements are more effective than "you" statements, which tend to put the other person on the offensive.
- Thank others for their feedback and suggestions as this recognizes they have been heard and supports further communication.
- Credibility is critical; trust can make or break how a message is received and interpreted.
- When difficult questions must be asked or there is a difficult discussion, it is important to select the time when the other person (receiver) might be more receptive.

The critical elements of effective communication include: talking, listening, exploring, and solving. Features of each element are described.

1. Talking
   - Present your ideas, views, goals, or feelings.
   - Explain your position.
   - Sell your view and rationale.
   - Make sure you are thoroughly understood.
   - Use nonverbal behaviors that show your reactions to what others are saying (e.g., nodding your head).
   - Ask leading questions.
   - Ask questions.

2. Listening
   - Work to understand other people's ideas, views, rationales, goals, and feelings.
   - Summarize their position.
   - Show that you understand all their main points.
   - Read body language and nonverbal messages.
   - Ask questions that encourage people to say more about what is really on their minds.
   - Demonstrate curiosity about other people's views.

3. Exploring
   - Attempt to understand the nature and scope of the problem.
   - Figure out what really matters to people, including yourself.
   - Suspend your judgment until the picture is clear.
   - Search for the root cause.
   - Check underlying assumptions.
   - Try to understand the real needs of all stakeholders.
   - Clarify the requirements for a mutually acceptable solution.

4. Solving
   - Find potential answers to the problem.
   - Make decisions about what to do next.
   - Choose a course of action.
   - Propose action steps.
   - Search for a solution that addresses the needs of all stakeholders.
   - Evaluate how different recommendations meet the specified requirement (Gebelein et al., 2000, pp. 508–509).

CURRENT ISSUES

Learn about events around the globe that relate to the chapter content.

Different people have different ways or styles of communication. Box 4-4 provides information about aggressive, passive, and assertive styles of communication. Recognizing ones style will help to improve communication and to use the most effective approach to communication.

Communication is complex and requires that staff use a thoughtful process to communicate effectively. It is something that is used daily in practice and management, and often is not viewed as important until there is a problem with it. Throughout this text, communication is a driving element for effective managers who are leaders.

CURRENT ISSUES

Learn about events around the globe that relate to the chapter content.

BOX 4-4   Aggressive, passive, and assertive styles.

Aggressive
- Loud, heated, arguing
- Physically violent encounters
- Blaming, name-calling, and verbal insults
- Walking out of arguments before they are resolved
- Being demanding: "Do this"

Passive
- Concealing one's own feelings
- Denying one's own anger
- Feeling that one has no right to express anger
- Avoiding arguments
- Being noncommittal: "You don't have to do this unless you really want to . . . "

Assertive
- Expressing feelings without being nasty or overbearing
- Acknowledge emotions but staying open to discussion
- Expressing self and giving others the chance to express themselves equally
- Using "I" statements to defuse arguments
- Asking and giving reasons: "I would appreciate it if you would do this, and here's why . . . "

Source: Katz, J. (2001). *Keys to nursing success.* Upper Saddle River, NJ: Prentice Hall, p. 267. Reprinted with permission.

THINK CRITICALLY

Try this exercise to apply what you have learned about this topic.

BENCHMARKS

Now let's take a moment to test your knowledge of the concepts you have studied in this section.

Chapter Wrap-Up

Now that you've reached the end of the chapter, you may wish to explore the concepts you've been reading about in greater detail, or test yourself to see how well you've comprehended the material.

SUMMARY AND APPLICATIONS

- Summary
- Practice Quiz
- Key Terms
- Tying It All Together
- Experiential Exercises
- Case
- Links

REFERENCES

Beard, E. (1999). Leading people through organizational transformation: The human side of radical change and transformation. In S. Smith and D. Flarey (Eds.), *Process-centered health care organizations* (pp. 103–111). Gaithersburg, MD: Aspen Publishers, Inc.

Boggs, K. (1999). Communication styles. In E. Arnold & K. Boggs (Eds.), *Interpersonal relationships* (pp. 195–239). Philadelphia: W. B. Saunders Company.

Comack, M., Paech, G., & Porter-O'Grady, T. (1999). From structure to culture: A journey of transformation. In S. Smith and D. Flarey (Eds.), *Process-centered health care organizations* (pp. 45–68). Gaithersburg, MD: Aspen Publishers, Inc.

Denning, S. (2001). *The springboard. How storytelling ignites action in knowledge-era organizations.* Boston: Butterworth-Heinemann.

Dessler, G. (2002). *Management.* Upper Saddle River, NJ: Prentice Hall.

Drucker, P. (1974). *Management.* New York: Harper & Row, Publishers.

Finkelman, A. (1996). *Psychiatric nursing administration manual.* Gaithersburg, MD: Aspen Publishers, Inc.

Flarey, D., & Smith, S. (1999). Management and organizational restructuring: Reforming the corporate structure. In S. Smith and D. Flarey (Eds.), *Process-centered health care organizations* (pp. 141–152). Gaithersburg, MD: Aspen Publishers, Inc.

Gebelein, S., et al. (2000). *Successful manager's handbook.* Minneapolis, MN: Personnel Decisions International Corp.

Institute of Medicine. (1999). *To err is human.* Washington, DC: National Academy Press.

Katz, J. (2001). *Keys to nursing success.* Upper Saddle River, NJ: Prentice Hall.

Marrelli, T. (1997). *The nurse manager's survival guide.* St. Louis, MO: Mosby-Year Book, Inc.

Milgram, L., Spector, A., & Treger, M. (1999). *Managing smart.* Houston, TX: Cashman Dudley.

Power, S. (1999). *Nursing supervision. A guide for clinical practice.* London: Sage Publications, Ltd.

Robbins, S., & Decenzo, D. (2001). *Fundamentals of Management.* Upper Saddle River, NJ: Prentice Hall.

Sullivan, E. (2004). *Becoming influential. A guide for nurses.* Upper Saddle River, NJ: Prentice Hall.

Watzlawick, P., Beavin, J., & Jackson, D. (1967). *Pragmatics of human communication.* New York: Norton.

ADDITIONAL READINGS

Beaudoin, L., & Edgar, L. (2003). Hassles: Their importance to nurses' quality of work life. *Nursing Economics, 21*(3), 106–113.

Brandi, C. (2000). Relationships between nurse executives and physicians. The gender paradox in healthcare. *Journal of Nursing Administration, 30*(7/8), 373–378.

Burech, B., & Gordon, S. (2001). *From silence to voice: What nurses need to know and must communicate.* Ottawa, Ontario: Canadian Nurses Association.

Mason, D. (2002). MD-RN: A tired old dance. *American Journal of Nursing, 102*(6), 7.

Salimbene, S. (1999). Cultural competence: A priority for performance improvement action. *Journal of Nursing Care Quality, 13*(3), 23–35.

Taylor, B. (2004). Improving communication through practical reflection. *Reflections on Nursing LEADERSHIP,* second quarter, 28–30.

DELIVERY SYSTEMS/NURSING MODELS

Nurses will aim to influence how health care is delivered through work with nurse educators, policy makers, and business leaders, armed with sound research on practice models.

Desired Future Statement (Vision)

Nurses unite to create integrated models of health care delivery through education, research, practice, and public policy partnerships that improve the health of the nation.

Five strategies were identified to achieve the vision; one of these was the primary or driving strategy. These strategies are:

Design integrated practice models. "Integrated" practice models are: interdisciplinary, nurse-led, or co-led; applied across the areas of nursing education, practice, research, and policy; and blended across practice settings. (Primary Strategy)

Nursing practice management is redefined and reshaped for positive change.

Strategic partnerships are created both within the profession and among influential outside groups.

Nurse leaders contribute to shaping both public and health policy.

Efforts are successful to advance the value and image of nursing.

Objectives to Support Primary Strategy

Secure a stable funding stream to support the design, implementation, and evaluation of new, creative, integrated practice models.

Develop strategic partnerships to advance the use of research findings and evidence-based practice to design, implement, and evaluate new integrated practice models.

Orchestrate and evaluate integrated practice model demonstration projects.

Integrate health care economics and financial principles/practices into basic, graduate, and continuing nursing education curricula.

Define, create, and evaluate nurse staffing and acuity models that demonstrate nursing's value to patient outcomes.

Organize a central database/clearinghouse/resource center for sharing best practice and integrated models.

SOURCE: American Nurses Association. (2002). *Nursing's agenda for the future. A call to the nation.* Washington, DC: Author. Reprinted with permission.

Organizational Structure for Effective Care Delivery

CHAPTER OUTLINE

MediaLink
www.prenhall.com/finkelman

The Interactive Exercises for this chapter can be found in the OneKey course at www.prenhall.com/finkelman. Click on Chapter 5 to select from the following activities: Test Your Understanding, Benchmarks, Current Issues, Your Opinion Counts, Think Critically, and Summary and Applications.

What's Ahead

Health care organizations have a long history of being centralized, hierarchical-controlled organizations that focus on centralized staffing, policies, and procedures; centralized budget control; daily variance reports; and that emphasize punishment when goals are not met. "Control is the easiest way to manage. You simply tell others what to do, how to do it, when it should be done, and then wait for them to comply. Although it may be the easiest way, it is certainly not the most effective" (Crow, 2002, p. 11). Changes in leadership approaches, as discussed in Chapter 1, have clearly affected organizational changes so that the hierarchical type of organization is slowly fading away. The growth of managed care is another reason for this change in the structure of health care organizations (Finkelman, 2001; Simpson, 1999). The traditional approach to department-focused organizations is no longer as effective in this new environment of change. There is also greater need for health care provider accountability for cost control due to managed care requirements that require extreme cost reductions and greater emphasis on outcomes. Another change is the move away from health care to wellness and more care provided in the community. Health care providers not only need to assist people to get better but also to keep them from getting sick. Health care organizations must now be change-oriented if they want to survive and be effective. This chapter addresses theories about organizational structure and process by describing some theories and an overall view of health care organizations. It also builds on content from earlier chapters about leadership and management, change and decision making, collaboration, coordination, and coping with conflict.

OBJECTIVES

Before you begin, take a moment to familiarize yourself with the key objectives of this chapter.

- Describe the key organizational theories.
- Distinguish between structure and process.
- Identify the key differences between for-profit and not-for-profit health care organizations.
- Identify the key health care providers and their services.
- Explain the purpose of nursing care models.
- Compare and contrast the different nursing care models discussed in this chapter.
- Describe the key advantages of shared governance for nursing staff.
- Describe what would be included in an organization analysis.

TEST YOUR UNDERSTANDING

Before we begin our exploration of this chapter, take a short "warm-up" test to see what you know about this topic.

Organizational Theories: Emphasis on Structure and Process

Organizational theories

Many theories exist about organizational process and structure. Some of these theories include classical theory, bureaucratic organization, systems theory, contingency design theory, integrated delivery system, and service integration. Theories about organization really cannot be considered without relating them to leadership theories as they are interconnected.

Classical theory

Classical organization theory was described by Henri Fayol in 1916. His theory, though quite old, has had an effect on many theories that came after it. This theory includes principles that provide guidelines for organization. Some of these principles are important in understanding other theories. Box 5-1 highlights the key principles.

- The first principle is **division of labor**, which is a method for identifying specialized jobs within organizations. The tasks of the job are described in the position descriptions and are used to determine the division of labor. There is a clear delineation of the organization's rules that are found in its policies and procedures. The goal of this specialization is to increase productivity. It is also easier to identify where there is a breakdown in productivity and who is responsible for tasks.

BOX 5-1   Classical theory: Key principles.

- Division of labor
- Unity of direction or command
- Centralization
- Authority and responsibility
- Scalar chain or chain of command

Source: Author.

- The second principle is **unity of direction or command**. Each staff member should report to only one supervisor.
- The third principle is **centralization**. This principle focuses on centralization with all decisions made by specific management levels. There should, however, be an optimum balance between centralization and decentralization, which is an organization structure that pushes decision making and activities into the smaller components of the organization (e.g., staff education is planned and implemented per unit rather than planned for the entire organization).
- The principle of **authority** and **responsibility** form the fourth principle. The ideal is that there is equality between these two—responsibilities of the manager and the authority to do the job. In larger jobs authority is sometimes more difficult to identify.
- The last principle in the classical organizational theory recognizes that the **scalar chain** or the **chain of command** is important. This is a vertical chain of command for decisions and communication, from top to bottom or bottom to top, though the former is the most common. This is a pyramid structure in that higher up in the organization structure there are less management staff and ultimately one person is responsible. Fayol's theory certainly has been modified, and new theories have taken its place. This theory, however, did emphasize the need to understand an organization's structure, function, and process, which has continued to be important (Robbins & Decenzo, 2001, p. 33).

Bureaucratic organizations

Bureaucratic organizations incorporate the key principles of classical theory. Weber's theory described the ideal type of organization as one that had a division of labor, a clearly defined hierarchy, detailed rules and regulations, and impersonal relationships (Robbins & Decenzo, 2001). Figure 5-1 highlights the key characteristics. All of these characteristics are directly related to classical theory.

FIGURE 5-1   Bureaucratic organizations and characteristics.

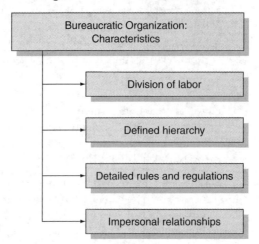

Source: Author.

One organization that is most commonly referred to as bureaucratic is the government. This form of organization can be described as the most predictable, but not necessarily the most effective. **Bureaucracy** is characterized by tight control, decreased uncertainty in the decision-making process, and very little individual staff choice. The goal is to ensure uniformity. Managers hold the authority, and staff are accountable to a manager. This type of organization appears impersonal, with decision making separated from staff who do the work. Seniority or gaining promotion is often based on the length of employment rather than skill or expertise. Positions are arranged in a hierarchy. Management, particularly top management, establishes the organization's philosophy or mission and its goals and objectives, making this centralized management. Control, however, is vested in top management.

What type of leadership is found in this type of organization? Decision making is in the hands of the leader, with staff not feeling comfortable or free to express their opinions. Staff lack confidence or trust in the leaders, and staff are not encouraged to use creative problem solving. The expectation from staff and from management is that the leader/manager will tell them what to do. This type of organizational structure is found less and less frequently as it does not meet the demands of today's health care delivery system or approaches to leadership, although some health care organizations still use it or have remnants of it left in their organizations. Many health care organizations tried to flatten their structure and eliminate their multiple layers (decentralizing), as will be discussed further in this chapter. Some of these organizations have been more successful than others with this change effort.

Systems theory

Systems theory views organizations as one entity with multiple elements or components that interact interdependently. Feedback is a critical process in a system. Input, process, and output rely on feedback, which is the dynamic process in which an organism learns from experiences within the environment. Systems are viewed from the perspective of closed and opened systems (Robbins & Decenzo, 2001). A **closed system** has limited or no interaction with its outside environment. It is isolated, and from a health care delivery perspective this system/organization would not be in tune with the needs of its consumers. In this situation consumers would not be involved in the organization other than to receive its services. Most health care organizations have discovered that this type of organization is ineffective and have turned more to developing organizations with **open systems**—systems that are "dynamically interacting with its environment" (Robbins & Decenzo, 2001, p. 41).

Within a hospital system, professional staff, administrative staff, equipment, supplies, and patients represent the system inputs. The process is the delivery of health care as patients work their way through the system to discharge. The outputs are the outcomes or results of that care. Adaptation, efficiency, and customer satisfaction are important in open systems, and criteria are used to determine system effectiveness. If an organization cannot adapt, it will cease to exist. **Adaptation** is the extent that the organization can and does respond to internal and external demands. Change drives the need for adaptation. Efficiency, which is the ratio of input to output, focuses on the amount of effort that is required to reach an outcome. Efficiency and productivity go hand-in-hand. Stakeholders (anyone who is affected by the organization's decisions and services) are very important, particularly in open systems. Thus, it is important to pay attention to stakeholder satisfaction by evaluating key player satisfaction. Who are the key players or stakeholders in the health care system?

1. **Customer.** Purchasers of care are employers and federal and state governments. They purchase care by contracting with insurers to cover some portion of health care costs for their employees.
2. **Third-party payer, insurer, or managed care organization.** They play an active role today in health care not only by financing care but often by direct involvement in medical decisions.
3. **Providers.** Providers include physicians, nurses, any health care professionals, unlicensed assistive personnel, ancillary therapists, hospitals, home care agencies, clinics, long-term care facilities, laboratories, radiological centers, city health departments, and so on, who deliver the care.
4. **Consumer.** The consumer is the patient and patient's family or significant others.

Contingency design theory

The **contingency design theory** recognizes that classical and bureaucratic approaches are not that helpful (Robbins & Decenzo, 2001). First, organizations vary widely so it is difficult to apply one theory to all organizations. Critical differences can be found in size, routines of task technology (impact on organization structure, leadership styles, and control systems), individual differences (leadership styles, job design), and environmental uncertainty (not stable or predictable anymore) (Robbins & Decenzo, 2001). Secondly, situations and factors that influence organizations need to be considered when organizations are developed, and they also affect their day-to-day functioning. These situational factors are particularly important as the organization responds to change or recognizes the need for change, which is similar to the Contingency theory and Chaos theory of leadership discussed in Chapter 1. The contingency design theory is a less rigid approach to organizations and how they function, although it certainly can cause more stress. Rigid approaches seem to be more reliable, and reliability decreases uncertainty. This decreases stress. This approach, however, does not necessarily mean that the organization can respond best to change and provide the best work environment.

Integrated delivery system

An **integrated delivery system** is an organizational structure that became very popular in the 1990s. "Integration means broadening the operational and production capabilities of an organization. It is a strategic move that will usually provide significant cost benefits" (Milgram, Spector, & Treger, 1999, p. 115). The development of this type of system is typically motivated by reimbursement changes and managed care. This system focuses on a continuum of care, provides a cost-efficient approach, and focuses on providing care to patients in the most appropriate setting (Spitzer, 2001). Integration can either be horizontal, vertical, or both.

- Horizontal integration merges several organizations doing the same type of work (for example, several acute care hospitals join together to form a horizontal health care organization). It is important to remember that these systems are complicated and difficult to manage. The organizations (or in the previous example, the hospitals that form one organization) may not be close to one another, which causes problems for coordination, collaboration, and communication. Distance between the various system components can make management more complicated. Horizontal integration has not always resulted in one seamless organization, but rather several organizations with a loose connection. This occurs when there is a limited unified identity and commitment to the larger organization. "When corporations merge, certain things usually result: a snappy new name, a single person running the show, consolidated departments. A big production is made of uniting the partners culturally and financially just as in a marriage. Except when the partners are hospitals" (Steinhauer, 2001, p. A1). It is not so simple to accomplish this merger and develop one organization out of several. Different competencies are required to manage a horizontal system as compared to a vertical system, and this difference is often neglected. Several organizations come together to form an integrated system, but there is limited change in leadership and management approaches. A major force in pushing health care organizations to become more integrated is managed care organizations (MCOs). Organizations are trying to better meet the MCO demands and outcomes required by managed care reimbursement.
- An organization that uses vertical integration is one that covers the continuum of care (for example, it might include an acute care hospital, a home care agency, a long-term care facility, a rehabilitation center, and an ambulatory care center). Diversification is one of the advantages of moving to vertical integration, which may provide more financial opportunities for the organization. As the organization has multiple services or products (e.g., wellness, prevention, acute and chronic care, disease management and rehabilitation, ambulatory care, long-term care, home care, and hospice care), there are increased opportunities to gain more reimbursement for services and thus increase revenues, or money that comes into the organization.

Regardless of the type of structure, vertical or horizontal, integrated systems need to have leaders who feel committed to all of the elements of the organization; use quantitative and qualitative innovation; are concerned with processes; use decentralized leadership; and design, support, and enhance organizational systems that drive performance (Spitzer, 2001). There has been criticism that the integrated delivery approach may not provide the best of services. Can one organization, the integrated organization, be an expert in all areas? What happens to individual entities that come together to form the integrated organization? Will they lose their strengths as they compete within the new organization (Campbell, Schmitz, & Waller, 1998)? Many questions remain unanswered about the advantages and disadvantages of this type of organization. Greater experience with this approach and analysis of its effectiveness is required to determine if this really is an effective way to organize a health care delivery system.

Service-line organization

The **service-line organization** groups activities according to product or service, such as women's health, emergency and urgent care, behavioral health care, and health and wellness. As an organization changes into a service-line structure, then the big question that arises is how to maintain a unified nursing presence within the organization and yet still experience benefits from this structure (Fitzpatrick, McElroy, & DeWoody, 2001). "Organizing nursing as a discipline into clusters for like areas of practice enhances the development of documentation tools, preprinted care plans, and orientation plans" (Fitzpatrick, McElroy, & DeWoody, 2001, p. 25). Interdisciplinary planning, which is emphasized more and more, enhances collaboration because it is easier to identify core health care provider groups that should be included; for example, if planning for behavioral health services, then behavioral health (psychiatric-mental health) nursing staff, psychiatrists, psychologists, social workers, and so on, would be involved. Even though an organization is structured around services/products there still needs to be some standardized features that continue to apply to all services/products. Job descriptions would have some content that is standardized along with specific content related to the service/product. A standardized nursing language may be developed for the entire organization. Some documentation forms would apply across all service areas, but there probably would still need to be some specialized documentation needs.

But what happens to the centralized functions such as the nursing department in a service-line organization? Fitzpatrick, McElroy, and DeWoody (2001) describe these functions in one organization that changed to product or service lines as follows.

■ Vice presidents, who were either physicians or nurses, directed the service lines. These vice presidents were responsible for fiscal management, marketing, physician relationships, quality of care, and growth of the service, and also assumed line accountability for the nursing units or other departments that were associated with the service.

■ Administrative responsibilities were assigned to the chief nursing executive, who was responsible and accountable for the centralized cost centers of staff development, patient education, float and per diem pools, and in-house nursing supervisors, which have typically been found in a nursing department. The chief nursing executive was responsible for the final approval of all centralized nursing policies and procedures.

■ A centralized director of nursing position coordinated the core elements of the discipline of nursing that support nursing practice. "This position had cross-campus reporting relationships for centralized staffing, house supervisors, employee education services, patient education services, and both campuses' nursing administrative offices" (Fitzpatrick, McElroy, & DeWoody, 2001, p. 25).

It is clear that this structure can be confusing for staff who have worked in more traditional nursing departments. It is even difficult to describe. In this type of structure, management and staff would need to learn more about the new structure and how it affects processes, staff, and management relationships. Staff should also be asked for input as the organization adapts to these changes.

This type of organization has become more common in health care. What are the advantages and disadvantages to this organization of the product/service-line approach to an organization's structure and process? The advantages are:

■ A single manager or director is responsible for ensuring that the service/product outcomes are reached. This means that from the beginning to the end of the service, all parts of the process are overseen, which should result in less fragmentation of care. Responses to problems that interfere with care should be timelier. If behavioral health is the service line, then all aspects that the organization provides from crisis intervention, inpatient to aftercare would be included in the service line (e.g., outpatient clinic, inpatient units, behavioral health emergency services, partial hospitalization, home care, and vocational therapy).

- ■ Performance can more easily be judged. Responsibility can also be more clearly defined, which can be a problem in performance evaluation. This may motivate staff to improve. An example related to the behavioral health service would be when a patient is discharged and then rehospitalized within a time period that is considered inappropriate. The patient's entire treatment process can be evaluated and then strategies can be developed within the service line instead of having to go to several different departments. A service line usually prevents one department from placing blame on another department (for example, the outpatient clinic blaming the inpatient unit). When they are both part of the same service line, this is more difficult to do. They would all participate together in planning and decision making and accept responsibility for ensuring that patients receive care in the service rather than respond as separate departments.

- ■ The director may be more motivated when the entire service is under the director's control.

- ■ Responsibility for giving continuous, undivided attention to the product or service leads to more sensitivity for the unique needs of the focus population that the service addresses. Staff can develop a better view of how all parts of treatment offered within the service relate to one another, can develop relationships with staff across treatment focus areas, and during evaluation staff can focus more on clearly analyzing problems rather than denying their responsibilities.

The disadvantages are:

- ■ There is duplication of effort, which may reduce efficiency.
- ■ Some services may become isolated from other services and their staff.
- ■ Increased communication about activities of the various service lines exists, which can result in confusion.
- ■ Organization-wide identity and commitment may be compromised as the service lines are emphasized (Dessler, 2002, pp. 137–139).

Each of the disadvantages can be limited if steps are taken early on to recognize these as potential problems and then staff respond proactively. For example, the organization as a whole can determine functions that cross all service lines (such as pharmacy) and decide the most effective way to ensure that resources that are needed in all the service lines are met.

Structure and process: Parts of organizational theory

Structure

Typically, organizations are described by their **structure** and their **process**. Why is it important to understand this? As organizational theories developed, they tended to focus on one of these aspects of organization, although some focus on both. Staff in organizations find that the organization's structure (what does the organization look like) and the process (how things are done) become important. For example, if a nurse does not understand to whom he/she reports, this can be a problem (structure), or if the nurse does not understand the communication process for reporting an error (process), this can lead to problems. What are the aspects of structure and process that are important to understand?

First, how would staff find out about an organization's structure? The best place to begin is with the organizational chart for the entire organization and the charts for its components, such as divisions and units. "An organizational chart is a graphical representation of an organization's hierarchical structure and the flow of responsibility within the organization. It should reflect the chain of command and illustrate the relationships between staff members" (Milgram, Spector, & Treger, 1999, p. 29). It provides a visual of the chain of command, centralization/decentralization approach, departments, and span of control. It is important that this chart is updated as changes are made in the organizational structure. When assessing an organization's structure, it is impor-

BOX 5-2   Elements of organizational
structure.

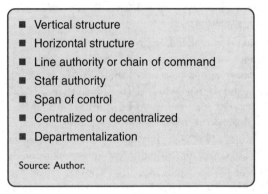

- ■ Vertical structure
- ■ Horizontal structure
- ■ Line authority or chain of command
- ■ Staff authority
- ■ Span of control
- ■ Centralized or decentralized
- ■ Departmentalization

Source: Author.

tant to remember that each organization has a formal and an informal aspect. How are these aspects demonstrated in an organization? The organization's organizational chart describes the formal positions and hierarchy; however, this does not reflect the informal structure. Staff who are leaders even if they do not hold a formal title in the hierarchy would not be indicated in the structure described in the organization chart nor would information about which managers are more powerful, although they all have the same authority due to their position as manager. A traditional structure uses vertical relationships or the chain of command that identifies to whom specific positions report. The view of organizational structure has been changing for many organizations as they move to greater emphasis on horizontal organization. Elements of the structure, which are highlighted in Box 5-2, that are important to consider are:

- ■ **Vertical structure.** Establishes line authority and uses centralized decision making. This is the type of structure found in bureaucratic organizations, with staff reporting "up the line" through the organization.
- ■ **Horizontal structure.** Departmentalization related to functions that uses decentralized decision making. Typically, a horizontal organization uses "a structure organized around customer-oriented processes (products/service lines), eliminates functional departments, and spreads functional specialists throughout the key process teams" (Dessler, 2002, p. 170).
- ■ **Line authority or the chain of command.** A more traditional approach to authority in organizations. This description identifies to whom each staff member reports up through the chain of command. For example, in line authority a staff nurse would report to the nurse manager, the nurse manager to the director of the service, the director of the service to the nurse executive, and the nurse executive to the chief executive officer.
- ■ **Staff authority.** Staff who function in an advisory capacity and cannot force other staff to do something but must use influence to make an impact. This can be a difficult position, but it has become more common. Staff authority is less clear because this relationship is advisory. An example is the director of nursing education in a hospital, who typically has no line authority over the nurse managers but rather a staff relationship. The director can suggest and advise nurse managers to initiate certain educational programs but cannot direct nurse managers to do this. Key skills for success in this type of position are effective communication, negotiation, and building collaborative relationships.
- ■ **Span of control.** Number of people supervised by one person/position. Span of control answers the question of how many staff report to one manager. This is a critical concern in the classical theory of organizations, which emphasizes that there are limits to the number of staff a supervisor can effectively direct. Issues that affect the number of staff are: (a) similarity and complexity of the jobs and functions, (b) geographic factors (for example, staff who are spread out in several clinics in a community as compared with staff who work on one unit in a hospital), (c) amount of direction and coordination required, and (d) amount of planning and time required to provide management. More efficient organizations usually have a shorter

span of control for their managers. "The result of the span of control that exceeds the capacity of any one manager affects decision making, resource utilization, interdepartmental relations, and patient care" (Alidina & Funke-Furber, 1988, as cited in Leitch, 1999, p. 9; Kolb, Rubin, & McIntyre, 1984).

■ **Centralized and decentralized organizational structures.** Used in health care organizations. A centralized approach focuses tasks and authority in one source. **Decentralized** spreads tasks and authority out over components of the organization. For example, how is staff education organized in a hospital? In a centralized approach there is a staff development department that is responsible for staff orientation and education throughout the hospital, whereas a decentralized approach gives this responsibility to the divisions or units. In the latter case, there may still be staff who provide some staff development services and also act as consultants to the units. In this case, they typically are also responsible for overall hospital orientation and education/training that is required for all staff, and nurse managers are responsible for their own unit's staff development. In a decentralized organization the nurse managers then have more independence in the management of their units in comparison to centralized organizations.

■ **Departmentalization.** Occurs when divided tasks are grouped. Functional departmentalization focuses on grouping related jobs while territorial departmentalization focuses on grouping jobs according to location within the organization. An example of a functional departmentalization, which is common in health care organizations, is the department of surgery, which might include the preoperative area, operating rooms, and post-anesthesia care unit (PACU). Another example is the obstetrics department composed of labor and delivery, postpartum, nurseries, and the neonatal intensive care unit. In some organizations the clinics for these specialty areas are also included in the department. This is very similar to a product/service-line approach. A different approach is to have all clinics, regardless of specialty, included in one ambulatory care department.

■ **Matrix organization.** Structures attempt to balance functional and service or product organizations. Staff belong to a functional department, such as a nursing department, and to a service or product department, such as women's health. Dual authority is part of this type of structure as staff report to two managerial systems. Why would this type of structure be used? It facilitates the efficient use of resources; allows for more flexibility during times of change with more timely response and interchange of information vertically and horizontally; encourages greater interdisciplinary interaction and innovation; improves motivation and commitment as staff have more responsibility for decision making; and it frees managers for greater opportunity to enhance planning (Dessler, 2002; Robbins & Decenzo, 2001).

THINK CRITICALLY

Try this exercise to apply what you have learned about this topic.

Process

Organizational process, the second critical descriptor of an organization, focuses on how the organization operates. Particularly important process factors are: communication, decision making, policies and procedures, organization performance and job performance, goal attainment and results, quality improvement, budget, marketing, and future plans. All of these factors are discussed in other chapters. Nurses participate in all of these aspects of organizational process whether they are staff nurses or in management.

The organization's vision, mission statement, and goals and objectives should be included in a review of an organization's process. The vision is important in describing the organization's beliefs and values. An organizational philosophy answers the question of "why" for an organization. "The values and principles of an organization set the parameters for decision making and determining what is critical to the organization. Thus, the organizational philosophy becomes the basis for operationalizing the mission of the institution" (Tuck, Harris, & Baliko, 2000, p. 180).

Tuck, Harris, and Baliko (2000) reviewed nursing philosophies that were written after 1982. In this review value statements were classified according to several categories: caring, professionalism, individualism, well-being or health, culture, need fulfillment, and adaptation. The results indicated that caring and individuation remain central concepts of nursing practice. Managed care, however, presents organizations and nurses with new challenges. How can organizations continue to incorporate these key concepts such as caring in their changing organizations? The responsibility for ensuring that values expressed in an organization's nursing philosophy or vision are implemented is the responsibility of the nurse executive. The mission statement clarifies the organization's purpose. It describes what the organization is while the vision describes what the organization wants to be. Goals and objectives identify how the organization plans to meet its vision and mission. An organization's mission statement is a "brief, concise expression of a company's (organization's) fundamental purpose and goals" (Milgram, Spector, & Treger, 1999, p. 62). All of the staff need to be committed to the organization's vision, mission, and goals and objectives.

Vision and mission statements, as well as goals and objectives, all help to define the organizational process—how things work to get the job done. What are other important elements of process? Box 5-3 highlights the key process elements.

- **Decision making.** Decisions are made frequently in all health care organizations: decisions about patient care, how they will be done, how the organization will run, and about the future of the organization. Decision making is a critical element of organizational processes (see Chapter 2).
- **Delegation.** Decisions should be made as close to the task or activity as possible, which has made delegation even more important in today's health care organizations. It is important to remember that delegation does not relinquish the person who is delegating from the responsibility over the task (see Chapter 8).
- **Coordination.** There needs to be "a clear framework of responsibility, the reporting relationships, groups of common products/functions, and mechanisms to link and coordinate all the elements" (Leitch, 1999, p. 10). Coordination is the process by which the parts of a process are synchronized or work together (see Chapter 3).
- **Communication.** As has been discussed in previous chapters and will be discussed in later chapters, communication is part of any organization's processes. Without communication nothing will get done in an organization; in fact, no one would know what to do without communication (see Chapter 4).
- **Evaluation.** Evaluation of the organization's performance and that of individual staff performance assists the organization in determining its needs in the planning process so that goals and objectives can be met. All processes are evaluated in some form, whether it be a formal evaluation or staff concluding that some action was successful on an informal basis (see Chapters 12 and 17).

BOX 5-3   Elements of organizational process.

Decision making
Delegation
Coordination
Communication
Evaluation

Source: Author.

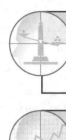

THINK CRITICALLY

Try this exercise to apply what you have learned about this topic.

BENCHMARKS

Now let's take a moment to test your knowledge of the concepts you have studied in this section.

Health Care Organizations

The following chapters contain more extensive discussion about the health care organizations such as acute care hospitals; however, before discussing these organizations further in other chapters, it is helpful to understand some key factors about the health care delivery system and its organizations. The health care system consists of all the agencies and professionals that are organized to provide health services. The three major purposes of the health care delivery system are to provide: (a) health promotion and illness prevention, (b) diagnosis and treatment of illness and injury, and (c) rehabilitation and health restoration. Box 5-4 highlights these purposes.

There are three levels of health care services based on the complexity of the care required.

1. **Primary care** includes health promotion and education, preventive care, early detection, and environmental protection.
2. **Secondary care** focuses on diagnosis and treatment in the primary settings of acute care and emergency care.
3. **Tertiary care**, the last level, focuses on long-term care, rehabilitation, and care of the dying. Health care systems are varied in the level of services they provide, and some provide a combination of services (for example, a large medical center might provide acute care, ambulatory care and primary care, emergency services, wellness center, home care, and also own a long-term care facility).

The second part of the health care delivery system is the public system, which provides care to those who experience health delivery access problems. Both the personal systems, which focus on care for individuals, and the public systems provide a variety of services including health promotion, prevention and early detection of disease, diagnosis and treatment of disease with a focus on cure, rehabilitative-restorative care, and custodial care. Managed care and other reimbursement approaches have had a major effect on both the personal and the public systems as discussed in Chapter 14.

Health care settings can be described by a variety of important characteristics, including the type of services offered, size, location (urban or rural), type of people served, and reimbursement for services. The following are examples of health care settings.

■ **Public health.** Government departments and agencies (federal, state, or local) funded primarily by taxes and administered by elected or appointed officials. Local health departments

BOX 5-4   Health care delivery system purposes.

Health promotion & illness prevention
Diagnosis and treatment
Rehabilitation and health restoration

Source: Author.

develop and carry out programs to meet the health needs of groups within the community and the community as a whole.

- Physicians' offices (or advance practice nurses' and nurse midwives' offices)
- Ambulatory care centers (e.g., one-day surgery centers, diagnostic centers)
- Clinics, which may be inside or outside a hospital and provide a variety of services
- Occupational health clinics, which provide health services at the worksite
- School health services, some of which may be full-service clinics
- Emergency
- Urgent care
- Crisis intervention
- Hospitals (acute care)
- Psychiatric hospitals and community mental health centers (behavioral health care)
- Substance abuse treatment centers (inpatient and outpatient)
- Extended care facilities, which includes skilled nursing (intermediate care) and/or extended-care (long-term care) facilities and may be part of a hospital system or freestanding
- Retirement and assisted-living centers
- Rehabilitation centers
- Home health agencies
- Hospice services, which may be provided in the home and/or in a freestanding facility

This list is not complete, but it does provide examples of the more common types of health care settings or organizations.

The U.S. health care system is complex, although it did not begin this way. In the past, care was primarily provided in the home and by visits to physician's offices. This gradually developed into a more complex system as the role of hospitals grew. Today, most care still comes through the personal health care system rather than through the public care system. Physician care is typically delivered in one of the following models:

1. The solo practice of a physician in an office, which continues to be present in some communities, although it is less and less common.
2. The single specialty group model, which consists of physicians in the same specialty who pool expenses, income, and offices.
3. Multispecialty group practice, which provides interaction across specialty areas.
4. The integrated health maintenance model that has prepaid multispecialty physicians.
5. Community health center—developed through federal monies in the 1960s—which addresses broader inputs into health such as education and housing (Finkelman, 2001, p. 189).

Health care organizations are confronted with many factors that influence how they are structured and how they operate. The following factors have had an impact or continue to have an impact on health care organization structure and processes.

- Problems with access to health care often resulting in disparity
- Increase in health care cost and cost containment
- Hospital mergers and closings
- Growth of managed care
- Shortage of health care providers (e.g., nurses, pharmacists, some specialty physicians)
- Increase in the number of uninsured and underinsured
- Improved technologic advances (e.g., computers, organ transplants, extension of life, genetics, telehealth/telemedicine)
- Increased specialization, which may increase fragmentation of care
- Growing consumerism
- Changes in demographics (e.g., single-parent families, immigrant populations, lack of nearby extended family, aging)

- Increase in homeless populations and other vulnerable populations
- Increase in availability of drugs, although many are expensive
- Lack of or limited coverage for prescriptions
- Uneven distribution of services (e.g., urban vs. rural areas)
- Lack of clear health policies
- Unequal treatment for some health problems (e.g., mental health services)

For-profit and not-for-profit delivery systems

Two terms that are often used in health care, for-profit and not-for-profit, can be confusing. They are nonetheless important terms as they identify an organization's characteristics that impact many aspects of the health care organization's structure and process. **For-profit health care organizations** have stockholders/shareholders who own stock in the business/organization. The organization is responsible to the stockholders, who expect to make a profit on their investment. If stockholders do not feel that they are making enough money on their investment, they may sell their stocks, and the organization will then have serious financial problems. Stockholders serve as an external control on decisions that are made by the organization. These organizations receive the same type of reimbursement for care as not-for-profit delivery systems, which are called voluntary or public health care organizations. In contrast, the **not-for-profit organization** does not have stockholders to whom it must report. Charitable institutions, government, and churches, as well as the typical reimbursement sources, fund not-for-profit health care organizations. Both types of organizations, for-profit and not-for-profit, must still make a profit to survive today. The not-for-profit organization does not share this profit with shareholders, as the for-profit organization does, but rather this type of organization reinvests its profit into its own organization to continue its services and maintain the organization. The for-profit organization, however, also does the same, but it must still share some profit with stockholders. Both financial approaches have direct effects on the organization's vision, mission, goals, budget, management and decision making, use of resources, types of services, relationships with other organizations and the community, and how quickly the organization responds to change that can make a financial impact on the organization. Some for-profit organizations have experienced ethical and legal problems because of their need for financial success, which are discussed in Chapter 10. Nurses need to be aware of their employer's status related to profits. It can affect why and how decisions are made.

YOUR OPINION COUNTS

Find out what others think about this topic. Post your response and check out other opinions.

Marketing

Marketing is a new area for most nurses, and for many it may arouse negative reactions because nurses may see it as too "business like" and not ethical. Why is it important for nurses to be aware of health care marketing and understand some aspects of it? The marketing process drives major decisions in health care as health care organizations compete with one another for patients and for third-party payer (insurer) contracts. Ineffective marketing may result in a health care organization cutting staff and services if it cannot attract enough patients. The marketing process includes three elements.

1. A determination of what is wanted and needed
2. A method(s) for reaching what is wanted or needed
3. An understanding of the patient, customer, or consumer and the need to serve

These elements should sound familiar because they are similar to those described in the nursing process. Like the nursing process, the marketing process is complex. It is dependent on data, interaction between people, problem solving, decision making, and evaluation of results. A **market** is an actual or potential consumer or customer who might need a product or service. For example, for a nurse-midwife, a market is the women in a specific community or geographic area who are of childbearing age. A more specific market would be the women in that community or geographic area who might use the services of a nurse-midwife. This is referred to as segmenting. Factors that help to identify segments of a market are age, sex, diagnosis, past medical treatment, geographics, accessibility, insurance coverage, and economic status. Selling is often confused with marketing, but selling is only one part of the marketing process. Nurses can be very helpful in the marketing process with their consumer skills: the ability to talk with patients, understanding of patient needs, their emphasis on health promotion and disease and illness prevention, understanding of the health care delivery system and the community, and problem-solving skills.

Marketing goals are established based on assessment data. The following are examples of goals that might be identified for a community clinic.

- To develop a practice that is accessible
- To increase the number of patients by 5%
- To provide health promotion and disease and illness prevention services
- To encourage active patient participation in their care
- To develop patient education support groups focusing on chronic illness (e.g., asthma, arthritis, hypertension)

Marketing is an integral part of providing direct patient care, quality assessment and improvement, risk management, utilization review, administration, decision making and planning, performance appraisal, staff development, and community relationships.

The four P's of marketing

The four P's of marketing are: product, promotion, price, and place. Box 5-5 highlights these principles.

- Products are the goods or services that meet the customer's needs. For a community clinic this would include physical exams, patient education, immunizations, well-child care, and blood pressure screening.
- Promotion is what is often referred to as advertising. How does the community clinic get the word out about the services or products that are provided? Informing local hospitals about its services and other community agencies to obtain referrals is promotion.
- Pricing focuses on identifying the cost of a product or service. Much of this is in the hands of third-party payers and the government, which determine their own reimbursement levels; however, if reimbursement does not cover expenses and provide some profit, this is a major problem for the health care organization.
- The fourth P is place or getting the product or service to the consumer. This includes such factors as physical location, type of location, accessibility to the facility, transportation, parking, handicap accessibility, and the type of setting, such as its "warmth," easy-to-locate offices, and so on.

BOX 5-5   The four P's of marketing.

Product

Promotion

Price

Place

Source: Author.

BOX 5-6   Marketing plan.

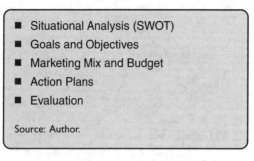

- Situational Analysis (SWOT)
- Goals and Objectives
- Marketing Mix and Budget
- Action Plans
- Evaluation

Source: Author.

The marketing plan

The marketing plan is a written description of the organization and what it wants to be in the future. The plan includes a description of the organization (for example, a group of nurse practitioners, an interdisciplinary group of practitioners, a clinic, hospital, and so on); the environment in which the organization operates, its potential and actual consumers; its competitors; and its plans for the future. A marketing plan should never be complete. Change is inevitable, and if the marketing plan does not change, it becomes just another piece of paper. A marketing plan contains five parts, as highlighted in Box 5-6.

1. Situational analysis is sometimes referred to as SWOT—the strengths, weaknesses, opportunities, and threats analysis of the organization. All of these elements are described with relevant data to support the ideas presented. Data from both internal and external environments are included in the analysis.
2. Marketing goals and objectives are identified that are reasonable and specific to the organization. A marketing goal might be to increase the number of patients from a specific geographic area by 20%. If this geographic area had a large number of professional women, single and married, a related objective would be to develop a special woman's health promotion program for women ages 30 to 40. Decisions like this need to be based on data.
3. Marketing strategy considers the marketing mix and the marketing budget. The marketing mix describes the specific combination of the four P's, focusing on how the combination of product, promotion, price, and place influence consumers to use the organization's services. As the marketing budget is developed, resources are allocated to each service area. For example, the budget identifies the amount of resources that will be allocated to market the health promotion program for women ages 30 to 40.
4. Action plans describe specifically how the marketing goals and objectives will be met. The written plan identifies actions to be taken, responsibilities and accountabilities, and time frames.
5. Evaluation is ongoing. It provides feedback as the plan is implemented and goals are achieved, as well as information that might indicate a need for a change in the plan. Any change must be carefully considered; however, no plan should be so sacred that it cannot be revised (Finkelman, 1996).

As the marketing plan is developed, consideration is given to several marketing expansion approaches: market penetration, market development, and diversification (Finkelman, 1996).

- Market penetration focuses on services that are already offered by the organization. This type of expansion is less risky as the organization knows that it has this market but wants to expand it. A group of advanced practice nurses that provides well-baby exams in a specific suburban area may decide to advertise more in this suburban area to increase the number of well-baby visits. This approach, however, may mean that the organization will miss opportunities to expand into new areas.
- Market development focuses on existing services but also on developing new markets for these services. For example, a group of nurse practitioners may already offer well-baby exams in an urban area, but they may decide to take this service into an adjacent rural area—in other words, it's the same service but an expanded market for it.

■ The third approach, diversification, focuses on developing new services for new markets. This is the riskiest approach. For example, a group of nurse practitioners may decide to develop a program for teens that focuses on health care promotion and contract with the local high schools to provide this service. The program may fail, and one of its goals to increase the number of teen referrals from this program to the practice for continued care may also fail. Time and money are required to develop the new service and market. Besides market expansion, the elimination of services must always be considered. Market assessment that includes budgetary issues may reveal that some services are not needed or that some services are not successful due to competition from other providers or for other reasons. Giving up services is always difficult but may be the best decision that can be made.

Health care providers

Health care providers can be classified as organizations such as a hospital or a clinic and individuals such as an individual nurse or physician. Both types provide care to individuals and groups of patients. There are many different types of health care provider organizations. The typical ones are hospitals, clinics, physician practices, ambulatory care centers, primary care, home health agencies, long-term care facilities, skilled nursing facilities, rehabilitation centers, hospice services, public health departments, school health clinics, birthing centers, ambulatory surgical centers, occupational health clinics, crisis clinics, and any other type of organization that provides care to the community.

The factors discussed earlier that have affected organization structure and process frequently cause these organizations to change. Managed care has been encouraging providers such as physicians to keep patients out of the hospital. Therefore, primary care is increasing in the community. In this case, when patients are admitted to hospitals they are often much more acutely ill, requiring more intensive care. At the same time hospitals are encouraged to discharge patients as soon as possible. These patients then return home still sick and often require care from family members or a home health agency. Home health services and hospice services have also increased. This shifting has had a major impact on physician practices, clinics, hospitals, home health agencies, hospices, and long-term care facilities, and certainly on nursing practice in all of these organizations. At the same time advanced practice nursing has grown, and advanced practice nurses are now found in many of these organizations.

The following provides a brief review of the major types of professional and non-professional members of the health care team.

■ *Registered nurse* **(RN).** This appears to be a simple designation; however, there are different types of educational routes to obtain a license to practice nursing. These include diploma, associate degree, and baccalaureate degree. In addition, many nurses now obtain master's degrees and doctorates. These advanced degrees provide them with the opportunity to practice more independently, teach, or to do research. Nurses practice in all types of health settings.

■ *Nurse practitioner* **(NP)** *and clinical nurse specialist* **(CNS).** Both of these types of nurses obtain education beyond a baccalaureate degree with special content either related to primary care (NP) or acute care (CNS). A nurse practitioner specializes in such areas as adult health, pediatrics, neonatal, gerontology, and psychiatric nursing. Nurse practitioners may work in clinics, the community, private practice, the home, the hospital, or long-term care facilities—any setting where health care is provided. A CNS typically works in acute care settings.

■ *Nurse midwife* **(NM).** This is a nurse who has completed an additional educational program that focuses on midwifery. Nurse midwives work in all types of settings in which women's health and obstetrical services are provided.

■ *Physician* **(MD).** A physician has a medical degree and typically specializes in a specific area of practice (e.g., internal medicine, surgery, pediatrics, gynecology, etc.). Due to managed care more physicians are specializing in primary practice than in the past. These physicians are designated as primary care providers. In this role they act as the gatekeeper by directing the patient's care. Some insurers are now allowing nurse practitioners and nurse midwives to act as primary care providers.

■ *Licensed practical/vocational nurse* (LPN or LVN). Licensed practical/vocational nurses perform some specific nursing functions and play a critical role in providing direct patient care. They have high school degrees and additional training. They work in all types of settings, typically under the direct supervision of a registered nurse or a physician.

■ *Unlicensed assistive personnel* (UAP). The increased use of UAPs on the health care team has caused some controversy in the last few years; however, a UAP is a critical member of the team. Aides and assistants have been in existence for a long time. Their responsibilities have changed over the years, and today they are providing more direct patient care. They are supervised by registered nurses, who must ensure that they are able to provide safe care to the patient. The home health aide functions fairly independently in the home, usually seeing the patient more than the home care nurse, who supervises the home health aide. The amount of education and training that all types of UAPs have is highly variable, and this has caused some of the concern about what they are able to do and the effect on the quality of care. Further information about UAPs and delegation is found in Chapter 8.

■ *Registered dietician* (RD). This health care professional assesses the patient's nutritional status and needs related to health status. A registered dietician may work in hospitals, long-term care facilities, clinics, community health areas, and in the home. Another similar health care provider is the nutritionist who has knowledge about nutrition and food in the community setting and recommends healthy diets and provides nutrition counseling and education.

■ *Social worker* (SW). Social workers assist patients and their families with problems related to reimbursement, access to care, housing, care in the home, transportation, and other social problems. They may also hold specialized positions as discharge planners and as case managers, particularly in acute care facilities or hospitals; however, they work in all types of settings.

■ *Occupational therapist* (OT). Occupational therapists assist patients with impaired functions to reach the patient's maximum level of physical and psychosocial independence. They work in all types of settings.

■ **Speech-language pathologist.** Speech-language pathologists assist patients who need rehabilitative services related to speech and hearing. They work in all types of settings.

■ *Physical therapist* (PT). Physical therapists focus on assisting patients who are experiencing musculoskeletal problems with rehabilitation and reaching maximum physical functioning. They work in all types of settings.

■ **Pharmacist.** Pharmacists are concerned with ensuring that patients receive the appropriate medication by preparing and dispensing medications. Pharmacists have become much more involved in patient education about medications and in monitoring and evaluating the effects of medications. They work in all types of settings including the local drug store, where they play a critical role in ensuring safe prescriptions and in providing consumer education.

■ *Respiratory therapist* (RT). Respiratory therapists provide care to patients with respiratory illnesses. They use oxygen therapy, intermittent positive pressure respirators, artificial mechanical ventilators, and inhalation therapy.

■ **Chiropractor.** Chiropractors are concerned with improving the function of the patient's nervous system with various treatment modalities (e.g., spinal manipulation, diet, exercise, and massage). Interest in using chiropractors has been increasing as the consumer has become more interested in nontraditional medical interventions.

■ **Paramedical technologists.** Paramedical technologists work in various medical technology areas (for example, radiology, nuclear medicine, and other laboratories) (Finkelman, 2001, pp. 195–196).

Other common providers are physician's assistants (PAs), who diagnose and treat certain diseases and injuries under the direction of a physician, dentists, case managers, and spiritual support persons (chaplains).

Nontraditional health care providers have become more important as consumers have increased their use of alternative or complementary therapies. There is great variation in how these services are accepted by health care professionals. In some communities some of these services can be found within traditional health care organizations, and traditional health care providers are also incorporating the use of alternative therapies into their practice. In other communities there is less integration of these services. Reimbursement for these services is still highly variable. Some of these therapies are massage therapy, herbal therapy, healing touch, energetic healing, acupuncture, acupressure, and so on. Some of the problem areas with these new therapies are: limited research to support their effectiveness, limited or lack of formal training and licensure requirements for practitioners, lack of standards, and limited or no reimbursement. The National Institutes of Health has established a center that focuses on alternative or complementary therapies and now funds research to determine the effectiveness of these therapies. These issues need to be addressed before these therapies and their practitioners will be fully accepted in the health care system.

Professional nursing practice within nursing care models

"The American Nurses Association (1995) broadly defines the professional practice of nursing as: (1) the attention to the full range of human responses to health and illness; (2) the integration of objective data with subjective data gained from the patient's experience; (3) the application of scientific knowledge to diagnosis and treatment; and (4) the provision of a caring relationship" (Ritter-Teitel, 2002, p. 31). Caring is a fundamental element within professional nursing practice, as was discussed earlier by identifying its frequent presence in nursing philosophies and in Chapter 4. Though caring is an important part of nursing practice, some experts have indicated that hospital nursing does not promote continuity of care, which is important in creating caring relationships with patients, through its organization (Scott, Aiken, Mechanic, & Moravcsik, 1995). The American Organization of Nurse Executives (AONE) emphasizes that professional nursing is evolving, and the nurse's role is particularly affected by empowerment, self-discovery, autonomy, independence, and partnership (AONE, 1996). AONE has identified elements of the evolving health care system that influence nursing practice.

- Networks of providers across the care continuum
- Collaboration among health professionals regarding interdependent functions
- Partnerships with consumers
- Collective accountability
- Advocacy for those who cannot advocate for themselves
- Leadership in cost-effective patient care

All of these elements have been discussed in earlier chapters or will be discussed in later chapters as they are critical aspects of leadership and management.

Intertwined within these critical elements is the recognition of the importance of autonomy, responsibility, delegation, and accountability.

- "Autonomy in clinical decision making occurs whenever a nurse makes an independent judgment about the presence of a clinical issue and then provides the resolution to nursing care" (Ritter-Teitel, 2002, p. 32). Autonomy requires competence and skills that focus on the nurse-patient relationship. It also means that there needs to be an organized assessment method to determine patient care needs and reassigning staff. Nurses also have the right to consult with others as professionals as they provide care or manage care. Autonomy, control, and decision making are related. "Professional practice implies control over the terms of the work but also control over its content and regulation of its standards" (Ritter-Teitel, 2002, p. 33). Nurses who feel that they have autonomy know that they have the right to make decisions in their daily practice and also participate in developing organizational policy and change. Staff autonomy, however, does not work in organizations in which leaders are authoritarian and when centralized decision making and control are key characteristics of the organization. This situation will quickly lead to conflict. In addition, the work environment must be conducive to collaboration with physicians, as is discussed in Chapter 3.

■ "Responsibility refers to being entrusted with a particular function" (Ritter-Teitel, 2002, p. 34). A nursing practice model that does not address responsibility will not be effective. Along with this is the need to clearly recognize the importance of delegation.

■ "Delegation involves transferring responsibility for the performance of the task from one person to another" (Ritter-Teitel, 2002, p. 34). Delegation is discussed in more detail in Chapter 8.

■ Accountability is a term that is typically found in job descriptions and descriptions of organizational structure. In nursing it is particularly important to recognize that "accountability is the acceptance of responsibility for the outcomes of care" (Ritter-Teitel, 2002, p. 34). Nurses need to know that what they do with patients needs to mean something—it must reach outcomes. Magnet hospitals are discussed in Chapter 6 as examples of organizations that exemplify these characteristics.

The AONE elements and these characteristics, such as accountability, need to be considered when nursing practice models are assessed. Models of care are developed to support or enhance professional practice, and by considering these elements and characteristics the models will be more effective. Within a health care organization, how do nurses provide nursing care? What is a model of care? Are these elements found in the model? "A model of care is a configuration of nursing practice or pattern of delivery" (Ritter-Teitel, 2002, p. 35). Models might also be called nursing or patient care delivery systems. These models have undergone major changes over the last several decades. Nursing practice models have been used to implement resource-intensive strategies with the goal of decreasing expenses and using staff more effectively. These practice models establish organizational frameworks that provide nursing staff opportunities to become more committed to their practice and to be more involved in decision making (Upenieks, 2000, p. 330). The following is a description of common models, some of which have undergone many changes over the years or are not used anymore though they have had an impact on other models. In addition, how models are used in an organization can be highly variable. The models are highlighted in Box 5-7.

Total patient care/case method

In this model, which is the oldest, the registered nurse is responsible for all of the care provided to a patient for a shift. A major disadvantage of this model is the lack of consistency and coordinated care when care is provided in 8-hour segments. This type of care is rarely provided today, except among student nurses who are assigned to provide all of the care for a patient during the hours that they are in clinical. Even in this case, the students frequently do not provide all of the care as they may not be qualified to do this. Home health agencies use a form of this model when nurses are assigned patients and provide all home care; however, even this has been adapted as more home care is provided by a team. An RN may coordinate the care and provide professional nursing services, but a home care aide may be involved as well as other providers such as a physical therapist, dietician, and social worker.

BOX 5-7 Nursing care models.

■ Total patient care/case method
■ Functional nursing
■ Care management model
■ Team nursing
■ Primary nursing
■ Care and service team models

Source: Author.

Functional nursing

Functional nursing is a task-oriented approach, focusing on jobs to be done. When it was more commonly used, it was thought to be more efficient. The nurse in charge assigned the tasks (e.g., one nurse may administer medications for all patients on a unit; an aide may take vital signs for all patients). A disadvantage of this model is the risk of fragmented care. In addition, this type of model also leads to greater staff dissatisfaction with staff feeling they are just grinding out tasks. Individualized care may also be compromised with patient care provided by different staff who may or may not be aware of other needs and the care provided by others. This model is not used much now. It can be found in long-term care facilities and in some psychiatric inpatient services, although in a modified form. In the latter situation a registered nurse may be assigned the task of medication administration for the unit, and psychiatric support staff may be assigned such tasks as vital signs and checks of all patients. In this situation, RNs would probably still be assigned to individual patients to coordinate their care.

Team nursing

Team nursing, developed after World War II when there was a severe nursing shortage as well as major changes in medical technology, replaced functional nursing. A team consists of an RN, licensed practical nurses (LPNs), and nurse aides. This team of two or three staff provide total care for a group of patients during an 8- or 12-hour shift. The RN team leader coordinates this care. In this model the RN has a high level of autonomy and assumes the centralized decision-making authority. Although the past approach to team nursing was thought to use decentralized decision making with decisions made closer to the patient, there actually was limited team member collaboration. In addition, these teams tended to communicate only among themselves and not as well with physicians. The team concept or model also focused on tasks rather than patient care as a whole. More current versions of the team model are different from this earlier type. Currently, the team model has been changed to meet changes in organizations and leadership corresponding to the needs for better consistency and continuity of care, as well as collaboration and coordination.

Primary nursing

In the late 1970s care became more complex, and nurses were dissatisfied with team nursing. In the **primary nursing** model the primary nurse, who can only be an RN, provides direct care for the patient and the family; an associate nurse provides care following the care plan developed by the primary nurse when the primary nurse is not working and assists when the primary nurse is working. The primary nurse needs to be knowledgeable about assigned patients and must maintain a high level of clinical autonomy. When primary nursing was first used and well-accepted it was easier to substitute RNs for other health care providers as cost was not as much of a focus as it is today. Because the shortage began to reoccur and salaries increased, implementing primary nursing became more difficult, and health care cost moved to the top of the concerns. There was, however, no research data to support that primary nursing was more expensive than team nursing, but many hospitals nonetheless felt it was (Gardner, 1991; Gardner & Tilbury, 1991; Glandon, Colbert, & Thomason, 1989; Shukla, 1983). Primary nursing is often viewed as a model in which the primary nurse has to do everything, limiting collaborative or team effort, although it does not have to be implemented in this way.

Second-generation primary nursing clarifies some of the issues about this practice model. One of the critical problems with primary nursing was whether or not it required an all-RN staff, which was thought to increase staff costs. The second-generation view of primary nursing noted that the mix of staff is more important than having an all-RN staff. Another concern with primary nursing was a need to develop a clear definition of 24-hour accountability, which was interpreted by some as 24-hour availability. This, of course, is not a reasonable approach, and it really does not apply to primary nursing. When the primary nurse is not working, the associate nurse provides the care. Primary nursing is a responsibility relationship between the nurse and the patient. The primary nurse is not the only caregiver but does have responsibility for planning the care and ensuring that care outcomes are met. Only registered nurses can be primary nurses. This role and the model requires RNs who are competent and possess leadership skills.

Care and service team models

In the 1980s, **care and service team models** began to replace primary nursing. These models are implemented differently in different hospitals, as is true of most of the models. Key elements of these models are: empowered staff, interdisciplinary collaboration, skilled workers, and a case management approach to patient care—all elements related to the more current views of leadership and management. Care and service teams introduced the different categories of assistive personnel (for example, multiskilled workers, nurse extenders, and UAPs). There has been some disagreement as to whether these new staff member roles were complementary or involved substitution of professional nursing care. **Complementary models** began in 1988 by using nurse extenders, such as a unit assistant, who would be responsible for environmental functions. The nurse would then have more time for direct patient care. Did this reduce costs? Certainly, when nurse positions were changed to nurse extender positions there was some cost reduction; however, some hospitals found that overtime, sick time, and on-call costs rose, particularly with nurse extender staff (Powers, Dickey, & Ford, 1990). Another example was Manthey's (1989) partners-in-practice. Technical assistants signed a partnership agreement to work with an experienced RN. Reduction in costs was initially seen with this model because each partnership could care for the same number of patients as two RNs. Staffing costs, however, continued to increase. Complementary models are not used as much today and have been replaced by substitution models in health care organizations. **Substitution models** tend to use multiskilled technicians to perform select nursing activities. The RNs supervise these activities.

Another more prevalent approach today is the use of **cross-training**. This involves training staff to work in different specialty areas or to perform different tasks. For example, a respiratory therapist may be trained not only to perform typical respiratory therapist tasks but also phlebotomy and basic nursing care. This offers much more flexibility in that staff can fulfill many different needs. They can then be used as staffing adjustments are needed for changes in patient census or acuity. It is critical that this cross-training meet patient needs so that staff will be able to deliver quality, safe care and not feel undue stress while delivering the care. It is also important that state practice act requirements are met, and this is not always easy to accomplish. It requires education staff to provide support, ongoing educational training, and documentation of competencies, as well as management staff who understand which staff members are qualified to move from area to area. Hospitals and other health care organizations are trying to find the best methods for using substitution without compromising quality and safety and yet control costs. As demands change, different models will be required, and nursing leadership to develop these models will be critical.

As with earlier team models, the RN must spend time coordinating care and the work. The focus of the team is on patient-centered care as opposed to the nurse-patient relationship. Case managers may also work with the teams to achieve outcomes, which increases shared accountability. Case management can be viewed as a nursing model when the case manager is a nurse; however, in some organizations nurses are not used as case managers but rather other health care professionals such as social workers are the case managers.

Care management model

The **care management model** focuses on the needs of the integrated delivery system. It has many similarities to case management, in that it includes planning, assessment, and coordination of health services. The patient focus, however, is population-based instead of based on an individual patient. The population might be the entire population, members of a managed care plan, or could be a specific group with similarities, such as patients with diabetes. The goal is to integrate a continuum of clinical services. Care management is not only concerned with medical care but also health promotion and disease prevention, costs, and use of resources. Case management is often used within the care management model. Typical tools used to facilitate care management are clinical pathways, disease management programs, and benchmarking.

Interdisciplinary and transdisciplinary practice models

The **interdisciplinary** practice model focuses on "team members who function independently, providing individualized care without benefit of collaboration with other team members.

While using the interdisciplinary approach, team consultation takes place among team members before care delivery, but after discipline-specific assessment. Responsibilities for care are delegated by specifics for each discipline" (Hebbert, St. Arnaud, & Dharampaul, 1994; as cited in Verdejo, 2001, p. 117).

A newer model of teams has been introduced in some health care organizations, which is a little more radical. This model is different from the interdisciplinary team model in which the "team is comprised of professionals from different disciplines who attempt to overcome traditional discipline boundaries. By crossing and re-crossing boundaries, there is a greater potential for team members to enhance communication and cooperation. This requires a pooling of knowledge and skills and commitment for each team member to teach, learn, and work across boundaries" (Woodruff & McGonigel, 1991; as cited in Verdejo, 2001, p. 117). An example of a transdisciplinary team would include an RN, LPN, and UAP, who would all serve as the primary caregivers on the team. The RN is the team leader or team manager, assuming accountability for the care. Up to this point the team appears to be a "normal" provider team, so how does it become a transdisciplinary team? A transdisciplinary team begins to unfold when other team members are added to the patient delivery team who are far from the traditional view of provider teams. Who might be added? Environmental service workers might assist patients with such activities as meals and ambulation, and ensure that the physical environment is therapeutic for the patient. This would all be supervised by the team leader. Before the environmental service workers are allowed to provide this care they would also receive training. In this model, volunteers, who also receive training, might assist with baths, feed elderly patients, and provide clerical services. "The model allowed a free flow of learned skills, among caregivers, to meet patient's needs. This new model provides new opportunities for staff and strengthens their communication and ability to work as a team. Sharing and exchanging roles within boundaries initially posed an element of distrust" (Verdejo, 2001, p. 117).

It is not difficult to imagine that some staff might be very concerned about boundaries and their jobs in the transdisciplinary model. It steps outside the traditional "way of doing things." This particular organization described by Verdejo (2001) used training and education, rewards, and recognition to promote staff change acceptance. The leader of a team that uses the transdisciplinary care model must be able to "affect change positively, the ability to communicate positively and effectively, the ability to empower staff, the ability to be a positive role model, the ability to be creative, the ability to be a risk taker, the ability to understand today's health care climate with a focus on future change" (Verdejo, 2001, p. 118). However, these competencies are not unique to this model as they are all critical for any leader to be effective in any type of organizational structure today.

YOUR OPINION COUNTS

Find out what others think about this topic. Post your response and check out other opinions.

Nursing care delivery models have changed over the years due to economic factors, staffing shortages or excesses, philosophy and goals, tasks that need to be accomplished, technology, information management, scientific advancements, and new leadership and organization theories and styles. Some models have disappeared for the most part (for example, functional nursing). Another example of a model that is used less often is primary nursing, which was popular in many areas of the country, but is not used as much now, primarily due to costs and the RN shortage. The total patient care or case method, although rarely used, may still be used in critical care settings and home care, although even here there is a movement toward interdisciplinary care. Why have the changes occurred? Some nursing care can be done by others more cost effectively and still be safe, quality care, and staff are available to do these tasks, such as LPNs/LVNs or UAPs. Typically, a hospital will use a combination of models.

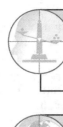

THINK CRITICALLY

Try this exercise to apply what you have learned about this topic.

CURRENT ISSUES

Learn about events around the globe that relate to the chapter content.

Shared governance

"Governance, or self-regulation, has long been recognized as a privilege given to professions that earn the public trust by demonstrating accountability for their specialized practices" (Crocker, Kirkpatrick, & Lentenbrink, 1992; as cited in Maas & Specht, 2001, p. 318). How does this relate to **shared governance**? As a nursing management form, shared governance "legitimizes nurses' decision-making control over the professional practice" (Hess, 1995, p. 14). It thus increases each nurse's influence over the organization, empowering staff. Literature on management, organizations, and professional nursing identifies six dimensions of governance. These dimensions are:

1. Control over professional practice
2. Influence over organizational resources that support practice
3. Formal authority granted by the organization
4. Committee structures that allow participation in decision making
5. Access to information about the organization
6. Ability to set goals and negotiate conflict

These dimensions were used by Hess to develop an instrument to identify and measure how nurses define governance and the distribution of governance. The sample in this study included 1,100 nurses from 10 hospitals (Hess, 1995). Shared governance can be viewed as a management philosophy, a professional practice model, and an accountability model that focuses on staff involvement in decision making, particularly in decisions that affect their practice. In doing this the model provides staff with autonomy and control over implementation of their practice—legitimizing control over their own practice. Nurses in these organizations usually feel less powerless and are more efficient and accountable.

A critical factor in shared governance is that accountability and responsibility are found in the same person. Accountability should rest in the person who is most likely to be the most effective person to complete the function. For individual staff to be accountable and responsible for a function or task, staff must also have the authority to make sure that the right decisions are made. "Within the professional context, then, the statement that the professional is accountable for her practice has meaning only when the necessary authority, which is part of that accountability, is transferred to the individual who assures compliance and who is capable of taking corrective action in the absence of compliance" (Porter-O'Grady & Finnigan, 1984, p. 80).

Shared governance is also a surrogate term for collaboration. "It is an organizational arrangement with a highly participatory staff empowered to function cooperatively with both management and colleagues, and leadership that empowers staff. The organization can be referred to as a learning organization" (Sullivan, 1998, p. 471). Transformational Leadership enhances shared governance. As was discussed in Chapter 1, an important element of leadership is self-awareness, and it is important in shared governance. In this type of organizational arrangement staff feel committed to the organization and consider themselves to be partners in meeting the goals of the organization. Staff should not feel that they are working alone, but rather working in teams and groups to meet specific goals (Sullivan, 1998).

In shared governance nurse managers are typically not directly involved in daily direct patient care, although there are some managers who are still involved in direct care. The typical responsibilities of the nurse manager are staffing, program evaluation, personnel evaluation, coordination, allocation of resources, financial activities, and long-range planning (Porter-O'Grady & Finnigan, 1984). If patient care outcomes are not met, it is the responsibility of the nurse providing the care to address this issue. The nurse manager may become involved, but it is the direct care provider who should take the lead. Clinical practice is the responsibility of the practitioners. When clinical problems occur, the nurse who provides direct care must be the one to solve these problems. The main factor in shared governance is that decision making is spread over a larger number of staff and is decentralized. Nurses are accountable for their practice. Health care organizations that use shared governance must have clear communication processes, or the organization will encounter problems and confusion in the decision-making process.

The key components of shared governance are practice, quality, education, and peer process/governance. How are these accomplished? As with any such change, some organizations change for "real" and others *appear* to change to this model, but in the latter situation very little has really changed in the decision-making process. Shared governance is associated with collaboration, horizontal relationships, and investment and need to be demonstrated in the organization. The change has to be real.

Organizations that use this model have some type of structure related to the shared accountability, such as councils, cabinets, committees, or a combination of these groups that make the decisions. The chain of command is not the same as in traditional organizations. In the shared governance model these groups make decisions about policies, procedures, and other aspects of getting the work done. How might shared governance be implemented?

Health care organizations have been working for several years to create leaner and more effective organizations. As organizations plan major organizational structural changes they need to consider the following elements (Evan et al., 1995).

1. The model selected must be integrated, and every level of decision making should reflect the character of the new care delivery system.
2. The medical staff need to be actively involved in all stages of planning and change. Nursing staff also need to be actively involved throughout the system.
3. Every level of authority in the organization needs to reflect the integration of decision making. "Each level of decision making would need to link with the other to create a seamless framework of restructuring the organizations and its members. The principles of partnership, equity, accountability, and ownership would form the foundation for building the structure" (Evan et al., 1995, p. 20). Applying this approach to an integrated system, Evan and co-authors (1995) describe one health care system's approach to shared governance, an approach that was dependent on various staff councils involved in organizational decision making. The following are examples of the councils used in this system.

   ▪ The Nursing Practice Council primarily focuses on nursing issues. It is composed of nursing representatives.
   ▪ The Physicians' Council focuses on medical staff issues and medical care. It is composed of physician representatives.
   ▪ The Patient Care Council focuses on issues that affect the delivery of patient care. The goal is to increase interdisciplinary decisions regarding patient care. The Patient Care Council has representatives from direct care provider groups including representatives from the Nursing Practice Council and the Physicians' Council.
   ▪ The Operations Council is the hospital-wide management group that is accountable for decisions that relate to the management of the organization's resources such as decisions affecting human resources and skills, support, and system resources. This council also makes decisions about organizational strategies, implementation of change, use of resources, and budgeting. The Operations Council does not make decisions for other councils, but it is responsible for overall review of their decisions so that overall organization goals are met.

■ The Governance Council focuses on the overall organizational direction and the orga-nization's vision and mission. It ensures positive relationships between internal and ex-ternal organizations, the effectiveness of the organization to get the work done, and maintenance of a continuing quality improvement initiative.

This particular organization learned that the following facilitates the shared governance model.

■ Shared governance and shared accountability do not mean management by committee as there must also be accountability in individuals and leaders within the organization.

■ The organization requires a learning curve to develop effective teamwork.

■ The organization requires that structures for group process are incorporated into the council work and decisions.

■ The focus of decisions must continually be directed to the point-of-service in the organization.

■ Roles need to be clearly defined so that accountability will be effective.

■ Staff who do not recognize the need for partnership in collaboration will limit success.

■ Managers who seem to only function in old roles and who worry about the loss of control will hinder successful integration.

■ Decision making and communication that limits or blocks newer strategies for dealing with problems will act to limit success.

■ Departments and professionals or disciplines within the organization who continue to act uni-laterally and are concerned about "turf" will limit integration (Evan et al., 1995, p. 24).

It is important to recognize that to move toward a shared governance model the organization must take a comprehensive change approach and not an incremental approach. All parts of the organization and all staff must be expected to change. This is very difficult to accomplish, but if shared governance is the goal, it is necessary.

Decentralized decision making is now found in many health care organizations, and it is frequently associated with participative management strategies such as shared government. This approach to organizational structure and process is associated with the economy, job sat-isfaction, and retention. It has been shown that job satisfaction influences an individual staff member's commitment to the organization and autonomy influences job satisfaction. "De-centralization has been linked to an increase in autonomy (Cox, 1980), job satisfaction (Przestrzelski, 1987; Ringerman, 1990; Shouksmith, 1994), and retention (Barhyte, Counte, & Christman, 1987; Shoemaker & El-Ahraf, 1983). Highly committed employees tend to per-form better than those who are not committed to the organization (Angle & Perry, 1981; Zahra, 1985). For decentralization to be effective staff must have autonomy to make deci-sions. All of this is intimately connected with shared governance. It requires staff who are committed to the organization's values and goals and demonstrate this by working to meet the goals.

Major studies that have focused on shared governance have highlighted critical outcomes that result from this practice model (Buckles-Prince, 1997; Hastings & Waltz, 1995; Kennerly, 1996; Lengacher et al., 1994; Radice, 1994; Upenieks, 2000; Westrope et al., 1995). Some of these outcomes are:

1. Nursing-based practice model had a significant effect on job satisfaction, task require-ments, and autonomy
2. Strong positive relation between job satisfaction and empowerment
3. Improved job satisfaction and organizational commitment, control, responsibility, praise, and recognition after implementation of the nursing-based practice model
4. Control over practice and opportunity to make decisions and enhanced job satisfaction and organizational commitment
5. Job satisfaction, turnover, and perceived effectiveness were not significantly influenced by the shared governance model; findings did suggest that the model did enhance team functioning
6. Significantly improved reliability with job satisfaction; also, enhanced awareness and em-powerment (Upenieks, 2000, p. 332)

CURRENT ISSUES

Learn about events around the globe that relate to the chapter content.

BENCHMARKS

Now let's take a moment to test your knowledge of the concepts you have studied in this section.

Organizational analysis

After reviewing some of the critical aspects related to organizations in this chapter, how would one go about analyzing an organization to better understand or assess its functioning? The following might be included in this analysis.

■ **Integration of vision and mission into organizational structure**

The vision and mission statements are the driving forces behind all decisions, or should be. They provide critical information about the organization's values and philosophy. It is also important to remember that many organizations have beautifully written vision and mission statements and yet never really make them come alive. When an organization is analyzed, the important issue is whether or not the vision and mission match what the organization and its staff actually do.

■ **Description of corporate culture, historical determinants**

The culture of a health care organization and its history have a major impact on the way that staff interact, communicate, work as teams, and feel rewarded and recognized or feel neglected. It also affects organization outcomes. The community in which the organization must survive also affects the organization's culture (see Chapter 17).

■ **Structural design of the organization**

Organizational structure varies, and structure affects how organizations communicate, work together, solve problems, or do not solve problems, which represent the organization's process. The structure of health care organizations is changing, and some of these efforts are resulting in positive outcomes.

■ **Decision-making patterns**

How does the organization handle decision making? This can be highly variable from one organization to another and even within an organization. Some nursing leaders and other organizational leaders have greater skill in this area than other leaders. All organizations need improvement in decision making. Do staff feel that decisions are handled well? Is there staff input? Is shared governance used and how effective is it? What is the response to accountability? How empowered are the staff (see Chapter 2)?

■ **Communication patterns**

Communication runs an organization. How is communication conducted? Who communicates with whom? What are the formal and informal aspects? How successful is communication? How is technology used? Do staff feel they are listened to when they speak up? How can it be improved? How are interdisciplinary, intradepartmental, and interdepartmental communication described? How have the communication patterns affected the change process? How does the health care organization communicate with the community and with other health care organizations (see Chapter 4)?

■ **Alignment of goals across subsystems**

Integrative systems and multiorganizations are more common organization structures today. Subsystems, whether they be subsystems of a multiorganization with multiple entities (one hospital in a system that has several hospitals) or the subsystems of one organization (departments and services) must be aligned. If goals of the subsystems are not in alignment with overall organizational goals, there will be conflicts, and it will be difficult to determine organization outcomes. This does not, however, mean that subsystems might not propose different goals; however, they then must convince the overall organization that this change is appropriate.

■ **Incorporation of quality and safety as a value**

There is no doubt that quality and safety are critical issues today in health care. All health care organizations are involved in quality improvement; however, some are much more successful than others. In analyzing an organization, its quality improvement effort needs to be assessed. When an organization's quality and safety are assessed, much can be learned about the organization's vision and mission, goals and objectives, structure and process, communication, decision making, utilization of resources, and what is really important to the organization. Is the organization using evidence-based practice? The key question is what are its outcomes (see Chapter 17)?

■ **Utilization of human resources**

Clearly, utilization of human resources is critical today. Some organizations are just sitting around worrying about the number of empty positions, but others are quite active in trying to find creative solutions. Understanding human resource needs and planning to meet them is a daily organizational concern (see Chapter 12).

■ **Effective financial and information infrastructure planning**

As organizations are analyzed, consideration must be given to their financial status and effective financial planning. Outcomes are always tied to financial issues and cannot be ignored. All health care organizations and providers are struggling with reimbursement issues and how these issues affect practice (see Chapter 14).

■ **Information management**

Information within the organization is also a critical component. What information is available? Who has it? How is it collected? Is it reliable and valid? How is the information used? How has technology impacted the collection and use of information? Is the organization in compliance with legal requirements (HIPAA)? All are critical questions. Throughout this text there is recognition of information and its importance (see Chapter 16).

■ **Organizational responsiveness to change**

Change is a running thread throughout all of the discussions in this text. Organizations that cannot change effectively will struggle, and many will disappear. Change cannot be avoided so the best approach is to learn how to effectively adapt—making sound decisions based on sound evidence and data. Health care organizations are at different stages of development in how they respond to change. Analyzing an organization should include an assessment of the organization's response to change. Leaders have a major impact on the organization's ability to change effectively (see Chapter 2).

■ **Organizational readiness for the multicultural world**

The United States and most of its communities are finding that they are now multicultural communities. Providers are caring for patients from many different cultures, and this affects their care. Staff who come from many different cultures are more common, and this impacts the organization's communication, staff relationships, problem solving and decision making, and morale. The United States is confronting many critical issues related to access of care and lack of insurance, and much of this has an impact on minority cultures (see Chapter 17).

■ **Effective leadership**

Effective leadership is critical to the success of any organization. As organizations are analyzed, its leaders should be identified and assessed. What is the leadership style? Does the leadership provide what is needed to help the organization succeed (see Chapter 1)?

■ **Assessment of future organizational challenges and opportunities**

Future needs should be considered in the assessment of an organization. Is the organization preparing for the future? Does it have a strategic plan? What is included in the plan? Is the plan reasonable? What is the process the organization uses to cope with future organization challenges and opportunities? Are the challenges and opportunities identified?

Chapter Wrap-Up

Now that you've reached the end of the chapter, you may wish to explore the concepts you've been reading about in greater detail, or test yourself to see how well you've comprehended the material.

SUMMARY AND APPLICATIONS

- Summary
- Practice Quiz
- Key Terms
- Tying It All Together

- Experiential Exercises
- Case
- Links

REFERENCES

Alidina, S., & Funke-Furber, J. (1988). First line nurse managers: Optimizing the span of control. *Journal of Nursing Administration, 8*(5), 34–39.

American Nurses Association. (1995). *Nursing's social policy statement.* Washington, DC: American Nurse's Publishing.

American Organization of Nurse Executives. (1996). The evolving role of the registered nurse. Retrieved on July 31, 2002, from www.aone.org/practiceresearch/evolvingroleregisterednurse.htm.

Angle, H., & Perry, J. (1981). An empirical assessment of organizational commitment and organizational effectiveness. *Administrative Science Quarterly, 26,* 1–14.

Barhyte, D., Counte, M., & Christman, L. (1987). The effects of decentralization on nurses' job attendance behaviors. *Nursing Administration Quarterly, 11*(4), 37–46.

Buckles-Prince, S. (1997). Shared governance: Sharing power and opportunity. *Journal of Nursing Administration, 27*(3), 28–35.

Campbell, C., Schmitz, H., & Waller, L. (1998). *Financial management in a managed care environment.* Albany, NY: Delmar Publishers.

Cox, C. (1980). Decentralization: Uniting authority and responsibility. *Supervisor Nurse, 11*(3), 25–38.

Crocker, D., Kirkpatrick, R., & Lentenbrink, L. (1992). Shared governance and collective bargaining: Integration, not confrontation. In T. Porter-O'Grady (Ed.), *Implementing shared governance: Creating a professional organization.* St. Louis, MO: Mosby.

Crow, G. (2002). The relationship between trust, social capital, and organizational success. *Nursing Administration Quarterly, 26*(3), 1–11.

Dessler, G. (2002). *Management.* Upper Saddle River, NJ: Prentice Hall.

Evan, K., et al. (1995). Whole systems shared governance. *Journal of Nursing Administration, 25*(5), 18–27.

Finkelman, A. (1996). *Psychiatric nursing administration manual.* Gaithersburg, MD: Aspen Publishers, Inc.

Finkelman, A. (2001). The health care system. In M. Nies & M. McEwen (Eds.), *Community health nursing* (3rd ed., pp. 183–203). Philadelphia: W.B. Saunders Company.

Fitzpatrick, M., McElroy, M., & DeWoody, S. (2001). Building a strong nursing organization in a merged service line structure. *Journal of Nursing Administration, 31*(1), 24–32.

Gardner, K. (1991). A summary of findings of a five year comparison study of primary and team nursing. *Nursing Research, 40*(2), 113–117.

Gardner, K., & Tilbury, M. (1991). A longitudinal analysis of primary and team nursing. *Nursing Economics, 9*(2), 97–104.

Glandon, G., Colbert, K., & Thomason, M. (1989). Nursing delivery models and RN mix: Cost implications. *Nursing Management, 20*(5), 30–33.

Hastings, C., & Waltz, C. (1995). Assessing the outcomes of professional practice redesign. *Journal of Nursing Administration, 25*(3), 34–42.

Hebbert, E., St. Arnaud, S., & Dharampaul, S. (1994). Nurses' satisfaction with the patient care team. *Canadian Journal of Rehabilitation, 8,* 87–88.

Hess, R. G. (1995). Shared governance nursing's 20th-century tower of Babel. *Journal of Nursing Administration, 25*(5), 14–17.

Ingersoll, G., Kirsch, J., Merk, S., & Lightfoot, J. (2000). Relationship of organizational culture and readiness for change to employee commitment to the organization. *Journal of Nursing Administration, 30*(1), 11–20.

Kennerly, S. (1996). Effects of shared governance on perceptions of work and work environment. *Nursing Economics, 14*(2), 111–115.

Kolb, D., Rubin, I., & McIntyre, S. (1984). *Organizational psychology*. Upper Saddle River, NJ: Prentice Hall.

Leitch, D. (1999). The administrative support team: Specialized support. *Journal of Nursing Administration, 29*(9), 9–11.

Lengacher, C., et al. (1994). Effects of the partners in care practices model on nursing outcomes. *Nursing Economics, 12*(6), 300–307.

Maas, M., & Specht, J. (2001). Shared governance models in nursing: What is shared, who governs, and who benefits. In J. Dochterman & H. Grace (Eds.), *Current issues in nursing* (6th ed., pp. 318–329). St. Louis: Mosby, Inc.

Manthey, M. (1989). Practice partnerships: The newest concept in care delivery. *Journal of Nursing Administration, 19*(2), 33–35.

Milgram, L., Spector, A., & Treger, M. (1999). *Managing smart*. Houston, TX: Cashman Dudley.

Porter-O'Grady, T., & Finnigan, S. (1984). *Shared governance for nursing*. Gaithersburg, MD: Aspen Publishers Inc.

Powers, P., Dickey, D., & Ford, A. (1990). Evaluating RN/co-worker model. *Journal of Nursing Administration, 20*(3), 11–15.

Przestrzelski, D. (1987). Decentralization: Are nurses satisfied? *Journal of Nursing Administration, 17*(11), 23–28.

Radice, B. (1994). The relationship between nurse empowerment in the hospital work environment and job satisfaction: A pilot study. *Journal of the New York State Nursing Association, 25*(2), 14–17.

Ringerman, E. (1990). Characteristics associated with decentralization experienced by nurse managers. *Western Journal of Nursing Research, 12*(3), 336–346.

Ritter-Teitel, J. (2002). The impact of restructuring on professional nursing practice. *Journal of Nursing Administration, 32*(1), 31–41.

Robbins, S., & Decenzo, D. (2001). *Fundamentals of management*. Upper Saddle River, NJ: Prentice Hall.

Scott, R., Aiken, L., Mechanic, D., & Moravcsik, J. (1995). Organizational aspects of caring. *Milbank Quarterly, 73*(1), 77–95.

Shoemaker, H., & El-Ahraf, A. (1983). Decentralization of nursing service management and its impact on job satisfaction. *Nursing Administration Quarterly, 7*(2), 69–76.

Shouksmith, G. (1994). Variables related to organizational commitment in health professionals. *Psychological Reports, 74*, 707–711.

Shukla, R. (1983). All-RN model of care delivery: A cost benefit evaluation. *Inquiry, 20*, 173–184.

Simpson, R. (1999). Changing world, changing systems: Why managed health care demands information technology. *Nursing Administration Quarterly, 23*(2), 86–88.

Spitzer, R. (2001). A case for conceptual competency in an integrated delivery system. *Nursing Administration Quarterly, 25*(4), 79–82.

Steinhauer, J. (2001, March 14). Hospital mergers aren't living happily ever after. *New York Times*, A1, A22.

Sullivan, E. (2004). *Becoming influential*. Upper Saddle River, NJ: Prentice Hall.

Sullivan, T. (1998). Transformational Leadership. In T. Sullivan (Ed.), *Collaboration: A health perspective* (pp. 467–497). New York: McGraw Hill.

Tuck, I., Harris, L. H., & Baliko, B. (2000). Values expressed in philosophies of nursing services. *Journal of Nursing Administration, 30*(4), 180–184.

Upenieks, V. (2000). The relationship of nursing practice models and job satisfaction outcomes. *Journal of Nursing Administration, 30*(6), 330–335.

Verdejo, T. (2001). Leading into the 21st century: Clarifying the vision and leading toward success. *Seminars for Nurse Managers, 9*(2), 115–118.

Westrope, R., Vaughn, L., Bott, M., & Taunton, R. L. (1995). Shared governance: From vision to reality. *Journal of Nursing Administration, 25*(12), 45–54.

Woodruff, G., & McGonigel, M. (1991). *Disabilities and gifted education*. Reston, VA: Council for Exceptional Children.

Zahra, S. (1985). Determinants of organizational commitment in a health care setting. *Journal of Health and Human Resources Administration, 8*, 188–208.

ADDITIONAL READINGS

Acorn, S., Ratner, P., & Crawford, M. (1997). Decentralization as a determinant of autonomy, job satisfaction, and organizational commitment among nurse managers. *Nursing Research, 46*(1), January/February, 52–58.

Coughlin, C. (2001). Care centered organizations, Part 2. *Journal of Nursing Administration, 31*(3), 113–120.

Creamer, J., Gaynor, S., Verdin, J., & Bultema, J. (1999). Building a 21st century facility. *Nursing Management, 30*(7), 28–30.

Curtin, L. (2001). Healing health care's organizational culture. *Seminars for Nurse Managers, 9*(4), 218–227.

De Ruiter, H., & Saphiere, D. (2001). Nurse leaders as cultural bridges. *Journal of Nursing Administration, 31*(9), 418–423.

Dixon, D. (1999). Achieving results through Transformational Leadership. *Journal of Nursing Administration, 29*(12), 17–21.

Dunham-Taylor, J. (2000). Nurse executive transformational leadership found in participative organizations. *Journal of Nursing Administration, 30*(5), 241–250.

Felgen, J. (2000). The patient as CEO passion in practice. *Journal of Nursing Administration, 30*(10), 453–456.

Ficaro, C., & Elberth, W. (2001). Reengineering patient care: A multidisciplinary approach intervention. *Seminars for Nurse Managers, 9*(2), 121–125.

Fisher, K., & Bonalumi, N. (2000). Lessons learned from the merger of two emergency departments. *Journal of Nursing Administration, 30*(12), 577–579.

Flarey, D. (1997). Managed care changing the way we practice. *Journal of Nursing Administration, 27*(7/8), 16–20.

Green, G. (2000). Clinical service lines bring patients into focus. *Nursing Management, 31*(3), 40–43.

Haigh, C. (2002). Using Chaos theory: The implications for nursing. *Journal of Advanced Nursing, 37*(5), 462–469.

Hepner, L., & Hopkins, L. (2000). Partnership 2000: A journey to the 21st century. *Nursing Administration Quarterly, 24*(2), 34–44.

Jones, K. R., & Redman, R. W. (2000). Organizational culture and work redesign: Experiences in three organizations. *Journal of Nursing Administration, 30*(12), 604–610.

Knight, K. (2004). AACN Model creates synergy in Indianapolis, *Nursing Spectrum/Midwestern Edition, 5*(5), 28–29.

Kotter, J. (1996). *Leading change.* Boston: Harvard Business School Press.

Malloch, K. (1999). A total healing environment: The Yavapai Regional Medical Center story. *Journal of Healthcare Management, 44*(5), 495–512.

Malloch, K. (2000). Health models for organizations: Description, measurement, and outcomes. *Journal of Healthcare Management, 45*(5), 332–345.

Marr, T. (1996). The healing community. *Physician Executive, 22*(6), 24–27.

McCullough, C., & Wille, R. (2001). Healing environments. In C. McCullough (Ed.), *Creating responsive solutions to healthcare change* (pp. 109–134). Indianapolis, IN: Center Nursing Press.

Miller, E. (2002). Shared governance and performance improvement: A new opportunity to build trust in a restructured health care system. *Nursing Administration Quarterly, 26*(3), 60–66.

Miller, J., Galloway, M., Coughlin, C., & Brennan, E. (2001). Care-centered organizations, Part 1: Nursing governance. *Journal of Nursing Administration, 31*(2), 67–73.

Moore, N., & Komras, H. (1993). *Patient-focused healing: Integrating caring and curing in healthcare.* San Francisco: Jossey-Bass.

Parker, M., & Gadbois, S. (2000). Building community in the healthcare workplace, Part 3. *Journal of Nursing Administration, 30*(10), 466–473.

Pinkerton, S. (1999). Integrated delivery systems: The chief nursing officers. *Nursing Economics, 17*(4), 219–221.

Porter-O'Grady, T. (2001). Is shared governance still relevant? *Journal of Nursing Administration, 31*(10), 468–473.

Porter-O'Grady, T. (1999). Quantum leadership: New roles for a new age. *Journal of Nursing Administration, 29*(10), 37–42.

Salimbene, S. (1999). Cultural competence: A priority for performance improvement action. *Journal of Nursing Administration, 13*(3), 23–35.

Seago, J. (2000). Registered nurses, unlicensed assistive personnel, and organizational culture in hospitals. *Journal of Nursing Administration, 30*(5), 278–286.

Shea-Lewis, A. (2002). Workforce diversity in healthcare. *Journal of Nursing Administration, 32*(1), 6–7.

Sleutel, M. (2000). Climate, culture, context, or work environment? Organizational factors that influence nursing practice. *Journal of Nursing Administration, 30*(2), 53–58.

Sorrells-Jones, J. (1999). The role of the chief nurse executive in the knowledge-intense organization of the future. *Nursing Administration Quarterly, 23*(3), 17–25.

Sullivan, E., & Decker, P. (2001). *Effective leadership and management in nursing.* Upper Saddle River, NJ: Prentice Hall.

Tornabeni, J. (2001). The competency game: My take on what it really takes to lead. *Nursing Administration Quarterly, 25*(4), 1–13.

Trofino, A. (2000). Transformational Leadership: Moving total quality management to world-class organizations. *International Nursing Review, 47*, 232–242.

Trossman, S. (2002a). Cultural crossroads. How nurses, healthcare meet the challenge. *American Nurse, 34*(4), 1, 16–18.

Trossman, S. (2002b). Envisioning a brighter future. *American Journal of Nursing, 102*(7), 65–66.

Ulrich, R. (1992). How design impacts wellness. *Healthcare Forum Journal, 20*, 20–25.

Weaver, D., & Sorrells-Jones, J. (1999). Knowledge workers and knowledge-intense organizations, Part 2: Designing and managing for productivity. *Journal of Nursing Administration, 29*(9), 19–25.

Webb, S., Price, S., & Coeling, H. (1996). Valuing authority/responsibility relationships. *Journal of Nursing Administration, 26*(2), 28–33.

Wells, G. (1990). Influence of organizational structure on nurse manager job satisfaction. *Nursing Administration Quarterly, 14*(4), 1–8.

Wolf, G. (2000). Vision 2000: The transformation of professional practice. *Nursing Administration Quarterly, 24*(2), 45–51.

Woods, D. (2002). Realizing your marketing influence, Part 1: Meeting patient needs through collaboration. *Journal of Nursing Administration, 32*(4), 189–195.

Acute Care Organizations: An Example of a Health Care Organization

CHAPTER OUTLINE

MediaLink
www.prenhall.com/finkelman

The Interactive Exercises for this chapter can be found in the OneKey course at www.prenhall.com/finkelman.
Click on Chapter 6 to select from the following activities: Test Your Understanding, Benchmarks, Current
Issues, Your Opinion Counts, Think Critically, and Summary and Applications.

What's Ahead

This chapter explores acute care hospitals, an example of a health care delivery organization. The health care delivery system depends more on community focused services; however, since most new graduates begin their careers in hospitals this is the appropriate place to begin to understand health care delivery settings. Though hospitals continue to be the centers of health care, a majority of health services may eventually be community focused. Despite this possibility, it is important to understand hospitals and how they relate to community health.

Hospital management is more complex than most businesses. As was discussed in Chapter 3, the hospital meets the criteria for an organization. It has a purpose or goals, people who work for it, and a systematic structure. Many hospitals continue to maintain a bureaucratic organization even if this is not the most effective type. Other hospitals, however, are undergoing restructuring and reengineering and thus changing into different types of organizations. Newhouse and Mills (2002) believe it is important for nurses to be informed about hospital organization factors and changes for the following reasons: (a) nurses coordinate the care of inpatients and play a major role in promoting continuity of care, (b) nursing is the largest labor source of health care services within the acute care organization, and (c) nursing is affected by each corporate decision to provide or discontinue selected services (p. ix).

This text also recognizes the critical need for nurses to understand some important elements related to hospital structure and functions to enable them to be more effective as care providers within this health care setting. The first part of the chapter focuses on the typical hospital organization and some issues related to it, and the second part discusses important information about acute care nursing services by exploring the Magnet Nursing Services Organization.

OBJECTIVES

Before you begin, take a moment to familiarize yourself with the key objectives of this chapter.

- Describe the development of U.S. hospitals and the role they play in the health care delivery system.

- Identify the key methods for classifying hospitals.

- Define the key departments found in most hospitals.

- Discuss the use of committees by describing the work done by a policy and procedure committee as an example of committees.

- Describe major changes that are occurring in hospitals and their impact on nursing.

- Describe the Magnet Recognition Program, its history, its process, and the impact it has had on nursing.

- Discuss why each of the forces of magnetism would be important to new graduates as well as to any nurse considering a job change.

TEST YOUR UNDERSTANDING

Before we begin our exploration of this chapter, take a short "warm-up" test to see what you know about this topic.

Development of U.S. Hospitals

The acute care hospital has long been the major focus in the U.S. health care delivery system. What is a **hospital**? This might sound like a strange question; however, the definition contains important descriptive criteria. It is an organization whose primary purpose is to deliver patient care, diagnostic and therapeutic, for certain medical conditions. These medical conditions may be highly specialized, such as those found in psychiatric or rehabilitation hospitals, or in general, such as a hospital that provides a variety of services, the general acute care hospital. There is an organized medical staff, and continuous nursing services are provided under the supervision of registered nurses, which is a critical component of 24-hour care. All hospitals must follow certain laws and regulations: federal, state, and local. **Accreditation,** which is discussed in Chapter 16, is also a criteria used to describe a hospital. From this description several critical criteria can be identified.

- Organization with purpose
- Medical and nursing care and professionals who must meet their own professional requirements and standards
- Standards established by laws, regulations, and accreditation
- A complex organization
- The consumer must play a role (see Chapter 11)

The health care system's goals are to provide services that focus on: (a) health promotion and illness prevention, (b) diagnosis and treatment, and (c) rehabilitation and health restoration and, if required, support during the dying process. To accomplish these goals the system is organized by the complexity of the services required to meet each of the goals: primary, secondary, and tertiary care. Some hospitals only focus on one of these goals (for example, a rehabilitative hospital or a hospice focusing on goal 3); however, others might meet all three goals. Hospital care is primarily secondary care, although other services related to primary care (such as clinic services and wellness programs) are also services hospitals might offer, as well as tertiary care, which may be found in a hospital organization (for example, when a hospital offers a hospital-based hospice program or a rehabilitation unit). The U.S. health care system is a multiprovider system, as is illustrated by the number of different providers identified in Box 6-1. These were discussed in Chapter 5.

BOX 6-1   U.S. multiprovider health care delivery system.

Acute care hospitals

Specialty hospitals

Physician offices: primary care and specialty

Advanced practice nurses and nurse midwives: practices

Clinics: Hospital and community

Dental offices/clinics

Urgent care centers

Ambulatory care centers
   (e.g., one-day surgery centers, diagnostic centers)

Industrial clinics as part of occupational health

Extended care facilities, including skilled nursing
   (intermediate care) and extended care (long-term care)

Retirement and assisted-living centers

Rehabilitation centers

Home health agencies

Hospice services

Psychiatric services and community mental health centers

Substance abuse treatment centers (inpatient and outpatient)

School health clinics

Public health includes government agencies, federal, state, and local, funded primarily by
   taxes and administered by elected or appointed officials.

Source: Author.

Hospitals can be described in many different ways, and are constantly changing. Some terms that are helpful to understand when trying to define "hospital" are: system, network, and organized delivery system, which describe organizational arrangements (Newhouse & Mills, 2002). A **hospital** system refers to a corporation that owns or manages health facilities, often using vertical integration as was described in Chapter 5. A **network** differs from a system in that it is a number of health care facilities that agree to deliver specific services, although each facility remains as an independent organization. The organized delivery system can be found in some communities, and it "provides or arranges to provide a coordinated continuum of services to a defined population and is willing to be held clinically and fiscally accountable for the outcomes and the health status of the population service" (Newhouse & Mills, 2002, p. 3).

As hospital organizations have been changing, mergers have become more common. A merger occurs when two or more organizations come together to form one organization. This is a challenge for all of the organizations and their staff. Organizations have cultures, and when a merger is created the various organizational cultures merge to form one organization. Otherwise, the organizations and their staff will continue to view themselves as separate organizations rather than one organization. (See Chapter 17 on organization culture.) The community also will need to change its view of the health care organizations, recognizing that individual organizations no longer exist and the merged organization is one organization. None of this is easy to accomplish, and some attempts at mergers have not been successful. Barriers to success are poor planning, lack of collaboration, territoriality, ineffective communication systems, lack of organization-wide leadership, and loss of control. All of this has a major impact on the organizations' nurses. Much work needs to be done to develop one organization. How this is accomplished and how much independence each organization in the merger can have is highly variable.

Acute care organization and governance

As acute care hospitals are described, three elements are important to consider: the system, the patient, and the outcome (Newhouse & Mills, 2002).

■ System characteristics include organizational, structural, and patient-focused characteristics. Each of these characteristics affect outcomes. Examples of **organizational characteristics** are governance (for-profit or not-for-profit), number of beds, teaching status, urban-rural location, technology level, **patient census** (both number admitted and length-of-stay), and operating expenses (The Nurse Executive Center, 1999). **Structural characteristics** are teaching status, urban density, and profit status (Van Servellen & Schultz, 1999). **Patient**-focused health care organizations are described by percentage of board-certified physicians, RN hours per patient day, volume of cases, technological availability, and operating expense (Van Servellen & Schultz, 1999).

■ In addition to these characteristics, some of which overlap, it is important to remember that each patient comes with individual characteristics such as age, gender, race, severity, illness, and health history, and experiences with the health care system, probably some of which are positive and some of which are negative.

■ All of these characteristics can affect outcomes, which "is the result of the affect of the system, patient characteristics, and intervention" (Newhouse & Mills, 2002, p. 13).

Levels of management in acute care include top management, middle management, and first-line management. Every hospital has a board of trustees or board of directors, which acts as the governing body. This board is responsible for developing the organization's mission and goals, as well as setting the overall hospital policies. The board ensures that the hospital provides the services that have been designated by the board. Typically, these boards are made up of community and business leaders. Top management includes the chief executive officer (CEO) of the hospital, who reports to the board and is hired by the board, and other key management staff. The chief nurse executive (CNE), who in some hospitals also reports to the board but more typically to the CEO, is also part of top management. The board has great influence over the functions and management of the hospital, and thus has a great impact on nurses and nursing care. It is important for the CNE to understand the board and develop strong communication mechanisms to get information to the board in order to ensure that patient care is of the highest quality and that nursing staff are supported. The chief financial officer (CFO), another member of top management, is responsible for the organization's financial management. Other high-level administrative staff may also be considered top management, but this can vary from hospital to hospital. If it is a hospital that has a CNE, the hospital may also have a director of nursing who may be included in middle or in top management. In this case the CNE may be responsible for more than just nursing. For example, the CNE may also be responsible for medical records, social services, laboratory, and so on. The inclusion of other services or departments can vary from hospital to hospital. Supervisory staff are middle management, while nurse managers are examples of first-line managers. Coordinating the work of the three levels is key to an effective organization. Many organizations are flattening their administrative or management staff levels by eliminating layers. When this occurs, there may be fewer than the three layers or levels described here.

The medical staff organization has great power in any hospital. This is a formal organization of the medical staff who provide services in the hospital, and it is part of the total hospital organization. These physicians may be on staff (paid by the hospital) or may have admitting privileges (which allows them to admit their patients and provide care within the hospital, although they are not paid directly by the hospital). In order to become a member of the medical staff, physicians have to complete a formal appointment process, which is described in the medical staff organization bylaws. References and credentials are checked as well as information about involvement in malpractice suits. "Credentialing and privileging are the most direct means for an organization to ensure that patients receive quality care from skilled practitioners" (Payne, 1999, p. 8). What is the difference between these two processes? **Credentialing** focuses on ensuring that practitioners meet certain qualifications. This is done by obtaining, verifying, and assessing qualifications. **Privileging** occurs when a health care organization "authorizes a specific scope and content of patient-care services for a licensed independent practitioner based on evaluation of the individual's credentials and performance" (Payne, 1999, p. 8). There would be a clear statement of what the physician is allowed to do within the hospital. For example, a physician who was not a qualified surgeon would not be allowed to perform surgery. The Joint Commission on Accreditation of Healthcare Organizations (JCAHO) requires that independent licensed practitioners go through these two processes. Advanced nurse practitioners (ANPs) and nurse midwives who want to practice and admit to a hospital must also go through this process. If the hospital is a university medical center, the medical school faculty also serve on the medical staff. House staff, interns, residents, and fellows can be found in all types of hospitals, not just university medical centers, but they provide care as "students," not as official members of the medical staff. They are paid by the hospital.

The medical staff is typically organized by committees, such as medical records, credentials, utilization review, infection control, and quality improvement committees. The committees focus on these areas to ensure that the patient care goals are met. A medical director or, in some hospitals, the chief of staff is usually elected by the medical staff to serve as their leader. In some hospitals, however, the medical director may be selected by the board of directors. Larger hospitals may also have service leaders or department heads for departments such as surgery, medicine, pediatrics, obstetrics/gynecology, psychiatry, emergency, pathology, and radiology. It is critical that the CNE develop a strong, positive relationship with the medical staff organization and its leaders. Collaborating together will allow for greater, positive outcomes for patients and nursing staff.

Although the formal organization is very important in a hospital, so is the informal organization. Recognizing the informal organization and using it to the fullest to reach desired outcomes is a sign of an effective leader. Nurses at all levels can benefit from a greater understanding of "what makes the organization run" other than the formal structure. There are many times when it is the informal organization that actually gets the job done, as sometimes the formal organization interferes or puts up barriers to effective functioning. Chapters 1 and 5 discussed leadership and organization in more detail, and this content is certainly applicable to this chapter's content.

Classification of hospitals

Hospitals are classified according to the following characteristics: public access, ownership, number of beds, length-of-stay, accreditation, licensure, teaching, vertical integration, and multi-hospital system organizations (Wolper & Pena, 1999).

■ **Public access**

Public access characteristics describe hospitals as community or non-community hospitals, determined by the amount of access that the public has to the hospital. Community hospitals are nonfederal, short-term, or other special hospitals, which the public may use. Non-community hospitals are characterized as federal, long-term, hospital units of institutions (prison hospitals, college infirmaries, psychiatric hospitals), hospitals for chronic diseases, (for mentally retarded, alcoholism, and other chemical dependency problems), or psychiatric/mental health.

■ **Ownership**

The owner of a hospital provides critical information about the organization—particularly who makes decisions and what is done with the profits. All hospitals need to make a profit to maintain financial stability and to maintain their physical plant and equipment. The following are different perspectives of ownership.

1. The **not-for-profit** hospital is funded by reimbursement, just as all hospitals are, and also with donations and endowments. It is important to remember that this type of hospital must also make a profit. The key difference with investor-owned (for-profit) hospitals is that the not-for-profit hospital invests its profits back into the hospital, and none of the profit is given to others outside the organization.

2. The **investor-owned or proprietary** organization is owned and administered by corporations who are shareholders or stockholders and own stock in the corporation. The hospital is responsible to the shareholders, and the shareholders expect that the organization will make a profit so that they can make money on their investment. As is true of hospitals in general, this type of organization will also have a board of directors or trustees that reports to the shareholders. This is the fastest growing type of ownership. Typically, the corporation is a large, national corporation. Examples are Hospital Corporation of America and Tenet. They own hospitals and other types of health care provider settings throughout the country, requiring them to meet their corporate standards and to provide profit for the corporation.

3. **Faith-based hospitals** are owned and administered by a faith-based group such as Catholic hospitals, Jewish hospitals, and so on. They maintain not-for-profit status.

4. **Government hospitals** are owned by the government. Examples of these hospitals are military hospitals; state psychiatric hospitals; hospitals owned and operated by states, counties, or cities; Veteran's Administration hospitals; National Institutes of Health Clinical Center; and hospitals on Indian Reservations, which are administered by the U.S. Public Health Service. Government hospitals maintain not-for-profit status.

■ **Number of beds**

The number of beds is another hospital characteristic that is considered. Typical bed number ranges that are used to classify hospitals are: 6 to 24, 25 to 49, 50 to 99, 100 to 199, 200 to 299, 300 to 499, 400 to 499, and 500 or more (Wolper & Pena, 1999).

■ **Length-of-stay**

Length-of-stay (LOS) is also used to classify hospitals. A hospital's average length-of-stay is used to determine if a hospital has a short-term (average LOS of less than 30 days) or long-term stay (average LOS of over 30 days). Length-of-stay has been decreasing for acute care hospitals and specialty hospitals such as psychiatric hospitals. This has been affected by pressure from managed care organizations/insurers, technological advances, scientific advancement, and more effective drugs and treatment, leading to more care provided in the community.

CURRENT ISSUES

Learn about events around the globe that relate to the chapter content.

■ **Accreditation**

Accreditation is another hospital characteristic, as hospitals are classified as accredited or non-accredited. JCAHO, which is discussed in more detail in Chapter 16, is the voluntary accreditation organization that accredits hospitals and other health care organizations. Hospital accreditation has been in existence for 60 years. A health care organization uses its accreditation status in marketing and communicating to consumers that it provides quality care, though accreditation does not guarantee quality. Managed care organizations (MCOs)/insurers want their members to receive care in accredited hospitals. For a school of nursing or medicine to use a hospital as a clinical site for students, it must be accredited.

■ **Licensure**

In addition to accreditation, licensure and certification are also important. Licensure of hospitals is done by states when the hospital meets certain state standards and requirements. To provide services a hospital must be licensed, although it does not necessarily have to be accredited (Shi & Singh, 1998). For a hospital to receive Medicare and Medicaid reimbursement it must be certified or given authority to provide this care by the Centers for Medicare and Medicaid Services (CMS), and it must be accredited. Accreditation, licensure, and certification all involve meeting specified standards and some type of inspection. This can consume much staff time and is costly, but it cannot be avoided.

■ **Teaching**

Hospitals are also classified as teaching or non-teaching. **Teaching hospitals** offer residency programs for physicians. These residency programs vary in size. Hospitals may be university-affiliated (with a major connection to a university) or freestanding (not connected to a university but still with a residency program). The latter might be a community hospital that has house staff or residents on their staff.

■ **Vertical integration**

Vertical integration is another hospital characteristic that considers whether or not a hospital focuses on primary, secondary, or tertiary care services. To be classified as a primary care hospital the hospital provides services on "an as needed basis to the public" (Wolper & Pena, 1999, p. 403). These services are part of a comprehensive health care system, providing outpatient or ambulatory care services. Secondary care facilities require greater sophistication in terms of equipment and skills. Examples are acute care hospitals and specialized outpatient services such as ambulatory surgical centers. Tertiary level hospitals require even greater skills and equipment, and are much more specialized in need. Examples of this level are university medical centers and specialty hospitals such as pediatric hospitals and burn centers.

■ **Multihospital system**

A multihospital system is a newer characteristic that is used to classify hospitals. "The previous cottage industry of individual, freestanding hospitals has become a complex web of systems, alliances, and networks" (Fottler & Malvey, 1999, p. 53). When large health systems or national health corporations first began, the emphasis was on horizontal integration or bringing together hospitals of like characteristics—similar size and purpose. After a time, these organizations have expanded, and diversification has occurred more and more. Now, these multihospital systems actually include more than just hospitals; they often also include other types of provider organizations. For example, a corporation might include acute care hospitals, home health agencies, long-term care facilities, hospice care, and various ambulatory care provider organizations.

THINK CRITICALLY

Try this exercise to apply what you have learned about this topic.

Typical departments found in an acute care hospital

Hospitals are complex organizations with many departments and services. Some departments provide direct care services to patients, and others provide support services to facilitate the provision of care. The following are examples of typical departments and services.

- **Administration**

  Administration may not be an official department but rather a description of administrative staff that support the work of the organization—it provides direction. Typically, administrative staff include the CEO, CNE, CFO, and other high-level management staff. Titles can vary from hospital to hospital.

- **Admissions**

  The admissions department ensures that patients are admitted in a timely and efficient manner, and reimbursement issues are resolved related to covered medical services during the admissions process. This department is involved in a great deal of paperwork and assigns patients to rooms and services. The department may be part of billing (financial) services or may work closely with these financial services.

- **Ambulatory care/outpatient services**

  This department or service provides services to persons who generally do not need the level of care associated with the more structured environment of an inpatient or a residential program. Typically, these services are organized by specialty (for example, medical, pediatrics, and orthopedics clinics). Usually these services are provided Monday through Friday during daytime hours although there is now a greater recognition that consumers/patients need access to these services in more nontraditional hours due to work, child care, and other scheduling issues.

- **Clinical laboratory**

  This department or service is equipped to examine material derived from the human body to provide information for use in the diagnosis, prevention, or treatment of disease; it is also called a medical laboratory. Some hospitals may contract out for these services to a company that would run the tests and then provide the hospital with the results. This may be more cost-effective for the hospital, although it can lead to communication problems if there are no clear policies and procedures for this service and it is less in the control of the hospital. The hospital is still responsible for the quality of the services, but some or all of the staff who deliver the services are not hospital employees. More hospitals are considering it to be more cost-effective to contract out for some services.

- **Clinical respiratory services**

  This department or service provides goal-directed, purposeful activity to patients with disorders of the cardiopulmonary system. Such services include diagnostic testing, therapeutics, monitoring education, and rehabilitation. Nurses are part of the staff.

- **Diagnostic procedures**

  This department or service provides laboratory and other invasive, diagnostic, and imaging procedures. Nurses are part of the staff (e.g., endoscopy services).

- **Dietetic services**

  This department or service delivers optimal nutrition and quality food services to individuals. This is a service that may be contracted out. Nurses need to work closely with this staff to ensure that patients' needs are met.

- **Finance and budget**

  This department ensures a financial plan (budget), financial analysis, and the financial solvency of the organization.

- **Housekeeping/environmental service**

  This department or service ensures the environment is clean. This is a service that may be contracted out.

■ Infection control program

This department or service ensures there is an organization-wide program or process, including policies and procedures, for the surveillance, prevention, and control of infection. Nursing is very involved in this area.

■ Infusion therapy services

This department or service provides therapeutic agents or nutritional products to individuals by intravenous infusion for the purpose of improving or sustaining an individual's health condition. Nursing is very involved in this area.

■ Inservice/staff development

This department or service provides organized education designed to enhance skills of staff members or teach new skills relevant to their responsibilities and disciplines. This department is critical for maintaining nurses' competencies (see Chapter 13).

■ Information management

This department or service is responsible for ensuring that information can be collected, linked, is accurate and reliable, monitors use of data, and ensures that legal regulations are met and ethical issues are addressed such as confidentiality and providing secure systems. Computer equipment is a major concern. It needs to be appropriate to the needs of the organization, as well as efficient and effective. This department must work closely with nursing and medical services as well as other clinical departments who require access to information. It also must input data into the system.

■ Material/resource management

This department or service ensures the hospital has the needed supplies by selecting, purchasing, storing, distributing, and obtaining reimbursement for their use when appropriate. This is another service that may be contracted out.

■ Medical equipment management

A component of an organization's management of the environment of care program designed to assess and control the clinical and physical risks of fixed and portable equipment used for the diagnosis, treatment, monitoring, and care of individuals. Nurses use equipment daily and need to be involved in monitoring safety issues and their application to the needs of patients.

■ Medical records

This department or service ensures that the documentation process is maintained, develops relevant policies and procedures, and provides availability of data as required. This is a department that works closely with clinical departments and medical records as well as quality improvement. Nurses are the staff who are responsible for most of the documentation, and they need to be very active in all aspects of medical records functions.

■ Nursing service/patient care

Nursing service is the key service in any acute care hospital as patients are admitted primarily for more intensive nursing care. This is not to say that patients do not receive other services that are important, but nursing care is critical to reaching patient outcomes.

■ Occupational therapy services

The department or service that provides goal-directed, purposeful activity to evaluate, assess, or treat persons whose function is impaired by physical illness or injury, emotional disorder, congenital or developmental disability, or the aging process. Nurses assist in referring patients for these services.

■ Pharmacy/pharmaceutical care and services

The department or service that is responsible for procuring, preparing, dispensing, and distributing pharmaceutical products and the ongoing monitoring of the individual to identify, prevent, and resolve drug-related problems. Nurses administer most of the medications and thus need to work closely with this department.

■ **Physical therapy services**

This department or service provides treatment with physical agents and methods such as massage, manipulation, therapeutic exercises, cold, heat, hydrotherapy, electric stimulation, and light to assist in rehabilitating individuals and in restoring normal function after an illness or injury. Nurses assist in referring patients for these services.

■ **Radiology**

This department or service provides diagnostic services such as x-ray, MRI, and CAT scans. Nurses prepare patients, and may provide care, during radiological procedures.

■ **Respiratory care services**

This department or service delivers care to provide ventilatory support and associated services for individuals. Nurses monitor these services and assist.

■ **Social work services**

This department or service assists individuals and their families in addressing social, emotional, and economic stresses associated with illness or injury. Nurses need to communicate, coordinate, and collaborate with social workers.

■ **Quality improvement performance**

This department ensures that the hospital meets standards (local, state, federal, and accrediting bodies) to ensure quality and safety of care. Chapter 16 focuses on this critical topic. Nurses must be active participants in all phases of quality improvement (Joint Commission on Accreditation of Healthcare Organizations, 2004, pp. 311–344).

This description of hospital departments and services is not complete; however, the descriptions identify some of the key departments found in many hospitals.

THINK CRITICALLY

Try this exercise to apply what you have learned about this topic.

Organizations and committees

Committees are used by organizations for planning, obtaining staff input, and getting some of the organization's work completed. Including staff from various levels and areas of the organization in committee membership offers greater opportunity for staff participation. Committees can also be very problematic—they can take time, can be unproductive and disorganized, and can lead to ineffective management. These problems need to be addressed so that committees can be productive. Nurses do not like working on committees that are unproductive, as they do not have the time. To prevent some of these problems the organization needs to consider the following.

■ Effectiveness of communication
■ Establishment of clear purpose and goals
■ Appropriate committee membership
■ Support from management/administration
■ Collaboration and sharing committee results
■ Recognition that some problems are not appropriate for committee decision making
■ Ensuring that appropriate data is used
■ Scheduling of committee meetings

Later in this chapter the work that the policy and procedure committee does will be described as an example of a committee and its process. This is a committee that is very important to nursing care.

Description of typical committees

Acute care hospitals typically have many committees. These committees may be within a department or service, professional group such as physicians or nurses, or hospital wide. The board of directors also has committees, which were described earlier. Committees are usually classified as standing or ad hoc.

- A standing committee is one that meets regularly for a particular purpose and submits reports to designated management staff. Examples of standing committees might be policy and procedures, medical records, and infection control. Hospitals may have different titles for committees, but the titles given here represent typical titles or focus areas.

- Ad hoc committees are established for a specific purpose with a specific time frame in mind. Some organizations may call these task forces. How long this type of committee exists can be highly variable and depends upon the focus and need. Examples of this type of committee might be a committee that is formed to address a major change in the information management system.

    Another characteristic of committees is they can be composed of members from one profession or be interdisciplinary. The latter type is best for any issue that crosses disciplines, which makes up the majority of issues today. Committees have designated meeting times, keep minutes, make decisions, and develop reports. Members need to prepare for meetings and attend regularly. There are two very common errors made with committees. The first error is having too many committees and too many meetings. When this occurs, staff get tired of committee work and feel that they are just attending meetings. The second error is meetings that are not effective. Both of these errors lead to problems—staff apathy, lack of effective results, loss of work time, lack of staff interest to participate, and so on.

Nursing roles on committees

Nurses need to be very active in the committee work in an acute care hospital, and in any health care setting in which they work. Depending upon how the hospital and its committee structure are set up, nurses may be selected or may volunteer for committee membership. Becoming involved in a committee provides a different perspective of the hospital and its needs. Nurses have much to add as planning is done and decisions are made that affect patient care. The CNE needs to take on the leadership of ensuring a nursing presence on hospital committees. Later in this chapter the work that the policy and procedure committee does is described as an example.

THINK CRITICALLY

Try this exercise to apply what you have learned about this topic.

Differentiated practice: Moving to a professional practice model

The profession of nursing has experienced a long struggle in defining who is a nurse. This struggle continues, probably because nursing has several entry points into the profession, although all who enter must meet the same licensure requirements. This confuses members of the profession, other health care professionals, and the public. There continues to be some diploma schools of nursing despite the fact that the American Nurses Association (ANA) agreed in 1965 to eliminate this entry point. **Differentiated practice** really focuses on three other levels, two of which are entry points—associate degree (AD) in nursing and the bachelor's degree in nursing (BSN)—and the third level is the master's of science in nursing (MSN). The profession has described key differences in these levels and needs to continue to communicate these to the consumers and employers. Do employers recognize a difference in the levels, particularly AD and

BSN? Not all do, and in fact probably the minority do not recognize a difference in their positions, job titles, salary, and so on.

Koerner and co-authors (1995) concluded after a literature review and discussions with nursing leaders that for nursing to develop a professional practice model four elements must be in place: (a) differentiated practice, (b) shared governance, (c) collaborative practice, and (d) case management. Shared governance is discussed in Chapter 5, and collaborative practice that improves interdisciplinary practice is discussed in Chapter 3. All three of these are found in more health care organizations today. Staff are involved in more decision making in many organizations. Collaboration is a constant theme today as noted in many recent Institute of Medicine reports, such as the reports discussed in Chapter 16. Health care organizations and health care education are discussing strategies to improve collaboration and interdisciplinary relationships, although this will not be easy to accomplish. Case management has been pushed by managed care and can be found in many types of health care organizations such as hospitals, home care agencies, and various community health services. Now, this leaves differentiated practice. What is it?

Boston (1990) defined differentiated nursing practice as "a philosophy that focuses on the structuring of roles and functions of nurses according to education, experience, and competence" (p. 1). This means that each nurse must be viewed or assessed from the perspective of the individual nurse's education, experience, and competence. "An evolutionary paradigm shift required of all nurses is the awareness that each nurse is not the whole of nursing, but rather each nurse contributes to the whole of nursing" (Koerner, 1992, p. 335). This goes beyond "a nurse is a nurse." It clearly recognizes that there are differences even though all nurses meet the same licensure requirements, which is a fact that has caused nursing some problems in resolving differentiation issues. It is important to note that differentiated practice does not mean that one nurse is better than another, but rather as noted in this discussion each nurse offers certain competencies that become part of the total nursing care provided. Nelson and Koerner (1994) identified the benefits of developing differentiated practice for nursing. "First, if properly carried out, it can serve to improve patient care and contribute to patient safety. Second, there is the benefit to be gained from a structure that enables the most effective and efficient utilization of scarce resources. Third, there is the opportunity to provide increased satisfaction for nurses themselves because they are better able to optimize their practice. Finally, differentiated practice provides the opportunity to compensate nurses fairly based on their expertise, contribution, and productivity" (Nelson & Koerner, 1994, p. 10).

The key question that could be asked is, "Is there a difference in nurses with AD, BSN, or MSN degrees that can be identified?" Blue et al. (1994) considered this question. They identified some clear differences. For example, when process is assessed the following differences are noted.

- AD graduates spend 40% of their time using technical skills, 40% on communication skills, and 20% on management skills.
- BSN graduates spend 20% of their time using technical skills, 40% on communication skills, and 40% on management skills. This view has expanded even further with the recent discussions about the need for greater leadership competencies for BSN graduates.
- MSN graduates spend 10% of their time using technical skills, 50% on communication skills, and 20% on management skills.

When structure is considered, the AD graduate works in a structured environment such as a nursing unit and requires well-defined boundaries. The BSN graduate requires less structure and boundaries, with the MSN graduate requiring even less. Box 6-2 compares and contrasts the ADN and BSN competencies.

What does all this mean for the new graduate? As new jobs are taken it is important to ask about differentiated practice. Is it recognized? How is it recognized? Is it an integral part of the organization's philosophy about nursing care? Certainly salary differences are important; however, it is more than just differences in pay between the ADN, BSN, and MSN graduates that is important. There must be recognition that what each type of graduate has to offer is different, but each is also important. This then affects how teams work and how care is assigned and delegated. It also affects efficiency and overall staffing guidelines.

BOX 6-2 AACN-AONE model for differentiated nursing practice.

Provision of Direct Care Competencies

The ADN provides direct care for the focal client with common, well-defined nursing diagnosis by:

A. collecting health pattern data from available resources using established assessment format to identify basic health care needs.
B. organizing and analyzing health pattern data in order to select nursing diagnoses from an establishment list.
C. establishing goals with the focal client for a specified work period that are consistent with the overall comprehensive nursing plan of care.
D. developing and implementing an individualized nursing plan of care using established nursing diagnoses and protocols to promote, maintain, and restore health.
E. participating in the medical plan of care to promote an integrated health care plan.
F. Evaluating focal client responses to nursing interventions to meet client needs.

The BSN provides direct care for the focal client with complex interactions of nursing diagnosis by:

A. expanding the collection of data to identify complex health care needs.
B. organizing and analyzing complex health pattern data to develop nursing diagnoses.
C. establishing goals with the focal client to develop a comprehensive nursing plan of care from admission to post-discharge.
D. developing and implementing a comprehensive nursing plan of care based on nursing diagnoses for health promotion.
E. interpreting the medical plan of care to nursing activities to formulate approaches to nursing care.
F. evaluating the nursing care delivery system and promoting goal-directed change to meet individualized client needs.

Management Competencies

The ADN organizes those aspects of care for focal clients for whom s/he is accountable by:

A. prioritizing, planning, and organizing the delivery of standard nursing care in order to use time and resources effectively and efficiently.
B. delegating aspects of care to peers, licensed practical nurses, and ancillary nursing personnel, consistent with their levels of education and expertise, in order to meet client needs.
C. maintaining accountability for own care and care delegated to others to assure adherence to ethical and legal standards.
D. recognizing the need for referral and conferring with appropriate nursing personnel for assistance to promote continuity of care.
E. working with other health care personnel within the organizational structure to manage client care.

The BSN manages nursing care of focal clients by:

A. prioritizing, planning, and organizing the delivery of comprehensive nursing care in order to use time and resources effectively and efficiently.
B. Delegating aspects of care to other nursing personnel, consistent with their levels of education and expertise, in order to meet clients' needs and to maximize staff performance.
C. maintaining accountability for own care and care delegated to others to assure adherence to ethical and legal standards.
D. initiating referral to appropriate departments and agencies to provide services that promote continuity of care.
E. assuming a leadership role in health care management to improve client care.

Communication Competencies

The ADN uses basic communication skills with the focal client by:

A. developing and maintaining goal-directed interactions to encourage expression of needs and support coping behaviors.
B. modifying and implementing a standard teaching plan in order to restore, maintain, and promote health.

The BSN uses complex communication skills with the focal client by:

A. developing and maintaining goal-directed interactions to promote effective coping behaviors and facilitate change in behavior
B. designing and implementing a comprehensive teaching plan for health promotion.

The ADN coordinates focal client care with other health team members by:

A. documenting and communicating data for clients with common, well-defined nursing diagnosis to provide continuity of care.
B. using established channels of communication to implement an effective health care plan.
C. using interpreted nursing research findings for developing nursing care.

The BSN collaborates with other health team members by:

A. documenting and communicating comprehensive data for clients with complex interactions of nursing diagnoses to provide continuity of care.
B. using established channels of communication to modify health care delivery.
C. incorporating research findings into practice and by consulting with nurse researchers regarding identified nursing problems in order to enhance nursing practice.

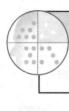

YOUR OPINION COUNTS

Find out what others think about this topic. Post your response and check out other opinions.

BENCHMARKS

Now let's take a moment to test your knowledge of the concepts you have studied in this section.

Framework for Effective Care

Chapter 16 discusses quality improvement in more detail. Quality improvement relies on standards as well as policies and procedures; however, the following provides information on these two topics as they relate to acute care hospitals and their operation and services.

Standards

Standards are used by hospitals to provide guidelines for care provided and professional responsibilities. They can have an impact on the quality of care, patient outcomes, and the workforce environment. The ANA and specialty nursing organizations have developed many standards. These standards may be used within a hospital and other health care settings such as a home health agency, city health department, behavioral health hospital, or a hospital that may use the standards to provide guidance that is specifically developed by the hospital. Many hospitals use a combination of both approaches to develop their internal standards. There typically are overall nursing standards and then standards for specialty areas. These standards, however, should be consistent with the professional standards. Other sources of information about standards are local, state, and federal laws and regulations and accreditation organizations. Evidence-based practice also emphasizes the use of standards and the development of standards based on what research demonstrates as effective care. Chapter 9 discusses the evidence-based approach as a tool that is used in health care.

Types of standards

There can be confusion about the different types of standards. A standard is an "authoritative statement by which the nursing profession describes the responsibilities for which its practitioners are accountable, reflecting the values and priorities of the profession" (American Nurses Association, 1996, p. 20). Clinical nursing standards include standards that focus on care and professional performance.

1. Standards of clinical nursing practice delineate professional responsibilities of registered nurses who work in any type of setting with any type of patient. Nurses who practice in a specialty area are held accountable for these standards, too. Standards of care identify what is expected for a competent level of care, which is demonstrated by the process of accurate assessment, diagnosis, outcome identification, planning, implementation, and evaluation.
2. The standards of professional performance focus on the competent level of professional behavior of the nurse in the areas of quality assessment, performance appraisal, education, collegiality, ethics, collaboration, research, and resource utilization appropriate to level of education, position, and practice setting.

Policies and procedures

Policies and procedures are found in every hospital and other types of health care organizations. They are the "formal, approved description of how a governance, management, or clinical care process is defined, organized, and carried out" (Joint Commission on Accreditation of Healthcare Organizations, 2004, p. 335). Policies and procedures provide guidelines for staff when decisions are made or procedures are done. This section describes the policy and procedure development process in some detail and is an example of how a health care organization develops its processes and how a committee might work.

In addition to the general overriding concerns of quality care, risk management, and cost containment, each hospital department within a general hospital and nursing department needs to consider eight factors that have an impact on policy and procedure development. When a hospital or department decides to develop or revise its policies and procedures, these factors should not be ignored, and they are also important for most major changes that nursing might consider in a health care organization. If a nursing department attempts to operate in isolation from other departments in the hospital, from the hospital organization itself, or from the external environment, this leads to communication problems and work performance barriers. Because change is inherent, each of these factors requires frequent review to maintain relevant policies and procedures.

■ Joint Commission on Accreditation of Health Care Organizations (JCAHO)

JCAHO provides accreditation surveys for health care facilities and details the requirements for accreditation in the *Accreditation Manual for Hospitals 2004*. It is the first resource for any nursing department to use in policy and procedure development; however, the detailed content of policies and procedures needs to be individualized. The JCAHO manual and its standards are not written to be used as an individual hospital's or a nursing department's policy and procedure manual. It does not include specific policies and procedures for hospitals, but rather it provides guidelines for content and direction.

■ Professional standards

Professional standards reflect a specific professional group's views on what is acceptable professional performance. The professional nursing standards, along with the JCAHO standards, identify many additional issues to consider in policies and procedures. For example, nursing standards describe the nurse's role in assessment. A hospital would use this guideline in the development of a policy and procedure related to the admission assessment.

■ State and federal legislation

State legislatures determine regulations that need to be monitored carefully, such as state nurse practice acts and rules and regulations, reimbursement requirements, safety requirements, facility requirements, and staffing level regulations. In the federal arena, the most important issue is reimbursement. It is particularly critical for hospitals reimbursed by Medicare and/or Medicaid to understand current reimbursement legislation and regulations. Emergency department issues, as discussed later in this chapter, are affected by laws, and these would have to be incorporated in policies and procedures about emergency admissions and transfers.

■ Court decisions

Court decisions have affected many areas of patient care, particularly when related to patient's rights, length-of-stay, commitment, discharge planning, patient and staff protection, and informed consent. The hospital's legal counsel often provides guidance in this area.

■ Reimbursement

Reimbursement governs or is a strong factor in many decisions made in hospitals, including decisions related to length-of-care and type of treatment as well as discharge plans. In addition, staffing cuts and increased stress to patients and families caused by concern about the cost of care and the duration of care that is covered by their personal health endurance directly affect the health care environment. Hospitals have policies and procedures about checking health coverage, what is covered, and other aspects related to reimbursement.

■ Patients' rights

Patients' rights are part of both the JCAHO standards and the ANA standards. These rights are identified in writing and shared with patients, families, and staff. In addition, the rights need to be incorporated into policies and procedures. For example, in a procedure that describes preoperative care, patients' rights would be included by identifying how informed consent should be obtained, by whom, when, and how it is to be documented.

■ **The Community**

The community in which the hospital is located must not be ignored. The hospital develops both a relationship with, and an image in, the community. Two areas of consideration are of particular importance. The type of support available to the patient and family in the community has a major effect on the hospital's ability to discharge patients and prevent complications and readmission. Examples of issues that need to be considered are availability of home care; medical supplies and equipment; general support such as Meals-on-Wheels, social services, case management, and so on; and ambulatory care clinics. With the increasing movement to care in the community, hospitals need to develop more strategies for connecting their services with the community.

■ **Research and literature**

The nursing department that is interested in maintaining an up-to-date department and providing quality nursing care will utilize research results and professional literature to develop and revise its policies and procedures. It is hoped that this external influence will also encourage the nursing department to support its own research and the development of literature for publication, and thereby share its experiences with other nurses. The continuing progress of nursing care depends on nursing research conducted in the clinical setting. For these reasons, policies and procedures related to nursing research should be included. Evidence-based practice, as discussed in Chapter 9, supports the need to have data to support decisions. This includes management decisions such as the development of policies and procedures. Figure 6-1 describes the key issues related to policy and procedure development.

After considering the major influences on policies and procedures, the policy development process has begun. Policy and procedure development is a complex process that ultimately affects both management of the nursing department and all of the care provided. The entire process takes place in the context of the critical concerns and influences previously described. It needs to involve all of the nursing staff. It is a process that flows from the chief nurse executive (CNE) to the nursing management staff, and then to staff at all levels in the department. Policy and procedure development is typically the responsibility of a committee designated for this purpose. The following discussion provides the objectives, definitions, and format of policies and procedures as well as the process of developing and implementing them. This is also a good example

FIGURE 6-1   Development of policies and procedures.

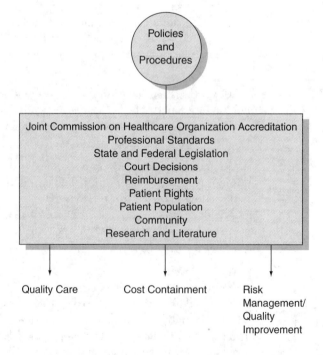

Source: Author.

of how committees function in organizations. As each nursing department is different, this information serves only as guidelines. It should be noted that the hospital has an organization-wide committee on policies and procedures; however, in some hospitals the nursing department also has its own policy and procedure committee that interrelates to the hospital-wide committee. Regardless of the type of structure, the process that is described applies to both types of committees.

The first step in developing policies and procedures for the nursing department is for nursing administration to identify the objectives for their development and their implementation. If this is not the first step, policy and procedure development will be neither organized nor helpful to the nursing staff. Each hospital and its nursing service are different, and objectives can therefore vary. The following is a list of possible objectives that can serve as guidelines for individual nursing departments.

1. To promote quality care.
2. To implement the hospital's and the nursing department's vision/mission and objectives.
3. To incorporate changes in health care into the hospital.
4. To increase the quality and quantity of work through consistent decision making and action.
5. To maintain cost containment through efficient use of staff, time, and supplies.
6. To meet accrediting agencies' requirements.
7. To maintain professional nursing standards.
8. To increase the quality of communication at all levels in the organization.
9. To promote a risk management program by preventing negligence and maintaining safety of patients, visitors, and staff.
10. To delineate lines of authority.
11. To increase interdisciplinary collaboration.
12. To assist in developing sound judgment.
13. To identify expectations for the staff and promote job security.
14. To promote the resolution of problems closer to the problem situation.
15. To act as a focus for discussion when differences occur and thus decrease the opportunity to personalize conflicts.
16. To decrease written communication regarding daily problems.
17. To decrease staff turnover due to poor communication and inadequate identification of expectations.
18. To assist with orientation for new, transferred, promoted, or temporary staff and for nursing faculty and students.
19. To assist with staff development for all nursing staff.

Each policy and procedure should relate to at least one of the objectives.

Definitions of policy and procedure

Many definitions for policy and procedure are found in the literature, but one consistent comment is that the terms are different from and yet related to each other. How are policies and procedures different or similar?

- A policy is a statement that communicates to staff the expectations and vision/mission of the organization, department, and management. It provides a guideline for decision making. A policy may exist without a related procedure if staff require no further specific guidance. Because policies relate to the hospital's and the department's objectives, which do not change very often, policies are revised less often than procedures. Review of a nursing department's policy manual should provide a total picture of the particular department's beliefs concerning its management and the nursing care it provides. Identifying a policy does not negate the need for individual judgment, nor does it negate the professional nurse's accountability for decision making.

- A procedure is a definite statement describing the step-by-step actions required for a specific outcome. It provides a recipe for reaching a specific goal and that goal is usually a completed treatment that is safe for the patient and efficient in the use of staff, time, supplies, and equipment. A procedure is more detailed than a policy, and changes in routine or treatment directly

BOX 6-3 Policy format.

DEPARTMENT OF NURSING POLICY MANUAL

POLICY NUMBER

_____

TITLE:
POLICY AREA:
EFFECTIVE DATE:
REVIEW SCHEDULE:
FINAL APPROVAL RESPONSIBILITY:
PRIMARY RESPONSIBILITY:

_____

PURPOSE:

POLICY:

Approved by:

_____

Date: _____   **Review Dates:** _____

Source: Author.

affect procedures, which then require revision. Written procedures support quality care and prevent errors that might be detrimental to the patient and to the department or hospital. Procedures and policies both help to maintain consistency and continuity; however, to do so, they need to be written in concise, easy-to-understand language and contain appropriate and up-to-date information. If policies and procedures are just words on paper, they will not be utilized by the staff, and all the effort, time, and money spent to develop them will therefore be wasted.

Policy and procedure formats

Formats for policies and procedures also vary greatly from hospital to hospital; however, certain elements always need to be included. These elements are the title, effective date, review date, purpose, and identification of the responsibility for final review. Boxes 6-3 and 6-4 describe examples of policy and procedure formats.

   More and more organizations are putting their policies and procedures online, moving away from hard copies or manuals. This makes the information more accessible as long as staff can access a computer and get into the hospital intranet. It is also easier to update the policies and procedures, and changes can be quickly communicated to staff. As changes are made, it is also easier to find related material that needs to be changed (for example, other policies and procedures) by searching for content.

BOX 6-4   Procedure format.

DEPARTMENT OF NURSING PROCEDURAL MANUAL

PROCEDURE NUMBER

TITLE:

PROCEDURE AREA:

EFFECTIVE DATE:

REVIEW SCHEDULE:

FINAL APPROVAL RESPONSIBILITY:

WHO MAY PERFORM:

PURPOSE:

EQUIPMENT AND SUPPLIES:

ACTION:

Source: Author.

Policy and procedure committee

The policy and procedure committee is a very active committee and requires members who are willing to do work that at times may be tedious. The committee does not have the ultimate authority for the approval of a policy or a procedure, but is an advisory committee. The final approval process and responsibility must be clearly defined. The best size for this committee is six to eight members with a chairperson. If the committee is too small, the members may feel burdened with work, and if it is too large, getting the members together efficiently becomes difficult. With at least a 2-year term of membership, the members will have time to be productive on the committee. Since it is also important to get new ideas from new members, committee membership should include both new and old members; therefore, it should have rotating changes in membership. This will ensure that there will be some experienced members on the committee at all times. The purpose of this committee is to develop the policies and procedures for the nursing service/department and to maintain a system for periodic review and revision of policies and procedures. This committee's work is never completed, and it thus requires active participation and an interest in this work from all members.

Role of nursing administration/management

The CNE typically does not serve on the committee but has many responsibilities related to this committee. Examples of these responsibilities include the following.

1. To clarify with hospital administration the nursing committee's relationship to the hospital policy and procedure committee and to provide written communication on this issue to the nursing committee.

2. To appoint a chairperson (unless the chairperson is to be elected).
3. To identify needs for policies and procedures.
4. To communicate specific policy and procedure issues to the committee.
5. To review and approve all new and revised policies and procedures.
6. To communicate to all nursing management staff and all nursing staff the importance of policies and procedures and encourage their input in the development process.
7. To ensure that policies and procedures are implemented and evaluated.
8. To review and respond to the committee's annual report.
9. To provide secretarial assistance for the preparation of the policies and procedures.

Through the fulfillment of these responsibilities, the CNE communicates the importance of policies and procedures and coordinates the committee's work both within the department and with other departments, acting as a facilitator.

Role of the committee chairperson

The chairperson should be a nursing staff member who can organize well and work effectively with others. The committee is very busy, and consequently, the chairperson should not have many responsibilities on other committees. The chairperson has the following responsibilities.

1. Select committee members using the designated approval process.
2. Establish a meeting schedule and attendance requirements.
3. Establish a process for electing a committee secretary, who will keep the minutes.
4. Maintain contact with secretarial assistance provided by nursing administration/management.
5. Ensure that all records are up-to-date (attendance, minutes, location of all manuals, annual reports, individual files on each policy and procedure, records of review dates for each policy and procedure).
6. Ensure that the committee selects appropriate methods for identifying need and content of policies and procedures.
7. Ensure that the committee develops the content for the policies and procedures and that the approval process is maintained.
8. Establish a system for review of each policy and procedure.
9. Select reviewers for policies and procedures and maintain a list of the reviewers, the policies and procedures reviewed, and deadlines.
10. Participate in staff development related to policies and procedures.
11. Prepare an annual report.

Role of the committee members

The policy and procedure committee's work will be more efficient and more responsive to actual needs if there is broad nursing representation on the committee. This representation allows for greater input and participation by nursing staff. Coming to the meeting prepared helps the committee do its work more efficiently and effectively. Committee members' responsibilities include:

1. Attend meetings regularly.
2. Complete designated work by deadlines.
3. Assist in selecting appropriate methods for identifying need and content of policies and procedures.
4. Collect data for policies and procedures.
5. Review policies and procedures for committee approval before moving the policy or procedure through the committee approval process.
6. Participate in staff development related to policies and procedures.

The process of policy and procedure development

It is important to remember that policies and procedures do not make robots out of the nursing staff. No two situations are exactly alike, and as a consequence, policies and procedures will be interpreted differently at different times. Professional nursing staff are taught and encouraged to think through their decisions using the policies and procedures as guidelines. They are developed to help the staff, not to freeze creativity. This flexibility does not negate the importance of implementing policies and procedures, but supports the idea that effective decision making requires more than just following a set of written rules.

1. Identification of need

After the committee structure is organized, the next step is to determine the policy and procedure needs of the nursing department. The best way to begin is to review existing policies and procedures. Some may require no changes, some may require changes, some may need to be eliminated, and some may need to be added. In addition, the major influences on policies discussed earlier in this section should be considered. A thoughtful evaluation of policies and procedures with input from nursing staff who use them is very helpful in making these decisions.

Many of the decisions in nursing departments are made in crisis situations. Health care is not static, and consequently, changes frequently occur suddenly and require immediate decisions. Decisions to develop a policy and procedure often are made during crises. However, responding to a crisis by saying "We need a policy on this" is not always the best approach and can result in many infrequently used policies or procedures. Too many policies and procedures can be just as harmful as too few. Staff may begin to see all policies and procedures as paper with little substance. If nursing administration and the committee are aware of changes occurring in the department, the hospital, the community, and health care, then policies and procedures will more likely be developed in non-crisis periods with a less harried approach. The critical word in policy and procedure development is change, a recurrent theme in this text. Changes may or may not affect policies and procedures, but it must always be considered. Changes in any of the following areas should be an indication for the committee to evaluate the policies and procedures.

- Hospital's policies and procedures
- Departmental organization
- Vision/mission and objectives for the department and the hospital
- Factors related to other departments that affect nursing
- Patient population and needs
- Medical procedures and treatment modalities
- Nursing routines
- Documentation
- Equipment changes
- Staffing
- Position descriptions
- Incidents and consultations with attorney and insurance carrier
- Reports from reviewing agencies and their criteria
- Reimbursement
- State and federal laws
- Current, relevant professional literature

There are many ways to obtain data that are useful in identifying policy and procedure needs. It is best to employ multiple methods and to evaluate these methods periodically to determine whether they provide relevant data. Staff interviews and questionnaires are two methods; however, they both require time to develop, collect, and analyze. A poorly conducted interview or poorly written questionnaire will not result in helpful information, and consequently, the committee's time and effort will be wasted. Nursing staff will also feel their time has been wasted. Surveys of other institutions may also be helpful, but again, surveys need to be well written and short. The response to a survey may not be great, so committees should not depend on this method for a major portion of the data.

Some methods of data collection do not require as much preparation as interviews and questionnaires but do require thoughtful analysis after the data are obtained. One of these methods is observation. One important reason for rounds by nursing management staff is to have the opportunity to observe, and committee members can also use this method. Not all that is observed is relevant to a policy or a procedure, so careful analysis of observations is important. Talking with nursing staff and physicians informally rather than using a structured interview can often reveal concerns and needs, but decisions cannot be made on what just a few people say. After informal discussion, further investigation will be necessary. Material that is already available, such as audits, incident reports, annual reports from nursing and other departments, requests for staff development on particular topics, and minutes from staff meetings, may reveal many needs for new policies and procedures or needs for change in existing ones. Another method that may provide data is interviewing new staff after their orientation to find out what information was difficult for them to obtain and what problems they encountered. Still another source is one that is often not considered: patients and their families, who frequently have concerns that relate to policies and procedures.

Need identification is a process. It does not happen once, and it is never complete. Communicating the nature of need identification to the nursing staff helps to emphasize that their input into the process is always useful. Staff should never put off communicating questions or concerns that they may have about policies and procedures. A committee or nursing management that does not listen to the nursing staff will soon encounter problems and will not have effective policies and procedures.

2. Development of content

Before developing the content for a particular policy or procedure, the committee identifies the policy or procedure's purpose. The committee asks, "What is the decision to be made?" and "Why make the decision?" At the same time, the committee identifies who will make the decision or perform the procedure. Policy and procedure content must support the vision, mission, and objectives of the department and the hospital, and the committee needs to be alert to conflicts between policies and procedures. It is important to compare new or altered policies and procedures with other policies and procedures and determine if there is conflict or overlap, or if the policy or procedure will cause problems with other departments.

In writing policies and procedures, there are several factors to keep in mind. First, terminology needs to be clear and concise. As lengthy, cumbersome statements do not communicate information quickly, short sentences are preferable. Abbreviations and acronyms may be used; however, when initially used, they need to be defined. Their meanings should be included for reference. Second, so that staff can make decisions efficiently, the information in a policy or procedure should be organized in logical steps. Committee members provide multiple checks of logical steps by asking questions such as the following: "Does this make sense? Can it be followed easily? Is it complete? Could it be stated more simply?"

3. Approval

After the content is developed, the approval phase begins. The approval process needs to be clearly designated. No policy or procedure should be implemented without written approval. This rule must be strictly enforced, particularly since there are probably copies of the draft that could be interpreted as official policy or procedure. All nursing staff should be told to check for the approval signature and date before applying a policy or procedure.

4. Implementation and communication

Implementation of a policy or a procedure requires planning and participation from the committee and nursing management. The goal of implementation is to make all nursing staff aware of the new or changed policy or procedure and to get them to apply it in appropriate situations. Implementation requires that staff know about the policy and procedure, understand it, and know when to apply it. All of these factors influence the implementation process. It is not always easy to get the nursing staff to use a policy or procedure. Management staff become important in this effort, but they need a thorough understanding of the purpose and the content of the policy or procedure. All of this makes communication a very important part of the implementation process to assure that nursing staff know about the policy or procedure content, when it is in effect, who may make the decision or perform the procedure, and what the process is for providing feedback about a policy or procedure.

A critical question about implementation that often arises is, "What keeps staff from using policies and procedures?" There are many answers to this question, and consideration of these answers will help to combat underutilization of policies and procedures. Some of the most frequent reasons for not using policies and procedures are that staff:

- Cannot find the policy and procedure manual.
- Do not know what is in the manual.
- Do not know how to use the manual.

- Do not know how to access the computer.
- Do not understand how policies and procedures reflect the philosophy of the department and the hospital.
- Do not feel the policies and procedures are practical or helpful.
- Do not like someone telling them what to do and how to do it.
- Do not understand how the policies and procedures protect the patient and staff and support quality care.
- Feel that poor communication in the department results in a poor relationship between the staff and administration.
- Feel policies and procedures represent more paperwork.

Staff may, however, have an appropriate reason for ignoring the policies and procedures. Each complaint needs to be discussed, and if necessary, resolved. It is, therefore, important to plan all steps of the development and implementation process. Anticipation of some of the possible problems before they occur may provide a better chance of successfully implementing a policy or procedure.

Staff development plays an important role in the implementation of policies and procedures. Staff development personnel frequently are directly involved in preparing staff for a new policy or procedure by providing programs about content related to a policy and procedure (for example, what happens during a code). As a consequence, staff development personnel need to be kept fully informed of changes. In fact, it might be helpful to have a member of this group on the policy and procedure committee. Staff development nurses frequently are the first to recognize that a policy or procedure requires a change or that a new one is needed. When all of this information is filtered through appropriate channels, the result is a more comprehensive, useful policy and procedure manual that is utilized on a daily basis by the staff.

Through staff development, nursing staff develop an understanding of why a policy or procedure exists and what the content means to their practice. It is clear that because the staff nurse cannot know everything, the nurse needs to know where to find information quickly. How can nurses be made to look in the manual or on the computer for the policies and procedures? Reminding them whenever situations occur that require implementation of a policy or a procedure is one way; however, more structured methods are also necessary such as written communications, inclusion of information in staff meetings, posters reminding staff of new policies and procedures, and staff development programs on these topics.

5. Evaluation and revision

In most departments evaluation and revision is probably the weakest part of policy and procedure development. It is, however, critical to the success of implementation. An outdated policy or procedure can be just as detrimental to care and to the organization as no policy or procedure. Changes never come easily and usually involve some risk, but a system designed to ensure that every policy and procedure is evaluated regularly and that records are kept on this evaluation can ease change. Box 6-5 provides an example of an evaluation form that can be used to get feedback from staff who are using the policies and procedures.

Why has so much content been presented about policies and procedures and the development process? They provide guidelines or expectations to assist staff as they make decisions and provide care. In addition, understanding one example of how an organization develops and provides direction to staff, such as through policies and procedures, helps in understanding project development—there is a problem and then the organization goes about solving it.

THINK CRITICALLY

Try this exercise to apply what you have learned about this topic.

BOX 6-5   Policy and procedure evaluation form.

**POLICY OR PROCEDURE NUMBER
TITLE:**

What is the problem(s) you encountered with this policy or procedure?

What recommendations do you have for changes?

**SIGNATURE:
UNIT:
DATE:**

Source: Author.

BENCHMARKS

Now let's take a moment to test your knowledge of the concepts you have studied in this section.

Changes That Affect Acute Health Care Delivery

With the change toward more community and primary care, emphasis on health care delivery and financial issues, such as growth of managed care and lower reimbursement rates for health care and reduced Medicare and Medicaid reimbursement, many hospitals have been downsizing, and some are even closing. This has caused problems for many communities (such as rural areas) when their hospitals close. Community members then have to travel longer distances to get health services. The key factors that have affected health care delivery and the acute care hospital system are:

- Problems with access (eligibility for government benefits such as Medicaid, transportation, hours of operation, number and type of providers, child care, cost of care)
- Managed care
- Increased number of the uninsured and underinsured
- Demographic changes (increasing age of population, single-parent families, immigrant growth, limited access to extended family members, diversity)
- Aging population with chronic illness and greater acuity and complications when hospitalized
- Improvement in technology that extends lifespan and increases costs
- Uneven distribution of health care services (for example, more services in urban areas as compared to rural areas)
- Increase in homeless population with limited health care access

BOX 6-6   Important change areas in acute care.

- Emergency services
- Patient access to services
- Patient education
- Expansion into new areas and approaches
- Use of hospitalists/intensivists
- Advance practice nurses, clinical nurse specialists, and nurse midwives
- Alternative/complementary therapies
- Financial issues and managed care: Impact on acute care
- Continuum of care and acute care
- Primary care
- Nurses and acute care hospital changes
- Staffing Issues

Source: Author.

- Increase in new drug therapies that are costly
- Increase in specialty usage leading to fragmentation of care and increased cost

Newhouse and Mills (2002) note that "Ackerman's (1992) description of the health care environment still rings true. Health care organizations are still engulfed in efforts to control spiraling costs, provide care for an aging population with increasing health demands, and obtain human resources to provide care. Technology has provided a means to affect the health of patients and reduce their length of staff, but has also increased the cost of care" (p. 6). The following is a discussion of some of the important changes affecting hospitals also highlighted in Box 6-6.

Emergency services

Emergency services are only provided in emergency departments that are part of hospitals, and also by urgent care centers, which may be freestanding, separate from hospitals, or part of a hospital organization. In hospitals with trauma centers the emergency services play a critical role in trauma services. "The scope of emergency nursing practice involves the assessment, diagnosis, outcome identification, planning, implementation or interventions, and evaluation of human responses to perceived, actual or potential, sudden or urgent, physical or psychosocial problems that are primarily episodic or acute, and which occur in a variety of settings. These may require minimal care or life-support measures, patient and significant other education, appropriate referral, and knowledge of legal implications" (Emergency Nurses Association, 1996, pp. 2–3).

Downsizing has also had a major impact on the emergency care services/department (ED). This service is one of the areas of care that has received much media attention, primarily focused on reimbursement denial when insurers consider the care non-emergent. Health plan benefits usually state that emergency care requires preauthorization and must be due to an emergency. Laypeople may consider many conditions an emergency, particularly when they are not sure what is happening to them. They go to the emergency room to have a health care professional diagnose their problem and need for treatment. Health plans, however, set their own standards for what constitutes an emergency; some plans do this more than others. Many providers of emergency services are experiencing adverse financial outcomes when some MCOs/insurers do not approve payment for their health plan members' emergency treatment (Haas, 1998). There has been concern for a long time that an increasing number of patients are using emergency services as their primary care provider. This is especially true for the uninsured. This is not the best treatment for continuity or for most medical problems. It also increases the patient load in the emergency department and provides less staff to treat true emergencies. Emergency staff also become frustrated with these patients who should receive care elsewhere, and their frustration spills over onto the patients and their families.

Not only are emergency services experiencing an increase in the number of patients who do not need emergency services, but in many hospitals the emergency room is often used to hold patients who are admitted and should be transferred to appropriate inpatient units. With decreased staff working on the inpatient units and some beds closed, patients cannot be transferred out of ED. Staff find this to be very frustrating, and these patients require staff time that should be used for patients who do need emergency services. Emergency room nurses need to be involved in recommending strategies for coping with these problems. This requires collaboration and an ability to assess these problems objectively. With the expertise that ED nurses have they should participate in the development of solutions. A place to begin is to consider some of the following questions: Do local HMOs need to extend their hours? Do patients know what care is available to them and how to access it? Could advanced practice nurses be used to assist with triaging patients or running urgent care clinics? Should the hospital develop urgent care centers or is it best for the hospital to collaborate with existing urgent care providers? There are many other possibilities, and with staff input hospitals can resolve these critical problems.

Herr (1998) recommends the following as strategies for emergency departments that are coping with reimbursement issues and the dilemma that is faced by both health care professionals in emergency rooms and by patients and families. When decisions are made about policies and procedures, their content must meet the requirements of the federal law, The Consolidated Omnibus Budget Reconciliation Act of 1984 (COBRA), or the hospital can be fined. In addition to the extension of coverage, COBRA established a federal requirement that all hospitals with emergency services that participate in Medicare—and this is most hospitals—must treat all patients requiring emergency treatment or who are in labor. Inability to pay cannot be used as a reason to deny treatment. This offers a major protection for the patient; however, the critical issue is the definition of an emergency and who defines it. Some patients use the local emergency department as their personal physician office. Insurers are concerned about this use, but the patients for whom this law is addressed often have no insurance. If hospitals meet these COBRA criteria, they cannot deny emergency services. How does this affect emergency service expenses? What is the hospital's moral obligation? Neither of these questions can be ignored, nor are they simple to answer. The following are aspects of this problem, which affects the ED, the entire hospital, and the entire health care delivery system in a community.

■ Triage

There are several issues pertinent to triage. The first is to perform a medical screening examination and to stabilize the patient. What constitutes a screening is not described by federal regulation. It could be as limited as taking vital signs and identifying a chief complaint to a complete workup or referral to a specialist. Clearly, the patient's condition should determine the type of screening that is required. Patients may refuse care at any point, and to protect the emergency room and its staff, this refusal should be obtained in writing. This prevents questions about the staff refusing treatment to the patient. The troubling issue arises when the managed care organization refuses to authorize the emergency care. The critical factor for emergency staff is the patient's condition and care should be provided if the patient accepts it. Patients may at times become upset with their insurer's response. Staff need to listen but avoid being judgmental, which is not easy to do. Emergency staff receive different directions about who is responsible for calling the patient's insurer to obtain authorization of emergency treatment. Hospitals need to have well-defined steps for this procedure because it can make a major difference as to whether or not reimbursement is covered. Many patients today are very aware of the need to contact their insurer and will bring it up themselves. Reaching the MCO or insurer with the information may vary depending on time of day and the MCO staffing level for authorization calls. These efforts to call should be documented by ED staff. Because this really is a financial issue, the patient is the best person to speak with the plan representative, but in many cases the patient is unable to do this due to his or her condition, and because family members may not be available.

■ Medical evaluation and therapy

There are times when the insurance plan representative insists that the patient be sent elsewhere for treatment or testing. This can cause a conflict for ED staff. The first priority is to stabilize the patient and ensure that the best care is provided. The physician may need to speak with the plan representative. MCOs want their patients seen and treated by contracted providers (e.g., physicians/hospitals who have been approved by the plan to treat the plan's members), something that is not always possible. When permission is given to use a non-contract provider, emergency staff must document this with details, such as authorization number, staff spoken to, time, date, and so on. Another treatment issue that occurs is the problem of reimbursement for specific medications. It is often easier to change the prescription to one that is covered than to argue about one that is not covered, unless there is no other appropriate medication available. Providers should never alter a diagnosis in order to ensure reimbursement. Any injury that occurred while the patient was working must be reported as an employment injury because this affects workers' compensation. If this is not done, it may be viewed as defrauding the patient's insurer.

■ Medical disposition and discharge

If patients are stable with little likelihood of deteriorating, they can be transferred. The patient must agree to the transfer; however, the patient must be legally competent to agree. Patients in this situation must realize that they can receive treatment regardless of their ability to pay. As is always true, transferring patients from one unit to another (or in this case to another facility) requires that the nurse and/or physician give a report to staff in the receiving facility or unit, and that the receiving facility or unit must have the resources to provide the care that the patient needs. The receiving admission office or ED staff must be notified of the transfer and time of arrival of the new patient.

Although use of urgent care can be a way to lower increasing usage of emergency services, it also can be a problem. Increased usage of urgent care is also a concern to managed care organizations (MCOs). A study focused on unscheduled patient visits to urgent care centers by health maintenance organizations (HMOs), which is one of the types of MCOs (Plauth & Pearson, 1998), indicated that HMO enrollees were not just using urgent care during nonoperational hours of their HMO, but they were also using urgent care during HMO office hours. Why was this occurring with 47% of the patients? The patients said that they were not able to get a primary care appointment, and if this had been possible, they would have preferred to see their own primary care provider (PCP) from the HMO within a day or two. Improvement in more rapid access to providers might alleviate the problem and increase patient satisfaction.

Emergency care is a specialty area that has been affected by recent legislation and will likely be important in health care legislation in the future. Questions related to denial of emergency services and the need for these services, the patient's view of emergency services, and emergency care provided outside the plan's geographic area need to be addressed and clearly described to consumers. Hospital staff frequently encounter problems such as the ones described with ED patients that then affect inpatient units and patient care.

Patient access to services

Patients have to get into and out of hospitals, and this process is one that can lead to problems for patients, their families, and the staff. As this content is discussed, consider how patients are admitted and discharged in local hospitals. What are the problems that occur? What can be done to improve the process for all concerned? It is not uncommon for staff who are responsible for the "paperwork" part of admission and discharge to be disconnected from the direct care providers, particularly nurses. This gap is where problems occur, and frustration increases. This is when nursing staff are heard saying, "Don't they realize we don't have a clean room yet?", "How many more admissions can we handle this shift?", "This patient should have been sent to another unit because he does not meet our admission criteria.", "Why is it taking so long to get those discharge papers?", and "Where is the transport staff to take the patient down to her car?" The comments can go on and on. In the meantime, admissions staff are also frustrated. They are saying: "Why can't they get those rooms cleaned up faster so that we can move these patients out?", "We don't have the doctor's order for discharge.", "This admission information is incomplete.",

"Where is the patient going after discharge?", and "The nursing home will not accept his insurance." As was mentioned earlier when committees were discussed, it is important to have interdisciplinary input for effective patient access services—admission and discharge. Transfers also cause problems, whether they are internal from unit to unit or external to other health care facilities. Transfers are also times of increase in errors, which can lead to complications for the patient. All of this can lead to less cost-effective care and to the patient. Admission and discharge problems take time, and this means additional costs to the organization. There is always the need to make sure that the admission is appropriate to ensure that reimbursement for care is approved. However, patients who stay too long may find that there is no or limited reimbursement for their care. These are major problems for hospitals.

Patient education

For many years acute care settings have been required to provide patient education to meet accreditation requirements. Nursing education and the profession also have a long history of emphasizing the role of nurses in providing patient education. Despite this emphasis on patient education, health care still has not been very successful in providing it. Managed care also recognizes the importance of patient education, believing that it will reduce costs and increase patient satisfaction. Patient education methods and evaluation of outcomes are still not fully understood. Providing patient education in acute care has become even more difficult with the decreasing length-of-stay. Patients are sicker when admitted because efforts are first made to keep the patient out of the hospital, and then they stay only a short time. Patients are then often too sick to absorb patient education content, and when they begin to improve, they have less time to absorb the information because they are quickly discharged. Family members also have similar experiences—they are unable to focus on education when their family member is acutely ill, and then when they can, it is time for discharge. Nurses are tired, stressed, and have problems including patient education with the rapid turnover of patients. Hospitals are turning more toward standardized patient education material, which they purchase. Nurses, however, need to assess these materials carefully and should participate in the development of these materials and their adaptation to meet individual patient needs. Standardized educational materials can be excellent resources if they meet the needs of the hospital and patients/families. These resources can also reduce staff preparation time and increase content consistency, which are both important factors in today's busy acute care hospitals. Rapid discharge also means that hospital nurses must develop effective communication and collaborative relationships with agencies and other providers who will care for patients after discharge. Patient education needs to continue, and hospital nurses must share what educational content has been provided and the response of the patient/family to ensure that additional patient education meets the needs of the patient/family.

Expansion into new areas and approaches

There are many changes in acute care services occurring almost daily, and due to the increasing use of outpatient surgery, surgical services have experienced major changes. Hospitals are increasing the size of their outpatient or ambulatory surgery departments and adjusting to the need of moving patients into and out of the surgical service in 1 day or even a few hours. This has affected many departments, particularly preadmission testing, admissions, nursing, clinical laboratories, pathology, radiology, pharmacy, anesthesiology, post-anesthesia recovery, and patient transportation. In some hospitals nurses call surgical patients at home prior to surgery to begin the nursing assessment and to give the patients brief preoperative education. Patients are coming in several days prior to surgery for their preadmission testing on an outpatient basis and then arriving at the hospital a few hours before their surgery for admission, which for some may be in the very early morning hours. Nursing staff may call patients a few days after surgery to assess their status. Surgical inpatient units are finding that their census has dropped because patients do not stay in the hospital after their surgery. Nurses have had to make adjustments in patient education that is typically provided after surgery because patients are now going home nauseated, barely recovered from anesthesia, and in pain. In these cases, family members receive the patient education.

Use of hospitalists/intensivists

Some hospitals have been using hospitalists or intensivists. These are physicians who focus on inpatient care and are employees of the hospital. **Hospitalists** are generalists in the sense that they serve as liaisons between the primary care provider in the office and specialists in the hospital. Primary care physicians trade off reduced income for fewer hospital visits to gain increased income for more billable time spent with patients in the office. "Hospitalists, therefore, attend to patients during hospital stays, rather than the primary care physicians who no longer visit their patients in the hospital. Hospitalists link specialists and coordinate care so that all physicians for one patient know the diagnoses, what has been ordered, and the patient's progress" (Milstead, 2002, p. 19). The goal in using hospitalists is to increase coordination and continuity of care. The **intensivist** works primarily in the intensive care unit in a similar role as a hospitalist. The idea is that the hospitalists and intensivists will be more up-to-date in hospital treatment than physicians in private practice since they provide hospital care daily.

How does the use of hospitalists and intensivists affect patients and their care? A study that focused on patient–physician relationships was conducted at Brigham and Women's Hospital (Simon, Lee, & Goldman, 1998). At the time of the study, the hospital did not use a designated hospitalist system; however, the study assessed patients with and without personal physicians in the hospital. The results indicated that patients who had the same physician in the hospital as in the ambulatory setting were less likely to report that they had communication problems with their physicians regarding tests and health habits. The relationship with the patient prior to hospitalization does influence communication with the patient while the patient is in the hospital. Patients feel less stress if they have had a prior relationship with their physicians. Entering the hospital means patients are turning over their care to strangers. At least having a prior relationship with the physician might provide some comfort and trust and establish communication. Nurses need to be aware of this because they will hear about it from their patients. In these circumstances, patients may also turn more to nurses for advice because they interact more with the nurses and have more of a relationship with the nurses.

Despite some concerns about the effects on the physician-patient relationship, however, the use of hospitalists has continued to grow. The benefits of using this method have been identified as:

1. Benefits for the patient due to expertise of the hospitalists/intensivists
   - Clear and timely explanations about care
   - Rapid access to physician to solve patient needs 24 hours/day
   - Rapid physician response to emergencies
   - Continued access to other specialists as needed
   - Reduction in the length-of-stay
   - Decreased utilization of resources, improving resources management
   - Enhanced coordination with other participants in an integrated delivery model
   - Reduced risk of untoward events
2. Benefits to the patient's personal physician
   - Enhanced economic security
   - Referral to specialists remain unchanged
   - Enhanced productivity/revenue gain for group practice
   - Improved clinical outcomes
   - Enhanced training programs
3. Benefits to care providers on the hospital team, including nurses
   - Increased communication and coordination among the care team
   - Cost containment by control of formulary, procedures, and purchased goods
   - Shared responsibility outcomes
   - Consistent approach to care with immediate response
   - Improved access to physicians
4. Benefits to the hospital and payers
   - Reduction in the variability of care
   - Reduction in the length-of-stay

- Decreased utilization of resources
- Enhanced coordination with all other participants of an integrated delivery model
- Reduced risk of liability (Noyes & Healy, 1999, p. 22)

Making the most effective use of hospitalists/intensivists requires planning, clear communication, identification and responsibilities, and education about the role and how other health care providers will relate with the hospitalist. It takes time to make changes, and this is one that requires thought and time. It can clearly be quite successful and reap benefits for many stakeholders, but if not handled well, may cause communication and coordination problems and patient dissatisfaction.

Advanced practice nurses, clinical nurse specialists, and nurse midwives

The roles of nurse practitioners, clinical nurse specialists, and nurse midwives have been expanding in many hospitals just as advanced practice nurses in primary care are increasing. Nurse practitioners who work in acute care are acute care nurse practitioners (ACNPs), but some of these nurse practitioners have completed educational programs that focused on hospitalized patients. Hospitals are also returning to using clinical nurse specialists (CNS) in areas such as neonatal units, cardiology, critical care, trauma, internal medicine, and psychiatry. Their duties might include ordering and interpreting laboratory studies, initiating discharge planning, interpreting chest x-rays, intravenous line management, wound care, and performing cultures (Hubbs, 1999). They work closely with families. Some hospitals are using ACNPs and CNSs in the same way they use house staff. Many of the decisions to expand the usage of these nurses are driven by costs and the pressure of managed care for hospitals to reduce costs.

Alternative/complementary therapies

Alternative/complementary therapies are now found in almost all types of health care settings. Acute care hospitals are no exception to this growth. MCOs/insurers are beginning to cover some of these services. Acute care hospitals might offer massage therapy, acupuncture, and other methods within the hospital setting, in their ambulatory care services, and in their wellness centers. It is not yet clear the direction this will all take so it bears watching. Nurses may find that they are more involved in these services.

Financial issues and managed care: Impact on acute care

Acute care has been greatly influenced by all financial issues related to health care and, of course, managed care. The financial impact of managed care on hospitals has led to downsizing, reengineering, and restructuring. As a result, nursing staff have experienced loss of jobs or changes in responsibilities. Hospitals have merged with others or acquired other hospitals or other types of health care facilities such as home health agencies, long-term care facilities, subacute services, and so on. Much of this has been motivated by financial needs to gain more revenue or reduce costs as well as a need to gain more patients. This reduction in staff has backfired with the major nursing shortage. Nursing staff have not only experienced the loss of jobs and addition of new responsibilities, but they have also experienced stress, burnout, and low morale (see Chapter 12). Later hospitals tried to rehire nurses when they needed to increase beds again, but this was not always so successful.

The financial status of many hospitals is precarious. "After a run of profitable years, hospitals across the country face cash-flow problems—squeezed, officials say, by slow-paying managed care companies, cutbacks in government programs, and rapidly growing numbers of uninsured patients. Pressured by rising costs, hospitals are aggressively trying to collect mountains of overdue bills for patient care" (Freudenheim, May 19, 1999). Hospitals say that managed care organizations are routinely delaying payments for 3 to 4 months, even in states where this is illegal. In 1998, in the 100 best-managed hospitals, the average wait for payment was 64 days, which was 5 more days than in 1997. This delay is extremely costly for hospitals. Hospitals then have less money to pay their own bills, and ultimately, this affects patient care and staffing levels. Medicare and Medicaid changes have also affected the amount of money hospitals receive when they provide services to these patients. The findings indicate that mandated cuts in 1999 Medicare spending had a major influence on hospital profits, particularly on the East and West Coasts. Hospitals most affected were those that were very successful in controlling costs. They had already made major changes necessary to reduce costs and have few choices left to reduce costs further. New strategies to reduce costs need to be used, and these have to be more radical (Mayer & Rushton, 1998). (See Chapter 14 for more information about financial issues.)

Continuum of care and acute care

Understanding and participating in the changing health care environment requires an appreciation of the importance of the continuum of care and its relationship to acute care. **Continuum of care** is "matching an individual's ongoing needs with the appropriate level and type of medical, psychological, health, or social care or service within an organization or across multiple organizations" (Joint Commission on Accreditation of Healthcare Organizations, 2004, p. 317). The goal is to avoid fragmented care, which only increases cost (Newhouse & Mills, 2002). The continuum includes health promotion, disease and illness prevention, ambulatory care, acute care, tertiary care, home health care, long-term care, and hospice care as it takes place within health care organizations and across organizations. Today, patients move into and out of the acute care setting quickly due to shorter lengths-of-stay. Acute care nurses are caring for sicker patients in shorter periods of time while they are overworked, short-staffed, and stressed. Nurses must become facilitators, actively using coordination skills to ensure that patients receive the care they need despite the shortened length-of-stay. Many nurses feel that they do not accomplish much with patients who often leave the hospital ill and in need of more care.

Using standardized operating procedures supports work processes to better ensure continuity (Newhouse & Mills, 2002). Case management has become common in many hospitals, and it is considered to be an important managed care strategy to reduce costs and ensure quality as the patient moves through the continuum of care. Hospitals have also found that case management is useful in assisting with care coordination and rapid discharge, which are both critical to cost reduction. The case manager is also used to ensure that quality care is provided throughout the stay. Nurses are frequently chosen to be case managers in hospitals. "Care coordination must include the following elements: a comprehensive plan of care; a multidisciplinary team approach for patients with complex needs; use of specialists as primary care providers (PCPs) as appropriate; collaboration with providers across the continuum of care; communication of post-discharge home and community arrangements; and medical record integration" (Newhouse & Mills, 2002, p. 87).

Primary care providers

Primary care has grown in the last decade, and it has affected acute care. This care is provided by a particular level of provider (for example, family medicine, general internal medicine, general pediatrics, obstetrical/gynecology, and advanced practice nurses). Managed care has pushed the use of primary care providers to reduce costs. The primary care provider should serve as the gatekeeper to the health care system, providing care at the primary care level, and referring the patient to others for specialty care. The primary care provider should be aware of the patient's entire treatment plan and monitor the patient's progress. Does this always happen? Not always, but the goal is to improve in this area.

Nurses and acute care hospital changes

Nurses in hospitals are members of the system, and they need to learn to be more assertive in order to ensure that nursing care is recognized as critical to successful acute care. Nurses have much to offer in acute care settings, although they do not always get recognized. They also need to use their leadership skills to improve their position and role in hospital decision making. As changes are made, three key issues need to be considered by nurses.

1. Will the approach help the nurse provide better care and ultimately improve patient outcomes?
2. Will the approach bring greater efficiency to the nursing operation?

3. Can the technique be implemented in such a way that costs are tightly managed and, if possible, lowered (Mayer & Rushton, 1998, p. 29)?

An unwillingness to change and the inability to explore new ideas that might be more cost-effective and yet provide quality care is a dangerous attitude. Nurses with this attitude will eventually find that they are not part of the team, feel left out of the health care system, and may be out of jobs. This victim mentality acts as a barrier to the roles that nurses could assume within health care organizations, acute care, and others.

Staffing issues

It is difficult to discuss acute care without discussing the major nursing shortage. Chapter 12 discusses this topic in more detail; however, it is important to recognize the problem in this chapter on acute care. Acute care hospitals are not only adjusting staffing levels but also the staffing mix to reduce costs. Registered nurses (RNs) are finding themselves supervising unlicensed assistant personnel (UAP) more and more. Many nurses have not been adequately prepared for the supervisory role and delegation. In some cases, patients are seeing fewer RNs and more UAPs. This has increased staff stress and concern for errors and potential legal consequences. UAP training and educational background is also a concern in some areas of the country; however, other areas require certification for UAPs. The trend of using UAPs will probably not change, and nurses must provide leadership and direction to ensure that quality, safe care is provided. UAPs are not only used in acute care but also in home care, skilled nursing facilities, rehabilitation, psychiatry, and long-term care.

Outcomes and staffing levels continue to be critical issues in acute care. Chapter 12 discusses some of the recent studies on this topic. If patients do not reach expected outcomes and then experience complications, this increases the cost of health care, and hospitals and managed care organizations do not like their patients/enrollees to experience complications that then require longer hospital stays, additional treatment, and extended care after hospitalization. Complications usually mean more medications are prescribed, and this is of particular concern since the cost of drugs is increasing. Nurses need data to demonstrate that decreasing nursing staff in hospitals will increase patient complications and affect outcomes negatively. Some of the studies that support the positive effect that nurses can have on patient outcomes are found in Chapter 12. Nurses need to gather more data about the positive effects that nursing care has on patient outcomes in the acute care setting.

Nurses who work in acute care settings have found that their work has changed. Skills that are more important now are advocacy, negotiation with a variety of internal and external staff, collaboration, coordination, delegation, and an understanding of the need to provide culturally appropriate care that considers language, religion, nutrition, and culture and family relationships. All of these are leadership competences and are discussed in this text.

BENCHMARKS

Now let's take a moment to test your knowledge of the concepts you have studied in this section.

Magnet Nursing Services Recognition Program

Today, "the public is inundated with media coverage of changes in health care that could adversely affect their access to and the quality of health care services. Public trust in hospitals is eroding and interest in the quality of care is increasing. . . . More than 80% of the public polled in a recent survey wanted to know how to evaluate the quality of hospital care" (Hensley, 1998; National Coalition on Health Care, 1997; as cited in Aiken, Havens, & Sloane, 2000, p. 27). It is important that nurses take active roles in determining the quality of care and the nurse's role in the process. Nurses run the risk of blame for some of the problems that are found in acute care today. "Politics in health care may not end at the bedside, but it certainly begins there. It would be a tragedy if patients and family members blamed nurses for system failures. But the more nurses detach from their patients, the easier it becomes for the rest of us (consumers) to lose sympathy" (Kaplan, 2000, p. 25). The Magnet program is one way to address this issue. What is the Magnet Nursing Services Recognition Program, its impact, and why is it important to new graduates? The following discussion explores some of the critical issues related to Magnet hospitals as an important consideration in any discussion about acute care hospitals in the 21st century.

Research: The pathway to the Magnet Nursing Services Recognition Program

The Magnet program was developed unexpectedly as a result of a study in 1981 conducted by the American Academy of Nursing entitled *Magnet Hospitals: Attraction and Retention of Professional Nurses* (McClure, Poulin, Sovie, & Wandelt, 1983). This study explored variables that helped some hospitals create a magnet or force that assisted in the recruitment and retention of nurses. The study considered the nursing practice and combination of variables that helped to create staff personal and professional satisfaction.

The Magnet Nursing Services Recognition Program began in the 1980s to recognize hospitals that provided quality nursing care or excellence in nursing care. At that time, the American Academy of Nursing conducted a study to identify hospitals that attracted and retained nurses and the characteristics that made these hospitals successful (Aiken, Havens, & Sloane, 2000). Throughout the country, 165 hospitals were nominated for consideration in the study, with 155 responding by submitting applications and information. From this group of hospitals, task force members reviewed the information and selected 46 hospitals. As five of the hospitals were unable to participate, this left 41 hospitals that were actually included in the sample, all predominately private, nonprofit institutions and all affiliated with some educational program in nursing (McClure, Poulin, Sovie, & Wandelt, 1983). Interviews were conducted to gather the data, creating one of the limitations of the study—self-reported data. In addition, interviews were conducted by different task force members, and staff nurses who participated were selected by their directors of nursing.

Results from this first study indicated that there were great similarities between how staff nurses and directors of nursing identified the variables that helped create the "magnet" so that the hospital environment was able to retain nurses or attract nurses to their hospital. These early results established the Foundation for the Magnet Recognition Program. When administration was described in these hospitals, the most common management style identified was participant management in which managers listened to staff and used two-way communication. Leadership was important, and leaders were able to describe the philosophy of care so that it meant something to the staff. These nurse leaders also supported nurses so that they received the resources and services they needed to do their job. This relates to content presented in earlier chapters about the most effective leadership styles and organization structure. Nurse managers were also critical to the success of these hospitals. Directors of nursing were of high quality and had high levels of education. When organization structure was discussed, decentralization was common, which led to more staff control. Nurses were also very active in hospital committees. Staffing, the ever present concern, was considered to be adequate, and they had a higher number of nurses who had baccalaureate degrees. Personnel policies are always important, and this study explored some of these policy issues. Work schedules often were innovative, and consideration was given to staff needs. Promotion opportunities not only included management tracks but also clinical tracks. Professional practice was also very important, and these hospitals were found to have higher levels of quality of care, autonomy, primary nursing, mentoring, professional recognition, respect, and the ability to practice nursing as it should be (McClure, Poulin, Sovie, & Wandelt, 1983). These hospitals also recognized the importance of professional development—orientation, inservice and continuing education, formal education, and career development. There were some differences between staff and manager viewpoints; however, there were "no instances of 'we versus they' dichotomy of employee-management relations" (McClure, Poulin, Sovie, & Wandelt, 1983, p. 20).

The original study led to six other studies that indicate hospitals that receive the Magnet recognition have better outcomes such as lower burnout rates, higher levels of job satisfaction, and higher quality of care than non-Magnet hospitals (Laschinger, Shamian, & Thomson, 2001). A critical study completed in 2001, *Staff Nurses Identify Essentials of Magnetism* (Kramer & Schmalenberg, 2002), included 14 Magnet hospitals and 279 staff nurses who worked in them. The study objectives were:

1. To update the variables staff nurses in Magnet hospitals today consider most important for nursing effectiveness in giving high-quality care.
2. To define what staff nurses mean by good nurse-physician relationships, control over nursing practice, and autonomy.
3. To quantify the preceding two variables empirically.
4. To ascertain the degree of relationship between these variables and nurse job satisfaction, effectiveness, and competence of co-workers.
5. To identify degree of value congruence among staff nurses, nurse managers, and chief nurse executives (Kramer & Schmalenberg, 2002, p. 27).

The results from this study identified eight variables that are important in providing quality care. Future research will undoubtedly further explore these variables. The following are the critical variables.

1. Working with other nurses who are clinically competent
2. Good nurse-physician relationships
3. Nurse autonomy and accountability
4. Supportive nurse manager-supervisor
5. Control over nursing practice and practice environment
6. Support for education
7. Adequacy of nurse staffing
8. Concern for patient is paramount (Kramer & Schmalenberg, 2002, pp. 53–55)

When these variables are reviewed it is easy to see how they connect to the results from the first study. These are the variables that create magnetism—the process of attracting nurses and keeping them.

YOUR OPINION COUNTS

Find out what others think about this topic. Post your response and check out other opinions.

Magnet hospital framework

As the research about Magnet hospitals has developed, a framework has guided the research based on work done about hospitals that recognizes hospitals are complex organizations with both bureaucratic structures and professional structures (Flood & Scott, 1987). "Nurses in hospitals, because of their employment status, are agents of the bureaucracy but hold professional values and seek peer relationships with other professionals and professional modes of organizing their work. Nurses are accountable to both the bureaucratic structure as headed by management and the professional structure as exemplified and headed by physicians" (Aiken, 2002, p. 62). This puts nurses in potential conflict situations. This conceptual framework considers the patient surveillance system that assists in identifying medical errors and adverse events. Nurses are the key players in the surveillance system. Other key factors are staffing, skill mix, and management decisions. Staffing looks at the total numbers of all types of nursing staff, and skill mix is the proportion of registered nurses compared to other nursing staff. The nurse work environment, which is a critical factor for any nurse in any type of health care setting, includes resource adequacy, administrative support, and nurse-physician relations. All of these variables come together in the implementation of the process of care that results in nurse and patient outcomes. Research results indicate that Magnet hospitals tend to provide quality care that leads to positive outcomes for patients and better work environments for nurses (Aiken, 2002).

There are other interesting results from recent research on Magnet hospitals. Cost is always a critical concern in health care, and so it is with Magnet hospitals. Since Magnet hospitals tend to have higher staff-patient ratios and staffing is the most expensive budget item, they do have higher nursing staff costs. Some research, however, does indicate that some patients have lower length-of-stay rates, which decreases health care costs (Aiken, 2002). There needs to be more research on this topic. As would be expected, these hospitals have better nurse outcomes or job satisfaction. There were also less needlestick injuries in the hospitals that were in the study. If nurses are more satisfied with their work, less frustrated, and work with the same staff over a longer period of time, then nurse workplace safety may improve. There is no doubt that further research about cost-benefit issues and Magnet hospital characteristics are needed and will be conducted. There also needs to be further exploration of nurse and patient outcomes (McClure & Hinshaw, 2002b).

Building magnetism

Forces of magnetism or organizational elements of excellence in nursing care are the critical elements that make a difference in whether or not a hospital receives Magnet status, and these forces or magnets seem to affect how a hospital attracts and retains nurses. How does a hospital get to the stage that it can demonstrate these elements? Hinshaw (2002) has described some of the strategies that might be used; however, a key point is to have competent nursing staff. Nurses want to know that they can count on their colleagues to know their job and what needs to be done to care for patients. This competency directly affects autonomy and control over nursing practice, which are part of the forces of magnetism. Hospitals need to ensure staff competence and provide educational opportunities—to maintain skills and enhance skills through staff education and to develop further (for example, by obtaining additional degrees or certification) (see Chapter 13). These hospitals are willing to invest in staff by providing education within the hospital, assisting staff in identifying the need to pursue formal education, providing flexibility with scheduling, and assisting with reimbursement of educational costs.

Staffing is, of course, critical, and this has been demonstrated in Magnet hospitals, which appear to have adequate staffing. Staffing includes not only numbers of staff but also their education, expertise, competence, and skill-mix. The goal is high-quality care, and this is supported with recent research indicating positive patient outcomes (Aiken, Havens, & Sloane, 2000; Havens, 2001; Kovner & Mezey, 1999; Sovie & Jawad, 2001). Magnet hospitals have used a number of strategies to improve their staffing such as establishing recommended levels of patient-staff ratios, limiting use of substitution (Sovie & Jawad, 2001), using teams of competent nurses that include agency or float nurses, and developing float teams that are used for particular types of patients (Kramer & Schmalenberg, 2002). Some states, led by legislation passed first in California, are establishing required nurse-patient ratios. There are pros and cons to this approach, which are discussed in Chapter 12. Magnet hospitals have higher RN-patient ratios, and more of the RNs have baccalaureate and master's degrees.

Autonomy is an important characteristic found in Magnet hospitals and in the forces of magnetism. Autonomy is "the freedom to act on what you know" (Kramer & Schmalenberg, 2002, p. 36). Responsibility and accountability are important components of autonomy. How is autonomy supported? Nursing leadership that is strong and visible is important, as is decentralization. Empowering staff to feel that they can make decisions and that they are competent is a strategy that helps to develop autonomy. It is difficult to separate autonomy from control over practice—to understand and participate in what needs to be done to ensure that nursing care meets nursing standards. Again leadership, empowerment, and decentralization are important, and hospitals have found that shared governance does make a difference. Communication at all levels is critical in providing care and for nurses to control their practice.

Finally, nurse-physician relationships are also important; typically, this can be problematic. The goal is to have positive relationships that are collaborative so that both work together to meet the needs of patients and reach positive outcomes for the patients. Interdisciplinary care is the norm today, and this requires communication and coordination to ensure that ongoing needs are met, plans are implemented, and that there is no unnecessary duplication of services. Information needs to be shared, clear, and reported in a timely manner. This also means that nurses and physicians need to respect one another and recognize the expertise of each other. Strategies that have been shown to be effective in improving nurse-physician relationships in Magnet hospitals are clearly defined communication procedures and structures, interdisciplinary committees, and the development of teams of nurses and physicians so that they can develop working relationships. Newhouse and Mills (2002) have identified some key points related to nurse-physician relationships and forming interdisciplinary teams.

- All teams are not created equal, but careful development of working relationships and clear goals can make all the difference.
- Successful teams are composed of competent team members with the necessary skills, abilities, and personalities to achieve the desired objectives.
- Teams composed of many professional disciplines are able to expand the number and quality of actions to improve health care systems.
- Interdisciplinary teams work collaboratively to set and achieve goals directed toward innovative and effective care and efficient organizational systems.
- The nurse team member represents the voice of nursing as a discipline responsible for the holistic care of patients.
- Positive relationships with physicians benefit the patient and enhance the work environment for nurses.
- Nurses must develop the skills to work collaboratively as a professional member of the interdisciplinary team (pp. 64–69).

There is no doubt that management is important. The content of this textbook is a testament to that as is the requirement of leadership and management content in nursing curricula. Magnet hospitals have demonstrated that nursing leadership needs to be strong and supportive of nursing staff—to be the advocate for the nursing staff and the care that they provide. Leadership provides the vision and ensures that it is implemented, ensures that staff have the resources needed to provide quality care, ensures that staff are competent, develops communication procedures and structures that work, provides information technology that supports the work that needs to be done, and ensures that nursing leaders play an important role in the organization of the hospital—thus representing the nursing staff.

In a study done by Havens (2001) that compared nursing infrastructure and outcomes in Magnet and non-Magnet hospitals, the results noted that there were some structural differences in the hospitals in addition to the characteristics that have been identified as part of Magnet hospitals such as autonomy, control of practice, quality care, and other critical elements. More of the Magnet hospitals had discrete departments of nursing. This might be more supportive of an organization that supports and respects nursing. Nursing was seen as visible—a distinct profession within the organization. The chief nursing executive also had more control of nursing practice and the nursing practice environment. These hospitals also had more doctorally prepared nurse researchers who supported staff participation in nursing research, affecting the quality of care. A critical difference was the Magnet hospitals had not responded to reengineering and restructuring in the same way (Havens, 2001). Whereas the non-Magnet hospitals had made major changes by eliminating the department of nursing, reconfiguring skill-mix, and reducing the number of RNs, the Magnet hospitals had taken different approaches. The result was actually an expansion of the chief nurse executive role to include non-nursing departments or services. The results of the study also re-confirmed the importance of applying the *ANA Scope and Standards for Nurse Administrators* (1996). "Based on research and grounded in professional standards (American Nurses Association, 1996), the Magnet Recognition Program may present a prescriptive model for administrative 'best practice' by recognizing excellence in four areas: (a) management philosophy and practices, (b) adherence to standards for improving the quality of care, (c) leadership of the CNE in supporting professional practice and continued nursing competence, and (d) attention to the cultural and ethnic diversity of patients, their significant others, and providers. The findings from this research further suggest that the ANCC Magnet Program may also offer an evidence-based approach to solve two crucial problems confronting hospitals: recapturing public confidence and recruiting and retaining high-quality employees" (Curran, 2000; Havens, 2001, p. 266).

The Magnet Recognition Process

The Magnet Nursing Services Recognition Program for Excellence, established in 1993, is administered by the American Nurses Credentialing Center (ANCC), the Commission on the Magnet Recognition Program. This program not only recognizes excellence in hospital nursing, but as of 1998, it also offers this recognition for long-term care facilities. The objectives of the program are to:

■ Recognize nursing services that utilize the *Scope and Standards for Nurse Administrators* to build programs of nursing excellence in the delivery of nursing care to patients.

■ Promote quality in a milieu that supports professional nursing practice.

■ Provide a vehicle for the dissemination of successful nursing practices and strategies among institutions utilizing the services of registered professional nurses (American Nurses Credentialing Center, 2002).

The recognition program is available to any size hospital that meets the standards. Its focus is on quality patient care and the nurses within the institution. How does a hospital receive Magnet Recognition? First, it is important to understand the difference between accreditation, certification, and recognition. The ANCC has defined "Accreditation as a voluntary process used to validate that an organization and an approval body meets established continuing education standards. Certification focuses on the individual and is a process used to validate that an individual registered nurse possesses the requisite knowledge, skills, and abilities to practice in a defined practice specialty. Recognition is a third credentialing process operationalized in ANCC to evaluate an organization's adherence to excellence-focused standards" (Urden & Monarch, 2002, pp. 102–103). The Magnet Program is a recognition program. The evaluation process uses the *Scope and Standards for Nurse Administrators* (American Nurses Association, 1996) and the forces of magnetism identified in Box 6-7 to determine excellence in nursing care.

When a hospital is interested in pursuing recognition, it must first conduct an environmental assessment. From the results of this assessment, the organization can determine if there are gaps between what exists and what is expected for Magnet status recognition. At this point, the hospital may decide that the gap is too large and more work needs to be done to improve before seeking recognition. If the hospital decides to seek recognition, the hospital must organize for the process, identify leaders for the process, make plans, and set timelines. Following this, there are four major phases (Urden & Monarch, 2002). Staff nurses need to be included in all phases.

1. The first phase is the application and designation process.
2. The second phase is documentation review when the hospital sends required documentation to ANCC for review. This material is reviewed and scored, which takes several months.
3. The third phase is the site visit. Several appraisers visit the hospital to meet with staff, administration, patients, families, and other critical people.
4. The final phase is review and decision. When Magnet status is awarded, the hospital maintains this status for 4 years. Then the hospital can apply for recognition again, but it must continue to meet the required standards.

What must a hospital do to maintain its Magnet recognition? The following is expected.

1. Submit annual monitoring reports.
2. Participate in the ANA's quality indicator study coordinated by the National Center for Nursing Quality.
3. Notify the Magnet Recognition Program office if any of the following occurs:
    ■ a significant increase in staff turnover
    ■ a significant increase in the nurse vacancy rate
    ■ a significant decrease in nurse decision-making positions/activities
    ■ a significant negative change in the organization's nurse-patient ratio
    ■ a significant negative change in the licensed/unlicensed ratio of the nursing staff
    ■ a significant increase in the organization's nurse absentee rate
    ■ a significant amount of mandatory overtime worked by nurses reporting to the Department of Nursing
    ■ Nursing-Sensitivity Quality Indicator data that fall significantly below the threshold established by the Magnet organization

BOX 6-7   Forces of magnetism: Organizational elements of excellence in nursing care.

Quality of nursing leadership—Nursing leaders were perceived as knowledgeable, strong risk-takers who followed an articulated philosophy in the day-to-day operations of the nursing department. Nursing leaders also conveyed a strong sense of advocacy and support on behalf of the staff.

Organizational structure—Organizational structures were characterized as flat, rather than tall, and where unit-based decision making prevailed. Nursing departments were decentralized, with strong nursing representation evident in the organizational committee structure. The nursing leader served at the executive level of the organization, and the chief nursing officer reported to the chief executive officer.

Management style—Hospital and nursing administrators were found to use a participative management style, incorporating feedback from staff at all levels of the organization. Feedback was characterized as encouraged and valued. Nurses serving in leadership positions were visible, accessible, and committed to communicating effectively with staff.

Personnel policies and programs—Salaries and benefits were characterized as competitive. Rotating shifts were minimized, and creative and flexible staffing models were used. Personnel policies were created with staff involvement, and significant administrative and clinical promotional opportunities existed.

Professional models of care—Models of care were used that gave nurses the responsibility and authority for the provision of patient care. Nurses were accountable for their own practice and were the coordinators of care.

Quality of care—Nurses perceived that they were providing high-quality care to their patients. Providing quality care was seen as an organizational priority as well, and nurses serving in leadership positions were viewed as responsible for developing the environment in which high-quality care could be provided.

Quality improvement—Quality improvement activities were viewed as educational. Staff nurses participated in the quality improvement process and perceived the process as one that improved the quality of care delivered within the organization.

Consultation and resources—Adequate consultation and other human resources were available. Knowledgeable experts, particularly advanced practice nurses, were available and used. In addition, peer support was given within and outside the nursing division.

Autonomy—Nurses were permitted and expected to practice autonomously, consistent with professional standards. Independent judgment was expected to be exercised within the context of a multidisciplinary approach to patient care.

Community and the hospital—Hospitals that were best able to recruit and retain nurses also maintained a strong community presence. A community presence was seen in a variety of ongoing, long-term outreach programs. These outreach programs resulted in the hospital being perceived as a strong, positive, and productive corporate citizen.

Nurses as teachers—Nurses were permitted and expected to incorporate teaching in all aspects of their practice. Teaching was one activity that reportedly gave nurses a great deal of professional satisfaction.

Image of nursing—Nurses were viewed as integral to the hospital's ability to provide patient care services. The services provided by nurses were characterized as essential by other members of the health care team.

Interdisciplinary relationship—Interdisciplinary relationships were characterized as positive. A sense of mutual respect was exhibited among all disciplines.

Professional development—Significant emphasis was placed on orientation, inservice education, continuing education, formal education, and career development. Personal and professional growth and development were valued. In addition, opportunities for competency-based clinical advancement existed, along with the resources to maintain competency.

Source: McClure, M., & Hinshaw, A. (2002a). *Magnet hospitals revisited, forces of magnetism: Organizational elements of excellence in nursing care*, Washington DC: American Nursing Publishing, pp. 106–107. Reprinted with permission.

■ Nursing-Sensitive Quality Indicator data that fall significantly below the national average as determined by the National Database of Nursing Quality Indicators (*The American Nurse*, 2002, p. 17)

This list of what a hospital must report provides a good example of the key acute care issues that should concern new graduates as they search for jobs.

Benefits of the program

Typically, hospitals that are recognized as Magnet hospitals publicize this in their marketing. Clearly, this recognition can affect patients' interest in receiving care in the hospital if they understand its significance. The information can also be used in the recruitment and retention of nursing staff. Hospitals that receive this recognition become models of excellence for other hospitals. Consumers want more and more information about the quality of their health care. The usual benchmark for hospitals has been receiving a high rating on JCAHO accreditation; however, the Magnet Recognition Program offers another method to determine quality—one that has been largely ignored and focuses primarily on nursing (Aiken, Havens, & Sloane, 2000). "The slow rate of ANCC Magnet hospital recognition is problematic. This potentially useful quality indicator must be propelled into the public domain" (Aiken, Havens, & Sloane, 2000, p. 33). More needs to be done to educate the public about the recognition, and hospitals that are designated as Magnet hospitals of nursing excellence need to publicize this status and explain what it means.

Why is this information about Magnet hospitals important to new graduates? The research over the last decade or more indicates that some hospitals are more successful than others in attracting and retaining staff. These hospitals also demonstrate critical positive outcomes for patients and for staff. As new graduates consider their first nursing positions, understanding Magnet hospitals, the related research results, and the forces of magnetism can help new graduates assess potential employers and decide if a particular hospital is the place for them. The description of a Magnet hospital via the forces of magnetism can provide a checklist when assessing hospitals and their nursing services.

CURRENT ISSUES

Learn about events around the globe that relate to the chapter content.

BENCHMARKS

Now let's take a moment to test your knowledge of the concepts you have studied in this section.

Chapter Wrap-Up

Now that you've reached the end of the chapter, you may wish to explore the concepts you've been reading about in greater detail, or test yourself to see how well you've comprehended the material.

SUMMARY AND APPLICATIONS

■ Summary
■ Practice Quiz
■ Key Terms
■ Tying It All Together

■ Experiential Exercises
■ Case
■ Links

REFERENCES

Ackerman, F. (1992). The movement toward vertically integrated regional health systems. *Health Care Management Review, 2*, 81–88.

Aiken, L. (2002). Superior outcomes for magnet hospitals. In M. McClure & A. Hinshaw (Eds.), *Magnet hospitals revisited* (pp. 61–82). Washington, DC: American Nurses Publishing.

Aiken, L., Havens, D., & Sloane, D. (2000). The magnet nursing services recognition program: A comparison of successful applicants with reputational magnet hospitals. *American Journal of Nursing, 100*(3), 26–35.

American Nurses Association. (1996). *Scope and standards for nurse administrators*. Washington, DC: American Nurses Publishing, Inc.

American Nurses Credentialing Center. Retrieved on January 28, 2002, from www.nursingworld.org/ancc/magnet.htm.

Blue, R., et al. (1994). Consultation. In J. Koerner & K. Karpiuk (Eds.), *Implementing differentiated practice: Transformation by design* (pp. 188–213). Gaithersburg, MD: Aspen Publishers, Inc.

Boston, C. (1990). Differentiated practice: An introduction. In C. Boston (Ed.), *Current issues and perspectives on differentiated practice* (pp. 1–3). Chicago: American Association of Nurse Executives.

Curran, C. (2000). Musing on magnets. *Nursing Economics, 18*(2), 57.

Emergency Nurses Association. (1996). *Position statements of the Emergency Nurses Association on healthcare and scope of emergency nursing practice*. Park Ridge, IL: Author.

Flood, A., & Scott, W. (1987). *Hospital structure and performance*. Baltimore, MD: Johns Hopkins Press.

Fottler, M., & Malvey, D. (1999). Multiprovider systems. In L. Wolper (Ed.), *Health care administration* (3rd ed., pp. 53–87). Gaithersburg, MD: Aspen Publishers, Inc.

Freudenheim, M. (1999, May 19). Insurers and uninsured put hospitals in a squeeze. *New York Times*, BU4.

Haas, S. (1998). Managed care's impact on emergency department workload. *Journal of Nursing Administration, 28*(11), 3–4.

Havens, D. (2001). Comparing nursing infrastructure and outcomes: ANCC magnet and nonmagnet CNEs report. *Nursing Economics, 19*(6), 258–266.

Hensley, S. (1998). VHA readies campaign. Proposed plan would play up local hospital's strengths. *Modern Healthcare, 28*(4), 2–3.

Herr, R. (1998). Managed care and emergency department: Nursing issues. *Journal of Emergency Nursing, 24*(5), 406–411.

Hinshaw, A. (2002). Building magnetism into health organizations. In M. McClure & A. Hinshaw (Eds.), *Magnet hospitals revisited* (pp. 83–102). Washington, DC: American Nurses Publishing.

Hubbs, L. (1999). Understanding the role of the acute care nurse practitioner. Retrieved on July 16, 1999, from www.nurse.com.

Joint Commission on Accreditation of Healthcare Organizations. (2004). *Hospital accreditation standards*. Oakbrook Terrace, IL: Author.

Kaplan, M. (2000). Hospital caregivers are in a bad mood. *American Journal of Nursing, 100*(3), 25.

Koerner, J., (1992). Differentiated practice: The evolution of professional nursing. *Journal of Professional Nursing, 8*(6), 335–341.

Koerner, J., et al. (1995). Differentiated practice: The evolution of a professional practice model for integrated client care services. In D. Flarey (Ed.), *Redesigning nursing care delivery*. Philadelphia: J.B. Lippincott Company.

Kovner, C. T., & Mezey, M. (1999). They just don't get it. *American Journal of Nursing, 99*(7), 9.

Kramer, M., & Schmalenberg, C. (2002). Staff nurses identify essentials of magnetism. In M. McClure & A. Hinshaw (Eds.), *Magnet hospitals revisited* (pp. 25–59). Washington, DC: American Nurses Publishing.

Laschinger, H., Shamian, J., & Thomson, D. (2001). Impact of Magnet hospital characteristics on nurses' perceptions of trust, burnout, quality of care, and work satisfaction. *Nursing Economics, 19*(5), 209–219.

Mayer, G., & Rushton, N. (1998). The hospital nurse's role in managed care. *Nursing Management, 30*(9), 25–29.

McClure, M., Poulin, M., Sovie, M., & Wandelt, M. (1983). *Magnet hospitals: Attraction and retention of professional nurses*. American Academy of Nursing Task Force on Nursing Practice in Hospitals. Kansas City, MO: American Nurses Association.

McClure, M., & Hinshaw, A. (Eds.). (2002a). *Magnet hospitals revisited*. Washington, DC: American Nurses Publishing.

McClure, M., & Hinshaw, A. (2002b). The future of magnet hospitals. In M. McClure & A. Hinshaw (Eds.), *Magnet hospitals revisited* (pp. 117–128). Washington, DC: American Nurses Publishing.

Milstead, J. (2002). Leapfrog group: A prince in disguise or just another frog? *Nursing Administration Quarterly, 26*(4), 16–25.

National Coalition on Health Care (1997). How Americans perceive the health care system: A report on a national survey. *Journal on Health Care Finance, 23*(4), 12–20.

Nelson, R., & Koerner, J. (1994). Context. In J. Koerner & K. Karpiuk (Eds.), *Implementing differentiated practice: Transformation by design* (pp. 1–21). Gaithersburg, MD: Aspen Publishers, Inc.

Newhouse, R., & Mills, M. (2002). *Nursing leadership in the organized delivery system for the acute care setting.* Washington, DC: American Nurses Publishing.

Noyes, B., & Healy, S. (1999). The hospitalist: The new addition to the inpatient management team. *Journal of Nursing Administration, 29*(2), 21–24.

Payne, D. (1999). Credentialing and privileging ensure skilled care. *Nursing Management, 30*(8), 8.

Plauth, S., & Pearson, D. (1998). Discontinuity of care: Urgent care utilization within a health care maintenance organization. *American Journal of Managed Care, 4*(11), 1531–1537.

Shi, L., & Singh, D. (1998). *Delivering health care in America.* Gaithersburg, MD: Aspen Publishers, Inc.

Simon, S., Lee, T., & Goldman, L. (1998). Improving communication with patient needs to be major focus for hospitalist systems. *Journal of General Internal Medicine, 13*(5), 836–838.

Sovie, M., & Jawad, A. (2001). Hospital restructuring and its impact on outcomes. *The Journal of Nursing Administration, 31*(12), 588–600.

The American Nurse. (2002, September-October). New law, JCAHO report recognize success of Magnet concept. *The American Nurse,* 16–17.

The Nurse Executive Center. (1999). *Understanding the impact of changes in nurse staffing: A review of recent outcome studies.* Washington, DC: The Advisory Company.

Urden, L., & Monarch, K. (2002). The ANCC Magnet Recognition Program: Converting research findings into action. In M. McClure & A. Hinshaw (Eds.), *Magnet hospitals revisited* (pp. 103–116). Washington, DC: American Nurses Publishing.

Van Servellen, G., & Schultz, M. (1999). Demystifying the influence of hospital characteristics on inpatient mortality rates. *Journal of Nursing Administration, 29*(4), 39–47.

Wolper, L., & Pena, J. (1999). History of hospitals. In L. Wolper (Ed.), *Health care administration* (3rd ed., pp. 391–405). Gaithersburg, MD: Aspen Publishers.

ADDITIONAL READINGS

AACN-AONE Task Force on Differentiated Competencies for Nursing Practice. (1995). *A model for differentiated practice.* Washington, DC: American Association of Colleges of Nursing.

Aiken, L., (2001a). Evidence-based management: Key to hospital workforce stability. *Journal of Health Administration Education, 19*(4), 117–124.

Aiken, L. (2001b). More nurses, better patient outcomes: Why isn't it obvious? *Effective Clinical Practice, 4*(5), 223–225.

Aiken, L., Clarke, S., & Sloane, D. (2000). Hospital restructuring: Does it adversely affect care and outcomes? *Journal of Nursing Administration, 30*(10), 457–465.

Aiken, L., & Havens, D. (2000). The Magnet Nursing Services Recognition Program. *American Journal of Nursing, 100*(3), 26–36.

Aiken, L., & Patrician, P. (2000). Measuring organizational traits of hospitals: The revised nursing work index. *Nursing Research, 49*(3), 146–153.

Aiken, L., & Sloane, D. (1998). Advances in hospital outcomes research. *Journal of Health Services Research and Policy, 3*(4), 249–250.

Aiken, L., Sloane, D., & Sochalski, J. (1998). Hospital organization and outcomes. *Quality in Health Care, 7*(4), 222–226.

Aiken, L., Sloane, D., Lake, E., Sochalski, J., & Weber, A. (1999). Organization and outcomes of inpatient AIDS care. *Medical Care, 37*(8), 760–772.

American Nurses Association. (2001). ANCC magnet criteria recognized in Senate. *Capitol Update, 19*(11), 3.

American Nurses Credentialing Center. (2002). *The Magnet Nursing Services Recognition Program for Excellence in Nursing Service, health care organization, instructions and application process manual.* Washington, DC: American Nurses Credentialing Center.

Anderson, R. (2000). Are our systems really integrated? *Nursing Administration Quarterly, 24*(4), 11–17.

Angelucci, P. (1999). Accept or divert? *Nursing Management, 30*(9), 16A–D.

Anonymous. (1990). The nurse doctor game: Are the rules changing? *Nursing 90, 20*(6), 54–55.

Beyers, M. (1999). About handing over medication administration to pharmDs. *Nursing Management, 30*(8), 56.

Brewster, L., Rudell, L., & Lesser, C. (2001). Emergency room diversions: A symptom of hospitals under stress. *Center for Studying Health System Change,* Issue #38 (May), 1–4.

Buchan, J. (1999). Still attractive after all these years? Magnet hospitals in changing health care environment. *Journal of Advanced Nursing, 30*(1), 100–108.

Burkhardt, J., Nardone, P., & Wandmacher, W. (1994). Nursing/pharmacy interface: A TQM project. *Nursing Management, 25*(3), 38–43.

Carr, J. (2000). Requirements management. *Journal of Nursing Administration, 30*(3), 133–139.

Conrad, D. (1993). Coordinating patient care services in regional health systems: The challenge of clinical integration. *Hospital & Health Services Administration, 18*(4), 491–505.

Conrad, D., & Dowling, W. (1990). Vertical integration in health services: Theory and managerial implications. *Health Care Management Review, 15*(4), 9–22.

Fagin, C. (1992). Collaboration between nurses and physicians: No longer a choice. *Academic Medicine, 67*(5), 295–303.

Forsey, L., Cleland, V., & Miller, C. (1993). Job descriptions for differentiated nursing practice and differentiated pay. *Journal of Nursing Administration, 23*(5), 33–40.

Fox, R., Fox, D., & Wells, P. (1999). Performance of first-line management functions on productivity of hospital unit. *Journal of Nursing Administration, 29*(9), 12–18.

Godchaux, C. (1999). Case managers drive care integration. *Nursing Management, 30*(11), 32B–C, 32F–32G.

Grady, C. (2001). Clinical research: The power of the nurse. *American Journal of Nursing, 101*(9), 11–13.

Havens, D., & Aiken, L. (1999). Shaping systems to promote desired outcomes: The Magnet hospital model. *Journal of Nursing Administration, 29*(2), 14–20.

Hess, R. (1995). Shared governance: Nursing's 20th century tower of Babel. *Journal of Nursing Administration, 25*(5), 14–20.

Hutchens, G. (1994). Differentiated interdisciplinary practice. *Journal of Nursing Administration, 24*(6), 52–58.

Institute of Medicine. (2001). *Crossing the quality chasm: A new health system for the 21st century.* Washington, DC: National Academy Press.

Jones, K., DeBaca, V., & Yarbrough, M. (1997). Organizational culture assessment before and after implementing patient-focused care. *Nursing Economics, 15*(2), 72–80.

Jones, K., & Redman, R. (2000). Organizational culture and work redesign. *Journal of Nursing Administration, 30*(12), 604–610.

Keating, C., & Morin, M. (2001). An approach for systems analysis of patient care operations. *Journal of Nursing Administration, 31*(7/8), 355–363.

Kennerly, S. (2000). Perceived worker autonomy: The foundation for shared governance. *Journal of Nursing Administration, 30*(12), 611–617.

Institute of Medicine. (1999). *To err is human: Building a safer health care system.* Washington, DC: National Academy Press.

Kovner, C., & Harrington, C. (2001). Acute care nurse practitioners. *American Journal of Nursing, 101*(5), 61–62.

Kovner, C., & Harrington, C. (2002). The changing picture of hospital nurses. *American Journal of Nursing, 102*(5), 93–94.

Kramer, M., (1990). The Magnet hospitals: Excellence revisited. *Journal of Nursing Administration, 20*(9), 35–44.

Kramer, M., & Schmalenberg, C. (1988a). Magnet hospitals: Part I: Institutions of excellence. *Journal of Nursing Administration, 18*(1), 13–24.

Kramer, M., & Schmalenberg, C. (1988b). Magnet hospitals: Part II: Institutions of excellence. *Journal of Nursing Administration, 18*(2), 11–19.

LaDuke, S. (2000). Top trends that support your stance. *Nursing Management, 31*(2), 40–42.

Laschinger, H., & Havens, S. (1996). Staff nurse work empowerment and perceived control over nursing practice: Conditions for work effectiveness. *Journal of Nursing Administration, 26*(9), 27–35.

Laschinger, H., Shamian, J., & Thomson, D. (2001). Impact of magnet hospital characteristics on nurses' perceptions of trust, burnout, quality of care, and work satisfaction. *Nursing Economics, 19*(5), 209–219.

Laschinger, H., & Wong, C. (1999). Staff nurse empowerment and collective accountability: Effect on perceived productivity and self-rated work effectiveness. *Nursing Economics, 17*(6), 308–316.

Marett, B. (2000). The time has come. *Journal of Emergency Nursing, 26*(4), 289–290.

Mason, D. (2000). Nursing's best kept secret. *American Journal of Nursing, 100*(3), 7.

Mastorovich, M., & Drenkard, K. (2000). Nursing future search. Building a community of nurses in an integrated healthcare system. *Journal of Nursing Administration, 30*(4), 173–179.

McBeth, A. (2000). Community care partnership: Planning with the community. *Seminars for Nurse Managers, 8*(2), 116–123.

Messmer, P., & Gonzalez, J. (2003). March to magnet: One hospital's experience in achieving Magnet status. *Reflections on Nursing LEADERSHIP,* fourth quarter, 14–15.

Miranda, D., Fields, W., & Lund, K. (2001). Lessons learned during 15 years of clinical information system experience. *Computers in Nursing, 19*(4), 147–151.

Monarch, K. (2003). Magnet hospitals powerful force for excellence. *Reflections on Nursing LEADERSHIP,* fourth quarter, 10–13.

Newhouse, R., & Mills, M. (1999). Vertical systems integration. *Journal of Nursing Administration, 29*(10), 22–29.

Page, L. (2002). Hospitalists save groups time, money. *Physician Practice Options,* (April 1), 10–11.

Pierson, P., Hesnard, D., & Haas, J. (2000). Intranet systems offer fast access to policies and procedures. *Nursing Management, 31*(1), 13.

Porter-O'Grady, T. (2003). Researching shared governance: A futility of focus. *Journal of Nursing Administration, 33*(4), 251–252.

Porter-O'Grady, T., Bradely, G., Crow, G., & Hendrich, A. (1997). After a merger: The dilemma of the best leadership approach for nursing. *Nursing Administration Quarterly, 21*(2), 8–19.

Rafferty, A., Ball, J., & Aiken, L. (2001). Are teamwork and professional autonomy compatible, and do they result in improved hospital care? *Quality in Health Care, 10* (Supplement II), 32–37.

Roye, J. (2001). More NPs are the answer for non-urgent ED patients. *Journal of Emergency Nursing, 27*(4), 321–322.

Rozich, J., & Resar, R. (2002). Using a unit assessment tool to optimize patient flow and staffing in a community hospital. *Journal on Quality Improvement, 28*(1), 31–41.

Schim, S., Thornburg, P., & Kravutske, M. (2001). Time, task, and talents in ambulatory care nursing. *Journal of Nursing Administration, 31*(6), 311–315.

Scott, J., Sochalski, J., & Aiken, L. (1999). Review of Magnet hospital research. *Journal of Nursing Administration, 29*(1), 9–19.

Schroeder, C., Trehearne, B., & Ward, D. (2000). Expanded role of nursing in ambulatory managed care, Part I: Literature, role development, and justification. *Nursing Economics, 18*(1), 14–19.

Shortell, S. (1988). The evolution of hospital systems: Unfulfilled promises and self-fulfilling prophesies. *Medical Care Review, 4*(2), 177–214.

Steefel, L. (2001). Magnets attract RNs. *Nursing Spectrum, 2*(10), 20MW.

Steefel, L. (2002). Is the safety net unraveling? *Nursing Spectrum Metro Edition Midwest Region, 3*(2), 16MW–17MW.

Tallon, R. (1996). Automated medication dispensing systems. *Nursing Management, 27*(8), 45–46.

Upenieks, V. (2000). The relationship of nursing practice models and job satisfaction outcomes. *Journal of Nursing Administration, 30*(6), 330–335.

Urden, L., & Rogers, S. (2000). Tips for successful merger integration. *Journal of Nursing Administration, 30*(4), 161–162.

Urden, L., & Walston, S. (2001). Outcomes of hospital restructuring and reengineering. How is success or failure being measured? *Journal of Nursing Administration, 31*(4), 203–209.

Walston, S., Burns, L., & Kimberly, J. (2000). Does reengineering really work? An examination of the context and outcomes of hospital reengineering initiatives. *Health Services Research, 34*(6), 1363–1387.

Whitcomb, R., et. al. (2002). Advanced practice nursing acute care model in progress. *Journal of Nursing Administration, 32*(3), 123–125.

Wolf, G. (2000). Vision 2000: The transformation of professional practice. *Nursing Administration Quarterly, 24*(2), 45–51.

Zander, K. (2000). Clinical integration at ground zero: Perceptions of patients and families. *Seminars for Nurse Managers, 8*(1), 10–15.

Zero waiting room time does not work when patients outnumber beds. *Journal of Emergency Nursing/Letters, 26*(5), 408–409.

Zhang, Z., Luh, W., Arthur, D., & Wong, T. (2001). Nursing competencies: Personal characteristics contributing to effective nursing. *Journal of Advance Nursing, 33*(4), 467–474.

Teamwork and Motivation

MediaLink
www.prenhall.com/finkelman

The Interactive Exercises for this chapter can be found in the OneKey course at www.prenhall.com/finkelman. Click on Chapter 7 to select from the following activities: Test Your Understanding, Benchmarks, Current Issues, Your Opinion Counts, Think Critically, and Summary and Applications.

What's Ahead

With an increasing outcome-oriented health care delivery system, synergy from teams can work to the system's benefit. Synergy is the "interaction of two or more agents or forces so that their combined effort is far greater than the sum of their individual efforts" (Mears, 1994, p. 4). Synergy requires good communication, particularly through listening and clarifying; supporting and encouraging one another; use of differing and confronting skills; a commitment to quality; acceptance of the value of teams and their collective contributions; and use of constructive feedback for the betterment of the team and outcomes. The content in this text is related to teams, how they function, and how they impact health care. This chapter specifically provides information about critical team elements and the team's functioning, or the structure process of teams that are important for nurses.

OBJECTIVES

Before you begin, take a moment to familiarize yourself with the key objectives of this chapter.

- Discuss the importance of teams in the health care delivery system.
- Describe the different types of teams.
- Describe team leader characteristics and how these relate to the team leader's tasks and responsibilities.
- Explain the important considerations related to team building.
- Compare and contrast a nursing team and an interdisciplinary team.
- Identify the stages of team development.
- Explain motivation and its relationship to teamwork.
- Identify three strategies that might be used to improve motivation.

TEST YOUR UNDERSTANDING

Before we begin our exploration of this chapter, take a short "warm-up" test to see what you know about this topic.

Teams in Today's Health Care Environment

No one person can do it all. This fact is even more relevant in today's health care environment with its dynamic and frequent changes. The information explosion has made it impossible for any one person to know it all. Expertise is developed over time, and some staff have different types of expertise. Teams improve skills, communication, participation, and effectiveness (Mears, 1994). All organizations desire to perform effectively, although clearly many do not. What is the relationship between high-performing teamwork and organizational effectiveness?

- Groups often make better decisions when issues are difficult.
- When tasks are complex, specialized, and changing, it is impossible for a leader or any one person to know all the relevant information.
- The likelihood of successful implementation can be improved through a well-coordinated team of people working together to help solve one another's problems.
- Quality will be higher when team members can confront each other about problems that are being hidden or information that is being withheld.
- Shared-responsibility teamwork sets the stage for further individual development, which occurs when the team is collectively performing many of the managerial functions involved in running meetings and projects, building the team effort, and managing problem-solving tasks.
- Teams help people learn through direct feedback, which is a valuable source of information and a powerful impetus for change (Mears, 1994, p. 3).

YOUR OPINION COUNTS

Find out what others think about this topic. Post your response and check out other opinions.

Teams and teamwork

What is the difference between teams and teamwork? "The team is a means rather than an end, while teamwork is about performance and how to achieve the primary objective" (Katzenbach & Santamaria, 1993; McCallin, 2001, p. 422). Another way of understanding the difference is to view **teamwork** as the way people work together (Manion, Lorimer, & Leander, 1996), whereas a **team** is a specific number of consistent people working together who have a common purpose and work toward common goals. All members of the team are mutually accountable for the team's success (Manion, Lorimer, & Leander, 1996). Shared governance, discussed in Chapter 5, might be confused with team-based organizations; however, it is different. "Teams are not models of shared governance. Both are structural entities designed to increase the involvement of employees in decisions relating to their work. But shared governance structures bring members of a specific discipline together to deal with the issues of the discipline, such as professional standards and credentialing. Teams are structures designed to accomplish specific day-to-day operations" (Manion, Lorimer, & Leander, 1996, p. 13). An organization could use the team model to provide nursing care and yet not use shared governance to empower staff and increase staff participation in overall organizational or departmental decision making.

Another area of confusion comes from comparing teams and working groups. Most assume that teams and working groups are synonymous, but they are not. "A group is a collection of individuals who are in an interdependent relationship with one another. A team goes beyond that, in that members are encouraged to share in the ownership of the team's function and direction in order to increase their confidence and commitment" (Mears, 1994, p. 98). A **working group** relies on individual contributions, but its members are not necessarily responsible for the group's outcomes other than their own (Manion, Lorimer, & Leander, 1996). There is less emphasis on a shared vision and mission with a working group as compared to a team. Teams typically feel committed to one another. Nurses participate in many group experiences as well as serve on teams. The following are some characteristics that help in distinguishing between teams and groups.

- Teams make decisions by consensus with all members participating. Groups usually have a majority and minority viewpoint.
- Disagreements certainly occur in teams, but the team makes a greater effort to examine them and resolve them constructively. There is less need to maintain the group than there is with a team.
- Teams have objectives that are shared by the members; however, group members may not always accept common objectives.
- Teams tend to demonstrate more free expression of feelings and listening as compared to groups.
- Team roles are clearly defined and understood whereas in groups there may be less clarification and individuals may protect their roles and niches in the group.
- Shared leadership may be required and is accepted when needed in a team, but in a group leadership is typically appointed (Mears, 1994, p. 99).

In reviewing these characteristics, one can see that there is a theme that distinguishes teams from groups—sharing, acceptance, and more openness to the team process. This, however, does not mean that some groups do not demonstrate team characteristics; if they do, they might better be defined as a team.

Types of teams

Teams have been classified in many different ways, although two broad categories for classifying them within organizations are formal and informal. Formal teams are created by the organization with a specific purpose in mind, even though the team may be permanent or temporary. Examples of formal teams are clinical teams, policy committees, nurses' councils, and quality improvement committees. Informal teams or groups are quite different in that they are formed by staff, and typically members share something in common. They may be simply a social or support group but can also serve as a real resource to resolve problems or provide a service. Other team classifications include the following:

■ **Suggestion teams.** These teams are usually temporary and work on specific assigned tasks.
■ **Problem-solving teams.** These teams research and develop solutions. An example is a quality circle, which is made up of staff who meet regularly to solve a problem affecting work. Typically, these teams receive problem-solving training so that they can more effectively arrive at solutions.
■ **Semi-autonomous teams:** These teams have influence and input into their job activities; however, they are still managed by a formal supervisor or manager.
■ **Self-managing teams:** These teams, also called self-directed teams, manage their daily work (e.g., setting their own schedules, identifying goals, hiring team members, and make operating decisions) (Dessler, 2002, pp. 280–283; Shonk, 1997, pp. 27–33).
        There are several common types of teams (Mears, 1994).

■ Task teams have a temporary assigned task(s), and its members are either appointed or elected. An example of a task team in a health care organization is a team that is directed to develop a new nursing admission assessment form.
■ Cross-functional project teams include interdisciplinary members and/or members from different units or services. They are assigned a task or project, so they might be described as a task and an interdisciplinary team. This type of team makes the most of a variety of expertise to reach a better solution. If members are not willing to step out of their own territory and participate as a team, the team's ability to reach its outcomes will be ineffective.
■ Functional teams include members from different departments or services and crosses departmental or authoritative lines. This team is more permanent than a task team.

There have been many changes in how teams are formed and how they are used in health care organizations. **Self-directed work teams (SDWTs)** often are associated with patient-focused care (McCullough & Sanders, 2000). This fairly new approach includes a focus on the patient, decentralized services, and use of a more efficient worker skill mix while maintaining or improving patient satisfaction. The goal is to move services as close to the patient as possible. Health care organizations that use this model—which can be found in inpatient as well as community health organizations such as ambulatory care—bring services to the patient. For example, laboratory services are provided at the bedside whenever possible, and if the organization is a clinic, these services would be provided onsite so that patients do not have to go to another site. It is thought that SDWTs decrease bureaucracy and improve staff motivation (McCullough & Sanders, 2000).

How is this model different from team nursing, which began during World War II? These teams were composed of nonprofessional nursing staff who provided most of the direct care with an RN team leader directing the team. The team leader planned and supervised the care delivered to a group of patients, which meant the team leader probably spent less time providing direct care. SDWTs are different from team nursing in that "employees are expected to be responsible for creating significant change in the way patient care is delivered and in the cost to the institution for the care delivered" (McCullough & Sanders, 2000, p. 93). These teams tend to accomplish more positive outcomes related to: (a) patient, staff, and physician satisfaction; (b) patient outcomes; (c) decreased costs with increased resource effectiveness; and (d) staff retention and productivity.

The critical assumptions related to the SDWT model are:

■ All team members are responsible for fulfilling their portion of the care.
■ All team members understand what is expected of them.
■ Managers relinquish control.
■ There are boundaries regarding autonomy.
■ Managers are responsible for the environment and culture that determine, in part, the success of the team (McCullough & Sanders, 2000, p. 94).

In addition to these assumptions, the team culture of SDWTs requires that the team have some characteristics that may not be typically found in health care teams.

■ The team defines specific responsibilities and boundaries for team members.

■ Roles within the team change because teams are structured around an entire process and everyone is equally responsible for the outcomes.

■ Education of the team members focuses on the technical, administrative, and interpersonal skills necessary for people to function within the SDWT.

■ Teams evolve into groups that work with less and less dependence on managers or other leadership.

■ Teams define their own performance measures to identify growth and accomplishments within the teams (Orsburn, et al., 1990, p. 53).

If management does not support the concept of SDWTs and their decisions, then this model will fail. It is also true that if team members do not accept the concept and their own responsibilities, these teams will also fail. The team and its members must learn how to set goals for the team and evaluate its performance. Teams need training and education so that they can be effective and obtain the skills that are needed to work together. Role transition may be very difficult and takes time. Over time, however, most teams develop into cohesive units.

THINK CRITICALLY

Try this exercise to apply what you have learned about this topic.

Team-based organizations

"In team-based organizations, the team is the basic work unit or element. Employees work together as a team, and do much of the planning, decision-making, and implementing required to get their assigned jobs done, while being responsible" for their typical job tasks (Dessler, 2002, p. 161). Changing to a team-based approach requires a total organizational change, and it is not something that a nurse manager can decide to do. It should be done organizationwide to have a positive effect on the work environment and outcomes. Critical aspects that an organization needs to consider when moving to a **team-based organization** include the following.

■ **Organizational philosophy.** From the top, the organization must commit to having employees involved in decisions and believe they can be trusted to do the best to meet the organizations goals.

■ **Organizational structure.** The basic work unit becomes the team. A flat organizational structure is required so that decisions can be made as close to the work level as possible, with authority delegated to the teams.

■ **Organizational systems.** Standard operating systems are necessary for organizations and continue to be important in team-based organizations. They need to be user friendly and not act as barriers to team success. One example of a change in a common system is the performance evaluation process. Organizations typically have the managers evaluate staff, but in a team-based organization "360-degree appraisals" may be used. This means that all team members provide feedback on co-team members as well as the manager.

■ **Organizational policies.** All policies need to reflect the philosophy and support the team-based approach.

■ **Employee skills.** Team members need to have the skills necessary to do their jobs, including specific job skills, interpersonal skills, team skills such as communication and decision making, and management skills such as planning, leading, and controlling. Competency is critical (Dessler, 2002, p. 163).

Many organizations use some teams; however, if an organization does not implement all of the previous criteria, it would not be a team-based organization.

The team leader

The **team leader** is very important to a team's effectiveness. RNs are the team leaders on many health care teams. Their leadership and management skills assist the team as it works toward its goals. This is a leadership role that new graduates typically assume early on in their careers: Who is the team leader; how does the leader function; and what are some issues that affect the team leader?

Team leader characteristics

In most organizations the team leader has less formal authority than those individuals in management; however, a team leader should have the necessary authority to meet the position requirements. Self-confidence and the ability to act as a role model for team members are important characteristics. Team leaders often must act as the "cheerleader" to move the team along with enthusiasm, but this should be done appropriately. No one wants to work with someone who is always "cheery." Team leaders need to demonstrate facilitative leadership, although how this is implemented may vary. This means that the leader leads with a vision and is willing to become a learner. A more "hands-off" approach seems to work best, but for this approach to be successful the team must be cohesive and demonstrate trust and open communication (Milgram, Spector, & Treger, 1999). If the leader is effective, the leader gradually relinquishes control as the team gains strength. Four types of approaches to team leadership exist:

1. Leadership is direct and dictatorial in nature, and there is limited input from team members, who are really subordinates.
2. Leadership is participative, with the leader as the central figure receiving input from team members.
3. The leader is open to receiving input from all team members, with the team leader functioning more as a team member. Team members are not viewed as subordinates, but rather as integral members of the team.
4. The group operates autonomously from the leader, with the leader using a true "hands-off" approach. The leader provides input and advice as needed (Milgram, Spector, & Treger, 1999, pp. 300–301).

The leader's role changes dramatically from the first approach to the fourth, as the leader gradually relinquishes direct control and becomes a facilitator. New RNs who are developing their leadership and management skills usually have more difficulty utilizing the third and fourth approaches due to a lack of self-confidence, lack of trust, and fear that it will go wrong if they do not make all decisions. They also have greater difficulty with communicating, delegation, and assessing team members. With time, experience, and mentoring, new RNs can further develop these important competencies.

The team leader focuses on the team's process as well as its outcomes. Process is how the team works together. The facilitative leadership approach offers coaching and development to members. Team leaders, as is true with other types of leaders, need to have an understanding of communication, psychology, change, problem solving and decision making, motivation, and systems. It is important to encourage team members to give honest feedback and to provide an environment in which members can feel comfortable and safe in doing so. By establishing open communication when the team meets, the team leader sets the stage for a comfortable work environment. In addition, the team leader moves the team from the use of first-person singular to words that focus on the team as a group with joint responsibilities; for example, "we" and "let us" to emphasize the team and interdependence rather than "I" and "me." Team leaders provide praise to the team and, during stressful times, support. This does not mean, however, that individual members should never be praised as there are clearly times when an individual team member shines through in the team.

Tasks and responsibilities

Team leaders who approach the position with an attitude of being different from team members or above the team members will not be successful. They must jump in and work too, although they must continue to see the whole—what needs to be done and how best to accomplish it. Guiding from above will not be effective, but guiding from within the team will. The organization needs to be clear about the decision-making boundaries for its teams. It is also important for the organization to discourage "we versus they" thinking between teams, which can be very destructive to individual teams and the organization (Gebelein et al., 2000). The key tasks and responsibilities of the team leader are to:

- Guide the team by helping to establish goals and objectives.
- Provide an environment where team members are active in all stages of team planning and feel comfortable in this role.
- Reinforce the focus on the patient, if that is the focus of the team.
- Ensure that the team's tasks are clear, planned, and accomplished in a timely manner.
- Ensure that standards and rules are established, and encourage team members to monitor their use.
- Link the team to key resources and with others in the organization.
- Assist the team to stay on task.
- Challenge the team to improve and develop.
- Remove barriers to collaboration.
- Follow-up on problems in a timely manner.
- Recognize and value contributions from team members.
- Minimize micromanaging, and encourage team members to assist in management issues.
- Use conflict management to benefit the team and help it reach its outcomes.
- Ensure that team self-evaluation occurs with an emphasis on outcomes.
- Accept feedback from team members.
- Provide appropriate and timely evaluation of team members' performance and team effectiveness.

Gender issues and team leadership

There can be no doubt that literature about leadership and theories of leadership have been more interested in masculine leadership than feminine leadership. Some of this can be understood in that historically women did not hold many leadership positions. Today, however, this is not true. Women are found in leadership positions in all major types of organizations, although clearly more are needed, as the majority of women are found in the lower ranks and in lower management positions. Health care is no exception. Leadership theory needs to catch up with changes in the gender of leaders.

How are masculine and feminine leaders described? Masculine leaders are described by the following terms: "dominance, independence, objectivity, rationality, competitiveness, aggressiveness, boldness, decisiveness, toughness, and being logical" (Grossman & Valiga, 2000, p. 116). These characteristics have come to be associated as only masculine and are also considered to be critical leader requirements. Consequently, they are not viewed as characteristics found in women, leading to the conclusion that women may not make good leaders. This viewpoint is not based on facts; therefore, it is important to understand that this viewpoint affects women getting leadership positions and how women in these positions are viewed. Female leaders are typically described with the following terms: "compliance, dependence, emotionality, weakness, being accepting, passivity, and nurturance" (Grossman & Valiga, 2000, p. 116). These terms are far from positive and certainly do not instill a great view of women as leaders. Women, however, can be effective leaders, even great leaders. Getting stuck in these two stereotypes of masculine and feminine characteristics is dangerous for health care organizations and certainly for nurses. Why is this gender view of leadership important? Some of the reasons suggested include "society does not expect and value leadership in women, women typically are not socialized as leaders, there are few women leader role models, and women who do try to exert strong leadership behaviors sometimes are discriminated against and not supported in those efforts" (Grossman & Valiga, 2000, p. 118).

Some experts have described the following as the female's approach to leadership (Helegsen, 1990; Rosener, 1990). Female leaders are usually more participatory and encourage others to be as well. Sharing power is seen as a positive characteristic, as is sharing information to reach the goals. Improving staff perceptions of themselves can improve the work environment and performance. Often female leaders focus more on process than on "the bottom line." They are concerned with broader issues. It is important to recognize that this description of female leaders can become a stereotypical viewpoint. The approach should also not be viewed as a negative or ineffective approach just because it is more commonly found in women. There are certainly men in leadership positions who have these characteristics, and there are female leaders who do not. Focusing too much on gender issues ignores the importance of individual differences in leaders regardless of gender.

YOUR OPINION COUNTS

Find out what others think about this topic. Post your response and check out other opinions.

Followership: A critical concept

Team leaders must recognize that teams do not exist without **followers,** the team members. Followers are critical to the success of any organization. "There can be no leaders without followers, and there can be no followers without leaders" (Grossman & Valiga, 2000, p. 44). As previously discussed in earlier chapters, followers have become more important as leadership theory has turned more and more to a participatory approach. Leadership means that followers are developed. Despite the importance of understanding this concept, it is still not a critical topic in many management and leadership publications, where the emphasis has been on leadership (Grossman & Valiga, 2000). In many publications, there is a direct and indirect message that **followship** is negative; however, when this is seriously considered, how could this be? Without followers there would be no work done and no need for leaders.

What does it take to be an effective follower? Every new graduate should consider this question, as it is a role that all will play. Even leaders experience situations when they are followers. Followers need to be "self-directing, actively participating, practicing experts [who work] on behalf of the organization and the mutually agreed upon vision and goals" (Sullivan, 1998, p. 469). It takes energy to be a follower, although some may think that following is just an automatic response. To be effective, it is not automatic nor is it a passive role that does not involve thinking. It requires use of expertise, development of expertise, sharing, understanding of problems and others, effective communication, and collaboration. "Followership also involves knowing when and how to assume the role of leadership when necessary" (Grossman & Valiga, 2000, p. 48). Sullivan (1998) also notes that "the organization is essentially a community of many leaders and many followers, frequently changing places depending on the particular activity that is occurring" (p. 477). It is important, however, to understand that followers do not exist just to become leaders. They exist because they are needed and have a critical role to play.

Not all followers are alike. One description of followers identifies four major types: effective or exemplary followers, alienated followers, "yes" people, and sheep (Grossman & Valiga, 2000; Kelly, 1992; Kelly, 1998).

1. Effective or exemplary followers are able to function independently and use critical thinking. They are not followers who simply do what they are told but rather add their own ideas to the process.
2. Alienated followers may use critical thinking but are not active. Passivity is common, and some may appear angry. Sometimes they are described as complainers, unhappy, and not involved. They do not like to invest energy.

3. "Yes" people will do what they are told with enthusiasm and support the leader. These followers do not like being in a position of decision making, preferring instead to complete tasks with little input. They like structure and are not the ones to suggest new ideas.

4. Some followers called sheep may sound like they would be "yes" people, but sheep are even more passive, dependent, and just do as told. This type of follower is the one that others can manipulate. They do not take initiative and must be given clear directions.

The last two types of followers are not team members who will challenge others, take on new projects, ask questions, or go beyond assignments. It is important for leaders to understand the types of followers that are on the team, and it is also important for followers to understand their co-workers and themselves.

There are other followership styles that are used in the work situation. Typical ones are partner, contributor, politician, and subordinate (Grossman & Valiga, 2000). What are some differences in these styles? The partner style demonstrates "positive, reciprocal relationships with leaders" (Grossman & Valiga, 2000, p. 50). Partners often become leaders later. Contributors are active in the work process and add to the process, working well with co-workers. When compared with partners, contributors do not align as closely with leaders or work to ensure that the leader's vision is met. The politician approach focuses on interpersonal skills and communication, but may not demonstrate the highest level of general work performance. The fourth style is subordinate. Here the focus is on doing the job but not necessarily with a strong commitment to improving. Considering the types and styles of followers, who are the effective followers? It may be surprising to note that the characteristics of effective followers are remarkably similar to the characteristics of effective leaders. The following are some of these follower characteristics.

- Strength and independence
- Critical thinking
- An ability and willingness to think for themselves
- An ability to give honest feedback and constructive criticism, particularly in a timely fashion
- A willingness to be one's own person
- Innovativeness and creativity
- Cooperativeness and collaborativeness
- A tendency to be a self-starter
- A tendency to "go above and beyond the call of duty" to go beyond job assignments
- A willingness to assume ownership
- A tendency to take initiative
- An attentiveness to what is happening in the environment
- A tendency to "hold up our end of the bargain"
- A sense of being energized by work and the organization (Grossman & Valiga, 2000, pp. 52–53).

Followers who are contributing to the team or the work environment are eager to add their ideas to the process, to participate actively in decision making, and to feel committed to the process and the vision. These followers trust the leader and recognize the importance of sharing feelings and concerns. They also feel comfortable discussing their own limitations. One should not view followers as insignificant or invisible because if they are, they are not effective followers. "Leaders and followers are therefore interdependent" (Grossman & Valiga, 2000, p. 54).

Team building: Development of effective teams

Teams do not just appear as fully functioning effective teams; rather, they develop through team leadership and team members who are committed to team goals. The team's structure and processes are gradually developed. Team leaders need to assess the individual team members and the team as a whole, considering styles of followers, communication team purpose, roles, and so on, to determine what needs to be improved to make the team even more effective. Box 7-1 identifies some characteristics of effective work teams.

BOX 7-1   Characteristics of high-performing work teams.

- Commitment to mutual goals
- Mutual accountability
- High level of trust
- Productive—get the job done effectively
- Self-manage
- Open and clear communication

Source: Author.

Team norms, roles, and communication

Typical service roles in teams besides the leader role are participant and service roles such as recorder, observer, resource person, and timekeeper (Mears, 1994). Participants are the real team workers when they focus on doing the job, whatever it might be. The leader is the team guide who facilitates the work of all members of the team. To ensure that there is documentation of team activities, the recorder or secretary records minutes from team meetings. Some teams also have an observer, who observes the process and shares this information with the team; a timekeeper to watch the time for specific discussions and meetings; and a resource person who is used to assist with specific content. The latter three roles are typically used for specific tasks or periods of time. An example might be when a team must produce a particular report or is having a thorough discussion that is conflictual. Clinical teams usually do not have all of these service roles, and the leader may have a more formal role defined in a specific organizational position description.

Teams that develop an identity are more successful. The team leader and members may actively move toward developing this identity. Some methods for developing identification are matching coffee mugs, t-shirts, and use of a team name. These may appear to be unimportant, but they do support the idea that "we are in this together." Informal interaction helps teams become more effective as they get to know one another and develop relationships (McCallin, 2001; Platt, 1994). Teams begin to develop inside jokes and stories that mean something to them. All of this develops team spirit, which affects outcomes and how team members pitch in to help one another. They will be more tolerant of one another and more able to recognize when team members need help. Team members will also feel more comfortable asking for help. Sharing knowledge and skills then becomes the norm in the team because the team feels connected and has a team identity. Box 7-2 describes some key team roles.

Team tasks and functions

"People typically attend meetings, voice comments, and feel they have made a contribution, but that's nonsense. Your contribution is not what you say or do, but instead how you are able to

BOX 7-2   Key team roles.

Coordinator: Pulls together the work of the team as a whole.
Critic: Guardian and analyst of the team's effectiveness.
Ideas Person: Encourages the team's innovative vitality.
Implementor: Ensures smooth-running of the team's actions.
External Contact: Looks after the team's external contacts.
Inspector: Ensures that high standards are maintained.
Team Builder: Develops the team spirit.

Source: Author and highlighted from Heller, R. (1999). *Learning to lead.* New York: DK Publishing, Inc., p. 42.

move the team forward. This is a difficult concept because we often think in terms of what we say or do, and not the effect our actions have on a team" (Mears, 1994, p. 107).

Teams exist to get a job done, and they need to be active. This involves both talking and doing. The major **group functions** are initiating, giving information, energizing, and evaluating or criticizing (Mears, 1994).

- Initiating occurs when the team proposes tasks, defines problems, coordinates its work, clarifies, and suggests ideas and strategies.
- Giving information occurs when team members provide facts or information that is needed for decision making.
- As the team is motivated, energizing occurs.
- Evaluating and criticizing is an important function as the team determines if its outcomes are met, and if not, why.
- Social support also is a team function, which occurs within teams as cohesion develops.
- Team cohesion results in a team in which members encourage and feel a bond with one another. Whenever possible it is best to have team members select their assignments; however, this is not always possible.
- Delegation is also a critical skill for team leaders and those team members who will be delegating (see Chapter 8). It can make a key difference in the effectiveness of the team.

The following guidelines are related to tasks and roles.

- Roles should be matched to personality rather than have the personality pushed into the role.
- If a team has only a few members, roles can be doubled or tripled up to ensure that the team's needs are covered.
- Once roles have been allocated, team members should be consulted to get their agreement on what needs to be done and how.
- Specific tasks should be allocated to each team member, complete with time frame and reporting responsibilities.
- Performance must be monitored at team meetings.
- It is important to concentrate on collective achievement.
- Individual contributions should be dealt with in a team context (Heller, 1999, p. 43).

The type of team affects its tasks and functions. A clinical team provides care, and thus, tasks and functions are centered on patient care. A team that is formed to complete a specific project such as change in documentation would include tasks and functions related to literature research and contacting other health care organizations to learn about their documentation review, development of forms and methods for ensuring that standards are met, planning staff orientation, and planning a pilot.

CURRENT ISSUES

Learn about events around the globe that relate to the chapter content.

Team size and composition

Team size is a common concern when teams are developed. In some situations, such as a clinical one, the size may be predetermined based on the number and types of staff required to provide care for a specific number of patients. A general principle related to size is that the team should include the smallest number necessary to do the assigned task. Size is directly related to the number of transactions that occur, with five being ideal and more than seven too many (Mears, 1994). The latter size becomes difficult to manage. Another issue that is related to team composition is whether or not participation in the team is voluntary or involuntary. Again, in a clinical situation if the team model is the delivery model then all clinical staff, such as RNs, LPNs, UAPs, and so on, would be assigned to teams. Volunteer team membership can be found in some organizational committees, while staff may be assigned to project teams or to committees. In these situations, volunteer membership is better as staff will hopefully then feel more committed, although this is not always clear. For example, a nurse may be told that participation on a committee will improve chances for a promotion although the nurse may select which committee team to join. Professional organizations are, for the most part, run by volunteers through committees. Again, this fact may not be so clear. A nurse may volunteer for a committee because this will "look good" on the nurse's résumé, although on the surface it appears the nurse volunteered. Commitment to the committee's work may thus be variable.

Examples: The nursing team and the interdisciplinary team

Nursing teams have been organized in a variety of ways over the years. One approach is the functional structure with work based on types of tasks to perform (Hansten & Washburn, 1994). This type of team might have a medication nurse, treatment nurse, and UAPs. Team members see patients based on the patients' need and related tasks. This approach can lead to segmented care if no one staff member reviews the patients' total care needs and may result in inadequate coordination. Total patient care is a second approach to organizing nursing teams. Most if not all UAPs are removed from the team, which then is composed of RNs, who provide all the care. The primary care team model was similar to this model but added an associate nurse to assist the primary nurse, and then they cared for all of their assigned primary care patients. The primary care nurse was responsible for 24-hour plans of patient care—although not providing all of the direct care for 24 hours.

In the literature, **interdisciplinary** teams and **multidisciplinary** teams are teams that can sometimes be confusing and used interchangeably. Sorrells-Jones (1997) has defined both of these terms. "Multidisciplinary refers to a team or collaborative process where members of different disciplines assess or treat patients independently and then share the information with each other. . . . Interdisciplinary describes a deeper level of collaboration in which processes such as evaluation or development of a care plan is done jointly, with professionals of different disciplines pooling their knowledge in an independent manner" (pp. 20–21). When the interdisciplinary approach is used, the focus is more on tasks that are part of an individual's profession and then blending these tasks with others. The interdisciplinary approach considers a more collective action and is process-oriented.

Primary nursing, which was begun in the 1980s, had a major impact on changing how nurses interacted with other professionals, altering interprofessional interactions from one of the physicians always deciding what should be done and how it should be done and nurses making decisions in the background (Lyon, 1993; Stein, 1967). In the 1990s, there was further development of these models and recognition of the need for greater teamwork (Minnen et al., 1993; Stein, Watts, & Howell, 1990). It is important to note that just decentralizing an organization will not automatically make different health care professionals more inclined to collaborate and become teams. It takes much more than this organizational change.

CURRENT ISSUES

Learn about events around the globe that relate to the chapter content.

BENCHMARKS

Now let's take a moment to test your knowledge of the concepts you have studied in this section.

Effective Teams

What is an effective team? Various characteristics have been used to describe effective teams, including the following:

- When one observes the team, the team members participate in discussions and work in an atmosphere that is relaxed with minimal competition.
- The team stays on track, and if it veers off track, the team is gently put back on track.
- The team task(s) can be clearly identified by all team members.
- Communication is clear, and a key strategy is listening, which is used by all of its members. The communication flows from one topic to another in a clear manner.
- Disagreement or conflict is not avoided but rather used to move the team forward and is seen as an opportunity to consider new viewpoints.
- Criticism is open and healthy so that all feel comfortable hearing it and considering pros and cons because people feel free to express their opinions. This is all done with respect.
- Decisions are reached by consensus.
- As the team plans, there are clear directions, actions to be taken, responsibilities, due dates, and evaluation methods.
- There is a balance between the leader and the team, with each adding and supporting one another.
- The team is willing and able to participate in self-evaluation (Mears, 1994, p. 5).

Stages of team development

Several approaches can be used to describe team development. The following method is commonly used (Mears, 1994; Milgram, Spector, & Treger, 1999; Tuckman, 1965). These stages are highlighted in Box 7-3.

1. Forming or the initial orientation

    During the first stage, **forming,** the team is learning about one another, and trust is not likely to be high at this time. If the task(s) is complex or unclear, anxiety may be experienced. As the team meets, it will focus on developing trust and team member working relationships, although this may not actually be stated. Team members begin assessing their roles in the context of the team. A leader is identified or may be identified prior to the first meeting. For a clinical team there is typically an identified person or position who is always the formal leader, such as the nurse team leader. Informal leaders, however, may develop within the team as time goes by.

2. Storming or the stage of conflict and confusion

    At the time of the second stage, **storming,** team members see themselves as individuals and will want to respond to the task in the manner that they would respond to tasks as individuals. Some members may be reluctant to really work as a team, and others will be restless with the need to get through the **team building** activities to the task. It may be noticed at this time that some members attempt to control the team and its communication. Other team members should step in to avert this move so that the team can function as a group. Conflict can arise from this process. As this stage begins to change into **norming,** the next stage, the team will formulate team rules that will guide

BOX 7-3   Stages of team development.

1. Forming
2. Storming
3. Norming
4. Performing

Source: Author.

team members in their performance, interaction, decision making, and how they accomplish their goals (Gebelein et al., 2000). Ideally, these rules are developed during the norming stage; however, during the storming stage these rules may be revised and then solidified. When rules are considered, one needs to factor in the organization's requirements that may affect team rules such as meeting requirements, minutes, and attendance. What might be included in these team rules?

- Definition of purpose
- Meeting schedule, days, time, and place
- Documentation requirements for meetings
- Attendance at meetings, requirements, and what happens if one does not attend
- Confidentiality
- Roles and responsibilities
- Assignment of tasks
- Sharing of information
- Collaboration and assisting one another
- Consensus process and decision making
- Evaluation of work

3. **Norming or the stage of consolidation around tasks**

As team members begin to work together, establish their roles, and help one another to see value in this, team cohesion develops. At this point, members must appreciate the strengths and limitations of one another.

4. **Performing or the stage of teamwork and performance**

When work is getting done, and the team feels positive about this, the **performing** stage has arrived. If interpersonal issues arise they can be worked through within the team. An important part of this stage is consensus building that occurs as decisions are made. Time is an important issue, which is dependent on the nature of the decisions that need to be made. Clinical decisions typically have the highest pressure for decision making. Many clinical decisions do not require consensus, or the consensus may be decided outside the team (for example, a clinical pathway has been developed that the team needs to apply). The team then decides when to use the clinical pathway, which is a tool developed by a team through research and consensus. Individual team members may need to make some decisions (for example, a physician may need to order a medical procedure or medication). Other issues on the clinical team that the patient may encounter, such as discharge problems, may be something the treatment team discusses before reaching a consensus to determine the best approach.

As the team members suggest ideas and approaches for the team to take there are some factors that need to be considered. When suggestions are made the reasons behind the suggestions and opinions should also be provided. It is important to ask others for information and their opinions. This would, of course, be other team members, but it may also mean seeking out others outside the team who have specific expertise. As one presents a suggestion or opinion, the team should be open to ideas and contributions made by others to make the team's work even better.

Conflict can arise when consensus is developed. However, this is not necessarily a negative situation as long as the conflict addresses the issues and does not focus on personalities of team members. The latter situation will be destructive to the team's work. Team members have the responsibility for suggesting alternatives when they disagree with other team members (Mears, 1994). Consensus is also not a unanimous agreement but rather a general agreement. All team members must agree to support the decision although all may not totally agree with it. All feelings or reactions to the decision should then be expressed appropriately. Box 7-4 identifies examples of strategies to build team performance.

Motivation

It is difficult to discuss any work issue without considering motivation. It relates to individual staff, teams, management, components of the organization (units, divisions, departments), and

BOX 7-4   Building team performance.

- Seek employee input
- Establish urgent, demanding performance standards
- Select members for skill and skill potential
- Pay special attention to first meetings and actions
- Set clear rules of behavior
- Move from "boss" to "coach"
- Set a few immediate performance-oriented tasks and goals
- Challenge the group regularly with fresh facts and information
- Use the power of positive feedback
- Shoot for the right team size
- Choose people who like teamwork
- Train, train, train
- Cross-train for flexibility
- Emphasize the task's importance
- Assign whole tasks
- Encourage social support
- Provide the necessary material support

Source: Dessler, G. (2002). *Management.* Upper Saddle River, NJ: Prentice Hall, pp. 288–289. Reprinted with permission.

the organization as a whole. Theories of leadership and management often address motivation. If one is a team member or a team leader, motivation will be important as it will affect whether or not the team works effectively. Given this, it is important to understand motivation. What is motivation, and how does it affect work? Figure 7-1 provides an overview of the motivation process.

Definition and motivation theories

The willingness to work and the ability to work go hand-in-hand. Knowledge about what drives a person to work is key for all who hold any leadership position and for those who work on teams.

FIGURE 7-1   The motivation process.

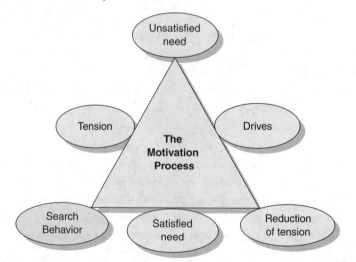

Source: Adapted from Robbins, S., & Decenzo, D. (2001). *Fundamentals of management* (3rd ed.). Upper Saddle River, NJ: Prentice Hall, p. 313. Reprinted with permission.

Motivation is related to behavior, performance, satisfaction, and rewards. Mobilizing the team to meet the outcomes is an important role for the team leader. "Motivation is the intensity of a person's desire to engage in some activity" (Dessler, 2002, p. 229). As was true with the theories discussed in Chapters 1 and 5 about leadership and management, theories about motivation vary, and there is no one correct or universally accepted motivation theory. The following is a brief historical review of some of the major motivation theories.

Maslow

Maslow's theory of motivation focuses on a need hierarchy (Maslow, 1943). These needs are physiological (the lowest level); safety and security; belongingness, social, and love; esteem; and self-actualization. People attempt to satisfy the lower needs first. His theory emphasizes that once a need is met then it no longer motivates the person. If a need is not satisfied, the person may feel stress, frustration, and conflict, which can affect performance.

Herzberg

Herzberg's two-factor theory of motivation, extrinsic (dissatisfiers) and intrinsic (satisfiers) (Herzberg, Mausner, & Snyderman, 1959) was originally based on research of engineers and accountants. It was thought to oversimplify the nature of job satisfaction, as it did not look at unconscious factors that might affect motivation. See Figure 7-2 for a description of the theory.

McClelland

McClelland's learned needs theory focuses on three needs: (a) the need for achievement, (b) the need for affiliation, and (c) the need for power (McClelland, 1962). The achievement need encourages a person to set goals, challenging oneself to achieve those goals. The affiliation need pushes a person toward social interaction, which affects motivation as few things can be achieved without others. The need for power focuses on the person's efforts to obtain and exercise power and authority. The theory supports the idea that people learn about these needs as they learn to cope with their environment. If they are learned, then behavior that is rewarded

FIGURE 7-2   Herzberg's Theory.

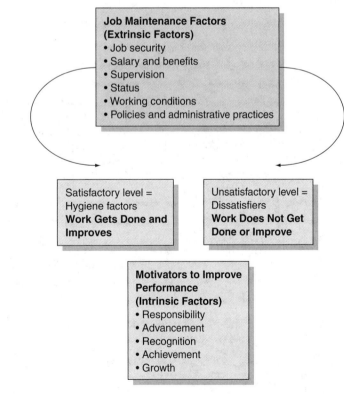

Source: Author.

will probably increase. This theory is different from Maslow's and McClelland's in that it focuses on socially acquired needs.

Skinner

Skinner's theory identifies reinforcement as its key factor. By accepting the importance of reinforcement, one can accept that behavior will continue if it is rewarded. Specific behavior will stop if punishment is received for the behavior (Dessler, 2002).

Equity theory

Equity theory emphasizes that staff make comparisons of their own efforts and rewards with those of others who work in similar jobs or situations. The critical question for the employees is "Are they equivalent" (Adams, 1963)? If inequity is felt, then staff tension rises, which affects motivation. This tension, however may work one of two ways. The staff member may feel that less work is required because some staff may be getting the same reward but with less effort. The staff may also feel that more work or effort are required if they recognize that others are working at a higher level and receiving additional rewards. This is a theory that most staff can probably relate to easily.

Theory X and Y and Theory Z

Theory X and Y and Theory Z are related and are theories that are mentioned when motivation is discussed. Box 7-5 highlights key issues with these motivation theories.

Assessment of the motivational climate

"Lancaster (1985) defines motivation as internal and unique to each employee. In other words, managers cannot motivate employees—they must be motivated from within, and what inspires motivation in one may not in another. Lancaster states that all employees are motivated, but those who appear to lack motivation are actually motivated in a different direction, or towards other outcomes, than a manager may desire. Because managers cannot directly motivate staff, they must work indirectly by creating an environment that tends to cause individual motivation towards the desired goals" (p. 16). Understanding a person's motivation is helpful in developing strategies to increase a person's motivation. The critical question is what makes a person work and also want to improve work performance. Methods that might be used to increase motivation include observation, asking staff, and comparing and contrasting outcome results with rewards that staff receive. When people are identified as having poor motivation, how are they usually described? Typical descriptors are:

BOX 7-5   Theory X and Theory Y premises.

Theory X

A manager who views employees from a Theory X (negative) perspective believes:
1. Employees inherently dislike work and, whenever possible, will attempt to avoid it.
2. Because employees dislike work, they must be coerced, controlled, or threatened with punishment to achieve desired goals.
3. Employees will shirk responsibilities and seek formal direction whenever possible.
4. Most workers place security above all other factors associated with work and will display little ambition.

Theory Y

A manager who views employees from a Theory Y (positive) perspective believes:
1. Employees can view work as being as natural as rest or play.
2. Men and women will exercise self-direction and self-control it they are committed to the objectives.
3. The average person can learn to accept, even seek, responsibility.
4. The ability to make good decisions is widely dispersed throughout the population and is not necessarily the sole province of managers.

Source: Robbins, S., & Decenzo, D. (2001). *Fundamentals of management* (3rd ed.). Upper Saddle River, NJ: Prentice Hall, p. 315. Reprinted with permission.

lack of energy, lack of initiative, poor communicator, lack of follow-through, low socialization at work, and no "get up and go." It is helpful to watch for changes in self and others. Motivation at work is also affected by personal problems and thus may interfere with staff motivation.

Strategies to improve motivation

Rewarding team members for achieved outcomes and effective performance is critical in developing the team and improving and supporting motivation. Recognizing effort should never be taken for granted. There will be times when team members or the team as a whole will excel, and it is particularly important to recognize these times. There will also be times when things do not go well, and these times cannot be ignored. The focus should be on improvement and moving forward, not on dwelling on errors (although they do need to be analyzed if improvement is to take place). The most common strategies used to motivate staff are: pay for performance, merit raises, spot rewards, skill-based pay, recognition awards, job redesign that results in greater job satisfaction, empowerment, goal setting because when people set goals they are more motivated to reach them, positive reinforcement, and lifelong learning that improves skills and demonstrates that the organization is committed to the employees (Dessler, 2002). The decision to use the reward method depends on the individual, situation, policies and procedures, roles and responsibilities, and timing.

Building team power and spirit

The development of effective teams does not just happen nor is there an end point as teams are always evolving and developing. One cannot just put a group of staff together, call them a team, and then assume that they will function as a team with very little change. As described in the stages of team development, it takes time and effort to really build a team. "Participation, empowerment, teamwork, and commitment hinge on one key factor: trust" (Mears, 1994, p. 117).

Empowerment was discussed in Chapters 3 and 5; however, it is also relevant to team functioning. "Empowerment is synonymous with authority" (Mears, 1994, p. 61). Another good definition of empowerment was developed by the Xerox Corporation: "An organization state where people are aligned with the business direction and understand their performance boundaries, thus enabling them to take responsibility and ownership for: seeking improvements, identifying the best course of action, and initiating the necessary steps to satisfy customer requirements" (Mears, 1994, p. 61). This is also a good description of what should be happening within a team. Empowerment means that some will lose power and prestige. In organizations that truly practice shared participation in decision making, middle management tends to lose the most, turning over power and authority to teams. Now, a key question that those who are empowered often ask and should ask is, "What am I empowered to do?" If this is not clear, then more questions need to be asked. Muddled empowerment is worse than no empowerment because this often increases errors and frustration.

Teams that are empowered will be involved in a process of self-control. They will be responsible for their own performance (Mears, 1994). Empowerment does not mean telling someone or a team exactly what they must do but rather giving some direction when required and giving the team authority to do the task(s) without having to wait for approval and other management control methods. More will be discussed about continuous quality improvement in Chapter 16, but it is also related to teamwork and empowerment. Empowerment is a "philosophy that involves sharing of power with employees working in empowered teams. It is getting everyone in the organization—management, employees, and support services—to focus on the consumer (patient, family, and other consumers)" (Mears, 1994, p. 65). In doing this, improvement of performance should occur. Teams can experience good times and bad ones. When a team is successful there is a connection between the quality of its members' relationships with one another (Crowell, 2000).

What does this tell a leader about this type of team? The development of team relationships is critical. Developing team spirit and a concern for one another will go a long way in setting up an environment in which the team can function effectively. Crowell (2000) has developed a five-stage process to build spirited teams.

1. Initiating, the first stage, is when team members get to know one another. It is important for the members to understand their differences and appreciate what each can offer as different

individuals and different professionals. Members need to learn more about the rules of behavior and values of the different members. Positive results are a sense of belonging and trust rather than disorientation, alienation, and mistrust.

2. Visioning, with the focus on sharing meaning and mission, is the second stage. At this time, the team will identify assumptions, which can be anxiety provoking, but this will help the team members to understand each other's work. From this will come a shared vision for the team.

3. Claiming, the third stage, is where the focus is on doing the work. These stages build on one another as it takes trust and a shared vision to help the team to do their work effectively. The positive results are establishment of goals, organizational support, and competence rather than incompetence and inability to reach outcomes.

4. Celebrating, the fourth stage, focuses on recognition, awards, and rewards. Taking things for granted is never helpful. The team and its members need to know they are valued and have been successful.

5. The last stage is letting go or really communicating. Team members may spend so much time trying to prove their point that they do not listen to one another or they are not open with feedback. It is particularly important that feedback is given by team members as they evaluate contributions given by one another. This may be done directly or indirectly. Subjective feedback often leads to negative feelings and may be destructive to the team. Objective feedback helps the team grow and do its job. Generalities and personal comments are not helpful. Mears (1994) suggests some guidelines for giving feedback. Being positive and thanking members is always important; however, it is also important not to give general praise but rather give specific praise. If a member is causing problems within the team, when this is addressed it is important to discuss positive feedback and specifics about concerns or problems. Keeping the feedback focused on issues rather than about things that are not important improves communication.

Emotions need to be experienced, identified correctly, and communicated. This relates to what was discussed in Chapter 1 about Emotional Intelligence leadership. It is important to be in tune with one's feelings as well as those of others. Team members do not have to always agree, and in fact, if this is so, then someone is not being open and honest. It is, however, important for members to listen and try to understand other members.

What happens to a team that feels empowered? Bennis and Goldsmith (1997) describe four critical themes that can be identified in empowered teams as well as empowered organizations.

1. People feel significant. They feel that they can make a difference.
2. Learning and competence matter. They are valued by the leader. "Leaders make it clear that there is no failure—only mistakes that give us feedback and tell us what to do next" (p. 165).
3. People are part of a community. "Where there is leadership, there is a team, a family, a unity. Even people who do not especially like each other feel the sense of community" (p. 165).
4. Work is exciting—stimulating, challenging, fascinating, and fun (p. 165).

Barriers to team success

As teams improve their functioning, which needs to be continuous improvement, teams do encounter barriers. Teams must address these barriers to become more effective, and this too should be a continuous process. Barriers come and go and are affected by many factors such as time, team member changes, leader changes, personal changes in members or leaders, organizational changes, and so on. The key barriers are:

- Lack of leadership.
- Lack of power: If the team is not given the authority it needs to do the task then the work will not get done in the manner expected.
- Poor communication.
- Territoriality and cliques.
- Role conflict.

- Sex-role stereotyping: Gender hierarchies, such as believing physicians are more important than nurses or nurses having the stereotype that all physicians are not collaborative (McCallin, 2001). It is important to note that generally today in most colleges of medicine more than 50% of the students are women. Nursing, however, still has few male students. Stereotyping or making assumptions about others can interfere with effective teams and communication. Separate educational experiences between nurses and physicians have led to increasing problems in this area (Beattie, 1995; Clark, 1997; Fagin, 1992; Stein, 1967).
- Conflict between the team leader and the team.
- Supervisor resistance: This may be in the form of resistance or disagreement and is often based on the purpose of the team; concern about loss of power and prestige; and inability to provide effective direction for the team. Managers need to offer support to teams and provide resources for the team to do its work. In addition, managers need to help staff develop skills to assist them in participating in teamwork.
- Collaboration vs. conflict among team members or with other teams.
- Lack of clearly defined purpose so that the team does not know what they are supposed to do or they feel unnecessary.
- Inability of team to incorporate new members effectively, which disturbs group cohesion and prevents the team from using each member's skills.
- Personnel issues: Common issues include wrong staff on the team, lack of specific expertise that is needed, and staff reluctance to participate on the team.
- Inadequate coping with difficult team members: Typical responses are use of scapegoating, denial of problems, anger, and conflict.

A team knows it is unproductive (Dessler, 2002; Varney, 1989) when it does not accomplish its goals. This is no different than evaluating patient care for an individual patient. A nurse knows there are problems with the patient's care when the patient outcomes are not met. Another indicator of unproductive teams is cautious or guarded communication, which indicates a low level of trust among team members or inadequate team communication with others in the organization. Lack of disagreement can also be used to evaluate a team, as it is not healthy. People do need to disagree sometimes, but it should not be frequent or interface with work.

Groupthink can be another barrier to effective team functioning. This occurs when the "members reach a unanimous agreement even when the facts point to another, perhaps more appropriate, conclusion" (Milgram, Spector, & Treger, 1999, p. 153). Why does this happen? The common reasons are:

- There is team pressure on each member to agree with everyone else.
- The group feels separated from the consequences of its actions.
- General closed-mindedness prevails.
- The team ignores suggestions, and its thinking is irrational.
- Members censor thoughts that go against group team ideas (Milgram, Spector, & Treger, 1999, p. 153).

This type of approach to decision making leads the team to poor judgment because the team is unable to consider alternative courses of action. To prevent groupthink, it is important to recognize the value of disagreement and the need for everyone to stretch themselves and consider alternatives.

Dysfunctional meetings can indicate a lack of enthusiasm, inability to reach decisions, control by some team members, or unclear communication. How might a staff nurse evaluate a team meeting? The following questions might be asked.

- Was it an effective meeting?
- Were the team goals for the meeting clearly understood?
- Did the team stay on track in working toward the goals?
- Did the team consider members' contributions?

■ Did members feel free to express their opinions?

■ Was the conversation balanced among the members?

■ Were members satisfied with the meeting (Mears, 1994, p. 106)?

THINK CRITICALLY

Try this exercise to apply what you have learned about this topic.

Getting the job done

The four major responsibilities of the team are to: "(1) set goals and priorities and get the task(s) done, (2) analyze the way the team is performing, (3) examine the way the team interacts in decision-making and communication, and (4) examine the relationship among the people doing the work" (Mears, 1994). The team's most important responsibility, however, is the need to make decisions.

Some decisions are minor and others are major. Asking the following questions will help improve the team decision-making process.

1. What is the problem we are trying to solve? What are the underlying causes? Before the team attempts to generate ideas, it is important that members fully understand the problem to be solved.
2. Who should be involved in this decision? Consider the following:
   ■ Who possesses the knowledge to ensure that the decision is logical and sound?
   ■ Who will be involved in implementing the decisions?
   ■ Who must approve the decision? (Approval may be easier to obtain if those in authority are invited to participate in the decision-making process.)
3. How should each person be involved? (Group/team members may be involved directly by actually making the decisions or consulted to provide information or opinions. Clarify in advance the roles group members will play in the process.)
4. When does the decision need to be made? (Set a time frame so people know when the decision is due.)
5. What are the steps that need to be taken to improve group problem solving, and what are the reasons for taking these steps (Let the team know about these steps.) (Gebelein et al., 2000, pp. 440–441)?

Personal accountability to develop critical-thinking skills should be recognized as a professional responsibility of every RN on a team. What might a nurse do to develop these skills?

■ Reflect on the way the nurse thinks, and review those steps most often missed.

■ Learn from mistakes and the mistakes of others.

■ Recognize personal indicators warning that thinking may be less than optimal, such as illness, short staffing, or stress at home that reduces focus on work issues.

■ Participate in or lead discussions of clinical scenarios.

■ Participate in mentorship or preceptor programs, as a participant or as a mentor.

■ Develop an individual educational plan based on what has been learned from reflection and feedback.

■ Trust intuition.

■ Use a model, such as the critical thinking model, for creative thinking and problem solving to habituate step-by-step critical thinking processes (Hansten & Washburn, 1999, p. 41).

Team members can support one another as they each develop their skills, including critical thinking. This in return makes the team more effective.

The charge nurse and the team

Methods used for selecting charge nurses vary from one organization to another. Common methods are permanent charge nurses per shift (who may be assistant nurse managers) or rotating charge nurses per shift. The charge nurse is typically not the nurse manager. The major responsibility of the charge nurse is to ensure that the unit is managed effectively and patient care is delivered in a quality, safe manner for a specific shift. A charge nurse needs to understand the organization, job responsibilities, and those who are supervised, and must also demonstrate clinical and managerial competencies. The charge nurse considers the broad unit perspective, and the team leaders focus on their individual group of patients. All nurses who hold the positions of charge nurse or team leader either permanently or temporarily need to practice self-evaluation. Nurses who are charge nurses or team leaders should be able to assess themselves by considering the following questions:

- Are you fair?
- Do you honor commitments?
- Are you consistent?
- Will you keep your word? (Miner-Williams, Connelly, & Yoder, 2000, p. 32)

Both the charge nurse and the team leader must spend a lot of time making decisions and ensuring that work gets done. Typically, a charge nurse is responsible for several teams who are providing care, and each team has a team leader. If teams are not used, the charge nurse supervises a large number of staff who have individual assignments. As has been pointed out in this text, the work will be easier and more effective if the charge nurse cultivates staff participation in decision making and encourages collaboration. Fostering teamwork by using staff strengths, developing awareness of what is going on, providing positive feedback, acknowledging the work of others, and also taking responsibility are critical concepts of leadership for the charge nurse and all team leaders (Miner-Williams, Connelly, & Yoder, p. 32). Interpersonal skills are constantly tested as work is assigned, evaluated, and staff coordinate care; therefore, it is important for nurses who hold either of these positions to be competent in these areas just as it is for a team leader. Both the charge nurse and team leaders hold similar positions with related required competencies; however, the charge nurse carries a larger responsibility for the unit or service during a specific shift while the team leader focuses on part of that unit or service.

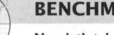

BENCHMARKS

Now let's take a moment to test your knowledge of the concepts you have studied in this section.

Chapter Wrap-Up

Now that you've reached the end of the chapter, you may wish to explore the concepts you've been reading about in greater detail, or test yourself to see how well you've comprehended the material.

SUMMARY AND APPLICATIONS

- Summary
- Practice Quiz
- Key Terms
- Tying It All Together

- Experiential Exercises
- Case
- Links

REFERENCES

Adams, J. (1963, November). Toward an understanding of inequity. *Journal of Abnormal and Social Psychology*, 422–436.

Beattie, A. (1995). War and peace among the health tribes. In K. Soothill, L. Mackay, & C. Webb (Eds.), *Interprofessional relations in health care* (pp. 11–30). London: Edward Arnold.

Bennis, W., & Goldsmith, J. (1997). *Learning to lead*. Reading, MA: Perseus Books.

Clark, P. (1997). Values in healthcare professional socialization: Implications for geriatric education in interdisciplinary teamwork. *Gerontologist*, 37(4), 441–451.

Crowell, D. (2000). Building spirited multidisciplinary teams. *Journal of PeriAnesthesia Nursing*, 15(2), 108–114.

Dessler, G. (2002). *Management*. Upper Saddle River, NJ: Prentice Hall.

Fagin, C. (1992). Collaboration between nurses and physicians: No longer a choice. *Academic Medicine*, 67(5), 295–303.

Gebelein, S., et al. (2000). *Successful manager's handbook*. Minneapolis, MN: Personnel Decisions International.

Grossman, S., & Valiga, T. (2000). *The new leadership challenge: Creating the future of nursing*. Philadelphia: F. A. Davis Company.

Hansten, R., & Washburn, M. (1994). *Clinical delegation skills*. Gaithersburg, MD: Aspen Publishers, Inc.

Hansten, R., & Washburn, M. (1999). Individual and organizational accountability for development of critical thinking. *Journal of Nursing Administration*, 29(11), 39–45.

Helegsen, S. (1990). Feminism and nursing—"Feminine principles" of leadership: The perfect fit for nursing. *Revolution: The Journal of Nurse Empowerment*, 2(2), 50–57, 135.

Heller, R. (1999). *Learning to lead*. New York: DK Publishing, Inc.

Herzberg, F., Mausner, B., & Snyderman, B. (1959). *The motivation to work*. New York: John Wiley and Sons.

Institute of Medicine. (2001). *Crossing the quality chasm*. Washington, DC: National Academy of Sciences.

Katzenbach, J., & Santamaria, J. (1993). *The wisdom of teams: Creating the high-performance organization*. New York: Harper Collins.

Kelly, R. (1992). *The power of followship: How to create leaders people want to follow and followers who lead themselves*. New York: Doubleday Currency.

Kelly, R. (1998). In praise of followers. In W. Rosenbach & R. Taylor (Eds.), *Contemporary issues in leadership* (4th ed., pp. 96–106). Boulder, CO: Westview.

Lancaster, J. (1985, January). Creating a climate for excellence. *Journal of Nursing Administration*, 14–17.

Lyon, J. (1993). Models of nursing care delivery and case management: Clarification of terms. *Nursing Economics*, 11(3), 163–169.

Manion, J., Lorimer, W., & Leander, W. (1996). *Team-based health care organizations*. Gaithersburg, MD: Aspen Publishers, Inc.

Maslow, A. (1943, July). A theory of human motivation. *Psychological Review*, 370–396.

McCallin, A. (2001). Interdisciplinary practice—a matter of teamwork: An integrated literature review. *Journal of Clinical Nursing*, 10, 419–428.

McClelland, D. (1962 July–August). Business drive and national achievement. *Harvard Business Review*, 99–112.

McCullough, C., & Sanders, D. (2000). Building self-directed work teams. In F. Bower (Ed.), *Nurses taking the lead* (pp. 89–118). Philadelphia: W.B. Saunders Company.

Mears, P. (1994). *Healthcare teams. Building continuous quality improvement*. Delray Beach, FL: St. Lucie Press.

Milgram, L., Spector, A., & Treger, M. (1999). *Managing smart*. Houston, TX: Cashman Dudley.

Miner-Williams, D., Connelly, L., & Yoder, L. (2000). Taking charge. *Nursing 2000*, 30(3), 32hn1–32hn2.

Minnen, T., et al. (1993). Sustaining work redesign innovation through shared governance. *Journal of Nursing Administration*, 23, 35–40.

Orsburn, J., et al. (1990). *Self-directed work teams, the new American challenge*. Homewood, IL: Business One Irwin.

Platt, L. (1994). Why bother with teams? An overview. In R. Casto & M. Julia (Eds.), *Interprofessional care and collaborative practice: Commission on interprofessional education and practice*. Pacific Grove, CA: Brooks/Cole.

Rosener, J. (1990). Ways women lead. *Harvard Business Review*, 68(6), 19–24.

Shonk, J. (1997). *Team-based organizations*. Chicago: Irwin.

Sorrells-Jones, J. (1997). The challenge of making it real: Interdisciplinary practice in a "seamless" organization, *Nursing Administrative Quarterly*, 21(2), 20–30.

Stein, L. (1967). The doctor-nurse game. *Archives of General Psychiatry*, 16, 699–703.

Stein, L., Watts, D., & Howell, T. (1990). The doctor-nurse game revisited. *New England Journal of Medicine*, 322, 546–549.

Sullivan, T. (1998). Transformational Leadership. In T. Sullivan (Ed.), *Collaboration: A health care imperative* (pp. 469–497). New York: McGraw-Hill.

Tuckman, B. (1965). Development sequence in small groups. *Psychological Bulletin, 63*(6), 334–399.

Varney, G. (1989). *Building productive teams: An action guide and resource book.* San Francisco: Jossey-Bass Publishers.

ADDITIONAL READINGS

Barter, M. (2002). Follow the team leader. *Nursing Management, 33*(10), 55.

Cohen, S. (2003). Motivation: Your key to IC ingredient. *Nursing Management, 34*(6), 52.

Cox, K., et al. (2003). The effects of intrapersonal, intragroup, and intergroup conflict on team performance effectiveness and work satisfaction. *Nursing Administration Quarterly, 27*(2), 153.

Dessler, G. (2002). *Management.* Upper Saddle River, NJ: Prentice Hall.

Drenkard, K. (2001). Team-based work redesign: The role of the manager when you are not on the team. *Seminars for Nurse Managers, 9*(2), 90–97.

Dumpe, M., & Ulreich (2001). Moving from parallel play to team play. *Seminars for Nurse Managers, 9*(2), 85–89.

Espin, S. (2001). Time as a catalyst for tension in nurse-surgeon communication. *AORN, 7*(11), 672–678.

Feara, C., & Elberth, W. (2001). Reengineering patient care: A multidisciplinary approach—an interview. *Seminars for Nurse Managers, 9*(2), 121–125.

Frelic, M., & Denby, C. (2000). Retooling the nurse executive for 21st century practice: Decision support systems. *Nursing Administrative Quarterly,* Winter, 19–28.

Hyakaas, M., et al. (2003). Continuous quality improvement through team supervision supported by continuous self-monitoring or work and systematic patient feedback. *Journal of Nursing Management, 11*(3), 177.

Makinen, A., et al. (2003). Organization of nursing care and stressful work characteristics. *Journal of Advanced Nursing, 43*(2), 197.

Marrelli, T. (1997). *The nurse manager's survival guide* (2nd ed.). St. Louis, MO: Mosby-Year Book, Inc.

O'Rouke, M. (2003). Rebuilding a professional practice model: The return of role-based practice accountability. *Nursing Administrative Quarterly, 27*(2), 95–97.

Pennington, K., Scott, J., & Magilvy, K. (2003). The role of certified nursing assistants in nursing homes. *The Journal of Nursing Administration, 33*(11), 578–584.

Stolzenberger, K. (2003). Beyond the Magnet award: The ANCC Magnet Program as the framework for culture change. *The Journal of Nursing Administration, 33*(10), 522–531.

Delegation for the Staff Nurse

MediaLink
www.prenhall.com/finkelman

The Interactive Exercises for this chapter can be found in the OneKey course at www.prenhall.com/finkelman. Click on Chapter 8 to select from the following activities: Test Your Understanding, Benchmarks, Current Issues, Your Opinion Counts, Think Critically, and Summary and Applications.

What's Ahead

With today's health care environment emphasis on teams and a more diverse workforce, any type of leadership position eventually requires the use of delegation to ensure that the job gets done. Not only do nurse managers need to use delegation, but nurses in staff positions must also use delegation daily. Delegation makes the best use of the talents and expertise of all staff as it facilitates the organization's work. To perform delegation effectively, nurses need to develop competencies in delegation and supervision. As has been discussed in several chapters in this text, no one person can do it all. Delegation is essential to productive organizations, and it is the most fundamental management process in organizations (Hill, 1993). Everyone eventually encounters a manager who refuses to delegate and tries to do it all. This will inevitably lead to problems for the staff and the manager. Hill comments in her work about new managers that the "consistent theme throughout their interactions with subordinates, both experienced and inexperienced, was how to achieve that critical, fine balance between delegation and managerial control" (Hill, 1993, p. 147). This critical topic of delegation is addressed in this chapter.

OBJECTIVES

Before you begin, take a moment to familiarize yourself with the key objectives of this chapter.

- Define delegation.
- Discuss the benefits of using delegation.
- Identify key legal issues related to delegation.
- Compare and contrast responsibility, authority, and accountability as they apply to delegation.
- Apply the delegation process in clinical situations when unlicensed assistive personnel are used.
- Discuss how to monitor and improve delegation.

TEST YOUR UNDERSTANDING

Before we begin our exploration of this chapter, take a short "warm-up" test to see what you know about this topic.

Delegation: What Is It?

It seems like there should be a simple definition for **delegation**, but it is not a simple process. First, delegation can relate to assigning a specific task, a range of tasks, a major job such as a project, or leadership of a team. Milgram, Spector, and Treger (1999) identify several key issues that relate to the definition of delegation:

- It is giving someone the responsibility and authority to do something that is normally part of the manager's (team leader's and so on) job. Delegation is not just a simple task assignment.
- It is not "dumping" problems on someone else. Employees should not feel that they are doing the manager's (team leader's and so on) work but rather that they have received an opportunity for growth.
- It is not abandonment. The manager (team leader and so on) retains ultimate accountability for the project and needs to establish check points to monitor progress.
- It is giving the employee the appropriate authority to act alone and providing the necessary tools for success. The manager (team leader and so on) should not dictate every detail about how the job should be done (p. 384).

Typically, what drives a leader or a staff nurse to use delegation is simply that he or she cannot do it all. "Delegation, in one sense, is a paradox: The manager who delegates and develops employees to make and take responsibility for decisions begins the process of eliminating the need for a manager" although typically it never gets to the point of no management (Grohar-Murray & DiCroce, 2003, p. 173).

YOUR OPINION COUNTS

Find out what others think about this topic. Post your response and check out other opinions.

Some key terms are important to consider as one discusses delegation (American Nurses Association, 1997). The **delegator** is the person who does the delegation, and the **delegatee** is the person who receives the delegation. **Supervision** plays a major role in delegation. This involves guidance or direction, including evaluation and follow-up, that is provided by the delegator to the delegatee. Although delegation involves delegating to many different types of staff including the **unlicensed assistive personnel (UAP)**, much of this discussion will focus on delegation to UAPs, who are "any unlicensed individual who is trained to function in an assistive role to the licensed nurse in the provision of patient/client activities as delegated by the nurse. The term includes but is not limited to nurse aides, orderlies, assistants, attendants, or technicians" (American Nurses Association, 1997, p. 3).

Benefits of delegation

Delegation offers many benefits to the organization and to the staff who work in the organization (Grohar-Murray & DiCroce, 2003). Cost-effectiveness is one benefit when resources, including staff, are used appropriately. There is a potential cost savings. Clearly, there can be time savings as activities are allocated among others, thereby multiplying the ability to get work done more efficiently. Professional growth can occur when staff are challenged to develop new skills as they take on new opportunities. The delegator, who might be a manager, team leader, or staff nurse, has the opportunity to grow as new skills are learned, more time is available to do other activities, and so on. When delegation is done in a thoughtful manner, the environment is typically one in which staff feel valued and trusted.

Delegation has always been present in nursing and, at different points in its history, it has been more important than others. With the increasing use of UAPs, delegation is now a skill that every nurse must have and use effectively. This includes newly licensed nurses, as it is difficult even for new nurses to avoid delegation in any health care setting. Delegation is "*transferring* to a *competent* individual *authority* to *perform* a selected nursing task in a *selected* situation. The nurse retains accountability for the delegation" (National Council of State Boards of Nursing, 1995b, p. 2). The italicized words in this definition are key to successful delegation. *Transferring* implies a process as well as indicates that it is something the nurse would do but is giving the responsibility to someone else. *Competent* means the person who will do the task has the required skills and experience. The nurse must be able to determine that the staff member can do the task. *Authority* or the power to act is given to the staff person. *Perform* means that some action must take place, and this action is described as a selected nursing task in a selected situation. The nurse must tell the staff member what is to be done. "Delegation, however, should not be confused with participation. In participative decision making, there is a sharing of authority. With delegation, employees make decisions on their own. That's why delegation is such a vital component of worker empowerment" (Robbins & Decenzo, 2001, p. 391)!

Legal issues related to delegation

Critical legal issues and factors that impact delegation are state boards of nursing, scope of practice and nurse practice acts, labor unions, and standards of care. Each one of these issues affects the "who," "what," "when," and "how" of delegation. Every nurse is responsible for knowing how these factors might affect delegation. The legal authority for delegation comes from state laws and regulations. The board of nursing in each state is established by statute or law. The nursing board in each state is the governing body that ensures the safe practice of nursing is provided to its citizens (Hansten & Washburn, 1995). Note that the focus is on the patient, not the nurse. The board in each state is also involved in approving the schools of nursing and granting and revoking licenses, which is discussed more in Chapter 10. Both of these functions are done to ensure the safe practice of nursing. The board regulates nursing practice, although states vary in how this is implemented. The critical issue is the state's nurse practice act. Disciplinary process and related actions are also taken by boards to ensure safe practice.

The nurse practice act of each state and its associated rules and regulations represent the law that every nurse needs to know. The law's associated rules and regulations are also important. The scope of practice is described in the practice act, providing the "legal framework of practice" (Hansten & Washburn, 1995, p. 50). The law itself may appear to be very general, and it usually is. This is why it is important to also be aware of the related rules and regulations, which tell how the law is to be implemented. Every registered nurse needs to know what is in the scope of practice and the legal limits. In addition, every registered nurse needs to know what certified and unlicensed personnel can do. Position descriptions within health care organizations are critical, but they cannot conflict with guidelines developed by the board of nursing. Nurses are responsible for knowing when a job description might conflict with board regulations. One cannot say "I followed the job description" when it does not meet state requirements related to what tasks can be developed, to whom, and when. The board of nursing is also responsible for clearly describing the principles related to delegation or what is expected of nurses in the state when they delegate.

THINK CRITICALLY

Try this exercise to apply what you have learned about this topic.

Nurses can contact their state board of nursing and request a copy of the state's nurse practice act. In addition, the Internet makes it easy to learn more about boards of nursing and related issues. What questions should registered nurses ask when learning about their state laws and regulations pertaining to delegation?

- Does it permit delegation?
- How is delegation defined?
- Does the nurse practice act specify certain tasks for delegation or list any that cannot be delegated?
- Does it authorize delegation based on certain circumstances?
- Does it describe the UAP role?
- What does supervision mean in the state?
- How much supervision must be given when delegation occurs?
- Does the nurse practice act indicate the consequences of inappropriate delegation?
- Does it provide guidelines for reducing delegation risks (Fisher, 2000, p. 58)?

Standards of practice are also important documents, although not legal documents. Why would standards be discussed under legal issues related to delegation? When delegation occurs, the tasks performed must meet the standards of practice, as well as the organization's policies and procedures. Nurses are expected to know what these are and how they apply. "The licensed nurse determines and is accountable for the appropriateness of delegated nursing tasks. Inappropriate delegation by the nurse and/or unauthorized performance of nursing tasks by unlicensed assistive personnel may lead to legal action against the licensed nurse and/or unlicensed assistive personnel" (National Council of State Boards of Nursing, 1995a). Registered nurses may delegate certain nursing tasks to licensed practical/vocational nurses (LPN/LVNs) and UAPs. Some states allow LPN/LVNs to delegate certain tasks within their scope of practice to UAPs. What happens if the nurse's employer wants tasks delegated when the nurse does not think that this delegation is appropriate (for example, the delegatee is unable to do the task safely)? Using professional judgment via application of the nursing process, the nurse must act as the patient's advocate by only taking action that is appropriate for the patient. This also means that the organization cannot just have a list of tasks that can be delegated, because nursing judgment and nursing process must also be applied to the delegation process. If the nurse does not use professional judgment and delegates when it is inappropriate, even if told to do this by supervisors, the nurse is still accountable for errors in delegation. This might result in disciplinary action from the board of nursing and increase liability concerns (American Nurses Association, 1997). Liability is being legally responsible for one's own professional practice and for those actions that are delegated. "Nurse managers have a legal duty to know what tasks are within the scope of their state's nurse practice act, the scope of practice of their staff members, and most important of the competency of the staff member to complete the assigned task. In addition, if nurse managers breach the standard of care for either of those duties, the nurse may be held negligent if any harm results from the acts of the subordinate" (Grohar-Murray & DiCroce, 2003, pp. 174–175).

One might ask if the organization itself has any liability when there are problems with delegation that is done by its staff? "The legal principle of corporate liability involves an agency's legal duty to provide appropriate facilities, staff, safety, and equipment in the delivery of a service offered to the public" (Grohar-Murray & DiCroce, 2003, p. 175). Therefore, so the organization does have some liability. In addition to this principle, the organization is also responsible based on the principle of *vicarious liability* or *respondeat superior*. This means the organization is responsible for the acts of its employees when they are performing their job. "The failure to delegate and supervise within acceptable standards of professional nursing practice may be seen as malpractice" (Guido, 2001, p. 340). "The degree of knowledge concerning the skills and competencies of those one supervises is of paramount importance. The doctrine of 'knew or should have known' becomes a legal standard in delegating tasks to licensed individuals whom one supervises" (Guido, 2001, p. 340). The delegator does need to determine if the staff member has the ability to do the job or task—known as assessment of competency. However, when staff delegate to UAPs or LPN/LVNs, the staff nurse as well as nurse manager need to supervise the work.

Supervision is the "active process of directing, guiding, and influencing the outcome of an individual's performance of an activity" (American Nurses Association, 1997, p. 3). Effective supervision strategies with UAPs include:

1. Know the UAP's role expectations, competencies, strengths, and weaknesses.
2. Allocate sufficient time for supervision, making rounds, opportunities for the UAP to bring up issues and concerns to the staff nurse, and evaluation of the progress of care delivery.
3. Develop and maintain clear channels of communication, including being available to UAPs as needed.
4. Adhere to patient care and work performance standards.
5. Give timely feedback, both positive and negative, and make time for sharing information with UAPs that will facilitate their work (Guido, 2001, p. 352).

Critical delegation issues: Authority, responsibility, and accountability

As was discussed in Chapter 5, organization structure illustrates how work is assigned and describes relationships among staff by identifying authority, responsibility, and accountability. The assignment of work and delegation are closely tied to the organization's structure. The scalar chain that describes the organizational chart with vertical lines and how employees are responsible to one another is an important resource to learn more about authority. "To delegate well, the manager (or staff such as a team leader) must share responsibility and authority with the delegatees and hold them accountable for their performance. The ultimate accountability, however, must still lie with the manager" (Milgram, Spector, & Treger, 1999, p. 304). **Accountability** identifies who is answerable for what has been done. How is this different from responsibility? "For example, the nursing assistant to whom you delegated the task of obtaining vital signs made an error in the procedure of taking the blood pressure. The nursing assistant is responsible for his or her performance, and you are accountable to the person for the decision you made to delegate the task and for taking action and correcting the error" (Hansten & Washburn, 1995, pp. 54–55). The delegator must take accountability seriously, and this involves identifying the best person for the task or job. Although this is not always easy to determine, it must be done thoughtfully. For example, can a UAP delegate to an RN or LVN? No, this cannot be done. A key question is whether or not the task or job is within the position description of the delegatee and whether the delegator is allowed to delegate the task or job. Overlapping accountability by having more than one person responsible often leads to problems unless this is very clear and both parties are aware of this potential overlap. There are, however, times when shared accountability is appropriate. When this is used, the same principles that are used for individual accountability need to be defined—"a clear and agreed definition and breakdown of tasks into very precise, individually allocated 'single-point' elements to eliminate any possible overlaps" (Heller, 1998, p. 27). Concern about autonomy or the right to make a decision and control can best be illustrated in the following two questions:

1. How much authority is the delegatee able to exercise when doing the task/job without referring back to the delegator?
2. How far should the delegator exercise direct influence over the work of the delegatee (Heller, 1998, p. 6)?

THINK CRITICALLY

Try this exercise to apply what you have learned about this topic.

Delegation requires thought, and also requires that the delegator use assessment and critical thinking. Applying responsibility, authority, and accountability to the delegation process is important (Fisher, 1996). Responsibility can be applied when delegation is assigned. The delegator is responsible for selecting the best person to do the job; explaining the task thoroughly; and validating that the delegator understands what needs to be done. When authority is given during delegation, knowledge about the job needs to be shared. Others within the organization who need to know which staff members are assigned the delegated task or job should also be told. Resources need to be assigned. Letting the delegatee control the job or task is part of giving the appropriate level of authority. In establishing accountability, the delegator provides deadlines, feedback time periods, and evaluation criteria, with emphasis on success. If the organization has labor unions, this will affect delegation. Why is this so? Union contracts typically cover issues that are important to delegation such as staffing, safety, work schedules, seniority, and a grievance procedure (Hansten & Washburn, 1995).

Delegation and unlicensed assistive personnel

There is no doubt that UAPs are used in many health care organizations; in fact, there are about 65 different job titles for this position, which only confuses the matter more (American Nurses Association, Task Force on Unlicensed Personnel, 1997; American Operating Room Nurses, 2002; Huber, Blegen, & McCloskey, 1994; Oncology Nurses Society, 2002; Zimmerman, 2002). In addition to title differences, there is no universal hiring, training, or job descriptions. Consistency is definitely a problem. As nurses move from setting to setting it is critical that they make sure they understand these differences. There can even be variations from specialty areas or units within the same organization.

With the increasing use of UAPs in all types of settings such as acute care, home health care, and long-term care, patients are encountering a variety of staff as they receive care. Lange and Polifroni (2000) conducted a study that focused on whether or not patients knew the difference between nurses and UAPs. Their sample included 100 patients. The results were not encouraging: 28% of the patients did not know the job title of their caregiver, 8% thought the UAP was an RN, and the 72% who did identify the title of the caregiver admitted to guessing at the title. A startling result was that neither RNs nor UAPs often introduced themselves by name or job title. With many staff wearing similar uniforms or there being so much choice about uniforms, uniforms are no longer helpful in identifying staff and their roles. Name badges are typically worn; however, there are problems with them such as too much information, poor readability, not enough information, and small type (patients may not be wearing glasses that they might need to read the badges).

Patients were also unsure of the roles even if they knew the job title. They were not able to describe the differences between the roles and responsibilities of an RN and a UAP. "Nursing has a social responsibility and moral mandate to provide care. Patients have a right to know who their caregivers are, by title and by name" (Lange & Polifroni, 2000, p. 513). The American Nurses Association marketing campaign, "Every patient deserves a nurse," implies a social responsibility to the public—to clearly identify who is a nurse, determine what are the caregiver roles, wear uniforms that can be used to identify differences in positions, and use name badges that are clear, informative, and readable (Lange & Polifroni, 2000).

A 1998 study surveyed 53 state and territorial boards of nursing staff that focused on the use of UAPs in acute care hospitals, state and jurisdictional authority, oversight and disciplinary action related to registered nurse delegation, and the future use of UAPs (Thomas, Barter, & McLaughlin, 2000). One conclusion from the survey indicated that 21 of the 53 boards did not use the definitions of delegation, supervision, and assignment that have been developed by the National Council of State Boards of Nursing (NCSBN) or by the American Nurses Association (ANA). These states developed their own definitions. Standards for education and training of UAPs are also of great concern. This survey indicated that 83% of the states did not have a standardized state curriculum for UAPs employed by acute care hospitals, and the hospitals that did not have curricula, 63% had no plans to develop curricula. This is in contrast to the fact that "U.S. federal regulators specify that Medicare-certified, skilled nursing facilities and home health agencies must hire nursing assistants or home health aides who are certified. Federal code mandates 75 hours of training for certified nursing assistants working in skilled nursing facilities as a condition of participation in the Medicare program" (Code of Federal Regulations, Section 483.152-156, Washington, DC; as cited in Thomas, Barter, & McLaughlin, 2000, p. 14). In addition, an Institute of Medicine report specifically addressed the possibility of potential adverse effects from the use of untrained UAPs as well as the need for RNs to be competent in delegation and supervision (Wunderlich, Sloan, & Davis, 1996). This survey also examined complaints against RNs for inappropriate delegation. Of the states in the survey, 61% reported complaints in this category for a 3-year period. The board actions ranged from warnings to reprimands for 233 RNs and probation to suspension for 13 RNs. There is no doubt that the use of UAPs is increasing across the country, a fact supported by the survey. The conclusions from the survey, however, also demonstrated the disparity between the educational and training requirements for UAPs in home health agencies, skilled nursing facilities, and acute care settings. There needs to be standards for these UAPs because home care and skilled nursing care are no less complex.

THINK CRITICALLY

Try this exercise to apply what you have learned about this topic.

The delegation process and the NCSBN guidelines

When delegation is considered, it is important to note that not all tasks or activities should be delegated. How does one determine what might be delegated? Typical management considerations are: "(1) What tasks are the manager doing that need not be done at all? (2) What is the manager doing that could be done by someone else? and (3) What tasks is the manager doing that can only be done by the manager?" (Heller, 1998, p. 17). Answers to these questions will provide a clearer picture of tasks to delegate. In each of the questions one could substitute "name" for "manager" because all these questions apply to all nurses (e.g., staff nurses, team leaders). In addition, the following key questions should be asked as the delegation process begins.

1. What is the task or job to be delegated? Consider the complexity and skills that are required for the task or job. Is it clear what needs to be accomplished?

2. To whom should the task or job be delegated? Consider if the delegatee has the skills and time to perform the task or job effectively.

3. How should the task or job be assigned? Consider how much information and explanation needs to be given to the delegatee.

4. How often and in what depth should the delegator follow-up to see that the task or job has been performed effectively?

What activities and tasks can be delegated? Activities and tasks that frequently occur, are considered technical by nature, are considered standard and unchanging, have predictable results, and have minimal potential for risks are the typical type of task that is delegated (National Council of State Boards of Nursing, 1998). Box 8-1 identifies the five rights of delegation.

Box 8-2 provides some criteria that can be used to determine when to delegate.

BOX 8-1 Five rights of delegation.

I. Right Task: One that is delegable for a specific patient or situation.

II. Right Circumstances: Appropriate setting, available resources, and other relevant factors considered.

III. Right Person: Right person is delegating the right task to the right person to be performed by the right person.

IV. Right Direction/Communication: Clear, concise description of the task, including its objective, limits, and expectations.

V. Right Supervision: Appropriate monitoring, evaluation, intervention (as needed), and feedback.

Source: American Nurses Association. (1995). Author and highlighted from content. *Delegation, concepts and decision-making process, national council position paper.* Retrieved from the National Council of State Boards of Nursing at http://www.ncsbn.org/public/regulation/delegation_documents_delegati.htm on November 2, 2002.

BOX 8-2 To delegate or not.

The following are some criteria that are used to determine if one should delegate an activity or a task.

■ Patient's condition, including complications and stability

■ Complexity of the assessment

■ Intricacy of the task

■ Repetitiveness of the task

■ Capabilities of the UAP

■ Amount of technology required

■ Infection control and safety precautions

■ Potential for harm

■ Level of supervision that the RN will need to provide

■ Predictability of outcome

■ Extent of patient interaction

■ Environment

Sources: Summarized by author from: Hansten, R., & Washburn, M. (1995). Knowing how to delegate. *American Journal of Nursing, 95*(7), 16H–161; Yoder-Wise, P. (1999). Delegation: An art of professional practice. In *Leading and managing in nursing* (2nd ed.). St. Louis, MO: Mosby; Zimmerman, P. Delegating to unlicensed assistive personnel. Retrieved from Nursing Spectrum Career Fitness Online at http://nsweb.nursingspectrum.com/ce/ce124.htm on November 5, 2002.

Hansten and Washburn (1995) describe delegation as a cyclical process, similar to the nursing process, which includes the following steps:

1. The assessment phase focuses on knowing your world, which includes your practice area and your organization; knowing yourself, your strengths and limitations; and knowing your delegatee. The last element requires that the delegator know the delegatee's competency level and motivation. Neither of these is easy to assess, but both are critical to ensure patient safety and quality of care.

2. The plan requires that you know what needs to be done. If you do not, you will not be able to clearly define the task for the staff member or delegatee. This requires that you have professional and technical skills as well as acknowledge the importance of customer service.

3. Intervention means that you are able to prioritize and match the job to the staff member. Communication, which includes the initial directions and follow-up, plays a critical role. If the delegator does not understand what needs to be done, when, where, to whom, and how, then the task will not be completed as expected. Conflicts may arise during the process, which require collaboration and negotiation.

4. Evaluation is ongoing throughout the delegation process. You need to know how to give constructive feedback as it can be a powerful motivator. Evaluation does require problem solving, particularly if the results or outcomes were not what you expected. Supervision is part of evaluation. This is "the provision of guidance by a qualified nurse for the accomplishment of a nursing task or activity with initial direction of the task or activity and periodic inspection of the actual act of accomplishing the task or activity" (Hansten & Washburn, 1995, p. 7).

Selection of staff or delegatee is an important part of the delegation process. Selecting staff who will be honest when they need help or if they have questions or concerns is paramount to successful delegation. Staff who take initiative can be good choices for some tasks. This demonstrates self-confidence and the ability to stand up and speak one's mind (Heller, 1998). Staff who are analytical, organized, and able to look at problems carefully will also be more successful. It is easy to fall into the trap of making decisions about delegation too quickly. Sometimes a situation calls for a quick decision; however, whenever possible, it is best to take time and be as objective as possible. Some tasks, activities, or projects may require that the selected staff obtain additional training to do the delegated work. If this is the case, it should be provided; this is an investment, and it will help the organization reach its goals. This training needs to be planned and directed at the needs.

Monitoring progress of a delegable task, activity, or project can be difficult. Too much or too little monitoring may get in the way of success. Heller (1998) identifies some "Do's" and "Don'ts" that can help during the monitoring phase of the delegation process.

Do's

Do encourage all delegatees to make their own decisions.

Do move from hands-on to hands-off as soon as possible.

Do intervene when absolutely necessary, but only at that time.

Do ask delegatees if they feel thoroughly prepared for the task.

Don'ts

Don't say or hint that you doubt the delegatee's ability.

Don't miss any stage in the briefing process.

Don't surreptitiously take back a task.

Don't place seniority above ability.

Don't deny a delegatee the chance to learn by interfering too much (p. 37).

Monitoring methods that might be used include observation, verbal feedback, written feedback, review of records such as medical records and other standard records, and e-mail. During monitoring it is important to praise and reward delegates. Finding something positive to comment on is important even when progress may not be all that was hoped for. Recognizing effort sometimes goes by the wayside because it is taken for granted. There are times when difficulties are identified during mentoring. How should these be handled by the delegator? The first step is to analyze the difficulties before jumping to conclusions. The focus areas of this analysis are: "(1) The delegator should look at his/her own role. (2) Assess the directions given to the delegatee as to clarity. (3) Assess the delegatee's strengths and limitations and how these might be affecting the problems. (4) Determine if the goals and the timelines were appropriate. (5) Determine if the delegatee has all the resources required to do the job or task. (6) Assess if the delegatee has the needed authority, and (7) Assess the accessibility of the delegator to the delegatee" (Heller, 1998, pp. 48–51).

THINK CRITICALLY

Try this exercise to apply what you have learned about this topic.

BENCHMARKS

Now let's take a moment to test your knowledge of the concepts you have studied in this section.

Effective Delegation

Assessment of the delegation process

The delegation process, like other procesess, is fluid and thus must be frequently assessed as to its quality. Are the steps followed? What are the outcomes—for the patient and staff members, the team, unit, and the organization? It is important to understand what is effective delegation. Box 8-3 provides a description of the decision-making process as it applies to delegation.

Characteristics of effective delegation

A critical factor about effective delegation is it "pushes authority down vertically through the ranks of the organization" (Robbins & Decenzo, 2001, p. 391). Effective delegation requires that the delegator have delegation skills as delegation is not simple. Milgram, Spector, and Treger (1999) describe some aspects of effective delegation that need to be considered in the assessment.

- Delegate when there is someone more skilled available or when the task can be completed by a subordinate whose time is less expensive.
- Do not give employees just menial tasks; include tasks that offer opportunities for learning and growth.
- Distribute tasks with an understanding of each employee's job status, abilities, and total workload.
- Use benchmarks to monitor progress along the way; having only a deadline can be overwhelming.
- Do not micromanage subordinates. Experienced employees usually have the skills necessary for managing complex tasks on their own. They can also provide a wealth of information that will help to better understand the functioning of the department or even of the entire organization.
- Establish what needs to be done, and then provide support for the employee as he or she decides how to accomplish the job (p. 245).

Effective delegation does not just happen. Every nurse has to learn how to delegate. It takes practice. Even if a nurse has the best intention, delegation may still be difficult. There are also barriers that can interfere with delegation.

Barriers to effective delegation

Barriers to effective delegation exist that require attention before, during, and after the process. Delegating may mean something different to different staff. Some staff even think that it means

BOX 8-3   Delegation decision-making process.

In delegating, the nurse must ensure appropriate assessment, planning, implementation, and evaluation. The delegation decision-making process, which is continuous, is described by the following model:

I. Delegation criteria
   A. Nursing practice act
      1. Permits delegation
      2. Authorizes task(s) to be delegated or authorizes the nurse to decide delegation
   B. Delegator qualifications
      1. Within scope of authority to delegate
      2. Appropriate education, skills, and experience
      3. Documented/demonstrated evidence of current competency
   C. Delegatee qualifications
      1. Appropriate education, training, skills, and experience
      2. Documented/demonstrated evidence of current competency

Provided that this foundation is in place, the licensed nurse may enter the continuous process of delegation decision making.

II. Assess the situation
   A. Identify the needs of the patient, consulting the plan of care
   B. Consider the circumstances/setting
   C. Assure the availability of adequate resources, including supervision

If patient needs, circumstances, and available resources (including supervisor and delegatee) indicate patient safety will be maintained with delegated care, proceed to III.

III. Plan for the specific task(s) to be delegated
   A. Specify the nature of each task and the knowledge and skills required to perform it
   B. Require documentation or demonstration of current competence by the delegatee for each task
   C. Determine the implications for the patient, other patients, and significant others

If the nature of the task, competence of the delegatee, and patient implications indicate patient safety will be maintained with delegated care, proceed to IV.

IV. Assure appropriate accountability
   A. As delegator, accept accountability for performance of the task(s)
   B. Verify that delegatee accepts the delegation and the accountability for carrying out the task correctly

If delegator and delegatee accept the accountability for their respective roles in the delegated patient care, proceed to V.

V. Supervise performance of the task
   A. Provide directions and clear expectations of how the task(s) is to be performed
   B. Monitor performance of the task(s) to assure compliance to established standards of practice, policies, and procedures
   C. Intervene if necessary
   D. Ensure appropriate documentation of the task(s)

VI. Evaluate the entire delegation process
   A. Evaluate the patient
   B. Evaluate the performance of the task(s)
   C. Obtain and provide feedback

VII. Reassess and adjust the overall plan of care as needed

Source: National Council of State Boards of Nursing. (1996–2001). *Nursing Regulation.* Retrieved on November 2, 2002, from the National Council of State Boards of Nursing, http://www.ncsbn.org/public/regulation/delegation_documents_delegati.htm. Reprinted with permission.

they are incapable if they delegate to others. This clearly indicates that the staff member does not understand delegation. Some staff may not even be aware of their inner feelings about delegation. The following are some of the typical barriers to effective delegation.

- The attitude of "I would rather do it myself" leads to the question of whether or not this is a good use of time and skills.
- Some staff or managers will think that to delegate means overburdening staff who are already overworked. In this case, the delegator is not going through all the delegation process, which requires an assessment of the delegatee's ability to do the job. This involves more than just knowing if the delegatee has the skills, but also if he or she has the time.
- Staff sometimes have a lack of knowledge and experience about delegation. Realizing they do not know how to do it is sometimes difficult for staff to recognize. There are often few resources for teaching and guiding staff who need further knowledge and delegation experience.
- Inexperienced delegators will hesitate to delegate, not knowing what to do. To prevent more problems, they avoid delegating. They try to do everything themselves, which will eventually lead to serious problems.
- Staff may not even think that delegation is a possibility or they may use denial (for example, a potential delegator may think that a certain task cannot be delegated when it can be).
- Staff fear loss of control, which is related to lack of trust in others to do the job right, insecurity, and suspiciousness. This interferes with delegation.
- The organization's policies and procedures can be helpful but also can be barriers if not updated or applied correctly.
- Position descriptions that do not state clearly responsibilities and accountability are a problem. This applies to both the delegator's and the delegatee's position descriptions.
- Concern about education and training of the delegatee is important. If the delegatee is expected to do a task and the delegatee is not prepared, the delegatee must receive appropriate training and education.
- Sometimes there does not seem to be enough time to consider delegation. Sometimes the situation is so complicated, and must move so quickly, it seems to the delegator that it would be easier and faster to do the task rather than delegating.
- Some delegators want staff to like them, so delegation is not used in order to lighten workloads.
- The Supernurse syndrome, or feeling that others cannot do what you can do so you try to do it all, is a major barrier.
- Lack of organization is always a barrier to effective work. The delegator needs to think through what needs to be done, by whom, when, and so on. This all takes organization.
- Changing staff does not allow time for developing trust and confidence in staff. Working with the same staff over time allows the delegator to get to know staff and feel more comfortable with delegation.
- Lack of role models to learn how to delegate effectively can be found in most organizations. Student nurses and new graduates need experienced RNs to act as role models.
- An RN supervising the delegatee may have little contact with the patient. This means the RN must trust the delegatee. It is better for the RN to have some patient contact.
- Poor communication interferes with all steps in the delegation process. Much sharing of information goes on in this process, which requires effective communication.
- If staff have difficulty taking a risk, delegation is difficult. Delegation involves some level of risk. If delegation follows the process, the risk level is less, but it can never be totally eliminated. Much more needs to be done to develop environments where risk taking is valued and not punished.
- Some staff experience the supermartyr syndrome by refusing to ask others to help. This is particularly important when the delegatee does not ask for help when needed.
- Lack of self-confidence interferes with the delegator's ability to delegate, and when experienced by the delegatee, this can interfere with effective completion of work that has been delegated.

■ Fear of criticism is a barrier, both for the delegator and delegatee. More needs to be done to help staff understand evaluation and feedback.

■ Poor relationships with staff will block effective delegation. Staff may not be motivated to respond appropriately or may not trust the delegator. Lack of respect for staff will be a major barrier, as everyone likes to be respected and appreciated (Grohar-Murray & DiCroce, 2003; Hansten & Washburn, 1995; Heller, 1998; Kopishke, 2002).

Additional barriers to effective delegation that need to be considered relate to delegator involvement. Delegators who get too involved in work details (called micromanaging) are not effective. This gets back to earlier comments about the delegator's ability to turn over control and to trust. This does not mean, however, that the delegator does not need feedback at regular intervals to monitor progress because this is an important step in the delegation process. Another barrier is when delegators only delegate the unpleasant or boring activities, keeping tight control over the more interesting activities or delegate the better tasks to certain staff. Empowering staff, which is done through delegation, requires that staff be given some responsibility for the more interesting activities, not just the boring or less important ones. It is also important to understand the reasons that staff are selected for tasks.

How can barriers be overcome? Heller (1998) recommends that the delegator consider several strategies. The first is to consider insecurity and lack of confidence in subordinates. Why are these responses experienced? What can be done to decrease insecurity and lack of confidence in others to get the job done? Clearly, recognizing the value of delegation will help the delegator appraise barriers and be motivated to remove them. Making sure that staff are prepared to do their jobs will decrease some of the insecurity in their ability to meet the delegation needs. Planning will help to focus on needs and to determine when delegation is necessary. Providing feedback and asking staff what help they need will also overcome barriers.

THINK CRITICALLY

Try this exercise to apply what you have learned about this topic.

Supervision and assignment

It is difficult to discuss delegation without considering supervision and assignment. All three can be confusing, particularly to new graduates. Supervision is defined by the American Nurses Association as "the provision of guidance or direction, evaluation and follow-up by the licensed nurse for accomplishment of a nursing task delegated to unlicensed assistive personnel" (National Council of State Boards of Nursing, 1995b, p. 2). An example of supervision is when a nurse visits all of the team's patients to ensure that the UAPs have completed an assigned task. Assignment is "designating nursing activities to be performed by an individual consistent with his/her licensed scope of practice" (National Council of State Boards of Nursing, 1995b, p. 1). Another definition provided by the American Nurses Association (1995b) is "the downward or lateral transfer of both the responsibility and accountability of an activity from one individual to another. The lateral or downward transfer must be made to an individual of skill, knowledge, and judgment. The activity must be within the individual's scope of practice" (p. 2). What does this mean in practice? A staff member is assigned to do an activity, which includes the responsibility and accountability for the activity. Assignment must be based on the staff member's skill, knowledge, judgment, and legal scope of practice (Zimmerman, 2002, p. 2). When a nurse is told to care for a group of patients by the nurse manager, this is an assignment. In this example, the nurse manager is accountable only for making the assignment and selecting who will be responsible for the care of the patients. The staff nurse is accountable and responsible for actually providing the care or ensuring that it is provided. In turn, the staff nurse can only delegate work to others, such as UAPs, but cannot assign work. "In comparison, delegation is the partial transfer of authority and responsibility regarding care activities, while accountability for completion and outcomes remains with the delegator" (Zimmerman, 2002, p. 2). The nurse manager expects the RN to complete the work assigned. Even if the RN delegates to other staff the RN must still ensure effective completion of the work. The RN as the delegator must analyze and evaluate the outcome of the delegated task or activity.

A key question that now becomes important is what activities can be delegated to the UAP. The ANA position statement, *Registered Nurse Utilization of Unlicensed Assistive Personnel* (1997), delineates between UAP direct patient care activities and indirect ones by describing them in the following manner.

- **Direct patient care activities:** These activities assist the patient/client in meeting basic human needs within the institution, at home, or other health care settings. This includes activities such as assisting the patient with feeding, drinking, ambulating, grooming, toileting, dressing, and socializing. It may also involve the collecting, reporting, and documentation of data related to the previous activities. Data are reported to the RN, who uses the information to make a clinical judgment about patient care.
- **Indirect patient care activities:** These activities support the patient/client and their environment, and only incidentally involve direct patient contact. These activities assist in providing a clean, efficient, and safe patient care milieu and typically encompass chore services, companion care, housekeeping, transporting, clerical, stocking, and maintenance tasks.

It is important to note that there are specific types of activities that cannot be delegated to UAPs. These include health counseling, teaching, and those activities that require independent, specialized nursing knowledge, skill, or judgment (pp. 2–3).

CURRENT ISSUES

Learn about events around the globe that relate to the chapter content.

It may seem clear as to what activities can be delegated and what activities cannot; however, this is a topic that is causing great discussion and debate in many state legislatures. Efforts have been made by various groups to change what certain health care providers can or cannot do. This is a great example of when it is important for nurses to become politically active, and many have done this in order to ensure that RNs have a voice in setting these parameters. Glazer (2000) noted that "the profession of nursing needs to develop consensus around what makes a nursing task or activity one that can only be performed by a registered nurse versus what nursing tasks and activities can be shared and delegated" (p. 1). She goes on to identify some key questions that need to be considered: "What is a nursing function? What criteria or logic dictates the functions that are specifically prohibited for unlicensed assistive personnel?" (Glazer, 2000, p. 2). This has become contentious as some nurses are against giving up some activities or concerned about the ability of others such as UAPs to do the job safely and provide quality care. Historically, although there are activities that only physicians did, some are now done by RNs. In addition, activities done by RNs are now done by LPN/LVNs or UAPs. There is, however, no consensus on this issue.

In conclusion, the following key guidelines are important in ensuring consistency and effective delegation (Zimmerman, 2002).

- **Start with a positive attitude.** This includes respecting staff and appreciating the work that they do. Good working relationships go a long way to ensure successful delegation; however, establishing a positive relationship cannot be done at the time of delegation. It needs to be ongoing.
- **Clarify availability.** In some situations, UAPs are assigned to several RNs at the same time with each of them delegating activities. This can clearly cause some confusion so it is important to determine what the UAP has time to do based on other activities. The UAP should not be in a position where RNs vie for the UAP.

- **Carefully consider how directions are given during delegation.** This relates back to respect in that directions should be given in a manner that respects the other staff member—avoiding sharp statements, giving directions on the run, talking down or patronizing, and other ineffective communication approaches.
- **Directions need to be clear.** Unclear directions can cause more problems for staff and patients. The delegator is responsible for making the directions clear and ensuring that the delegatee understands them. As discussed earlier, directions should include what needs to be done, by whom, how, and when. If the activity is complex, directions should also include reportable parameters and rationale. An example of this activity would be telling the UAP what blood pressure range should be reported to the RN immediately.
- **Be fair about undesirable activities.** Nursing is not immune to activities or tasks that are unpleasant or even boring. When these activities are delegated, they should be delegated fairly so that the same person is not always chosen for these activities.
- **Indicate priorities.** Direction implies that the delegator identifies priorities, what activities are more important, or what should be done first. This should be clear to the delegatee. The RN may work with the UAP to consider all activities that need to be done and prioritize the approaches to be taken.
- **Give and receive feedback.** The RN gives feedback to the UAP during delegation. This should be ongoing and not just provided when something goes wrong. Feedback needs to be seen as a time for teaching and learning. The RN must also be able to receive and actually seek out feedback from the UAP related to delegation and supervision that the RN provides to ensure that the delegated activity is completed effectively. Is the RN providing clear directions? How does the UAP feel about the activities that are delegated? Is the UAP respected? These are just a few of the questions to consider.

CURRENT ISSUES

Learn about events around the globe that relate to the chapter content.

BENCHMARKS

Now let's take a moment to test your knowledge of the concepts you have studied in this section.

Chapter Wrap-Up

Now that you've reached the end of the chapter, you may wish to explore the concepts you've been reading about in greater detail, or test yourself to see how well you've comprehended the material.

SUMMARY AND APPLICATIONS

- Summary
- Practice Quiz
- Key Terms
- Tying It All Together

- Experiential Exercises
- Case
- Links

REFERENCES

American Nurses Association. (1997). *Position statement: Registered nurse utilization of unlicensed assistive personnel.* Washington, DC: Author.

American Nurses Association, Task Force on Unlicensed Assistive Personnel. (1997). *Registered professional nurses and unlicensed assistive personnel.* Washington, DC: American Nurses Association. Retrieved on June 25, 2002, from American Nurses Association at www.nursingworld.org/readroom/position/uspuse.htm.

American Operating Room Nurses. (2002). *AORN official statement on unlicensed assistive personnel, standards, recommended practices, and guidelines.* Denver, CO: Author.

Code of Federal Regulations, Section 483:152–156, Washington, DC.

Fisher, M. (1996). *Redesigning the nursing organization.* Albany, NY: Delmar Publishers.

Fisher, M. (2000). Do you have delegation savvy? *Nursing 2000, 30*(12), 58–59.

Glazer, G. (2000). What makes something a nursing activity or task? Retrieved on June 23, 2003, from *Online Journal of Issues in Nursing,* at http://www.nursingworld.org.

Grohar-Murray, M., & DiCroce, H. (2003). *Leadership and management in nursing* (3rd ed.). Upper Saddle River, NJ: Prentice Hall.

Guido, G. (2001). *Legal and ethical issues in nursing* (3rd ed.). Upper Saddle River, NJ: Prentice Hall.

Hansten, R., & Washburn, M. (1995). Knowing how to delegate. *American Journal of Nursing, 95*(7), 16H–16I.

Heller, R. (1998). *How to delegate.* New York: DK Publishing Inc.

Hill, L. (1993). *Becoming a manager.* New York: Penguin Books.

Huber, D., Blegen, M., & McClosky, J. (1994). Use of nursing assistants: Staff nurse opinion. *Nursing management, 25*(5), 64–68.

Kopishke, L. (2002). Unlicensed assistive personnel: A dilemma for nurses. *Journal of Legal Nurse Consultant, 13*(1), 3–7.

Lange, J., & Polifroni, E. (2000). Nurses and assistive personnel. Do patients know the difference? *Journal of Nursing Administration, 30*(11), 512–513.

Milgram, L., Spector, A., & Treger, M. (1999). *Managing smart.* Houston, TX: Cashman Dudley.

National Council of State Boards of Nursing. (1995a). *Delegation. Concepts and decision-making process, national council position paper.* Retrieved on November 2, 2002, from the National Council of State Boards of Nursing at http://www.ncsbn.org/public/regulation/delegation_documents_delegati.htm.

National Council of State Boards of Nursing. (1995b). *Delegation: Understanding the concepts and decision-making process.* Retrieved November 2, 2002, from the National Council of State Boards of Nursing at http://www.ncsbn.org/files/publications/positions/delegate.asp.

National Council of State Boards of Nursing. (1998). Delegation concepts and decision-making process, National Council position paper. *Insight, 7*(1), 6.

Oncology Nursing Society. (2002). Position on the role of unlicensed assistive personnel in cancer care. Revised October 2000. Retrieved on June 19, 2002, from Oncology Nursing Society at http://www.ons.org/publications/positions

Robbins, S., & Decenzo, D. (2001). *Fundamentals of management.* Upper Saddle River, NJ: Prentice Hall.

Thomas, S., Barter, M., & McLaughlin, F. (2000). State and territorial boards of nursing approaches to the use of unlicensed assistive personnel. *JONA's Healthcare Law, Ethics, and Regulation, 2*(1), 13–21.

Wunderlich, G., Sloan, F., & Davis, C. (Eds.). (1996). *Nursing staff in hospitals and nursing homes: Is it adequate?* Washington, DC: National Academy Press.

Zimmerman, P. (2002). Delegating to unlicensed assistive personnel. Retrieved November 5, 2002, from Nursing Spectrum Career Fitness Online at http://nsweb.nursingspectrum.com/ce/ce124.html.

ADDITIONAL READINGS

Anthony, M., Standing, T., & Hertz, J. (2000). Factors influencing outcomes after delegation to unlicensed assistive personnel. *Journal of Nursing Administration, 30*(10), 474–481.

Anthony, M., Standing, T., & Hertz, J. (2001). Nurse's beliefs about their abilities to delegate within changing models of care. *The Journal of Continuing Education in Nursing, 32*(5), 210–215.

Badovinac, C., Wilson, S., & Woodhouse, D. (1999). The use of unlicensed assistive personnel and selected outcome indications. *Nursing Economics, 17,* 194–200.

Barter, M., McLaughlin, F., & Thomas, S. (1997). Registered nurse role changes and satisfaction with unlicensed assistive personnel. *Journal of Nursing Administration, 27*(1), 29–38.

Barter, M., McLaughlin, F., & Thomas, S. Use of unlicensed assistive personnel by hospitals. *Nursing Economics, 12*(2), 82–87.

Blouin, A., & Brent, N. (1995). Unlicensed assistive personnel: Legal considerations. *Nursing Management*, 23(11), 7–8, 21.

Fisher, M. (1999). Do your nurses delegate effectively? *Nursing Management*, 30(5), 23–25.

Hansten, R., & Washburn, M. (1994). *Clinical delegation skills. A handbook for nurses*. Gaithersburg, MD: Aspen Publishers, Inc.

Hansten, R., & Washburn, M. (1996). Why don't nurses delegate? *Journal of Nursing Administration*, 26, 24–28.

Hopkins, D. (2002). Evaluating the knowledge deficits of registered nurses responsible for supervising nursing assistants. *Journal of Nurses Staff Development*, 18, 152–156.

Hurley, M. (2000). Workload, UAPs, and you. *RN*, 63(12), 47–49.

Huston, C. (1996). Unlicensed assistive personnel: A solution to dwindling health care resources or the precursor to the apocalypse of registered nursing? *Nursing Outlook*, 44(2), 67–73.

Keeling, B., Adair, J., Seider, D., & Kirksey, G. (2000). Appropriate delegation. Uncovering opportunities for improvement. *American Journal of Nursing*, 100(12), 24A, 24C–24D.

Krapohl, G., & Larson, E. (1996). The impact of unlicensed assistive personnel on nursing care delivery. *Nursing Economics*, 14(2), 99–110.

McCloskey, J., Bulechek, G., Moorhead, S., & Daly, J. (1996). Nurses' use and delegation of indirect care interventions. *Nursing Economics*, 14(1), 22–33.

McClung, T. (2000). Assessing the reported financial benefits of unlicensed assistive personnel in nursing. *Journal of Nursing Administration*, 30(11), 530–534.

McGillis-Hall, L. (1998). Policy implications when changing staff mix. *Nursing Economics*, 16(6), 291–297, 312.

National Council of State Boards of Nursing. (1996–2001). *Nursing regulation*. Retrieved November 2, 2002, from the National Council of State Boards of Nursing at http://www.ncsbn.org/public/regulation/delegation_documents_delegati.htm.

Russo, J., & Lancaster, D. (1995). Evaluating unlicensed assistive personnel models: Asking the right questions, collecting the right data. *Journal of Nursing Administration*, 25(9), 51–57.

Salmond, S. (1995). Models of care using unlicensed assistive personnel—Part I: Job scope, preparation and utilization patterns. *Orthopaedic Nursing*, 14(6), 47–58.

Sikma, S., & Young, H. (2001). Balancing freedom with risks: The experience of nursing task delegation in community-based residential care settings. *Nursing Outlook*, 49(7), 193–201.

Stanek, B. (1995). Preparing competent assistive personnel for ICU. *Nursing Management*, 26(5), 48J–48L.

Zimmerman, P. (2000). The use of unlicensed assistive personnel: An update and skeptical look at a role that may present more problems than solutions. *Journal of Emergency Nursing*, 26(4), 312–317.

Tools to Manage and Evaluate Care

CHAPTER OUTLINE

MediaLink
www.prenhall.com/finkelman

The Interactive Exercises for this chapter can be found in the OneKey course at www.prenhall.com/finkelman. Click on Chapter 9 to select from the following activities: Test Your Understanding, Benchmarks, Current Issues, Your Opinion Counts, Think Critically, and Summary and Applications.

What's Ahead

Using methods or tools to manage care, such as clinical pathways, practice guidelines, and disease management programs, requires collaboration—from providers, case managers, third-party payers, patients, and families. Collaboration is important within clinical settings and between organizations. Because health care is complex, working together to reach goals is more successful and usually more efficient. As was discussed in Chapter 3, collaboration is "a dynamic transforming process of creating a power sharing partnership for pervasive application in health care practice, education, research, and organizational settings for the purposeful attention to needs and problems in order to achieve likely successful outcomes" (Sullivan, 1998, p. 255). Collaboration is needed to develop the tools to manage care, and it is also critical in implementing the tools. This chapter discusses these tools, their development and implementation, and the benefits to the patient, health care providers, health care delivery systems, and third-party payer/managed care organizations (MCOs). The content focuses on a variety of examples of tools used by different health care settings and providers to assist in managing care for individuals, families, and communities. These tools or strategies are: clinical pathways, practice guidelines, disease management, demand management, standards of care, utilization review/management, benchmarking, evidence-based practice, and health promotion and disease and illness prevention. In order to gain an understanding of the process used to develop many of the tools, clinical pathways will be discussed in more detail to provide a model for understanding the development process.

OBJECTIVES

Before you begin, take a moment to familiarize yourself with the key objectives of this chapter.

- Define clinical pathway.
- Identify the purpose of clinical pathways.
- Describe the pathway development process.
- Identify liability and ethical issues related to the use of clinical pathways.
- Illustrate how clinical pathways might be implemented in a clinical setting, and both the positive and negative consequences.
- Explain why variance analysis is an important component of clinical pathways.
- Discuss the importance of practice guidelines.
- Compare and contrast the use of practice guidelines and disease management in managed care.
- Explain the difference between disease management and demand management.
- Explain why standards of care, utilization review, benchmarking, and evidence-based practice are considered tools to increase collaborative care.
- Discuss the reasons for including health promotion and disease and illness prevention in this content.

TEST YOUR UNDERSTANDING

Before we begin our exploration of this chapter, take a short "warm-up" test to see what you know about this topic.

Clinical Pathways

"The survival of health care institutions depends upon a delivery system focusing on appropriate use of resources and controlling length-of-stay while monitoring clinical progress toward identified outcomes. Using a clinical path as a tool for managing resources, research activities, continuous quality improvement, and increased collaborative practice can enhance the professional practice environment and benefit patient care" (Clark, Steinbinder, & Anderson, 1994, p. 230). Collaborative care and interdisciplinary care are intertwined, as the development of clinical pathways and their implementation requires interdisciplinary collaboration. This section describes definitions, historical background of clinical pathway development, purpose, the clinical pathway development process, implementation, the effect of pathways on outcomes, and providers' responses to clinical pathways.

Definition of clinical pathway

There is no universally accepted definition of **clinical pathways** even though pathways have been used for more than 10 years. Reviewing a variety of definitions is helpful in appreciating their differences and similarities. The following are some examples of clinical pathway definitions.

■ An optimal sequencing and timing of interventions by physicians, nurses, and other staff for a particular diagnosis or procedure, designed to minimize delays and resource utilization and to maximize the quality of care (Coffey et al., 1992)

■ A visualization of the patient care process (Coffey et al., 1992)

■ A timeline that identifies expected patient outcomes and associated interventions for a specific diagnosis or class of cases, often defined by a diagnosis-related group (DRG) (Griffin & Griffin, 1994)

■ A tangible method for linking the patient, family, and the achievement of definable outcomes to the direct caregivers, interdisciplinary team, and continuous quality improvement (Zander, 1992)

■ Tools to define practice and guides for patient care activities; delineate the best/ideal practice (Cesta, Tahan, & Fink, 1998)

■ Tools for managed care that provide the interdisciplinary team with desired outcomes and identified time frames in which they should be accomplished; predict the critical targets a patient will achieve within specific time intervals, coupled with efficient use of resources (Flarey & Blancett, 1996)

■ A proactive set of daily prescriptions that has been prepared following a particular timeline to facilitate the care of a specific patient population from preadmission to postdischarge (Cesta, Tahan, & Fink, 1998)

■ Important tools to link patients, clinicians, and managed care organizations and other payers to achieve both high-quality and cost-effective care; effective tools to improve the planning, coordination, communication, and evaluation of care foster collaborative goal setting among multiple care providers for specific case types (Coffey et al., 1996)

One can conclude from these definitions that there are some common characteristics, including:

■ Provide guidelines for practice
■ Define outcomes
■ Focus on timelines
■ Use resources efficiently
■ Emphasize the need for coordination, communication, and collaboration
■ Include the patient and family
■ Provide interdisciplinary effort
■ Collaborate

Evolution of pathways

Why have health care organizations developed clinical pathways? Oil and chemical refineries were the first industries to use pathways as a method for defining their work processes, and then pathways were adopted by engineering, construction, and computer industries, as they discovered that it was a good tool for managing projects. Karen Zander, a nurse, then borrowed the idea in the mid-1980s and adapted it to the acute care setting. These early clinical pathways focused on nursing interventions and use of technology to provide care, as problems with these typically led to hospitalization. Zander was interested in decreasing the cost of care without decreasing quality. The process to develop clinical pathways was very similar to the nursing process and the nursing care plan. As is true of all new ideas, they grow and change, and hopefully improve.

The initial efforts to use pathways were restrained by limitations. Because of the generic nature of these plans, they did little to control the use of resources, types of medications, route of administration, or other factors related to cost and quality. Although the pathways did suggest the appropriate number of hospital days to allocate to a diagnostic-related group (DRG), they did little beyond that to control the kinds of product resources applied to the particular broad groupings of patients (Cesta, Tahan, & Fink, 1998). Pathways, however, have changed and improved as they no longer focus only on nursing interventions. Instead, they focus much more on interdisciplinary treatment and the effect of interventions on cost and quality.

An unresolved issue with the evolution of pathways is their name. Initially, they were called critical pathways. Now, pathways may be called care paths, CareMaps®, case management plans, anticipatory recovery plans, care guides, collaborative plans, coordinated plans, integrated plans, plans of action, and, probably the most common name, clinical pathways. This does cause confusion, as some health care professionals think that each of these represents a unique tool, and yet they are all basically the same. As is discussed in later sections of this chapter, there are other tools that add to this confusion (for example, algorithms, practice guidelines, practice parameters, and the newest, disease management programs). How are pathways different from these other tools? The following four characteristics have been attributed to clinical pathways rather than to the other types of clinical management tools:

1. Comprehensiveness through their emphasis on interdisciplinary care
2. Timeliness through their use of specific timelines for interventions
3. Collaboration through joint development by an interdisciplinary team
4. Case management, frequently used with pathways (Coffey et al., 1992, p. 46)

Practice guidelines focus on general treatment for a specific illness or condition, whereas pathways are more specific and unique to the health care agency or managed care organization (MCO) in which they are used. Pathways are also individualized for patients and meet the practice concerns of the providers. These characteristics make it more difficult to use pathways developed by other institutions and organizations. Pathways need to be adapted to meet the individual needs of the institution, its providers, and its patient population.

A common misperception is that clinical pathways and case management are the same. How did this come about? The case management plan used by case managers confuses the issue, as it focuses on case manager responsibilities, while the clinical pathway focuses on shared accountability of the interdisciplinary team. More case managers are using pathways as they coordinate care with the interdisciplinary team.

Purpose of pathways

Pathways provide direction in the coordination of care and ensure that outcomes are met within a designated time frame. The emphasis is on efficient use of resources and controlling costs (Ireson, 1997). Pathways have an interdisciplinary focus, and thus include all aspects of the patient's care that are critical to meeting outcomes. They can be used to demonstrate compliance with standards of care, accreditation, and regulatory requirements. These tools assist staff during orientation and in teaching nursing and medical students and others. Some institutions have developed patient versions of pathways that are given to the patient/family on admission or when treatment begins. They can be used to help the patient and family understand the patient's care and what to expect (Cesta, Tahan, & Fink, 1998).

What are the advantages and disadvantages of using clinical pathways? Because they have been used for some time, there is considerable information about their use and difficulties in using them. Figure 9-1 identifies some of the advantages of using clinical pathways. These advantages relate to all of the major aspects of patient care delivery and help to explain why clinical pathways have become so common.

FIGURE 9-1 Advantages of clinical pathways.

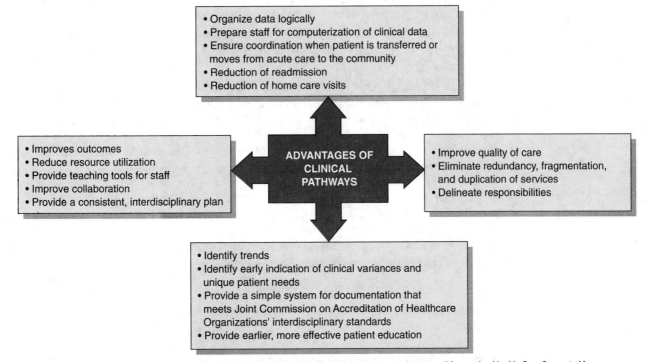

Sources: Author, content summarized from Griffin, M., & Griffin, R. (1994). Critical pathways produce tangible results. *Health Care Strategic Management,* *12*(7), 1, 17–23; Critical paths concept evolves into more comprehensive system. (1992). *Hospital Peer Review, 17*(2), 27–30; Hague, D. (1996, May). Clinical pathways: The careplans of the 90s. *Ohio Nurses Review,* 15–19; and Cesta, T., Tahan, H., & Fink, L. (1998). *The case manager's survival guide: Winning strategies for clinical practice.* St. Louis, MO: Mosby-Year Book, Inc.

Critics of pathways question why pathways are not rigid requirements and allow for limited individuation. This could be a major disadvantage; however, health care organizations have considered this potential problem. They usually require that pathway content is assessed each time it is used with a patient to ensure that individual patient needs are met. There is a temptation to make this into a "cookbook" treatment, to follow the pathway without thinking about the individual patient (Clark, Steinbinder, & Anderson, 1994). The physician, nurses, and other providers need to document changes or adaptations. Another disadvantage is the cost and time required to develop and implement pathways. For any health care organization, the development of its first pathway is the most expensive part of the project. It takes time to develop the process, policies and procedures, and forms, and then conduct the research that is required to get started as well as time to educate the project committee, interdisciplinary teams, and all of the staff. This process is described later in the chapter.

Selection of the illnesses or conditions that require pathways should be done carefully (Clark, Steinbinder, & Anderson, 1994). If there are few patients in a category (illness or condition), it may not be cost-effective to spend time on developing pathways that may make little difference in care, outcomes, and expenses. For example, if a hospital does not do transplants of any kind, developing a pathway for transplant care is not useful. A negative staff attitude toward pathways can also be a major disadvantage. If staff view the development of pathways as another project with excessive paperwork, redundant documentation, and a new gimmick to endure, then the process of implementing pathways will be an arduous one. Staff will be waiting for it to pass and will not feel committed to the project. This is particularly problematic in organizations that have instituted many "new projects" only to have them fall by the wayside due to a lack of commitment, a lack of knowledge about their use and implications to practice, or a lack of funding to complete the project. If care and systems do not change as a result of pathway outcomes, staff will wonder about all the effort that is expended on the project. If staff are fearful that pathways may be used to identify individual staff performance problems rather than assessment of process and systems to improve care, they will be reluctant to participate. Health care organizations that spend time considering these disadvantages and staff concerns, resolving them, and increasing staff commitment and participation will be much more successful.

Pathway development and implementation process

The pathway development process is a long one that requires administration and staff commitment and patience (Dykes, 1998a; Hofmann, 1993). Typically, a project committee develops the framework that will be used for all pathways and oversees the project. This committee should have a broad-based representation. Some of the departments or services in an organization or agency that might be included are nurses, physicians, and representatives from social service, case management, admissions, finance, administration, medical records, utilization review, quality improvement, risk management, and materials management. Laboratory, radiology, claims processing, and other specialized areas, such as respiratory therapy and physical therapy, may also be on the interdisciplinary teams that develop the content for specific pathways.

Before any specific plans are made for this project, the organization's environment for change needs to be assessed. As is true of all change efforts, the commitment of key staff is the critical element for the success of pathway development. Change has become an all too common experience in health care today, and it is unlikely to go away. There are steps that can be taken, however, to make it easier on the staff and to maintain an environment that is supportive of change. If pathways are to be used, the organization's leaders must support the effort, communicate this support to all staff, and ensure that the project is completed. Too frequently, projects are begun but never seem to be completed. A lack of commitment to complete projects affects future projects in the organization. Staff are then not enthusiastic or supportive, knowing the organization's history of failure with new projects. Open and consistent communication assists staff as they adjust to new requirements.

Because instituting the use of pathways or any of the other tools or strategies highlighted in this chapter is a major undertaking, beginning other major projects at the same time needs to be considered carefully. Too much stress at one time may affect the success of all new projects. There must also be a clear definition of the goals and identification of those staff who will have leadership responsibilities in instituting clinical pathways. Because this is not a quick fix, a reasonable timeline is required, with identified key points for reassessment of progress. With these decisions made, the project committee can begin work on specific pathways. The first phase of the project is the development of the pathways, and the second is implementation. Evaluation is incorporated throughout the project.

Development team

Pathway development requires an interdisciplinary team/committee that is: (a) willing to openly discuss issues and research information, (b) receptive to change, and (c) committed to the project. It is, however, helpful to have some staff who are skeptical as they provide the "other viewpoint" that is critical in the development of realistic pathways. Hopefully, these team members will not be so negative that they are destructive to the process, but rather they will identify issues and concerns that staff will undoubtedly experience. The committee works its way through the phases highlighted in Box 9-1.

The project committee and interdisciplinary teams need education about project development, change, and clinical pathways. It is helpful to provide this education prior to beginning the project or in the initial stages. Content should include:

- Project development and organizational change
- Definition and purposes of a pathway
- Advantages and disadvantages of pathways
- Implementation of pathways
- Research resources
- Variances and variance analysis
- Project evaluation

BOX 9-1 Pathway development process.

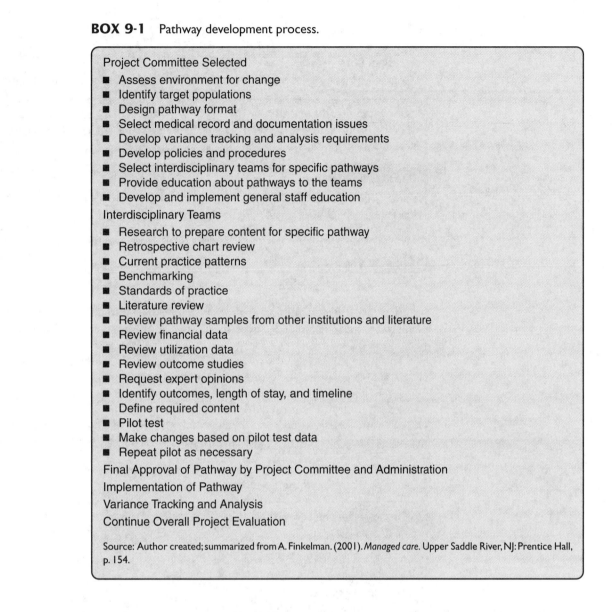

Project Committee Selected
- Assess environment for change
- Identify target populations
- Design pathway format
- Select medical record and documentation issues
- Develop variance tracking and analysis requirements
- Develop policies and procedures
- Select interdisciplinary teams for specific pathways
- Provide education about pathways to the teams
- Develop and implement general staff education

Interdisciplinary Teams
- Research to prepare content for specific pathway
- Retrospective chart review
- Current practice patterns
- Benchmarking
- Standards of practice
- Literature review
- Review pathway samples from other institutions and literature
- Review financial data
- Review utilization data
- Review outcome studies
- Request expert opinions
- Identify outcomes, length of stay, and timeline
- Define required content
- Pilot test
- Make changes based on pilot test data
- Repeat pilot as necessary

Final Approval of Pathway by Project Committee and Administration

Implementation of Pathway

Variance Tracking and Analysis

Continue Overall Project Evaluation

Source: Author created; summarized from A. Finkelman. (2001). *Managed care.* Upper Saddle River, NJ: Prentice Hall, p. 154.

Providing committee members and teams with resources such as current articles on pathways, books, and even sample pathways from similar organizations is a good way to begin. The project committee and the teams that develop the content for specific pathways need access to data such as length-of-stay (LOS), common admission diagnoses, laboratory tests, and incident data. Some staff may not know what data are available within the organization, so including information management system (IMS) staff who can assist the committee and the teams is very helpful.

Development of the pathway format

It is best if there is a standard pathway format that will be used throughout the organization. Reviewing formats used by other organizations is a good way to understand what can be done, and many examples are found in the literature. The committee may also want to contact similar organizations and ask about their pathway formats as well as their experiences with using clinical pathways. The format that is chosen needs to be easy to use, clear, and should not seem so overwhelming that staff will immediately complain that it will only add more work for them. Staff appreciate brevity, relevance, and conciseness.

What is included in the clinical pathway format? The scope of clinical pathways can vary; for example, a pathway might focus on inpatient care, a complete episode of care, specialized applications, or life and health management. Box 9-2 describes the scope in more detail.

BOX 9-2   Scope of clinical pathways.

Inpatient Care

Focus is on admission to the inpatient setting to discharge. This is the most common.

Complete Episode of Care

Focus is on the time that care is requested at the physician's office to termination of post-hospitalization treatment.

Specialized Applications

Focus is on the patient's special needs (e.g., renal dialysis, ambulatory surgery, management of outpatient treatment of a problem).

Source: Author created; summarized from A. Finkelman. (2001). *Managed care.* Upper Saddle River, NJ: Prentice Hall, p. 158.

Specific pathway content may also vary among organizations; the most common categories of information that are included in pathways are identified in Box 9-3 ; however, a pathway does not have to include all of these categories.

The committee selects the categories of information that are important to include for specific patient populations and organizational audit providers.

Key indicators are a very important part of the pathway. These indicators are the interventions that must be implemented in order to attain specified outcomes. During the development phase of pathways, it is important to understand the key indicators; however, overemphasis on indicators can be a problem. This usually happens when staff are concerned about missing some-

BOX 9-3   Pathway content categories.

Assessment and monitoring

Psychosocial assessment

Actual and potential problems

Treatment interventions: prevention and therapeutic

Tests and procedures

Expected outcomes

Consults

Required observations

Predetermined length-of-stay

Timeline with trigger points

Key indicators

Medications

Patient activity

Nutrition

Intravenous therapy

Patient/family education

Variance tracking

Delineate responsibilities of interdisciplinary team

Source: Author created; summarized from A. Finkelman. (2001). *Managed care.* Upper Saddle River, NJ: Prentice Hall, p. 158.

thing important. "In today's short health care stay, the question to be asked about key indicators is: What is absolutely necessary for me, as the caregiver, to attend to the patient to meet the outcome" (Hague, 1996, 16)? Nurses and other health care providers need to continuously remind themselves to focus on the most important care needs. This is not easy to do in today's stressful health care environment with its complex patients.

Documentation is also a very important issue that must be considered throughout the planning and development phases (Hague, 1996). The organization must make a decision about whether or not the pathways will be a permanent part of the medical record. If it is optional, confusion and inconsistency often occur. Accrediting agencies may question records that are not consistent. Pathways that are not part of the medical record may be viewed as less important by the staff. In the past nurses experienced this with nursing care plans when some hospitals included them in their medical records and others did not. If staff are concerned that using the pathways does not really cover documentation needs, they may over-document. As the interdisciplinary teams develop specific pathway content, it is essential to review the present documentation system and how it relates to the specific content and use of pathways. How will documentation need to change in the medical record and on the clinical pathway? Organizations or providers that use computerized information management systems need to incorporate their pathways into these systems. These are critical questions that need to be repeated for each new pathway that is developed. In addition, the following questions are helpful to consider as documentation needs are reviewed.

- Is the pathway replacing existing forms?
- Will the pathway meet the documentation needs of the organization, accreditation bodies, and third-party payers?
- Will documentation result in duplication, thereby possibly contributing to a decrease in compliance?
- Who will be documenting on the pathway?
- Do policies and procedures need to be revised to reflect the changes in the documentation process (Mateo, Newton, & Kanatas, 1996, p. 81)?

Including medical records staff on the project committee is critical. Their participation and input will prevent many future documentation problems.

Identification of target population

Identification of the target population is a critical decision for the project committee, as time should not be wasted on the wrong population. It is costly and will only aggravate staff. A typical way to approach classifying diagnoses for pathway development is to use the International Classification of Diseases, Version 9 Conversion Manual (ICD-9-CM) (Dykes, 1998a). This is the primary resource for medical diagnoses and third-party payer reimbursement coding. Those diagnoses with the highest cost are the best ones to select. In addition, the committee considers the following as it reviews the typical illnesses or conditions in its patient population (e.g., patients in the hospital or home care agency, enrollees in an MCO, etc.):

- High volume
- High risk
- Complex care requirements
- High cost
- Variations in length-of-stay compared with the "norm" or benchmarks
- Variations in practice patterns
- Payer request or interest in the illness or condition
- Opportunity for improved care

Development of the content

Interdisciplinary staff teams who are selected to develop specific pathway content need to be qualified in the particular clinical area or some aspects of the delivery of care (Dykes, 1998a). For example, a pathway for a surgical condition should include surgeons, registered nurses from surgical units, operating room, and recovery room, and might include representatives from anesthesia, transportation, pharmacy, laboratory, medical records, admission, finance, utilization review, quality improvement, risk management, and IMS. The team begins by brainstorming but must focus on the routine, not the exceptions. Developing a flowchart often provides a helpful picture of the steps required from the routine care for the identified illness or condition. The team considers all aspects of care, a timeline that corresponds to the LOS goal, outcomes, and the key indicators for reaching the outcomes. As the team prepares to develop content, they review medical records of cases with the same diagnosis or condition, literature, outcome data, current practice, and local practice patterns (both internal and external), and seek expert opinions. Identification of outcomes is a critical aspect of the process. Outcomes need to be specific, objective, and quantitative, and they should be reviewed periodically to ensure that they are current with new research, technology, medications, and clinical practice. There is now a greater emphasis on evidence-based practice, and pathways need to be evidence-based.

It is important, and yet often difficult, for staff to question current practices within their own organization as they often feel that they are criticizing their colleagues or themselves. Serious questions, however, need to be asked.

- What criteria are really necessary for the patient to meet for discharge?
- What care can be provided at home or on an outpatient basis?
- What intermediate patient care objectives or outcomes are really necessary to accomplish the desired long-term outcomes?
- What activities contribute to meeting outcomes?
- What activities are unnecessary or not directly related to the key discharge criteria?
- Do different practices really result in different outcomes (Coffey, Richards, Wintermeyer-Pingel, & LeRoy, 1996, p. 310)?

These questions certainly apply to nursing and all types of care that is provided in any setting. With the increasing emphasis on care in the community, acute care hospitals need to consider what is the best setting in which to deliver the care and how to better collaborate with community providers and resources. The development of pathways is a good time to consider these questions.

Another approach to the development of pathways is to use pathways that have been developed by other health care or professional organizations or are found in the literature. It is critical that all selected pathways are then adapted to the specific provider organization. Questions that the team considers as they review these external pathways to use in their own organization include:

- Does the provider base its pathways on national standards and large national studies?
- Does the pathway define a population that fits our patients?
- Does the pathway consider long-term outcomes?
- Does the pathway contain information about long-term services that may be required?
- Does the author (organization) have a reputation of honesty and integrity ("Algorithms and paths," 1995, pp. 146–147)?

The reviewers must also consider how current the references are that were used to develop the pathway's content. Outdated references can be a problem in reflecting the currency of the pathway content. "One of the most significant criticisms of critical pathways is that they are rarely evidence-based. According to Bailey, Litaker & Mion (1998), the prevailing method of critical pathways development is the use of internal, institution-specific 'expert knowledge' of health care professionals to devise the approaches for patient care. If critical pathways are to be an effective means of controlling costs while promoting optimal patient outcomes, health care practitioners must work systematically to build scientifically based pathways. Unfortunately, these critical pathways are rarely evaluated after their initial development" (Renholm, Leino-Kilpi, & Suominen, 2002, p. 201).

Many drafts of the pathways are required as the team works through the content, discusses it with other staff, and reviews the literature. The project committee identifies the final review process that should be followed for all pathways that are developed. This process includes key persons in the organization and the project committee. Consensus is critical for successful implementation, but it is not always easy to reach. Negotiation and collaboration often are needed to reach consensus.

Initiation of the pilot testing

Clinical pathways need to be pilot tested prior to their final approval. The project committee determines the pilot testing process, including its length, number of times the pathway is implemented with patients, and data collection procedures. Issues that are important to consider during pilot testing are pathway quality, feasibility of use, appropriateness of timeline and LOS, delays or variations in care practice patterns, and compliance (Cesta, Tahan, & Fink, 1998). Undoubtedly, changes need to be made, and some of these may be major. If so, another pilot may be required. Obtaining staff feedback as they use the pathway in the pilot is critical for obtaining helpful information. If this feedback is ignored, staff feel left out and less inclined to support the pathways when they are implemented. Once pathways are approved, implementation begins; however, there are two issues that are important throughout the development and implementation phases: collaboration with other health care organizations that might require the use of clinical pathways (MCOs and other third-party payers) or receiving patient referrals for additional services and the liability and ethical issues related to the use of pathways.

Collaboration with managed care organizations

Clinical pathways have been helpful in meeting MCO demands that health care organizations provide quality care that is cost-effective and meets outcomes. "As shoppers and buyers of health care, managed care companies demand to know whether the services that they are paying for will have the effect that providers claim" (Dykes, 1998c, p. 3). Some health care organizations and MCOs have been collaborating in the development of pathways. MCOs are requesting more and more data about their enrollees and the care that they receive. Pathways can be used to collect these data. Variances that occur can then be addressed quickly, thereby reducing costs and hopefully improving care. In addition, MCOs review variances and ask questions about them. When managed care contracts are renewed with providers, MCOs evaluate the providers' variances and improvement. Providers who can show that they are identifying variances and actively pursuing changes to resolve variances will have an easier time with contract renewal. Even though demonstration of improvement is important, there is no doubt that variance review is often seen as accusation or finding fault. Providers worry that these data will be used against them and limit their access to patients, decrease their revenue, or cause them to lose MCO contracts. Variance analysis is not always viewed as a method for improving care but rather limiting care or providers. Collaboration, however, can occur only if the MCO–provider relationship focuses on sharing and helping one another rather than fear, competition, and conflicts.

Liability and ethical issues

Clinical pathways can be introduced as evidence in court to demonstrate a standard of care or what the outcomes or timelines should be for a patient. There are two areas of concern. The first is liability for staff who develop pathways, and the second is provider liability for those who use the pathways. Pathway developers have been named in liability cases. These accusations typically allege that the committee used inadequate and outdated content and did not seek adequate expert advice (Sheehan & Sullivan, 1998). What can be done to prevent this experience? The committee should be an interdisciplinary team, with representatives who have expertise in the pathway focus area. Their résumés should be kept on file in case questions arise later. Written policies and procedures about the pathway development process and implementation, including a clear description of how pathways are individualized and how this is to be documented, should also be kept on file. It is important that all of this material is dated. A file should be kept for each pathway that includes the pathway tool, all of its major drafts, reference material, pilot testing data, and evaluations. All relevant organizational policies and procedures need to be evaluated to ensure that there is no conflict with new pathways. It is best that risk management staff and legal counsel review final pathways, policies, procedures, types of records that should be kept, and the like. Staff who develop and use the pathways need to have appropriate education about them, and attendance needs to be documented. The evaluation process should be clearly defined, and compliance with the process documented.

What is the liability for the provider? There are four provider responses to pathways that may lead to liability problems.

1. The provider follows the clinical pathway but delivers negligent care.
2. The provider follows the clinical pathway, but the clinical pathway outlines substandard care to be delivered to the patient.
3. The provider does not follow the clinical pathway and fails to document the variance and the reason for noncompliance.
4. The provider misinterprets the clinical pathway or applies it incorrectly (Sheehan & Sullivan, 1998, p. 118).

An important point to make is that the provider is at risk if a pathway is blindly followed. If a pathway contains errors or represents substandard care, the provider is still responsible for the care provided. Nothing relieves the professional, such as a nurse, of the responsibility for using professional judgment. If pathways are used, every health care professional who uses them must be responsible for learning how to use them correctly in the best interest of individual patients or take the risk of making an error. Variances are tracked and used to assess achievement of outcomes. Comments about general variance data should never be documented in individual medical records. Disclaimers may be used with pathways. General disclaimers should state that the pathway provides guidance for the plan of care, but staff recognize that each patient requires individualized care. The disclaimer should convey that treatment decisions are made by the practitioner after an assessment of the patient's condition. The patient's version of the pathway should contain a statement that the guidelines are provided to inform the patient and that, because every patient is different, treatment and outcomes differ (Sheehan & Sullivan, 1998).

Pathway implementation

Implementation of clinical pathways requires time and patience. Staff will be uncomfortable and have concerns about how their use will affect their practice. Pathways should not be seen as a method for improving all of an organization's problems. For example, using clinical pathways probably will not improve overall communication in an organization that has a long-standing problem of poor communication. During the implementation of pathways, problems are often encountered that need to be resolved to prevent project failure. The following are examples of potential problems that may interfere with pathway implementation.

- There is concern that pathways represent cookbook medicine in that they standardize care without regard to individual patient needs or individual provider practice. Pathways ignore practice pattern differences that occur when physicians and nurses care for the patients with the same diagnosis. Staff education is required to ensure that clinical staff understand the purpose of pathways and that they appreciate the need for individualizing pathways to meet individual patient needs.

- Pathways can become just one more record to keep or follow, particularly if the documentation system is not evaluated at the time of pathway development. Duplication is a frequent complaint and serves only to frustrate staff and increase documentation errors. Consolidating the progress notes often helps. In addition, there is a tendency to include too many indicators or too much detail in the pathways. This makes them cumbersome to use. If a pathway is long, staff may assume that using it is a complex process that will only increase their workload.

- If pathway outcomes are based only on data from within the institution and do not consider relevant external information and outcomes, the pathways may represent only the internal current standards rather than the optimal. In this case, patient care may not improve.

- Turf battles may become very serious, particularly if they were present prior to implementing pathways. Who is in charge of the pathways? Utilization review? Nursing staff? Case managers? Job boundaries need to be reviewed prior to implementation. When project leadership is defined, staff need to be included in discussions. Gaining consensus is an important part of the implementation process for all levels of staff. As has been experienced many times, staff "did not understand the vision or the 'why' of this new strategy. Some perceived that the program was being imposed on them rather than feeling a sense of ownership in this important and worthwhile undertaking. They see the CPM (pathways) as the creation of more rework and 'paper trails'— just an administrative strategy to keep down the hospital length-of-stay" (Hofmann, 1993, p. 236). Clearly defining purpose and responsibility will help to prevent many future problems.

- A common problem in pathway development is to overestimate or underestimate the expected LOS. This can lead to increased staff stress. Using pathways is the best way to assess the LOS, and their use helps to determine the best expected LOS.

- **Comorbidities** are also problematic. Pathways usually are developed for one illness or condition; however, patients often have more than one. How should staff use the pathways for these patients? This needs to be clarified before implementation. One way to resolve this problem is to develop co-paths. This prevents confusion and problems with increased documentation. The co-path is usually used across departments, as typically these are problems that are experienced with different types of patients. Co-paths typically include only an outline of the outcomes that need to be met rather than an extensive description of interventions (Dykes, 1998b; Griffin & Griffin, 1994; Hague, 1996).

Physicians usually are concerned about pathways, as they need to be reassured that pathways do not replace physician orders. They are also concerned about losing their autonomy. To decrease this fear, physician input is absolutely necessary during pathway development, implementation, and evaluation. Some institutions have even gone so far as to require a physician's order for the use of a pathway. Others allow a physician to rescind a pathway and add or delete interventions to the pathways (Coffey et al., 1992). Of course, these approaches could defeat the purpose of the pathways, and the health care organization would need to monitor the use of these alternatives to ensure that pathway implementation is not sidetracked. Data obtained from the pathways about patient outcomes may also be affected by these physician options.

Staff resistance to the use of pathways must be dealt with directly. Often, recognizing that it might be a problem and taking steps to alleviate staff concerns can prevent it. Cesta, Tahan, and Fink (1998) have discussed examples of such measures and advantages to emphasize.

- Increase staff involvement in all phases of development and implementation
- Share critical literature with staff
- Identify pathway benefits to specific health care professionals
- Ensure that pathways are recommendations, not rigid requirements
- Emphasize that pathways affect the quality of care: coordination, collaboration, patient/ family education, outcomes, and data assessment
- Decrease costs, achieve expected LOS, increase consistency and improved care, and decrease risk management issues
- Increase compliance with accreditation and regulatory requirements
- Increase marketing ability to attract more plans and MCO contracts
- Provide data for research
- Serve as staff education tools

Pathway evaluation

Pathway evaluation should not be made into a complicated process. The areas of most concern are whether costs are changing per patient diagnosis and for itemized costs, such as laboratory tests, pharmacy, physical therapy, and radiology, and whether the quality of care is compromised. Are outcomes met? Evaluation also focuses on the LOS or the length of treatment. Particularly important in evaluation process is variance analysis.

Variances are deviations from the expected or that which is defined in the clinical pathway. They may be positive or negative. Negative variances indicate that the patient has not achieved expected outcomes or that activities have not been completed. A positive variance indicates that the patient achieved an outcome or activity prior to the expected deadline. If the trend is toward more positive variances, it may mean that the deadlines need to be reviewed and could be shortened. Negative variances are typically categorized as system or operational, caregiver/provider, or patient focused (Cohen & Cesta, 1993; Windle & Houston, 1996). System or operational variances focus on hindrances in the system or the organization that prevent the achievement of patient outcomes. Examples are delay in laboratory results, lack of bed space, hours of service, delayed transfers to a long-term care facility, lack of supplies, and so on. Provider variances focus on the variances that may be caused by the provider. Examples include:

- The physician does not respond to a telephone call from a nurse about a patient's condition.
- A mislabeled medication is given to a patient.
- A staff member is unable to do a procedure due to lack of experience or knowledge.
- Orders are misread, and a patient is sent for the wrong procedure.
- Inadequate nursing staff decreases the time a nurse has to review a patient's history.

A patient variance identifies factors related to the patient that prevent the achievement of patient outcomes; for example, a patient refuses medication; a patient experiences complications (e.g., elevated temperature that interferes with proceeding with treatment); a patient experiences inadequate pain relief; or a patient arrives late for his admission for ambulatory care surgery.

It is important to avoid blame when assessing variances but rather to look at reasons and resolution; this is a key recommendation from many of the Institute of Medicine reports about quality and patient safety. Staff need to consider all aspects of an issue (for example, a patient's medication problem). Why is the patient refusing medication? Is the patient afraid of the medication and its side effects? Does the patient lack understanding of the purpose of taking the medication? Does the patient not have the money to pay for the medication? Does the patient lack transportation to pick up the medication or feel that the medication will not help? Jumping to conclusions is not helpful and limits true understanding as to the reason for the variance. Variance data are most critical in understanding outcome achievement or lack of achievement and also provide direction for change. Data should be shared with the pathway development team and relevant staff. Involving them in resolution development is also important.

Variance analysis assists in identifying patterns of concern or problems that are seen in a number of patients. These problems may require more intensive action for every patient who experiences these problems. It might, however, be due to a repetitive problem in the system. Algorithms are created to resolve these variances and prevent future variances. Generally, algorithms are not developed until variance data indicate a need. Algorithms are developed in the same way as pathways. Typically, they are formatted as decision-making trees. "The pathway provides an overview of the entire production process from start to finish, not just pieces of the process, and can be used to reduce variation in the production process. . . . Conversely, algorithms often guide clinicians through the 'if, then' decision-making process, such as a variation from a pathway" (Schriefer, 1994, p. 136). For example, if a patient experiences an elevated temperature, then specific treatment is begun.

Documenting these variances can be problematic due to liability risk. Staff need to avoid blaming a staff member in the medical record; for example, to state in the medical record that because a physician did not respond to a call from the nurse about the patient's condition the patient developed a complication. Documenting variances must be done with care. Reasons for the variance, if known, need to be identified but should be based on factual data. When treatment that is not in the pathway is added or deleted, this must be documented. Nurses document most of the variances because they have the most contact with patients, particularly in acute care, home care, and long-term care. Variance documentation requires accurate and complete documentation. The health care organization develops documentation policies and procedures and prepares staff in their use.

Patient and staff satisfaction are also critical evaluation issues. Patient satisfaction is a very important factor in the evaluation of the use of pathways and should consider three key questions:

1. Does the patient/family feel involved in the care?
2. Were the patient's goals met?
3. Did staff discuss the patient's progress with the patient?

Patients need to first understand what a clinical pathway is and how it is used. Individual nurses best provide this explanation because they interact more with patients and families. Several studies have indicated that the use of pathways seems to increase patient satisfaction (Goode, 1995; Leibman et al., 1998; Polit & Hungler, 1997; Renholm, Leino-Kilpi, & Suominen, 2002). Other issues that have been discussed as factors that might be affected by the use of pathways are patient education, continuity of information, continuity or care, quality of care, length-of-stay, and reduction of costs. All these appear to be affected positively by the use of pathways, although additional research is clearly necessary (Renholm, Leino-Kilpi, & Suominen, 2002).

Staff satisfaction should also not be overlooked in pathway evaluation. Important questions to consider include:

■ Do you understand the reasons for using pathways?
■ Did you feel prepared to use the pathways?
■ If you participated in the development of the pathways, do you feel that your input was respected?
■ How has the use of pathways affected your daily practice/work?
■ How has the use of pathways affected your relationship with your patients/families?
■ Do you think that pathways support interdisciplinary collaboration? If so, how?
■ How has the use of pathways affected your documentation?
■ What would you like to see changed with pathways and their implementation?

Are staff using the pathways and using them correctly? These questions are particularly important for health care organizations that use temporary nurses, part-time staff, and travel nurses, which may make it difficult to ensure that all staff are knowledgeable about the pathways and are committed to using them. Full-time staff may carry the burden of ensuring that pathways are used correctly. This can lead to increased staff stress and affect patient care delivery.

There are many questions that can be asked in the evaluation process. Health care organizations need to develop questions relevant to their environment, patients, and staff. Gathering data can be overdone, so question selection and related data should be carefully considered. When evaluation is complete, a summary of the results and any pathway revisions must be shared with the staff. In many organizations, staff find out about changes when they are affected by them, but this is too late. Staff should not pick up a copy of a pathway when they need to use it and find out it has been changed. This does not allow time for staff to understand the changes and how they affect patient care delivery.

THINK CRITICALLY

Try this exercise to apply what you have learned about this topic.

BENCHMARKS

Now let's take a moment to test your knowledge of the concepts you have studied in this section.

Other Tools Used to Manage Care

A number of tools other than clinical pathways are used to manage care. Some of the tools that are described in this section include practice guidelines, disease management, demand management, standards of care, utilization review/management, benchmarking, evidence-based practice, and health promotion and disease and illness prevention. How these tools are used, type of setting, and type of patients can vary.

Practice guidelines

Managed care organizations are interested in practice guidelines. Other types of health care provider organizations, the federal government, and health care professional organizations have become involved, too. This interest in tools to manage care stems from the need to decrease costs and yet provide quality care. Guidelines have been used in conjunction with clinical pathways. The goal is to narrow the gap between an organization's current care and optimal care. **Practice guidelines** are used to assist with treatment decision making and to evaluate care. The Joint Commission on the Accreditation of Healthcare Organizations (JCAHO) does not require the use of practice guidelines but does require that hospitals consider their use and application to the hospital's services and processes. Several questions about practice guidelines that could also be applied to disease management programs include the following.

- Are clinical practice guidelines (or disease management programs) a means for improving the quality of health care?
- Are clinical practice guidelines (or disease management programs) a means for saving money in the health care system?
- Are clinical practice guidelines (or disease management programs) a means for solving the malpractice problem?
- Are clinical practice guidelines (or disease management programs) a means for making the health care system work better for all?
- Or are they a recipe for disaster (Lohr, 1995, p. 51)?

The last question is of concern, but for now, there is no answer to this question. As with all new changes, such as these and clinical pathways, experience data will help to answer these questions. Early studies on the use of clinical pathways indicate that this patient care management tool has had some positive impacts on cost containment and quality (Lohr, 1995). There has been less research on practice guidelines and disease management programs, so less is known about their effect.

Definition and purpose

Practice guidelines are "systematically developed statements that assist practitioners in making decisions about appropriate health care for specific clinical conditions" (General Accounting Office, 1996). As with clinical pathways, practice guidelines are called by many names. Some of the more common ones are appropriateness indicators, practice parameters, medical review criteria, and standards. Their purpose is to pull together research information from the literature, evaluate these results, and access expert opinion about the clinical condition. They should be evidence-based. This information is then prepared in a usable form. Practice guidelines are different from standards of care in that guidelines do not define treatment but rather provide information and options.

Managed care interest practice guidelines

Managed care organizations support the use of practice guidelines. The common reasons for this support are to:

- Reduce health care costs
- Improve the quality of care
- Ensure consistency of care

■ Provide performance data for comparison with other MCOs, as well as comparison of individual provider performance levels

■ Comply with accreditation and regulatory requirements

In 1996, the General Accounting Office reported to the House Subcommittee on Health on the use of practice guidelines within the managed care environment (General Accounting Office, 1996). Interviews were conducted with medical directors from 19 managed care plans representing multiple states, with a combined enrollment of 7 million people. In addition, professional literature was reviewed, and interviews were conducted with representatives from health care organizations, condition-specific organizations, and the Agency for Health Care Research and Quality (AHRQ). What did this report tell the health care community about the use of practice guidelines? The first important fact is that by March 1996, 2000 practice guidelines had been developed, and this number is even higher today. This indicates potential problems because many of these guidelines are on the same topics. Some of these guidelines may also offer conflicting guidance. As providers and MCOs consider the many different practice guidelines, conflicts do arise. The report's conclusions identified the following.

1. Clinical practice guidelines promote greater uniformity within physician networks, encourage improved efficiency and clinical decision making, and eliminate unnecessary care.
2. Several health care plans have adopted clinical practice guidelines to control costs, improve performance on standardized measures, receive accreditation, and comply with regulatory requirements.
3. Due to time and fiscal constraints, many health care plans customize published clinical guidelines rather than generate original guidelines.
4. Physicians are more likely to use a clinical practice guideline if local health providers develop it.
5. Managed care plans customize existing clinical practice guidelines to suit alternative treatments, available resources, population needs, and format and currency concerns.
6. While health care plans modify existing clinical practice guidelines to varying degrees, extensive changes could jeopardize the guidelines' effectiveness.
7. Some health plans would prefer that the federal government publish and update evidence on medical conditions and services, develop useful practice guideline tools, and perform outcomes research and medical technology assessments that would help them to develop, modify, and update their guidelines. Since the time of this report the federal government has developed many more practical guidelines.

Typically, MCOs select practice guideline content based on services or conditions that have high cost, high liability risk, and a high incidence in their particular enrollee population, which are the same key criteria used to select pathway focus. If an MCO has few enrollees with renal problems, it does not make sense for it to expend efforts to institute the use of practice guidelines for renal problems. The MCO must reduce its costs but also must consider the expenses that are incurred to make changes that might reduce costs.

In addition to cost reduction and quality issues, another force that is pushing MCOs to use practice guidelines is accreditation. The National Committee on Quality Assurance (NCQA) standards require that MCOs who apply for NCQA accreditation use practice guidelines that focus on preventive services. JCAHO also has these standards for the MCOs it accredits. The MCO must not only use guidelines, but the guidelines must be:

■ Based on reasonable medical evidence

■ Developed by or adopted by the MCO providers

■ Reviewed on a regular basis

■ Applicable to the enrollees

Most MCOs, however, do not develop their own practice guidelines. They review guidelines that have been developed by professional organizations, the AHRQ, or other resources. Guidelines are then selected and adapted to meet the needs of the MCO. This is less costly, expedites the development process, and, more importantly, the final product meets the individual needs of the MCO, its providers, and its enrollees. For example, lengthy guidelines—and there are many that are quite long—have not been found to be as helpful to the provider. Many providers do not even take the time to read them. Some guidelines may make recommendations that the MCO considers too costly. The MCO must recognize that once it adapts a practice guideline, it is no longer the same guideline and thus loses the integrity of a published guideline as agreed upon by the publishing organization or authors. The MCO must then take the responsibility of periodic evaluations to ensure that the content is current and accurate.

Development of practice guidelines

Public and private sector organizations develop practice guidelines, including professional organizations, health care organizations, and researchers. Condition-specific organizations (e.g., American Heart Association, Arthritis Foundation) have also developed guidelines. As members of these various organizations, nurses have been active in the development of guidelines. Governmental agencies that have been involved in the development are the AHRQ through the National Guideline Clearinghouse, the National Institutes of Health, the Centers for Disease Control and Prevention, the U.S. Preventive Services Task Force, Centers of Medicare and Medicaid Services, and the Department of Health and Human Services. Active participation from many types of organizations indicates the level of interest in practice guidelines. The AHRQ guidelines are well-known sets of statements that may be used to assist practitioners and/or patients in making health care decisions for specific clinical problems. Interdisciplinary panels of experts develop these guidelines. The guidelines include:

- Supporting materials, such as methodology, scientific evidence, and comprehensive bibliography
- A desktop reference, the Clinical Practice Guideline, for the practitioner that includes recommendations, algorithms, flowcharts, tables, figures, and references
- A quick reference guide for practitioners that is an abbreviated version of the Clinical Practice Guideline
- The Patient's Guide, which provides information for the patient about the clinical problem and treatments

Physicians are using practice guidelines but the level of use is variable. How might physicians and other providers such as advanced practice nurses use these guidelines? Examples of their purposes that are important for practitioners are to:

- Establish schedules for immunizations.
- Develop screening programs (focus, content, timeline) for specific needs, such as glaucoma, hypertension, and breast cancer.
- Determine when to use or not use diagnostic tests (e.g., complete blood count, serum lipid tests, mammography).
- Improve case findings and treatment of depression among patients seen by primary care providers.
- Understand how to manage patients with diabetes mellitus (Lohr, 1995, p. 50).

What are the problems or factors that are keeping providers, such as physicians and nurse practitioners, from using practice guidelines? One major problem is the accessibility of the information while the provider (such as a physician, nurse, or nurse practitioner) is with the patient. If the provider has access to a computer in the examining room, then this information could be discussed with the patient in the examining room. This would save time and be more relevant to the patient. This is, however, an expense. With so many guidelines in existence, making decisions about which ones to use is problematic. Information overload is a major complication today, and it can actually increase stress rather than decrease it or control it. A common approach made by providers is to amalgamate the guidelines by considering providers' personal experiences and approaches with the specific condition.

Non-adherence to guidelines can often be traced to limited provider input in guideline development, after which the provider does not accept the guidelines. Change that is instituted from outside is rarely successful. In addition, change that brings limited rewards often fails. Some MCOs encourage guideline use by paying incentives to providers who use them and by tracking their use when they evaluate provider performance. A final concern with practice guidelines is coverage of comorbidities, which is also true with clinical pathways. For example, what does the provider do when a patient has a cardiac condition and diabetes? There are guidelines for the cardiac condition and also guidelines for diabetes. The guidelines may not consider the impact of one illness on the other and may actually offer conflicting treatment options. Often, the provider chooses not to use any practice guideline rather than deal with conflicting and confusing recommendations.

Nurse practitioners also encounter the same problems with practice guidelines as they use them in their practice. As more nurse practitioners enter private practice and clinics, they will need to review these guidelines and determine their relevance to advance practice nursing. Nurses who work in the community can make use of the guidelines to help plan community health education and services that focus on specific problems. Examples of U.S. Preventive Task Force Guidelines that might be used in the community are:

- Treating tobacco use and dependence. (2000)
- Developing vaccines for preventable diseases: Improving vaccination coverage in children, adolescents, and adults. (2000)
- Using behavioral counseling in primary care to promote a healthy diet: Recommendations and rationale. (2002)

Informatics can be used to support implementation of guidelines as well as assist with evaluation of their use and outcomes (Duff & Casey, 1998). First, informatics can provide quick access to the guidelines. Within the information system staff should be able to get to the guidelines when they are needed, review them, and then apply them to planning and patient education. The information system can also be set up to remind staff to use guidelines and integrate these guidelines into the documentation system. Information systems also allow for easy updates of guidelines, but for this to be successful it must be built into the system to ensure that it gets done.

Evaluation of the implementation of practice guidelines is important, and the key questions are:

- How does the guideline improve practice?
- Is the guideline still scientifically based?
- Does the guideline continue to meet the needs of the patient population?
- Are clinicians implementing the guidelines as designed (Poniatowski, 2000, p. 13)?

Disease management

Definition and purpose

There is no universally accepted definition for disease management and, as is true of many of the tools that are used to manage care, there are a number of terms used to describe it. Common terms, besides disease management, are population-based care, continuous health care improvement, and disease state management. Disease management is "an integrated system of interventions, measurements, and refinements of health care delivery designed to optimize clinical and economic outcomes within a specific population" (Gurnee & Da Silva, 1997, p. 8). Another definition describes it as the "systematic, population-based approach to identifying persons at risk, intervening with specific programs of care, and measuring clinical and other outcomes" (Epstein & Sherwood, 1996). Examples of illnesses that are often targeted for disease management are asthma, arthritis, cancer, diabetes, hypertension, osteoporosis, high-risk pregnancy, congestive heart failure, depression, high cholesterol, and human immunodeficiency virus/acquired immune deficiency syndrome (HIV/AIDS).

The purpose of disease management programs is to provide patients with education and preventive care that improves the quality of their lives and prevents complications that may increase health care costs. "Disease management plans target that high resource utilization sub-population for more deliberate, integrated management. This is not to suggest that a disease management plan will not benefit all patients. . . . The DSM plan, however, hopes to first identify and intervene on behalf of those patients at greatest risk" (Tallon, 1995, p. 24). Examples provided in the previous paragraph are problems that are of higher risk.

How does a disease management program really work? The MCO groups its enrollees into disease-specific populations and, based on the numbers within a specific disease category, it then focuses its disease management program on this population, and it usually is one whose care incurs higher costs. Disease management programs focus on prevention and health maintenance for the selected disease-specific groups. Usually, the physician's role is to continue to provide appropriate interventions for the patient; however, other health care professionals—often nurses—provide education that focuses on prevention and health maintenance based on the disease and individual needs of the patient. The major goal is to prepare the patient to understand the disease and increase the patient's self-management of the disease.

Managed care interest in disease management

Many MCOs are developing or using disease management programs (Dalzell, 1998). Disease management characteristics that are attractive to MCOs include:

- Targets high volume DRGs (such as congestive heart failure) or disease processes important to the patients served (such as breast cancer and treatment).
- Facilitates the creation of clinical pathways, which leads to early identification of individual patient variance and, when this variance is noted, to rapid intervention (guidelines provide evidence-based content for use in pathways).
- Simplifies patient management across the continuum of care.
- Identifies patient subgroups that may be optimally managed by a specialty team approach, as in the case of patients with sickle cell disease, hemophilia, or cystic fibrosis.
- Facilitates the objective, valid comparison of alternative plans of care between different physicians, hospital systems, and/or specialties.
- Keeps the focus of care at the patient/health provider level (Tallon, 1995, p. 23).

MCOs are focusing many of their disease management programs on the diseases listed in Box 9-4.

Population-based care is similar to a community or public health approach. It does not deny the need for individualized care and interventions but rather looks at aggregate health care issues. The criteria that are often used to identify the disease focus include:

- High-prevalence chronic disease states
- High-dollar-volume or high-velocity drug use
- Potential for wide variation in treatment approach
- Potential for lifestyle modification to improve outcomes

BOX 9-4   Disease management programs: Common diseases.

Asthma

Cardiovascular diseases (e.g., coronary artery disease, congestive heart failure, angina, lipid irregularity)

Depressive disorders

Diabetes

Ambulatory infectious diseases (e.g., otitis media, urinary tract infection, community-acquired pneumonia)

Pain

Upper gastrointestinal disease (e.g., peptic ulcer disease, reflux esophagitis)

Women's and children's health

Source: Author; content summarized from Gurnee, M., & Da Silva, R. (1997). Constructing disease management programs. *Managed Care, 6*(6), 8–16.

■ Therapies with many treatment options

■ Diseases with high risk of negative outcomes (Gurnee & Da Silva, 1997, p. 3)

In focusing on these aggregates, Knight (1998) identifies the goals as to:

1. Reduce the incidence of disease through targeted preventive care.
2. Detect members at risk for developing the selected disease.
3. Minimize the medical complications associated with the disease.
4. Improve the health and functional status of patients with the disease (p. 219).

Development of disease management programs

Developing disease management programs takes time and is costly. Many MCOs are turning to other groups or organizations that have developed these programs or contract with experts to design a customized program. Health care organizations, insurers, and health care businesses, such as consulting businesses, have developed disease management programs that are then sold as a package or contracted to providers and MCOs. Disease management also provides an opportunity for partnerships between MCOs and other organizations to create innovative programs. For example, 150 health plans are collaborating with the American Diabetes Association in a 10-year disease management program to decrease blindness and foot amputations among diabetics by 40% and kidney failure by 30% (Kilborn, 1998). Another innovation that has resulted from disease management is the use of "circuit-riding" nurses who specialize in specific chronic diseases. These nurses go out and teach patient classes and counsel new patients. These nurses also make follow-up calls to the patients (Kilborn, 1998).

Some of these programs offer nurse call lines and nurse-led education programs and support, consider readiness to learn and behavior modification, encourage partnerships that are formed between the patient and the primary care provider, and track critical data such as hospital admissions and use of emergency services and prescriptions. These programs offer great opportunities for nurses.

Another program that was developed at the National Jewish Medical and Research Center for asthma management demonstrates how successful these programs can be (Lawrence, 1998). This program is used by patients at the medical center and also has been sold as a product to other health care organizations. The program focuses on the patient–physician partnership and includes an individual action plan and regular telephone contact. The action plans consider symptoms and respiratory parameters such as peak flow. The program encourages the entire health care team to communicate consistently in an open manner with the patient and the patient's family. The educational program includes a wide range of topics such as anatomy and its relationship to the use of controllers, triggers, and monitoring flows with the use of inhalers. Patients are instructed to use peak flow to determine when to call the physician or nurse practitioner. Outcome evaluation indicates that this program does affect patient response and costs. Anxiety about their asthma, which can exacerbate asthma, was found in 57% of the patients prior to the program; however, after attending the educational programs, 90.3% of the patients experienced no asthma-related anxiety. Six months later, 75% of the patients experienced no asthma-related anxiety. Because employers are concerned about missed work time, the evaluation also assessed changes in work habits. Prior to the implementation of the program, 68.3% of the patients had work-related problems, but 6 months after joining the program this percentage decreased by almost half. Clearly, this disease management program has demonstrated positive outcomes.

Even though it seems that disease management programs could be highly effective programs for patients, there are reasons for not developing a disease management program. As an MCO makes decisions, it must always consider their costs and long-term benefits. Employers usually give their employees the option to change their enrollment in health plans annually, and many employees continue to change their health plans due to costs and also benefits offered. This flux in enrollment means that an MCO may go to considerable lengths to identify the needs for disease management. These programs are based on enrollment data collected at a specific time only to find out that there are changes in the data as enrollees move in and out of various benefit options. The other problem is that an MCO could develop a reputation for providing excellent management of a particular disease, and this might draw more enrollees with this disease. Treatment for chronic illnesses costs money, and they are difficult to resolve (Knight, 1998). Does the MCO want to attract more enrollees who are sick? No, it does not, so this presents a dilemma for MCOs as they develop disease management programs.

Provider response to disease management programs

Provider concerns about disease management programs are similar to those with practice guidelines and clinical pathways. Is this "cookbook" health care with little regard for the individual? Program supporters and developers insist that these programs offer individual assessment of needs and an opportunity to incorporate individual treatment needs. Some providers do not understand the concept, and thus they have problems accepting disease management programs. Others are concerned that this is an effort to take over their treatment. Supporters of disease management emphasize that the programs augment the provider's treatment and help patients better accept treatment and encourage compliance. Comorbidities continue to be a problem, particularly with older patients. To increase physician support, physicians need education about the program and its purposes. They need to be recognized as coordinators of patient care and understand that disease management programs offer support to their treatment.

In addition to physicians benefiting from disease management programs, advanced practice nurses can benefit by using these programs, but they must also understand disease management and its application to their practice. Including the nurses and physicians, as well as other health care providers, in the development or adaptation of these programs is critical for their success. MCOs collect data on the outcomes, and then use these data to demonstrate results to physicians and other providers. Nurses can play major roles in the development and implementation of these programs because they are highly suited to teaching patients and monitoring progress.

Pharmacists have also taken an active role in disease management programs. Pharmacy costs are a major MCO concern. Disease management programs can focus on the use of medications and medication education for specific diagnoses in order to decrease costs. Pharmaceutical companies are also developing disease management programs that they sell or contract to MCOs. The danger with these programs is the potential of pushing specific drugs on the MCO and its providers. This could result in ethical dilemmas. The companies are, however, providing a variety of services that could be very helpful. These include expertise, analysis of care processes, organization of databases, development of clinical information systems, and development of patient education materials and programs (Terry, 1993).

Demand management

Demand management, also called **care management**, is an approach that might be used by an MCO to decrease member demand for health services and to encourage members to maintain good health. The MCO wants its members/enrollees to make informed health decisions as well as participate in healthy lifestyle behaviors. Managed care organizations have tried to focus more on care management to reduce costs, but whether or not this will have a long-term effect on health care is still unknown.

Why is personal health management so important to MCOs? All MCOs are concerned with health care problems that might increase their costs; for example:

- Lifestyle-related illnesses are present in all populations.
- The number of emergency room visits that are non-urgent continues to be a problem.
- Sixty percent of physician office visits are unnecessary.
- Sixty-five percent of tests and procedures are unnecessary (Blue Cross/Blue Shield, 2002).

Some MCOs refer to demand management programs as wellness programs or personal health management. The goal is to provide self-management tools that the patient can use. The demand management programs may include some or all of the following.

- Health education classes and seminars
- Self-care books and other written materials
- Personal health assessments
- Shared-decision-making videos or software programs
- Triage call centers or nurse hotlines
- Targeted member outreach programs (Knight, 1998, p. 59)

The MCO may also send reminders for annual exams, such as Pap smears and mammograms. Enrollees may be taught how to recognize complications as well as how to change nutrition styles, exercise, and use of preventive care such as immunizations. Triage health centers and nurse hotlines are methods that are used to reduce the use of unnecessary health services. MCOs have also entered the world of the Internet. Enrollees can access information about their MCO and its benefits as well as educational materials related to health. The MCO wants this information to assist its enrollees to maintain healthy lifestyles. As use of the Internet has expanded, there is no doubt that MCOs are using the Internet to share health education information with enrollees. E-mail has become more useful in sharing educational information. In addition, MCOs are using videos, CD-ROMs, and computer programs to educate enrollees. With a focus on patient education and advocacy, these strategies provide opportunities for nursing, which has always emphasized these approaches.

Standards of care

Standards of care provide minimal descriptions of accepted actions expected from a health care organization or professional with specific skill and knowledge levels. They are important in establishing expectations (Finkelman, 1996). Standards are developed by professional organizations, legal sources such as nurse practice acts and federal and state laws, regulatory agencies such as accreditation bodies and federal and state agencies, and health care facilities, and are supported by scientific literature and clinical pathways. Standards act as guides for care (for example, the nursing process is part of professional nursing standards). Chapter 16 discusses standards and their implications in more detail.

Utilization review/management

Utilization review/management (UR/UM) is the process of evaluating necessity, appropriateness, and efficiency of health care services for specific patients or patient populations. UR/UM has been used in acute care settings for a long time; however, it is also very important in other types of delivery settings and to MCOs. Nurses are frequently hired as UM staff. They have the clinical skills and knowledge necessary to evaluate patient needs and services to determine necessity, appropriateness, and timeliness of services. MCOs are particularly interested in UR/UM because it is primarily used to control costs. UR/UM data are used when tools are developed to access outcomes. Chapter 16 discusses UM in more detail.

Benchmarking

Although there is no universally accepted definition for benchmarking, it is a tool that identifies "best practices." "Clinical benchmarking is a tool and a process of continuously comparing the practices and performances of one's operations against those of the best in the industry or the focused area of service and then using that information to enhance and improve performance and productivity" (Fitzgerald, 1998, p. 23). Another definition describes it as "an ongoing search for best practices that produce superior performance when adapted and implemented in an organization" (Berendt, Schaefer, Heglund, & Bardin, 2001, p. 71). It is also a tool that links standards of care, guidelines, documentation, quality assurance programs, and clinical pathways. The process allows organizations to compare their performance both within the organization and with other organizations. In doing this it identifies benchmarks or "measurement to gauge the performance of a function, operation, or business relative to others" (Berendt, Schaefer, Heglund, & Bardin, 2001, p. 71). "Benchmarking focuses not only on comparative data, but also on an in-depth analysis of the processes and practices that drive data results" (Karpiel, 2000, p. 54). The goal is to find new opportunities for cost and quality improvement. As a tool, it creates value in four ways:

1. Focusing the organization and individuals on key performance gaps
2. Bringing in ideas from external organizations and identifying opportunities
3. Rallying the organization around the findings to create a consensus to move forward
4. Implementing ideas to yield better-quality products and services (Czarnecki, 1995, p. 2)

Benchmarking as a process uses data to improve. It requires that staff use data-driven, decision-making processes, and makes the organization and its staff aware of options. "Benchmarking results in real introspection and the development of a new vision for health care—a vision that is built on the detailed redesign of basic processes" (Czarnecki, 1995, p. 3). It begins with identifying the areas of greatest need and those for which there is comparable performance data. Time should not be wasted on correcting problems that will not have an impact or for which it is difficult to obtain data.

When data are collected for benchmarks, there are typically three possible broad focus areas: literature, internal, and system (Rudy, Lucke, Whitman, & Davidson, 2001). Literature-based benchmarking can be done, but there may not be enough relevant literature that matches the focus of the benchmarking, specific patient population, problem, and so on. There is uncertainty in matching. The second type, internal or using only organization-specific data, causes problems because the organization is comparing itself with itself. A system approach, which would apply to an integrated hospital or other types of health care organizations, can be more useful; however, there still needs to be careful considerations of data and characteristics. The key is to compare organizations that are similar to avoid the problem of comparing "apples with oranges." The fourth type occurs when a hospital or other health care organization selects similar organizations and compares its data with them.

There can be confusion about benchmarking when it is compared with other similar tools. Benchmarking does not establish rigid goals that must be met by the organization. It does not focus on variances. "It is not a precise analysis of work flow, bottlenecks, waste, or redundancy. It is not a reflection on current or past management staff practices" (Fitzgerald, 1998, p. 25). Benchmarking is a catalyst for change by demonstrating where the organization is compared with others, but it will not say what the organization needs to do. The organization must then use data and analysis to make a plan for improvement.

A key component of benchmarking is sharing, and this has not always been easy for health care organizations. If information is shared, it will benefit all, but this requires some trust. Any organization that participates in benchmarking will undoubtedly want its legal advisors to review policies and procedures related to this project. Competition has not disappeared—in fact, it has increased. Acknowledging competition and also participating in benchmarking can be a complex endeavor.

Evidence-based practice

Evidence-based practice (EBP) is being incorporated into more and more health care delivery systems. The recent Institute of Medicine reports on quality and safety emphasize the need to apply EBP in practice. Evidence-based practice has been defined as "developing changes and improvements with a firm foundation of the best data that exist at that time from the science, the individual performing the services, and the consumer of the service" (DePalma, 2002, p. 55). Another definition that focuses on nursing is, "Evidence-based nursing emphasizes ritual, isolated, and unsystematic clinical experiences, ungrounded opinions, and tradition as a basis for nursing practices, and stresses instead the use of research findings and, as appropriate, quality improvement data, other operational and evaluation data, the consensus of recognized experts, and affirmed experience to substantiate practice" (Stetler et al., 1998, pp. 48–49). Evidence-based practice (EBP) helps to identify and assess high-quality, clinically relevant research that can be applied to clinical practice as well as the development of health policy. As one travels from one area of the country to the other, or even within one community, there can be great variation in practice and delivery. Problems are approached differently and often with no rationale that is based on sound evidence.

EBD synthesizes results found in professional research so that they can be used to improve care or the delivery of health care services. These systematic reviews:

■ Estimate the effect of health care interventions.
■ Provide generalizable answers, because they are based on a number of studies in different settings and include a variety of participants.
■ Identify the individual, clinical, and contextual factors that influence effectiveness.
■ Identify uncertainties and gaps in research (Dickson & Entwistle, 1997, p. 3).

Two key goals of evidence-based practice and also evidence-based policy development that are important for organizations to consider are to: (a) challenge others to provide evidence for their practice or their policy decisions and (b) critically assess to find and use evidence (Mooney, 2001, 9, 17). Today, patients are more knowledgeable about their illnesses and treatment. Technology has brought much more information to consumers. Information increases control, and now more and more patients want the best. Evidence-based care looks for the best (Cope, 2003). Management needs to keep these two goals in mind. In order to meet these goals, management and staff will need to know how to:

■ Frame a clinical question (delivery, or policy question).
■ Search for the evidence.
■ Evaluate the evidence.
■ Implement the evidence (Mooney, 2001, p. 17).

Evidence-based practice requires that information is available for specific questions. The research literature is reviewed using explicit scientific methods and includes all relevant research. This valuable information is then available to practitioners and should be helpful in directing their care decisions. An obvious question is how does one get to this information and then how does one know what information is valid and reliable? Evidence-based reviews act as gatekeepers of the knowledge (Evans & Pearson, 2001). Clearly, criteria need to be used to determine what type of evidence will be useful, too. The hierarchy of evidence can be described in three levels (DePalma, 2002; Rutledge & Grant, 2002).

1. The highest level is published research differentiated by methodology such as randomized, controlled studies, and then qualitative studies.
2. The middle level is theoretical evidence, which is based on propositions that may not have been tested.
3. The lowest level is non-research evidence. Examples of this type of evidence are: benchmarking data, cost analyses, regulatory and legal opinions, ethical principles, case reports, quality and risk data if systematically obtained, principles of pathophysiology, standards of care, and infection control data, if systematically collected.

Mooney (2001) recommends that not only do staff or the reviewers need to evaluate the information based on its scientific merit, as is indicated in the hierarchy described, but also the following must be considered: Have the results been replicated? This helps to establish credibility. Are the results relevant to the practice, policy, or delivery? What are the risks and benefits of incorporating the results into practice, policy, or delivery? Just adopting ideas without considering these factors can be costly. What is the feasibility of incorporating the new evidence? This is tied to the previous question as it can increase costs or limit benefits. Now, what happens after evidence is collected? It could be overwhelming, as the result is often a large amount of information, and some may conflict. Typically, a panel of stakeholders is selected to review the information and come to a consensus about the information (DePalma, 2002).

Pearson (2002) describes a framework developed in Australia that is used for qualitative data and development of systematic reviews. It focuses on feasibility, appropriateness, meaningfulness, and effectiveness, and is called FAME. Evidence is ranked according to these terms by using the following criteria.

1. Feasibility
   - Immediately practicable
   - Practicable with limited local training or modest additional resources
   - Practicable with extensive additional training or resources
   - Practicable with significant national reforms
   - Impracticable
2. Appropriateness
   - Acceptable and justifiable within ethical guidelines
   - Acceptable after minor revisions to ethical guidelines
   - Acceptable after major revisions to ethical guidelines
   - Acceptable after development of new ethical guidelines
   - Ethically unacceptable
3. Meaningfulness
   - Provides a rationale for practice development
   - Provides a rationale for local, regional, or national reform
   - Provides a rationale for practice-related research
   - Provides a rationale for advocating change
   - Evidence unlikely to make sense to practitioners
4. Effectiveness
   - Extensively validated and contradictory findings limited
   - Limited triangulation of convergent findings and no contrary findings
   - Descriptive accounts of application
   - Systematization of concepts
   - Concept identification and development (Pearson, 2002, p. 21)

Participating in evidence-based evaluation of information to arrive at the best view of practice, policy, or delivery requires some skills. The following are some critical skills that are needed to be effective.

- Big-picture thinking
- Critical thinking
- Flexibility/willingness to try new things and be a continuous learner
- Advanced communication and relationship-building skills
- Interdisciplinary influence and team-building skills
- Outcomes orientation and the ability to demonstrate value added
- Commitment to an evidence-based practice
- Research and data interpretation skills
- Computing and technology skills
- Leadership competency (Mooney, 2001, p. 18)

Mooney (2001) also emphasizes the importance of the knowledge worker, which relates to content in Chapter 1 on knowledge and leadership. "Transitioning to an evidence-based practice requires a different perspective from the traditional role of nurse as 'doer' of treatments and procedures based on institutional policy or personal preference. Rather, the nurse practices as a 'knowledge worker' from an updated and ever-changing knowledge base, contributing to the oncology [or can be any type] health care team as knowledgeable clinical colleague" (Mooney, 2001, p. 17). Others have also commented on the need for nurses to see themselves as knowledge workers. "Clinical scholarship is value-driven—a demonstration of willingness to test creativity, courage, and autonomy because of the love and belief in the work. It is also about intellectual problem solving, activating and disseminating practice innovations, and being collaborative. Acquiring, analyzing, synthesizing, and applying evidence to inform the practice process become key components to being a clinical scholar" (Dickenson-Hazard, 2002, p. 6). Blind acceptance of research results that are then applied to patient care is clearly not what nurses should do. Nurses are able to do more than this. They can play a role in assessing and selecting information to apply to the care. This, however, requires that nurses demonstrate the skills identified by Mooney (2001).

Finding sources of data to support evidence-based practice in nursing may not always be easy. Clearly, well-designed research is the best; however, there may be none available on a particular problem area. The U.S. Preventive Services Task Force, which is an interdisciplinary group that works under the AHRQ, evaluates research and publishes guidelines based on their reviews. This can be a source of information to support evidence-based practice. "The AHRQ Evidence-Based Practice Center (EPC) Program sponsors and disseminates state of the art systematic reviews on important topics that provide the evidence bases for guidelines, quality improvement projects, quality measures, and insurance coverage decisions. They sponsor both methodological investigations and publications of systematic reviews" (Cronewett, 2002, p. 4). Twelve evidence-based practice centers in the country produce reports that include the critical appraisal of the literature using explicit grading systems (Lohr & Carey, 1999). Cronewett (2002) notes that EBP reports from AHRQ are typically developed by scientists from single disciplines, thus providing one point of view rather than an interdisciplinary view, which is a disadvantage. Clinicians, patients, and advocacy groups are not usually involved, but when the development of clinical practice guidelines was begun these groups usually did participate. The EBP reports include analyses, evidence tables, references, and search strategies. Cronewett (2002) has some criticisms of the AHRQ evidence-based practice reports due to the incomplete literature, possible database publication biases, and the emphasis on using evidence from randomized controlled trials, which can skew the information, and making the conclusions only relevant to the patient populations included in the studies.

CURRENT ISSUES

Learn about events around the globe that relate to the chapter content.

The *American Journal of Nursing* estimates that only 35% of nurses subscribe to a professional journal (Mason, 2002); however, with the availability of online access to many journals this may not be an accurate account of the percentage of nurses who have access to professional literature. If nurses need to use an EBP approach, nurses will need to be more aware of the professional literature.

Professional nursing organizations have also become more involved in EBP. An example is the effort that the Association of Women's Health, Obstetric and Neonatal Nurses (AWHONN) began in 1996 to participate in evidence-based practice and thus promote its mission of promoting excellence in nursing practice to improve the health of women and newborns. "Developing an evidence-based practice is a journey of continuous improvement for clinicians and organizations. It is a process which challenges us to shift our approach to providing patient care from reliance on expert opinion and consensus, to the development of clinical practice guidelines grounded in science" (Association of Women's Health, Obstetric and Neonatal Nurses, 1996). AWHONN believes that clinical nursing practice should be based on the best available scientific evidence, and therefore designed a process for clinical practice guideline development that is based on the American Nurses Association and the AHRQ frameworks for evidence-based guideline development. The AWHONN evidence-based clinical practice guidelines reflect an expansion of those presented in their standards, *Standards and Guidelines for Professional Nursing Practice in the Care of Women and Newborns*. Each of the AWHONN evidence-based clinical practice guidelines includes:

- Clinical practice recommendations, referenced rationale statements, and a quality of evidence rating for each statement.
- Detailed background information describing the scope and importance of the clinical issue addressed by the evidence-based clinical practice guidelines.

■ A Quick Care Guide, which serves as a quick reference to the guideline for the clinician.

Some examples of nursing EBPs, including those developed by AWHONN, are:

■ Continence for Women (2000)
■ Nursing Management of the Second Stage of Labor (2000)
■ Breastfeeding Support: Prenatal Care through the First Year (2001)
■ Nursing Care of the Woman Receiving Regional Analgesia/Anesthesia in Labor (2001)
■ Neonatal Skin Care (2001)
■ Promotion of Emotional Well-Being During Midlife (2001)
■ Cardiovascular Health for Women: Primary Prevention (2001)

How would the evidence-based approach be applied to nursing management or administration? Titler, Cullen, and Ardery (2002) addressed this question, and they emphasized the importance of interdisciplinary collaboration, which seems to be a key issue with so much of what is happening in health care today. They identify that it must be a continuous process and takes commitment. The key factors in the process are:

1. Incorporating evidence-based practice terminology into the mission, vision, strategic plan, and performance appraisals of staff
2. Integrating the work EBP into the governance structure of nursing departments and the health care system
3. Demonstrating the value of evidence-based practice through administrative behaviors of the chief nurse executive
4. Establishing explicit expectations about EBP for nursing leaders (e.g., nurse managers and advanced practice nurses) who create a culture that values clinical inquiry (Titler, Cullen, & Ardery, 2002, p. 26)

From this description it is clear that to be successful, EBP has to be incorporated into all aspects of the organization structure, culture, and systems. Examples that are given to implement these four factors are: integrate EBP in all staff education; monitor and act upon results of key indicators for selected EBPs; select a specific number of EBPs each year that have been identified from operational or quality improvement data; establish a documentation system that supports EBP and allows for tracking or monitoring of application; provide routine staff education on EBP; incorporate EBP into orientation, and so on. EBP does have much to offer management and the delivery of nursing care to improve care and the way the nurses work, but the organization has to make a commitment to implement it.

Health promotion and disease and illness prevention

Health promotion and **disease and illness prevention** are strategies that focus on encouraging people to become partners in maintaining their own health. These are also critical strategies used by MCOs, primary care, and community health. Medicare is also providing more reimbursement for these strategies. Education is a key method for accomplishing this partnership. Each time an MCO develops health promotion and disease and illness prevention services, it reassesses the costs and benefits of these services. The HMO is the managed care model that is more likely to cover preventive services, such as immunizations, well-baby care, and physical examinations. Many of the other types of managed care organizations do not provide preventive care or do so minimally. The three major health promotion and prevention methods used by health care organizations, community health, and MCOs are:

1. **Screening.** This method includes periodic physical examinations and laboratory tests based on the patient's medical history and risk assessment, such as family history and smoking and exercise habits.
2. **Counseling.** The primary care doctor or other medical professional explains the relationship between risk factors and health. Through counseling, the health plan assists patients in obtaining knowledge and skills, and developing the motivation to adopt and maintain healthy behavior.
3. **Immunization and chemoprophylaxis** (Korczyk & Witte, 1998, p. 128).

The goals of health promotion are to help people modify their lifestyles and make choices to improve their health and quality of life. Health education is very important in helping enrollees/patients to accomplish this goal. There are three types of disease and illness prevention strategies: primary, secondary, and tertiary.

1. Primary prevention focuses on wellness behaviors and prevention of illness or prevention of the natural course of an illness. Examples of interventions are prenatal clinics, stress management courses, AIDS prevention education, nutrition education, safety for children, smoking clinics, alcohol usage, and seat belt safety.
2. Secondary prevention focuses on early diagnosis of symptoms and treatment after the onset of disease or illness and recognizes that early treatment may decrease complications. Examples of interventions are mammograms, parent education, and screening for diabetes or glaucoma.
3. Tertiary prevention focuses on rehabilitative strategies to decrease disability from a disease or illness. Examples of interventions are chemotherapy education for a cancer patient and bladder training for a stroke patient.

What methods are used to determine what services or interventions to offer? National guidelines are frequently used. For example, *The Guide to Clinical Preventive Services* (U.S. Preventive Services Task Force, 1996) is used to determine which interventions should be provided. This resource provides information about preventive services categorized by age and sex. It also identifies screening for the following health care problems:

- Cardiovascular diseases
- Neoplastic diseases
- Metabolic, nutritional, and environmental disorders
- Infectious diseases
- Vision and hearing disorders
- Prenatal disorders
- Congenital disorders
- Musculoskeletal disorders
- Mental disorders and substance abuse (U.S. Preventive Services Task Force, 1996)

Preventive services are frequently inadequately provided. Some of the reasons for this are: inadequate reimbursement, fragmentation of health care delivery, and insufficient time with patients that limits time for assessment of these needs, interventions, and patient education. Even when these factors have been removed, the services are often not provided. This is partially due to a lack of knowledge about what to provide and questions about their effectiveness. Patients may also be unaware of their needs for preventive services, and thus do not request them. Patient adherence is a critical factor for success. Some preventive services are best provided on a community basis as opposed to an individual focus in a clinical setting, and this may become more common in the future. In addition, MCOs, as well as other health care providers, may develop their own clinical guidelines for preventive services, which increases the variability of these services. MCOs use newsletters, personal letters, information provided at the worksite, and the Internet to share information with their enrollees. Health care organizations such as hospitals, clinics, school nurses, and others use many of these same methods.

As decisions are made about which preventive services to offer, cost-effectiveness is an important consideration. Cost-effectiveness analysis is a method for assessing and summarizing the value of a medical technology, practice, or policy. Underlying the methodology is the assumption that the resources available to spend on health care are constrained, whether from the societal, organizational, practitioner, or patient point of view. Cost-effectiveness information is intended to inform decisions about health care investments within the finite budget. The cost-effectiveness ratio summarizes information on cost and effect, allowing interventions to be compared on the basis of their worth and priority to the patient, society in general, or some other constituency. Although the cost-effectiveness ratio takes the form of a price—that is, a dollar cost per unit of effect—it is generally interpreted in the inverse manner, as a measure of the benefit achievable for a given level of resources (U.S. Preventive Services Task Force, 1996). There is a need to allocate resources efficiently or to get the most out of the resources. For example, if it costs $1,000 per person to do a screening test and the chance of identifying a problem is quite small, is it worth it to provide this screening to all patients? An MCO may also be hesitant to provide coverage for screening to identify major medical problems that may require costly treatment, such as using HIV screening (Rosenthal, 1997). MCOs need to factor into the cost-effectiveness analysis the value of providing services that will keep enrollees healthy when the long-term benefit will be reaped by another MCO. Why is this a concern? It is common for enrollees to change health plans, and thus an MCO's membership is rarely constant over a long period of time. Some authorities believe that the most cost-effective services are immunizations and smoking cessation for pregnant women. Other preventive services can be questioned when their cost-effectiveness is considered (Rosenthal, 1997). Clearly, this is a highly controversial area for health care providers and health plans (Brody, 2000).

CURRENT ISSUES

Learn about events around the globe that relate to the chapter content.

BENCHMARKS

Now let's take a moment to test your knowledge of the concepts you have studied in this section.

Chapter Wrap-Up

Now that you've reached the end of the chapter, you may wish to explore the concepts you've been reading about in greater detail, or test yourself to see how well you've comprehended the material.

SUMMARY AND APPLICATIONS

- Summary
- Practice Quiz
- Key Terms
- Tying It All Together
- Experiential Exercises
- Case
- Links

REFERENCES

Algorithms and paths: Use them to monitor, improve quality care. (1995). *Case Management Advisor*, 6(11), 145–146.

Association of Women's Health, Obstetric and Neonatal Nurses. (1996). Retrieved from internet. June 6, 2004, from http://www.awhoan.org.

Bailey, D., Litaker, D., & Mion, L. (1998). Developing better critical paths in healthcare: Combining 'best practice' and the quantitative approach. *Journal of Nursing Administration*, 28(7/8), 21–26.

Berendt, M., Schaefer, B., Heglund, M., & Bardin, C. (2001, April). Telehealth for effective disease state management. *Home Care Provider*, 67–72.

Blue Cross/Blue Shield. Retrieved on May 6, 2002, from http://www.bluecross.com.

Brody, J. (2000, March 14). A big maintenance problem at the HMO. *New York Times, 28.*

Cesta, T., Tahan, H., & Fink, L. (1998). *The case manager's survival guide: Winning strategies for clinical practice.* St. Louis, MO: Mosby-Year Book, Inc.

Clark, C., Steinbinder, A., & Anderson, R. (1994). Implementing clinical paths in a managed care environment. *Nursing Economics, 12*(4), 230–234.

Coffey, R., et al. (1992). An introduction to critical paths. *Quality Management in Health Care, 1*(1), 45–54.

Coffey, R., Richards, J., Wintermeyer-Pingel, S., & LeRoy, S. (1996). Critical paths: Linking outcomes for patients, clinicians, and payers. In P. Kongstvedt (Ed.), *The managed health care handbook* (pp. 301–317). Gaithersburg, MD: Aspen Publishers, Inc.

Cohen, E., & Cesta, T. (1993). *Nursing case management: From concept to evaluation.* St. Louis, MO: Mosby-Yearbook, Inc.

Cope, D. (2003). Evidence-based practice: Making it happen in your clinical setting. *Clinical Journal of Oncology Nursing, 7*(1), 97–98.

Cronewett, L. (2002, February 19). Research, practice and policy: Issues in Evidence Based Care. *Online Journal of Issues in Nursing,* available http://www.nursingworld.org/ojin/keynotes/speech_2.htm.

Czarnecki, M. (1995). *Benchmarking strategies for health care management.* Gaithersburg, MD: Aspen Publishers, Inc.

Dalzell, M. (1998, September). Just what the devil is population-based care. *Managed Care.* Retrieved from Internet on January 4, 2004, from http://www.managedcaremag.com.

DePalma, J. (2002). Proposing an evidence-based policy process. *Nursing Administration Quarterly, 26*(4), 55–61.

Dickenson-Hazard, N., (2002). Evidence-based practice, 'the right approach'. *Reflections on Nursing LEADERSHIP, 28*(2), 6.

Dickson, R., & Entwistle, V. (1997, February). Systematic reviews: Keeping up with research evidence. *Systematic reviews: Examples for nursing (2)*, 3.

Duff, L., & Casey, L. (1998). Implementing clinical guidelines: How can informatics help? *Journal of the American Medical Informatics Association, 5*(3), 225–226.

Dykes, P. (1998a). The process of clinical pathway development. In P. Dykes (Ed.), *Psychiatric clinical pathways: An interdisciplinary approach* (pp. 11–18). Gaithersburg, MD: Aspen Publishers, Inc.

Dykes, P. (1998b). Psychiatric algorithms and copathways: The key to success with comorbidity. In P. Dykes (Ed.), *Psychiatric clinical pathways: An interdisciplinary approach* (pp. 85–90). Gaithersburg, MD: Aspen Publishers, Inc.

Dykes, P. (1998c). The role of clinical pathways in health care and psychiatry: An overview. In P. Dykes (Ed.), *Psychiatric clinical pathways: An interdisciplinary approach* (pp. 3–9). Gaithersburg, MD: Aspen Publishers, Inc.

Epstein, R., & Sherwood, L. (1996). From outcomes research to disease management. A guide for the perplexed. *Annals of Internal Medicine, 24*(9), 830–835.

Evans, D., & Pearson, A. (2001). Systematic reviews: Gatekeepers of nursing knowledge. *Journal of Clinical Nursing, 10,* 593–599.

Finkelman, A. (1996). *Psychiatric nursing administration manual.* Gaithersburg, MD: Aspen Publications, Inc.

Fitzgerald, K. (1998). Clinical benchmarking: Implications for perinatal nursing. *Journal of Perinatal Nursing, 12*(1), 23–30.

Flarey, D., & Blancett, S. (Eds.). (1996). *Handbook of nursing case management: Health care delivery in a world of managed care.* Gaithersburg, MD: Aspen Publishers, Inc.

General Accounting Office. (1996). Practice guidelines: Managed care plans customize guidelines to meet local interest. (GAO/HEHS-96-95). Washington, DC: Author.

Goode, C. (1995). Impact of a care map and case management on patient satisfaction and staff satisfaction, collaboration, and autonomy. *Nursing Economics, 13*(6), 337–349.

Griffin, M., & Griffin, R. (1994). Critical pathways produce tangible results. *Health Care Strategic Management, 12*(7), 18–23.

Gurnee, M., & Da Silva, R. (1997). Constructing disease management programs. *Managed Care, 6*(6), 8–16.

Hague, D. (1996, May). Clinical pathways: The care plans of the 90s. *Ohio Nurses Review, 71*(5), 15–19.

Hofmann, P. (1993). Critical path method: An important tool for coordinating clinical care. *Joint Commission Journal of Quality Improvement, 19*(7), 235–246.

Ireson, C. (1997). Critical pathways: Effectiveness in achieving patient outcomes. *Journal of Nursing Administration, 27*(6), 16–23.

Joint Commission on Accreditation of Healthcare Organizations. Retrieved on August, 2002, from http://www.jcaho.org.

Karpiel, M. (2000, May). Benchmarking facilitates process improvement in the emergency department. *Healthcare Financial Management, 54*(5), 54–59.

Kilborn, P. (1998, December 17). Managers of care, not cost: HMOs find that treating chronic diseases can pay off. *New York Times*, A12.

Knight, W. (1998). *Managed care: What is it and how it works*. Gaithersburg, MD: Aspen Publishers, Inc.

Korczyk, S., & Witte, H. (1998). *The complete idiot's guide to managed care*. New York: Alpha Books.

Lawrence, J. (1998). Asthma programs show progress, not just promise. *Managed Care, 7*(2), 3–7.

Leibman, B., et al. (1998). Impact of a clinical pathway for radical retropubic prostactectomy. *Urology, 52*(1), 94–99.

Lohr, K. (1995). Guidelines for clinical practice: What they are and why they count. *Journal of Law, Medicine & Ethics, 23*, 49–56.

Lohr, K. N., & Carey, T. S. (1999). Assessing "best evidence": Issues in grading the quality of studies for systematic reviews. *Joint Commission Journal on Quality Improvement, 25*, 470–479.

Mason, D. (2002). Who says it's 'best practice'? *American Journal of Nursing, 102*, 10, 7.

Mateo, M., Newton, C., & Kanatas, K. (1996). Developing and implementing critical paths in case management. In D. Flarey & S. Blancett (Eds.), *Handbook of nursing case management: Health care delivery in a world of managed care* (pp. 80–99). Gaithersburg, MD: Aspen Publishers, Inc.

Mooney, K. (2001). Advocating for quality cancer care: Making evidence-based practice a reality. *ONF, 28*(2 Supplement), 17–21.

Pearson, A. (2002). Nursing takes the lead. *Reflections on nursing LEADERSHIP, 28*(4), 16–20.

Polit, D., & Hungler, B. (1997). *Essentials of nursing research: Methods, appraisal, and utilization* (4th ed.). Philadelphia: Lippincott-Raven.

Poniatowski, L. (2000, February). Clinical practice guidelines: Consider, adopt, or do your own. *Nursing Management, 31*(2), 13.

Rehnholm, M., Leino-Kilpi, H., & Suominen, T. (2002). Critical pathways: A systematic review. *Journal of Nursing Administration, 32*(4), 196–202.

Rosenthal, E. (1997, March 16). When healthier isn't cheaper. *New York Times*, A1, A4.

Rudy, E., Lucke, J., Whitman, G., & Davidson, L. (2001). Benchmarking patient outcomes. *Journal of Nursing Scholarship, 33*(2), 185–189.

Rutledge, D., & Grant, M. (2002). Introduction to evidence-based practice in cancer nursing. *Seminars in Oncology Nursing, 18*(2), 1–2.

Schriefer, J. (1994). The synergy of clinical pathways and clinical algorithms. *Journal of Quality Improvement, 20*(9), 485–499.

Sheehan, J., & Sullivan, G. (1998). Psychiatric clinical pathways, documentation, and liability. In P. Dykes (Ed.), *Psychiatric clinical pathways: An interdisciplinary approach* (pp. 115–124). Gaithersburg, MD: Aspen Publishers, Inc.

Stetler, C., et al. (1998). Evidence-based practice and the role of nursing leadership. *Journal of Nursing Administration, 28*(7), 45–53.

Sullivan, T. (1998). Concept analysis: Part I. In T. Sullivan (Ed.), *Collaboration: A health care imperative* (pp. 3–42). New York: McGraw-Hill.

Tallon, R. (1995). Devising and delivering objectives for disease state management. *Nursing Management, 26*(12), 22–24.

Terry, K. (1993, April). Disease management: Continuous health care improvement. *Business & Health* (4), 64–72.

Titler, M., Cullen, L., & Ardery, G. (2002). Evidence-based practice: An administrative perspective. *Reflections on Nursing LEADERSHIP, 28*(2), 26–27, 46.

U.S. Preventive Services Task Force. (1996). *The guide to clinical preventive services*. Alexandria, VA: International Medical Publishing.

Windle, P., & Houston, S. (1996). Documentation to achieve patient outcomes through critical pathways. In D. Flarey & S. Blancett (Eds.), *Handbook of nursing case management: Health care delivery in a world of managed care* (pp. 100–135). Gaithersburg, MD: Aspen Publishers, Inc.

Zander, K. (1992). Quantifying, managing, and improving quality. Part II: The collaborative management of quality care. *The New Definition, 7*(3), 1–2.

ADDITIONAL READINGS

Barnsteiner, J., & Prevost, S. (2002). How to implement evidence-based practice. *Reflections on Nursing LEADERSHIP, 28*(2), 18–21.

Bensing, J. (2000). Bridging the gap. The separate worlds of evidence-based medicine and patient-centered medicine. *Patient Education and Counseling, 39*, 17–25.

Blackmon, T. (1999). Disease management: When is it the right time? *Managed Care Quarterly, 7*(2), 65–68.

Bolger, A., Colone, M., & Crane, J. (1998). The clinical path project at Northwestern Memorial Hospital. In M. Parsons, C. Murdaugh, & R. O'Rourke (Eds.), *Strategies for improving patient care: Interdisciplinary case studies in health care redesign* (pp. 308–323). Gaithersburg, MD: Aspen Publishers, Inc.

Caramanica, L., et al. (2002). Evidence-based nursing practice, Part 1: A hospital and university collaboration. *Journal of Nursing Administration, 32*(1), 27–30.

Coffey, R., & LeRoy, S. (2001). Clinical pathways: Linking outcomes for patients, clinicians, payers, and employers. In P. Kongstvedt (Ed.), *The managed health care handbook* (pp. 521–538). Gaithersburg, MD: Aspen Publishers, Inc.

Couch, J. (1998). *The health care professional's guide to disease management*. Gaithersburg, MD: Aspen Publishers, Inc.

Czarnecki, M. (1996). Benchmarking: A data-oriented look at improving health care performance. *Journal of Nursing Care Quality, 10*(3), 1–16.

DeWoody, S., & Price, J. (1994). A systems approach to multidimensional critical paths. *Nursing Management, 25*(11), 47–51.

Diamond, F. (1998). You can drag physicians to guidelines . . . but you can't make them comply (mostly). *Managed Care, 7*(9), 10–13.

Donovan, T., & Sanders, M. (1998). Care path design in the neonatal intensive care unit: Case study for the extremely low birthweight infant. In M. Parsons, C. Murdaugh, & R. O'Rourke (Eds.), *Strategies for improving patient care: Interdisciplinary case studies in health care redesign* (pp. 222–238). Gaithersburg, MD: Aspen Publishers, Inc.

Doran, K., Sampson, B., Staus, R., Ahern, C., & Schiro, D. (1998). Clinical pathway across tertiary and community care after an interventional cardiology procedure. In C. Mullahy (Ed.), *Essential readings in case management* (pp. 284–295). Gaithersburg, MD: Aspen Publishers, Inc.

Duff, L., Kitson, A., Seers, K., & Humphris, D. (1996). Clinical guidelines: An introduction to their development and implementation. *Journal of Nursing Administration, 23*(3), 887–895.

Dykes, P., & Wheeler, K. (Eds.). (1997). *Planning, implementing, and evaluating critical pathways into the 21st century*. New York: Springer Publishing Company.

Frink, B., & Strassner, L. (1996). Variance analysis. In D. Flarey & S. Blancett (Eds.), *Handbook of nursing case management: Health care delivery in a world of managed care* (pp. 194–223). Gaithersburg, MD: Aspen Publishers, Inc.

Gardner, K., Allhusen, J., Kamm, J., & Tobin, J. (1997). Determining the cost of care through clinical pathways. *Nursing Economics, 15*(4), 213–217.

Garry, R. (2000). Benchmarking: A prescription for health care. *Journal of Nursing Administration, 30*(9), 397–399.

Glanville, I., Schirm, V., & Wineman, J. (2000). Using evidence-based practice for managing clinical outcomes in advanced practice nursing. *Journal of Nursing Quality, 15*(1), 1–11.

Handley, M., Stuart, M., & Kirz, H. (1994). An evidence-based approach to evaluating and improving clinical practice: Implementing practice guidelines. *HMO Practice, 8*(2), 75–83.

Howe, R. (Ed.). (1996). *Clinical pathways for ambulatory care case management*. Gaithersburg, MD: Aspen Publishers, Inc.

Hronek, C. (1995). Redesigning documentation: Clinical pathways, flowsheets, and variance notes. *MEDSURG Nursing, 4*, 157–159.

Huber, D., et al. (2000). Evaluating nursing administration instruments. *Journal of Nursing Administration, 30*(5), 251–272.

Jennings, B., & Loan, L. (2001). Misconceptions among nurses about evidence-based practice. *Journal of Nursing Scholarship, 33*(2), 121–127.

King, M., McDonald, B., & Good, D. (1995). Redesigning care using total quality management and outcomes/variance analysis. *Aspen's Advisor for Nurse Executives, 41*(7), 73–78.

Klenner, S. (2000). Mapping out a clinical pathway. *RN, 63*(6), 33–36.

LaLatini, E. (1998). Trauma critical pathways: A care delivery system that works. In C. Mullahy (Ed.), *Essential readings in case management* (pp. 233–236). Gaithersburg, MD: Aspen Publishers, Inc.

Lichtig, L., Knauf, R., & Milholland, D. (1999). Some impacts of nursing on acute care hospital outcomes. *Journal of Nursing Administration, 29*(2), 25–33.

Lohr, K. N., Eleazer, K., & Mauskopf, J. (1998). Health policy issues and applications for evidence-based medicine and clinical practice guidelines. *Health Policy, 46*, 1–19.

Massey, B., Prevost, S., & Warren, M. (1998). Case management for capitated contracts. In M. Parsons, C. Murdaugh, & R. O'Rourke (Eds.), *Strategies for improving patient care: Interdisciplinary case studies in health care redesign* (pp. 170–182). Gaithersburg, MD: Aspen Publishers, Inc.

Melnyk, M., & Fineout-Overholt, E. (2002). Putting research into practice. *Reflections on Nursing LEADERSHIP, 28*(2), 22–25.

Metzger, J., Haughton, J., & Smithson, K. (1999). Improvement-focused information technology for the clinical office practice: A patient registry for disease management. *Managed Care Quarterly, 7*(3), 67–72.

Mullahy, C. (Ed.). (1996). *Essential readings in case management.* Gaithersburg, MD: Aspen Publishers, Inc.

Nelson, M. (1994). Critical pathways in the emergency department. *Journal of Emergency Nursing, 19*(2), 110–114.

Parsons, M., Murdaugh, C., & O'Rourke, R. (Eds.). (1998). *Strategies for improving patient care: Interdisciplinary case studies in health care redesign.* Gaithersburg, MD: Aspen Publishers, Inc.

Plocher, D. (1996). Disease management. In P. Kongstvedt (Ed.), *The managed health care handbook* (pp. 318–329). Gaithersburg, MD: Aspen Publishers, Inc.

Schriefer, J. (1998). Managing critical pathway variances. In C. Mullahy (Ed.), *Essential readings in case management* (pp. 128–141). Gaithersburg, MD: Aspen Publishers, Inc.

Shendell-Falik, N., & Soriano, K. (1996). Outcomes assessment through protocols. In D. Flarey & S. Blancett (Eds.), *Handbook of nursing case management: Health care delivery in a world of managed care* (pp. 136–169). Gaithersburg, MD: Aspen Publishers, Inc.

Simpson, L., Kamerow, D., & Fraser, I. (1998). Pediatric guidelines and managed care: Who is using what and what difference does it make? *Pediatric Annals, 27*(4), 234–240.

Sperry, S., & Birdsall, C. (1994). Outcomes of pneumonia critical path. *Nursing Economics, 12*(6), 332–345.

Spiers, L., & Editorial Board. (1998). *International classification of diseases, 9th revision, clinical modification* (5th ed.). Salt Lake City, UT: Medicode Publications.

Stone, P., Curran, C., & Bakken, S. (2002). Economic evidence for evidence-based practice. *Journal of Nursing Scholarship, 34*(3), 277–282.

Villaire, M. (1995). Putting critical pathways on the map. *Critical Care Nurse, 15,* 106–113.

Wagner, E., Davis, C., & Austin, B. (1999). A survey of leading chronic disease management programs: Are they consistent with the literature? *Managed Care Quarterly, 7*(3), 56–60.

Weingarten, S., & Krumholz, H. M. (2001). Can practice guidelines be transported effectively to different settings? *Joint Commission Journal on Quality Improvement, 27,* 42–51.

Whitman, G., Davidson, L., Rudy, E., & Wolf, G. (2001). Developing a multi-institutional nursing report card. *Journal of Nursing Administration, 31*(2), 1–7.

Windle, P. (1994). An integrated documentation tool: Critical pathways and desirable patient outcomes. *Nursing Management, 25,* 80F–80P.

LEGISLATION/ REGULATION/POLICY

New collaborations will increase nursing's role in shaping public policy.

Desired Future Statement (Vision)

As leaders in the health and public policy process, nurses are unified in the implementation of standards of nursing education and practice. Nurses develop evidence-based health policy (e.g., legislation, regulation) in collaboration with consumers to ensure access to health care services and safe, competent nursing care.

Five strategies were identified to achieve the vision, and one of these was identified as the primary or driving strategy. They are:

Nurses are policy makers at the local, state, national, and international levels. (Primary Strategy)

Nursing collaborates with all stakeholders for the development of public policy.

Reliable data support all health policy formulation.

Universal access is ensured through the delivery of outcome-driven quality health care services.

Health policy is congruent with standards for nursing education and practice.

Objectives to Support Primary Strategy

Establish a Web-based network among nursing organizations that would scan current legislative and regulatory issues and issue alerts when support or opposition is required.

Cultivate a cadre of nurse experts to serve in key federal, state, and institutional positions, including internships.

Identify existing databases and begin developing workforce and patient outcome databases that are shared and utilized for policy making.

Form a nationwide grassroots system to educate all nurses about the public policy process. Nurses' basic educational curricula and annual/membership professional organizational meetings will include education about the public policy process.

Hold a health policy-planning summit with key consumer organizations, including minority groups, to plan collaborative efforts.

SOURCE: American Nurses Association. (2002). *Nursing's agenda for the future. A call to the nation.* Washington, DC: Author. Reprinted with permission.

Health Care Policy, Legal Issues, and Ethics in Health Care Delivery

CHAPTER OUTLINE

MediaLink
www.prenhall.com/finkelman

The Interactive Exercises for this chapter can be found in the OneKey course at www.prenhall.com/finkelman. Click on Chapter 10 to select from the following activities: Test Your Understanding, Benchmarks, Current Issues, Your Opinion Counts, Think Critically, and Summary and Applications.

What's Ahead

Nurses in one medical center, who recognized the need for change and the roles of nurses in the change process, made the following statement: "To preserve the quality of care while becoming cost competitive, and to strengthen nurses as integral players in this evolving market, we must become a part of the solution—for our patients, ourselves, and the institutions in which we practice. Our goal is to improve the quality of care provided by nurses, increase both job and patient satisfaction, and strengthen our institution's position in a highly competitive market" (Nokleby et al., 1998, p. 34). These nurses were very wise. When nurses assume a leadership role in policy development, this better ensures that both nurses' and patients' needs are included in critical health care policies, legislation, and regulation, all of which are directly connected to ethical decision making in the health care environment. This chapter presents content about health care policy and legal and ethical issues. Nurses need to understand policy development, ethics, and legal concerns while they provide care and when they are in leadership roles.

OBJECTIVES

Before you begin, take a moment to familiarize yourself with the key objectives of this chapter.

- Explain why nurses should be involved in health care policy.
- Identify the difference between private and public policy.
- Describe the policy-making process.
- Discuss how nurses can be involved in the policy-making process.
- Identify how federal and state laws can affect health care.
- Discuss malpractice and how it relates to nursing practice.
- Describe ethical decision making.
- Discuss the impact of health care fraud on the health care system.
- Identify how nurses can become involved in reducing health care fraud and cope with ethical dilemmas presented by fraud.

TEST YOUR UNDERSTANDING

Before we begin our exploration of this chapter, take a short "warm-up" test to see what you know about this topic.

Health Care Policy

Why is health policy relevant to nurses? Nurses should not avoid active participation in health policy and pretend it has nothing to do with nursing. An isolationist approach is never helpful, and for nursing it may actually be a destructive approach. Nurses practice in the health care environment, and health policy and its effects on health care services and the profession are part of that practice. Health policy impacts changes that affect nursing practice and education, staffing, roles, and responsibilities. Legislation and regulation on the state and federal levels affect nursing practice daily. In order to become active participants in the health care environment and the changes that are inevitable, nurses as leaders must become involved in policy development at the local, state, and national levels. Health care policy is critical as it determines what health care services are provided, who provides the services, who can receive services, reimbursement, quality care, improvements, and requirements. Nurses have always been concerned about consumers. This concern for and understanding of consumers and their needs is an important component of successful policy development. As patient advocates, this is an ideal time to take a leadership position to protect patient rights, ensure that patient needs are met, and ensure that the profession of nursing retains its strength. Figure 10-1 provides a view of the importance of health policy to nurses.

This section of the chapter focuses on health care policy. **Policy** and how it is developed are addressed to provide background for the specific policy issues that are discussed. There are many health care policies that could be discussed, so those included are only some of the possibilities. Legislation is also discussed in this section because it plays a critical role in health policy. Box 10-1 provides a list of the critical issues found in the rapidly changing health care environment that either become health policy issues or are related to policies.

FIGURE 10-1   Why is health care policy relevant to nurses?

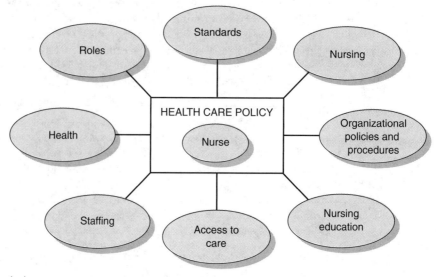

Source: Author.

Key health care policy issues

There are many important health care issues. The following examples of these issues are discussed: increasing cost of health care, disparity in health care delivery, commercialization of health care, and consumers. Solutions for these issues are typically related to policies.

BOX 10-1   The changing health care environment: Critical issues.

- Changing practice patterns and the physician
- Cultural diversity
- Federal and state governments
- Growth of advanced practice nursing
- Diagnosis-related groups
- Health care consumerism
- Health care organization mergers and acquisitions
- Health care role changes
- Immigration
- Legislation
- Managed care backlash
- Managed care models
- Medical–industrial complex: Privatization and corporate health care
- Managed competition
- Minority health
- Move from acute care to ambulatory care
- Quality care
- Reimbursement
- Restructuring and reengineering
- Uninsured and underinsured

Source: Author.

Increasing cost of health care

"The United States operates a health care system that is unique among nations. It is the most expensive of systems, outstripping by over half again the health care expenditures of any other country. By many technical standards, U.S. medical care is the best in the world, but leaders in the field declared in 1997 at a national round table that there is an 'urgent need to improve health care quality'" (Broder, 1997, p. 1). This view has been further supported by the Institute of Medicine (IOM) reports published from 1999 to 2003. (See Chapter 16 for more about these critical reports.) Rising medical costs have driven many of the changes in health care in the last few decades.

What are the causes of increasing health care costs (McIntosh, 2002)?

■ As insurance coverage expanded, it became available to more people. There was little incentive not to use health insurance coverage when the patient was required to pay limited out-of-pocket expenses. This, however, changed as employers and insurers recognized that this system led to overuse, and eventually the expansion, of managed care.

■ In the past, health care professionals often paid limited attention to the costs of care (e.g., ordering tests and procedures, using supplies, extending hospital stays) and were not concerned about the relationship of treatment appropriateness and costs.

■ Technological advancement has had both a positive and negative impact. Clearly, these advancements have led to more effective diagnostic approaches and treatment; however, advancements also increase costs. The development of new equipment, procedures, and drugs is expensive, and these costs are passed on to the customer or the employer who covers some of the insurance costs and the consumer (patient).

■ The increasing use of prescription drugs and their costs are difficult problems that are increasing. New drugs usually mean improved treatment, but there is a cost. Whether or not it is a reasonable cost is a critical question.

■ Defensive medicine, which is making medical decisions in order to protect oneself from lawsuits (for example, ordering diagnostic tests to make sure nothing is missed), also affects health care costs. Cost-containment and cost-effectiveness efforts have been tried for many years, some with more success than others. This will undoubtedly continue, and it is important for nurses to understand the problems and possible solutions so that they can participate actively in resolving cost issues.

In 1997, only one-third of the health maintenance organizations (HMOs) recorded a profit. This lack of profit continues to be a problem today, and is only one piece of bad news for the future of health care expenditures. The U.S. health bill is expected to double to over $2.1 trillion by 2007. Efforts to control costs led to decreases until 1997, but now they are increasing again. "Although managed care is credited with helping hold the line on increases in recent years, 85% of working Americans are now enrolled in such plans and the savings from the one-time shift to managed care have already been realized" (Broder, 1997, p. 1). In addition, prescription costs are expected to more than double by the year 2007.

What will happen now with health care costs? There is no doubt that they are going up. In 2002 health care spending per privately insured person increased 9.6%, which represented a slight reduction from the 10% increase in 2001 (Strunk & Ginsberg, 2003). Many experts believe that all of the "fat" has been removed, or rather the easier, more obvious methods to reduce costs have been used. To decrease costs further or even to just maintain the cost level so that it does not go up will now require more serious, difficult decision making.

The increasing costs and limited access to health care have led to major problems with the number of uninsured and underinsured in this country, estimated to be around 44 million (U.S. Census Bureau, 2004). In 2003 there was a national effort to focus on this critical problem called "Cover the Uninsured Week." Universal health coverage is still not a reality for this country, although the state of Maine has moved to ensure that all of its residents receive coverage. What might universal coverage offer to an expensive system where so many yet go uncovered?

■ Insuring everyone under one national health program would spread the insurance risk over the entire population—ensuring access to all.

- The cost of prescription drugs would decrease.
- Billions of dollars in administrative costs would be saved—health costs relate to all of the costs required to provide coverage. (The number of health plans available in the United States increases administrative costs. For example, a physician in practice has multiple health plans to understand and requires more support staff to administer reimbursement for the physician's patients. The same is true for other types of providers such as hospitals and clinics.)
- "Competition" could focus on quality, safety, and patient satisfaction.
- Resources would be redirected toward patients (Coffey, 2001, p. 11).

Disparity in health care delivery

Disparity in health care delivery is certainly related to the number of uninsured and underinsured, but it is also more than this. The Institute of Medicine report, *Unequal Treatment: Confronting Racial and Ethnic Disparities in Health Care* (2002), addressed factors that might provide causes of disparities in health care. The report indicates that bias, prejudice, and stereotyping on the part of health care providers might be major factors in explaining differences in care. In addition, the report identified clinical uncertainty as an important factor. This was described as any degree of uncertainty a physician may have relative to the patient's condition, which leads the physician to depend on inferences. "The doctor can therefore be viewed as operating with prior beliefs about the likelihood of patients' conditions, 'priors' that will be different according to age, gender, socioeconomic status, and race or ethnicity. When these 'priors' are considered alongside information gathered in a clinical encounter, both influence medical decisions" (Institute of Medicine, 2002, p. 3). Disparities were particularly found in cancer, cardiovascular disease, HIV/AIDS, diabetes, and mental illness. What can be done to improve the problem? There needs to be more cross-cultural education for health care professionals to improve awareness of how cultural and social factors affect health care, which should focus on attitudes, knowledge, and skills. Nursing education has included more content and learning experiences related to cross-cultural issues. There also needs to be greater standardization of data collection to gain more understanding of the problem. Nurses need to be leaders in providing direction for this data collection as these are data that affect their practice. A third strategy that needs consideration is the development of policies that look at the entire health care system to decrease fragmentation in the delivery system and education of health care professionals. Fragmented delivery affects nursing care (for example, patients may be more acutely ill when admitted to a hospital or when they come to a clinic because previous care was not coordinated effectively).

CURRENT ISSUES

Learn about events around the globe that relate to the chapter content.

Commercialization of health care

The United States has struggled for some time to determine the best way to "achieve reasonably equitable distribution of health care, without losing control of total spending on health care, and without suffocating the delivery system with controls and regulations that inhibit technical progress" (Reinhardt, 1994, p. 106). This struggle continues today. Most industrialized countries have chosen to focus on equitable distribution of health care by providing universal coverage; however, the United States continues to vacillate between equity and innovative dynamism. The result has been one of limited success on both sides.

A definite result of this struggle has been the development of the **medical–industrial complex**. Health care has changed from a social good to a product. Health care delivery has become commercialized, and health care professionals, such as hospitals and physicians, have turned more toward business techniques, such as advertising and tighter control of costs, to survive. The rapid growth in hospitals and other types of health care facilities has at times put pressure on all providers to find patients. This pressure has led to economic problems, increasing costs, and new health care delivery approaches. Not all of these factors have been negative as some changes have resulted in improvement with better management and increased focus on community care. In most communities competition is high among all types of health care organizations. After efforts for health care reform failed during the Clinton Administration, implemented reform is based in the private sector. It is the private sector focus that set the stage for the rapid growth of managed care and the tremendous change experienced by the health care delivery system.

As managed care has grown, it has experienced more criticism. Inevitably, blame has become an issue. Many questions arose as managed care became more complex. Who started managed care? Who wanted it? Was it the employers, who experienced accelerating health care costs for their employees? Was it the government, who also experienced this cost acceleration? Was it the consumer, who wanted better access to care and also decreased personal costs? What does the provider want? What were these groups willing to give up? What was managed care supposed to be? These questions have not been easy to answer as the health care system turned more to business methods and managed care. The fact is that the health care delivery system is very complex, with many players, and there is no easy solution for the problem of increasing health care costs.

Consumers

There is no doubt that consumers are also greatly troubled by many of the changes that have occurred in the health care delivery system. Of particular concern to consumers are:

- Increasing access problems
- Increasing costs
- Decreasing quality
- Confusion over the role of third-party payers
- Caregiver competence and ethics
- Impersonal care
- Decreased communication

Consumers can no longer rely on having the same physician to care for them over time. Communities are finding that their local hospitals are merging, disappearing, or being purchased by large for-profit health care corporations. Hospitals often lose their community identification with these changes. Consumers are losing their trust in the health care system and its providers, physicians, nurses, and the like.

Managed care has been a driving force during these changes. The last few years have revealed a backlash against managed care, as illustrated later in this chapter in the discussion about **anti-managed care legislature**. The media have been important players in this response. What can be heard on the television or the radio about health care and consumers' concerns? What articles are published in the newspapers and magazines that focus on health care and health policy? The responses to both of these questions probably indicate that it is a "hot topic" in most of these media sources. Congress has turned its legislative activity into looking at the issues of health care consumer rights, and cases related to managed care have found their way to the U.S. Supreme Court. Employers are even feeling the backlash from their employees, who are requesting more health care plan options and insisting on their right to choose their own health care providers. There is increasing concern that care has been managed too tightly.

Recent legislative activity has finally addressed the growing concern of prescription coverage for seniors, and yet even before the legislation was passed there were criticisms about the proposed coverage (for example, the amount of out-of-pocket costs seniors would still have to pay). As the program is implemented problems will arise that may require further policy development, or this policy may have effects on other health care policy. It is clear that consumers are playing a greater role in health care policy and that this will continue. Chapter 11 discusses health care consumerism in more detail as it is something that nurses need to be aware of since nurses often take on the role of patient advocate.

Health care policy effects on the community

The Center for Studying Health System Change (HSC) provides information about changes in the health care system at both the local and national levels to health care providers. In 1998 HSC addressed a critical question: Are the changes underway in the health care system going to result in better or worse care for Americans (Center for Studying Health System Change, 1998)? To study this question, HSC initiated a community tracking study that focused on 12 communities. This study posed several questions:

1. How are the different components of the health system changing?
2. What forces are driving these changes?
3. How do these changes affect the care people are receiving with respect to access, cost, and perceived quality?

Surveys and site visits are used to collect data about these communities. The effect of changes on consumers, particularly related to access, cost, quality, and service use, are examined. Round one surveys included 33,000 families who were interviewed about access to care, satisfaction, service use, and insurance coverage to determine if their access to care is improving or declining. In all, 12,000 practicing physicians were interviewed to determine how they were paid, changes in their practices, and their assessment of their ability to provide quality care to all of their patients. In addition, 22,000 employers were interviewed, and they were asked about their health plans, how they control health coverage costs, the amount of employee health contributions, and the quality of information that they provide their employees. Other surveys will be conducted. Results thus far indicate that:

- Access to care has been compromised for the medically indigent. There are also differences among communities as to employers who offer insurance and the ability to use specialists.
- Costs vary across communities. Reasons for these variations require further study.
- Use of services requires further study. Particularly important are the use of preventive services and less use of intensive services, frequency with which patients are seeing physicians, and the types of services that patients are receiving in the various health plans.
- Quality of care varies from the perspective of patient satisfaction. Reasons for this variation require further investigation.

This type of study, which uses large samples covering a long-term time perspective and includes many communities, is important in understanding the effects of change and provides guidance for future health policy changes. This approach also indicates the increasing interest in understanding recent health care changes and the use of this knowledge to improve health care for communities rather than just focusing on individuals. Nurses must be involved in these types of studies to ensure that nursing care is also considered.

The policy-making process

A policy is a course of action that affects a large number of people and is stimulated by a need (Bodenheimer & Grumbach, 1998). Policies may include a mixture of laws, regulations, interpretations, court decisions, and other information relevant to the policy content. What does health care policy do? It can answer questions such as:

- What health care services are reimbursed?
- What is the reimbursement for a particular health care service?
- Who can obtain reimbursement for a service?
- How are health care resources allocated?
- Who is eligible for specific health care services?
- Who may provide a service?
- What are the educational requirements and competencies required for specific health care professionals?
- Who pays for health care services?

BOX 10-2 Examples of organizations important to the health care delivery system.

- National Association of Children's Hospitals and Related Institutions (NACHRI)
- American Academy of Hospice and Palliative Medicine (AAHPM)
- American Association of Homes and Services for the Aging (AAHSA)
- American Association of Retired Persons (AARP)
- American Home Care Association (AHCA)
- American Hospital Association (AHA)
- American Nurses Association (ANA)
- Nursing Specialty Organizations
- American Public Health Association (APHA)
- Disease-focused organizations; for example, Arthritis Foundation (AF), American Diabetes Association (ADA)
- Joint Commission on the Accreditation of Healthcare Organizations (JCAHO)
- National Association of Private Psychiatric Hospitals (NAPPH)
- National Association of Public Hospitals (NAPH)
- National Committee on Quality Assurance (NCQA)
- National Health Council (NHC)

Source: Author.

These are all critical questions in today's health care environment, and they demonstrate the impact that policy has on health care delivery. Why are these questions important for nurses? Input from health care professionals is important during the **policy-making process** as they have expertise that may affect policy outcome, and nursing practice is often directly affected by health care policy.

There are two categories of policies: private and public. Private policy is health care policy that is developed by either health care organizations or a profession, such as nursing. Some examples of organizations that participate in health care policy development are identified in Box 10-2.

Despite the active involvement of these organizations and others in the United States, the federal government is the major influence on the financing, structure, and delivery of health care services. One might conclude that because of the major role of the federal government that the United States would have an overall health care policy. This, however, is not the case, and this is a problem. The lack of a coordinated federal and state view of health care delivery often results in different, sometimes conflictual, approaches to health problems; for example, the purposes of some health care policies are not always easy to understand (Bodenheimer & Grumbach, 1998).

- Some policies are poorly written and designed. Others are purposely vague so that many groups can feel they are represented by the policy.
- Not everyone will be a winner with every policy. This is particularly important to understand with health care policy.
- Some groups are represented and receive the services they need, and in the same policy, others are denied services due to lack of funds, resources, and the like.

Box 10-3 identifies some of the key federal government departments and agencies that participate actively in developing public policy in an effort to address these complex issues, and Figure 10-2 describes the U.S. Department of Health and Human Services.

Public policy should reflect the needs of the public, but politics influence and shape many policies, sometimes to the detriment of the policy. "The unacceptable options are that you cannot ask people to reduce their own quality of care so more people will have care; you cannot displace them from private coverage to enter a government program; and you cannot ask them to voluntarily go into a government program if it's less generous than the private coverage they

BOX 10-3   Important federal government departments and agencies.

- Agency for Healthcare Quality and Research (AHCQR)
- Center for Medicare and Medicaid Services (CMS)
- Centers for Disease Control and Prevention (CDC)
- Consumer Product Safety Commission (CPSC)
- Department of Health and Human Services (DHHS)
- Food and Drug Administration (FDA)
- National Institute of Occupational Safety and Health (NIOSH)
- National Institutes of Health (NIH)
- Occupational Safety and Health Administration (OSHA)
- Veteran's Administration (VA)

Source: Author.

already have" (Toner, 1999, p. A1). It is difficult to develop public policy because there are often conflicts that must be considered, such as the example described by Toner. It is also impossible to meet all needs for all people. This means that choices will be made, and this is where politics have an effect. Deals will be made. Compromises will be required. **Cost-benefit analysis** is used to determine the costs and benefits of the various alternatives and then to select the best choice. Figure 10-3 describes several types of public policies that are relevant to health care policy.

The policy-making process should be very familiar to nurses because it is the problem-solving process, similar to the nursing process. The policy process steps are described in Figure 10-4.

To begin this process it is critical to assess the problems in order to arrive at the best solution. Part of this assessment must include the impact the policy might have "on people, the economy, the environment, technology, and the health care system as a whole" (Ferguson, 2001, p. 547). **Policy criteria** are identified during the policy-making process to be used as policy issues are analyzed. Today, typical criteria identified for health care policy are:

- Cost–benefit analysis
- Efficiency
- Equity

Generally, people think of policy as providing the greatest good for the greatest number of people, but not all policies do this. Political feasibility must be considered when policies are developed because it can make the difference between a successful policy and a failed one. If a policy is developed and legislation is proposed that supports the policy but there is limited political support for it, the policy and its legislation will never be accepted.

Today, outcomes have become a more important consideration in policy development. Outcome delivery analysis allows for more informed decision making. Reasons for this interest are:

1. Payers are demanding information about the results of care delivery.
2. Outcomes are an integral part of accreditation.
3. Consumers have a right to know about outcomes.
4. Regulatory agencies demand information about outcomes.
5. Outcomes represent the basic reason for providing care (Jones, Jennings, Moritz, & Moss, 1997, p. 261).

Outcome data are then used to assist in the development of health care policy by either improving policy, deleting policy, or creating new policies.

FIGURE 10-2 U.S. Department of Health & Human Services.

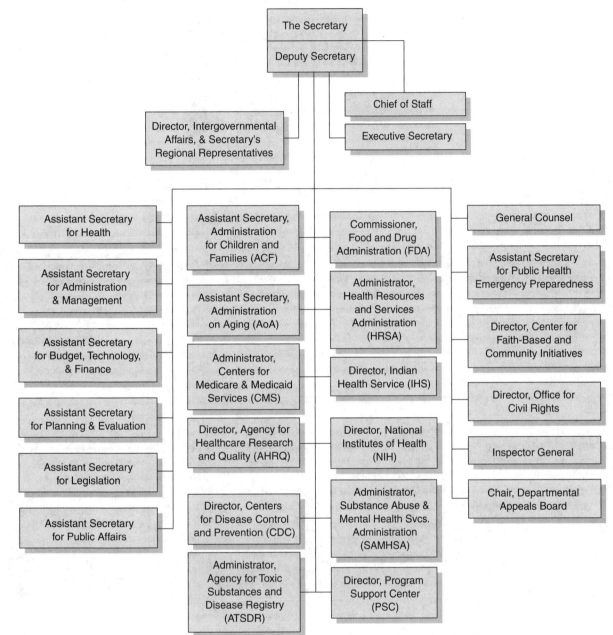

The political process

Since most health policy comes through the legislative process, politics cannot be ignored. "Generally, health policies influence groups and organizations. Health policies express decisions made by legislators and regulators or other judicial and governmental entities" (Ferguson, 2001, p. 547). Nurses, as has been noted, get involved in the **political process** to provide input in the direction that health policy will take, how it will be implemented, and how best to evaluate the results or outcomes. Nurses need to understand the process and the system so that they can influence these decisions. More nurses have been assuming leadership roles in policy making by holding elected public offices in state legislatures and Congress and holding positions in many government agencies. This gives nursing more voice in policy making at all levels. Lobbying is another important

FIGURE 10-3   Types of public policy.

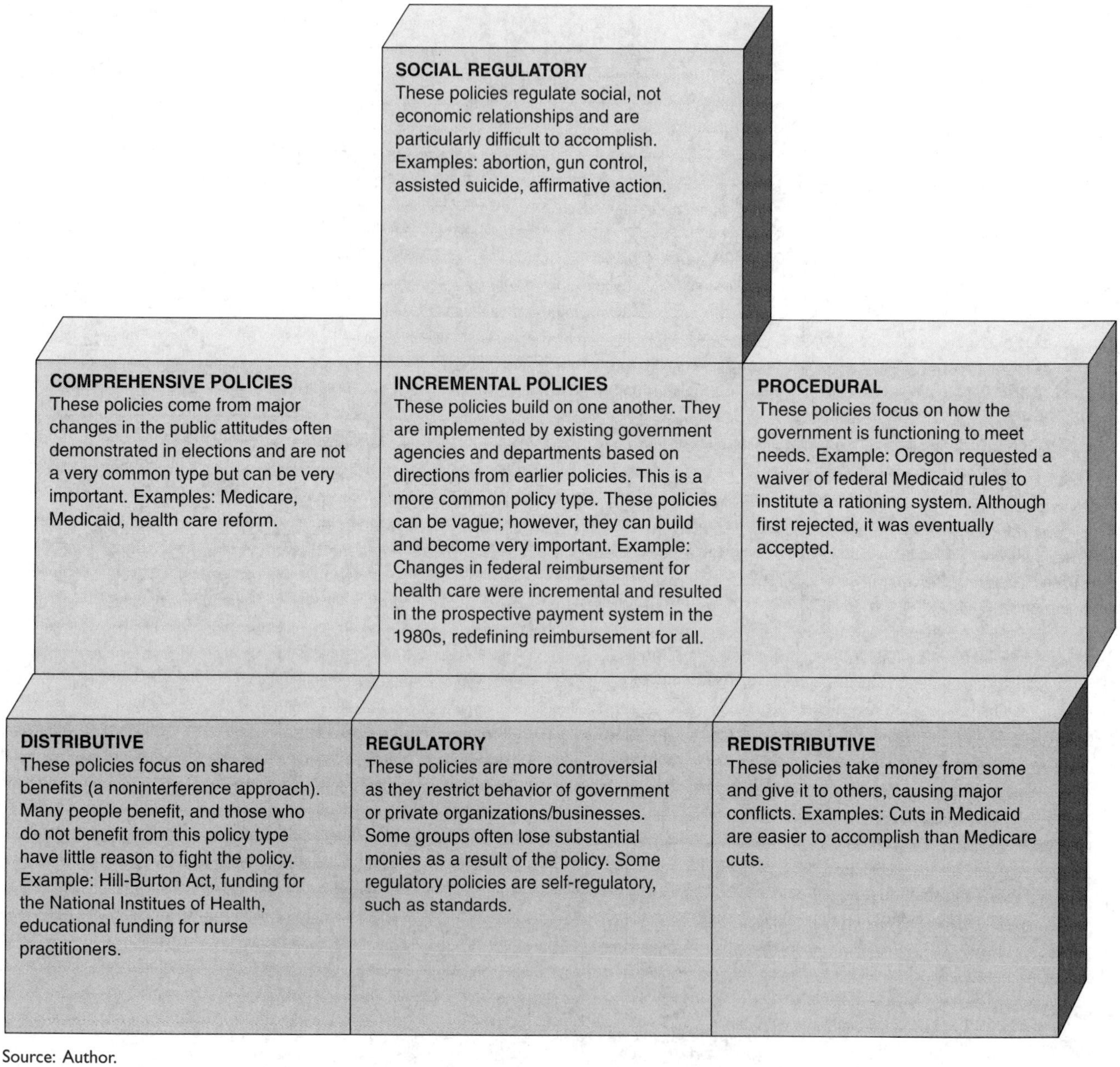

SOCIAL REGULATORY
These policies regulate social, not economic relationships and are particularly difficult to accomplish. Examples: abortion, gun control, assisted suicide, affirmative action.

COMPREHENSIVE POLICIES
These policies come from major changes in the public attitudes often demonstrated in elections and are not a very common type but can be very important. Examples: Medicare, Medicaid, health care reform.

INCREMENTAL POLICIES
These policies build on one another. They are implemented by existing government agencies and departments based on directions from earlier policies. This is a more common policy type. These policies can be vague; however, they can build and become very important. Example: Changes in federal reimbursement for health care were incremental and resulted in the prospective payment system in the 1980s, redefining reimbursement for all.

PROCEDURAL
These policies focus on how the government is functioning to meet needs. Example: Oregon requested a waiver of federal Medicaid rules to institute a rationing system. Although first rejected, it was eventually accepted.

DISTRIBUTIVE
These policies focus on shared benefits (a noninterference approach). Many people benefit, and those who do not benefit from this policy type have little reason to fight the policy. Example: Hill-Burton Act, funding for the National Institues of Health, educational funding for nurse practitioners.

REGULATORY
These policies are more controversial as they restrict behavior of government or private organizations/businesses. Some groups often lose substantial monies as a result of the policy. Some regulatory policies are self-regulatory, such as standards.

REDISTRIBUTIVE
These policies take money from some and give it to others, causing major conflicts. Examples: Cuts in Medicaid are easier to accomplish than Medicare cuts.

Source: Author.

tool. Chapter 13 discusses some of this as it relates to professional development. Coalition building, which helps nurses join together with other groups that have similar interests, also serves to get nursing's message across. Networking and collaboration require some compromises so that the end result will be as effective as possible. All of this is related to leadership and the skills of communication, planning and decision making, collaboration, responding to change effectively, and encouraging participation of nurses on all levels.

Political factors need to be factored in when the possible solutions to policy issues are identified, and also when the selected solution is implemented. Selecting a solution that does not have a chance of succeeding due to politics is not helpful and only leads to frustration. When legislation is enacted, then rules or regulations must be developed to assist with the implementation of the law or the policy (Longest, 2002). As policy is implemented, it should be monitored, which may lead to additional changes. This entire process is cyclical in that evaluation data lead to other policies or reshaping of current policy, and it is also dynamic as it is affected by many factors throughout the process. Table 10-1 describes this process.

FIGURE 10-4 The policy-making process.

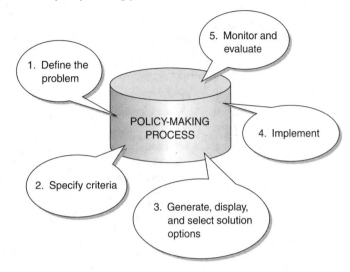

Source: Author.

Health care policy and nursing

As changes occur in the health care environment, health care policy, legislation, regulation, and ethics, it is important for nurses to understand and participate in the legislative process and consider how policy may affect ethical decision making. Active involvement of nurses in all of these areas must occur at the local, state, and federal levels. What are some examples of issues that have affected nursing?

1. An example of a policy issue that has offered nursing many opportunities and substantial risks is managed care. Nurses recognize that there are aspects of managed care that demonstrate positive changes in health care delivery, such as preventive services and a greater emphasis on the continuum of care rather than episodic care. Nurses are also confronted with staffing shortages, shortened hospital stays, increasing patient acuity both in the hospital and in the community, less staff, and a complex reimbursement system. These changes have made it difficult for nurses and other health care professionals to deliver what they believe is quality care. Hadley (1996) identifies four challenges that must be resolved and are important to nursing:

   ■ Demonstrate that nurses provide cost-effective, high-quality, measurable care. This requires data related to outcomes and costs that specifically address nursing care.

   ■ Adopt uniform licensure and educational requirements for the profession and establish fewer, simpler titles. This has been and continues to be a conflictual topic for nursing. If nursing does not resolve this problem for itself, who will?

   ■ Overcome the mentality of an oppressed minority. Nurses have moved into more leadership positions in health care organizations, as clinicians and administrators, and in government, both as staff and elected officials. In addition, nurses need to hold more leadership positions in managed care organizations (MCOs) and in all types of insurer organizations.

   ■ Sustain a commitment to lifelong professional learning. This is important as nurses take on new roles and participate in policy development. Credibility requires knowledge. As discussed in other chapters, nurses have the opportunity to move into new roles and even develop them, but this means that nurses must develop new competencies and acquire new knowledge.

2. Understanding health policy and its implications for leadership and management is a journey through the health care delivery system, its players, its successes and its limitations, and its future.

   If there is acceptance that the health care environment has changed and continues to be reshaped, critical questions are: what will be the role of the nurse in this process and

TABLE 10-1   Applying the policy development process.

POLICY PROCESS	APPLIED TO LEGISLATIVE PROCESS	EXAMPLE
Policy issue develops	Senator learns about consumer concern about a health issue and has staff work on the issue.	Staffing levels in acute care hospitals are affecting the quality and safety of care. Examples of errors and lack of quality are provided from various hospitals that have led to patient deaths and to complications that have extended the need for treatment.
Gather data about issue	Legislative staff gather data about the issue; some data may come from federal departments or agencies, which act as resources for legislative activity. Criteria are developed to evaluate the data (e.g., cost, efficiency, equity, and political feasibility).	Testimony may be provided from experts, patients, insurers, hospitals, nurses, physicians, and so on. Data related to errors, quality, and access will be used to further understand the problem. Data about enrollment and graduation rates in nursing schools would be important to obtain. Costs would be critical to obtain related to lack of staff: costs for the hospitals, insurers, employers, and patients (consumers).
Coalition building	Senator will form coalitions to back the legislation with other Senators, Congressmen, and stakeholders.	Stakeholders that would be interested in this problem and solution would be health care professionals and their organizations (nurses, physicians), American Hospital Association, insurers, employers, consumer groups, nurse educators, and others. Building a coalition from these groups would help to get the bill passed.
Identify possible solutions	Apply cost-benefit analysis of data to determine possible solutions; testimony from experts, lobbyists input and pressure; arrive at list of possible solutions.	Cost data would be used to help assess cost-benefit for each of the possible solutions. Some examples of solutions might be: do nothing, require every hospital to have a specific number of staff, require hospitals to use a patient classification system or require that every hospital use the same system, require minimum ratios, and many others.
Select a solution	Federal (or state) written law will probably repeat some of the activities described as part of "identify possible solutions" to gather more data or clarify. Coalition building also continues throughout the process.	For this example, requiring a minimum ratio is selected as the solution. (This does not indicate that it is the best solution but is just used for an example in this scenario.) A law is drafted by the Senator based on information gathered during the first phases of the process. The Senator will need to gain additional support in the Senate and then in the House of Representatives to get the law supported by a Representative(s). The law will wind its way through the legislative process.
Implement policy	Rules and regulations are developed; staff receive feedback on rules and regulations; and implement rules and regulations to apply the law.	DHHS develops draft of rules and regulations that will be used to implement the law. Professional organizations respond to them by providing feedback. The American Hospital Association submits criticisms. Rules and regulations are revised and may be posted for additional comments. By specific date, rules and regulations are effective and required by law. Hospitals will have to get this information and make appropriate changes to meet requirements (e.g., increase staffing or alter ratios, recruit more staff, and so on).
Monitor outcomes: evaluation	Federal department or agency responsible for implementation develops evaluation plan and monitors outcomes. The department may have to report to Congress at specific times, and may recommend and implement changes as long as within framework of the law. Otherwise, the department will need to recommend legislative changes (new law or amendments to law).	Outcomes analysis is ongoing. What are the outcomes of the plan to establish a minimum staffing ratio? Are hospitals able to meet the requirement deadlines? If not, what are the barriers? Can the barriers be addressed and how?

Source: Author.

what will be the end product? The new health care environment demands that providers take responsibility for whole populations. The focus is not just on curing patients but also preventing illness and providing care across the health care continuum. High-quality care must be provided in all types of settings and by all providers, and it must be cost-effective. Health care professionals need to develop new skills, competencies, and attitudes toward their work in order to reinvent their professional culture. Nursing has recognized this change by including more content about community health in nursing education.

3. The increase in direct reimbursement for care provided by advanced practice nurses is an excellent example of the impact of legislation and government on nursing practice.

4. The federal government provided additional funding for nursing education, something that is a major concern each year as the federal budget is developed, when they passed the Nurse Reinvestment Act of 2003. State legislation has also had a major impact on nursing practice. This legislation offers many opportunities to pilot new programs in education and delivery.

A recent example of a health policy change that has had a major impact on health care delivery in California is the passage of legislation that requires California hospitals to meet fixed nurse–patient ratios (Purdum, 1999). This policy is affecting health policy in other states and on the federal level, as similar legislation is considered. Health care issues that are affected by nursing, and few are not, require nursing input if nursing is to remain a viable health care profession in the health care environment.

Nurse participation in health care policy development

How can nurses participate in health care policy development? Active participation in nursing organizations gives every nurse a voice, as nursing organizations are often represented on committees that develop health care policy or provide input (for example, the President's Advisory Commission on Consumer Protection and Quality in the Health Care Industry, 1996–1998, and the recent Institute of Medicine reports on quality and safety in health care (see Chapter 16). Nursing organizations use **lobbyists** to make regular contact with elected officials, both state and federal, in order to influence policy development. In fact, some of these lobbyists are nurses. Each year, the American Nurses Association (ANA) identifies key issues that it will focus on as it lobbies Congress. Typical issues include: nurse staffing plans and ratios, mandatory overtime, nurse education incentives and funding, needlestick protection, advanced practice Medicaid reimbursement, whistleblower protection, ergonomics, nursing workforce data, latex allergies, continued competence, unlicensed assistive personnel, violence in the workplace, and immigration and the nursing workforce. These issues have a direct impact on practice.

CURRENT ISSUES

Learn about events around the globe that relate to the chapter content.

Individual nurses are encouraged to contact their own elected representatives by mail, e-mail, or telephone and provide them with important information about nursing and health care needs in their communities. Nursing expertise has been very beneficial to policy makers, but if nurses do not speak out, they will not be recognized for their expertise. ANA testimony was provided in 1998 to the National Bipartisan Commission on the Future of Medicare, a commission designed to identify how to strengthen Medicare (Gross & Reed, 1999). Nursing expertise was also provided when the president of the ANA testified before a Senate committee about the relationship between staffing decisions and patient safety (Gross & Reed, 1999). This testimony was related to the release of the government-initiated report, *To Err Is Human. Building a Safer Health System* (Institute of Medicine, 2000). There are many examples of nurses representing many nursing organizations by providing testimony on the local, state, and federal levels.

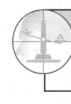

THINK CRITICALLY

Try this exercise to apply what you have learned about this topic.

Understanding consumer needs and acting as the patient's advocate have been important elements of nursing for a long time. Nurses can help consumers understand health care policy, legislation, regulation, and their effect on health care delivery. There should be no doubt that every nurse has a role to play. It may be in writing a letter to a member of Congress, calling a senator, attending a nursing organization meeting, providing expert testimony, serving on a local or state health care planning committee, or participating in other types of activities to influence policy development.

Importance of collaboration in health care policy

Concern over health care changes, policy, and managed care has even brought nurses and physicians closer as they work collaboratively for a common goal: better-quality care. This is a positive result of managed care—nurses and physicians talking with one another to solve problems such as staff cutbacks, quality issues, patients' rights, and ethical concerns. An example of a collaborative effort is one that began in Massachusetts in 1997 (American Nurses Association, 1998). Nurses and physicians formed the Ad Hoc Committee to Defend Health Care Plans. This group provides an arena for dialogue. They have held teach-ins, conferences, and other events to stimulate debate among health care professionals and the public, and are united against the corporatization of health care. This collaboration is an opportunity for nurses to provide their valuable input and to serve as leaders in this effort to improve patient care. The Ad Hoc Committee identified the following principles for health care reform.

- Medicine and nursing must not be diverted from their primary tasks: the relief of suffering, the prevention and treatment of illness, and the promotion of health. The efficient deployment of resources is critical but must not detract from these goals.
- The pursuit of corporate profit and personal fortune have no place in caregiving.
- Potent financial incentives that reward "overcare" or "undercare" weaken doctor–patient and nurse–patient bonds and should be prohibited. Similarly, business arrangements that allow corporations and employers to control the care of patients should be proscribed.
- A patient's right to a physician of choice must not be curtailed.
- Access to medical and nursing care must be the right of all (Himmelstein & Lown 1997, p. 1738).

Reviewing some of the key policy issues that have been discussed in this chapter indicates that these health care reform principles are related to many of the policy issues.

Nursing has been in the forefront of consumer education, so the principles for health care reform as described should not be foreign to nursing. An example of nursing's role in consumer activism is the ANA's initiative, "Every Patient Deserves a Nurse," which provided the public with information about the critical staffing issues in health care organizations and the role of nurses. The ANA also collaborated with Johnson & Johnson to develop a media campaign to address the need for more nurses. Nurses recognize the need to further develop the image of nursing and that combining communication skills, consumer education, and media expertise will help to improve the image. Sometimes this will mean collaborating with others such as physicians to initiate a broader media impact that affects the profession's image as a member of the interdisciplinary team, and at other times, it will mean focusing just on nursing and what nurses can do. Collaboration will be needed as health care professionals participate in health care changes. New ways to support collaboration need to be created.

Legislation: Impact on health care delivery and policy

What is the important health care legislation, both federal and state, and how has this legislation affected health care delivery? Legislation is a part of health policy and also has a direct impact on legal and ethical issues in health care delivery. Legislation occurs at three levels in the government: federal, state, and local. Most health care legislation is found at the federal and state levels, so these two levels will be the focus in this chapter. Nurses should, however, be aware of relevant local legislation that might be passed by cities or counties.

Federal level

The federal legislative process is clearly defined and is important to nursing. The American Nurses Association (ANA) website includes a description of the process so that it can be used by nurses as they become involved in policy development (http://www.nursingworld.org). The political action component of the ANA is very active in influencing health policy and monitoring legislation.

When legislation passes into law, the work is not done. Most legislation establishes or modifies federal or state programs. When this occurs, the administrative responsibility of a federal or state law becomes the responsibility of a federal or state agency, program, or department. An example is the Department of Health and Human Services (DHHS), which is responsible for implementation of Medicare law. Before a law is implemented, regulations are developed. Regulations are critical because they describe how the law will work, and they can make a difference in the success of the law's implementation. In the federal arena, draft regulations are published in the *Federal Register*, which makes the regulations available for public comment. In some cases, public hearings are held to discuss the regulations. When health care legislation and its regulations are important to nurses, representatives from nursing organizations often comment on regulation drafts. In addition, nurses may have participated earlier in the health care policy development, such as by providing expert testimony to Congressional committees, lobbying efforts, and so forth. Regulations can affect staffing, health care organization policies and procedures, access to care, and other delivery issues. All comments about regulations are considered, and then the agency/program/department releases the final regulations. This occurs at least 30 days prior to the effective date of application. After that date, the law and its regulations are in effect.

Understanding the history of critical health care legislation, relationships between laws, and their effect on the delivery system is very important for all health care professionals who hope to participate in future health care policy development and implementation. There is no doubt that remaining current with federal legislation can be a time-consuming activity, which is why nursing organizations have lobbyists who follow legislation and provide input, as well as political action committees (PACs), to influence the policy making and election processes. There are many more options that could be explored. As nurses enter practice, relevant laws to their practice should be understood. With access to the Internet, it is easier to keep current with health care legislation.

What are the critical federal legislation and regulation actions related to health care delivery in the United States? The two pieces of legislation and their amendments that have had the most impact on the health and welfare system in the United States are the Social Security Act of 1935 and the Public Health Act of 1944. The changes and additions to these laws demonstrate the long-term effect that laws can have on society. "The financing and delivery of health care is so connected with the public interest that there also must be public accountability. Government has a basic responsibility to ensure that health plans and providers are qualified and operate in the public interest" (Zatkin, 1997, p. 33). Passing legislation should not be taken lightly because it may not be easy to reverse and has a major impact on citizens/consumers. Accountability and responsibility are critical components of the legislative process.

CURRENT ISSUES

Learn about events around the globe that relate to the chapter content.

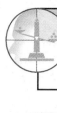

THINK CRITICALLY

Try this exercise to apply what you have learned about this topic.

THINK CRITICALLY

Try this exercise to apply what you have learned about this topic.

State level

States play an active role in health care policy, legislation, and regulation. Generally, they are involved in financing, delivery of services, and oversight of insurance. The latter has become very important as managed care has grown. There are five typical health care areas in which the states have major input.

1. **Public health and safety.** States are responsible for protecting public welfare, including services related to such areas as prevention and treatment of communicable diseases, monitoring of environmental health conditions, harm from violence, and workplace accidents.
2. **Provision of indigent care.** Most state constitutions require that the state, either alone or with local governments, provide health care to those who cannot pay for it. This is usually done through state or local government-run facilities and the Medicaid program. This care changes as health care policy, delivery, and reimbursement change.
3. **Purchase care.** Many states have been changing from providers of health care to purchasers of care. This is particularly relevant for the Medicaid program and for state public employees for whom the state provides insurance coverage. This requires that states monitor the care they purchase from MCOs.
4. **Regulation.** States are responsible for licensing and/or credentialing facilities and professionals to ensure quality and for regulating insurers. There is increasing regulation of health care services, including quality assurance, utilization review, solvency, benefits, marketing, access to services, provider contracting, rating, grievances and appeals, organizational structure, reporting, and confidentiality (Knight, 1998). These activities demonstrate the major role that states have in the regulation of insurers.
5. **Resource allocation.** Typically, states have not been responsible for funding of medical and nursing education because this has been in federal hands, although this does not exclude greater state involvement in the future due to the growing staff shortage. States are, however, more involved in identifying state health care delivery needs (e.g., number of health care professionals that a state needs to graduate to meet state health care needs). Some states still assist in funding some public health care facilities. Due to the California legislation in 2002 that directed the California state health department to develop staffing guidelines, many other states are considering doing something similar, which means the states will be more involved in health resource allocation (Robert Wood Johnson Foundation, 1997, p. 20).

States have their own process for developing, passing, and implementing their laws and procedures related to its regulation process, although this process is usually similar to the federal process. Nurses need to understand their own state process and participate when content is relevant to nursing. Nurses are usually even more involved in the process at the state level than at the federal level. The state nurses' association is often the major player. State activities are more accessible to nurses for lobbying, support of candidates, involvement in committees, and personal contact with legislators. Often nurses feel less intimidated by the state level than the federal level.

In conclusion, Table 10-1 provides a description of the relationship between the policy process and the legislative process.

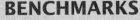

BENCHMARKS

Now let's take a moment to test your knowledge of the concepts you have studied in this section.

Legal Issues and Nursing

Each nurse confronts legal issues daily in practice, although often it may not be done obviously. Administering medication, restraining patients, protecting patients from falls, or observing a patient on suicide precautions all have a legal component. Documentation is critical to any legal issue that may arise in the clinical setting. The statement "if it isn't documented it didn't happen" is highly relevant to any malpractice suit. What do nurses need to know about the legal issues? They certainly do not have to be attorneys, and they should seek the advice of an attorney whenever they are involved in a serious legal issue. Some issues, however, bear some review so that nurses have a basic understanding of the critical issues. Prior to reviewing these issues, it is important to distinguish the difference between law and ethics. Law is the formal organization of societal values that are demonstrated through laws that are passed and then implemented on the local, state, and federal level, and in some cases, even internationally. Ethics focuses on what ought to be done in relation to what is done. This chapter also discusses some aspects of ethics in relation to health care delivery in a later section. Understanding legal issues is important for any nurse in practice and for nurses who are leaders.

Basic legal terminology

Laws are developed and implemented through organizations within society. State legislatures or the Congress, as well as state and local governments, develop these laws. They are then implemented by state and federal law enforcement agencies or other agencies such as the state board of nursing. There are several types of laws.

1. Common laws are rules and principles that were derived from past legal decisions that were developed in England and then brought to the United States.
2. Criminal law concerns offenses against the general public, and response is directed at deterrence, punishment, and/or rehabilitation of the person who committed the crime. Examples of behavior or actions that relate to this law would be murder, robbery, and rape. Criminal law can also apply to health care situations as it covers assault and battery, which can occur in the health care setting.
3. **Civil law** concerns the rights of individuals, and remedies typically involve payment of money or some type of compensation. An area of civil law that most concerns nurses is tort law as it includes negligence, personal injury, and medical malpractice.

The following provides information about basic legal terms that are important for the nurse to understand.

1. Negligence and malpractice are terms that are not uncommon for nurses to hear. What is the difference between malpractice and negligence?
   - "**Negligence** is a general term that denotes conduct lacking in due care. Thus, negligence equates with carelessness. . . . **Malpractice** is a more specific term and looks at a professional standard of care as well as the professional status of the caregiver . . . the failure of a professional person to act in accordance with the prevailing professional standards or failure to foresee consequences that a professional person, having the necessary skills and education, should foresee" (Guido, 2001, p. 79). Negligence is the failure to act as an ordinary prudent person would under similar circumstances. This is based on that person's education and training.
   - The standard in negligence is average level of care. A variety of sources for standards exist (for example, expert witness testimony, accreditation requirements, publications by experts, clinical practice guidelines or pathways, statutes and regulations, advertising for services, contracts, and professional standards).

BOX 10-4   Elements of negligence.

> 1. There was a duty owed to the patient.
> 2. There was a breach of duty or standard by the health care professional.
> 3. There was harm caused by the breach of duty or standard.
> 4. The person (plaintiff) experienced damages or injuries.

- To prove negligence there are four elements that must be met, which are described in Box 10-4.
- Damages or injuries may be physical, emotional, loss of job, loss of present and/or future earnings, disfigurement, disability, pain and suffering, loss of enjoyment of life, and so on.
- Negligence can be unintentional (when no harm was intended) or intentional (for example, invasion of privacy or false imprisonment are examples of intentional acts, although these are rare in health care). Both of these examples can occur in health care when a patient's privacy is not maintained or when a patient is held against his/her wishes without legitimate medical reasons.
- The elements that must be met for malpractice are the same as those for negligence with the emphasis on what would be expected from a professional. Some of the examples of potential risks for nurses are failure to adequately assess, monitor, and communicate; failure to act as the patient's advocate (for example, not providing patient education to a patient who has diabetes); or failure to protect a patient when the patient is suicidal or when at risk for falls. Every nurse needs to consider these risks when care is provided or when holding management positions.
- As noted earlier there are certain elements that must be proved by the plaintiff; however, there is an exception, which is called the **doctrine of *res ipsa loquitor***, which means that the "thing speaks for itself." This rule of evidence indicates that although one may not be able to prove that an individual did something to cause harm or injury, because there is harm or injury, the negligence can be inferred.
- A question that often comes up with nurses is who is responsible for negligence: the nurse or the nurse's employer? ***Respondeat superior*** is the doctrine that says the employer may also be responsible if the nurse was functioning in the employee role at the time of the negligence in a situation where the employer controlled the nurse (Guido, 2001). This means that both the health care organization and the nurse could be sued. This is also referred to as ***vicarious liability***, which extends liability.
- Other terms of interest are assault and battery, although many nurses may not see how these apply to nursing care. **Assault** does not require physical contact, but only that the patient fears harmful contact may occur. There has to be some consideration given to timing and the fear that results, as one could not call a threat that happens several days earlier assault. **Battery** requires actual physical contact. Both of these are considered intentional torts. They are good reasons for obtaining informed consent from patients before procedures are performed, which could be assault or battery if the patient does not consent.

2. Consumer rights issues have become more and more important in health care. Consent, living wills, durable powers of attorney, and assisted suicide are some of these issues.
   - **Consent** "may be either oral, implied by law, or apparent" (Guido, 2001, p. 109). This can be as simple as the patient orally consenting to being touched by a nurse; in this case, there is no risk of battery.
   - **Consent implied by law** is consent that may occur in emergency situations when, even though the patient may not be able to provide consent for emergency treatment, emergency treatment can be given. The following elements must be met to be consent implied by law: "(1) An immediate decision is made to prevent loss of life or limb; (2) The person is incapable of giving or denying consent; (3) There is no reason to believe that consent would not be given if the patient were capable of such; and (4) A reasonable person in the same or similar circumstances would give consent" (Guido, 2001, p. 109).

■ **Informed consent** "mandates to the physician or independent health care practitioner the separate legal duty to disclose needed material facts in terms that patients can reasonably understand so that they can make an informed choice" (Guido, 2001, p. 129). It is an interactive process in that the practitioner is required to tell the patient who will perform the procedure or treatment, discuss available alternatives to the recommended treatment, and identify possible harm in language the patient can understand. Patients must be informed that they have the right to refuse treatment. If there is no informed consent, the practitioner is at risk for negligence. Informed consent can be given orally or in writing, and it can also be implied by the patient's behavior, or as noted earlier, in emergency situations it can be presumed. The physician or the independent practitioner is accountable for obtaining informed consent. So where does this leave the nurse who is not an advanced practice nurse functioning as an independent practitioner? The nurse is not accountable for obtaining the consent for every nursing action, as most routine nursing interventions are implied or there is oral consent (for example, the patient agrees to take the medication). The critical elements for the nurse are to "continually communicate with the patient, explaining procedures, and obtaining the patient's permission. What it also means is that the patient's refusal to allow a certain procedure must be respected" (Guido, 2001, p. 135). A nurse is not required to obtain informed consent for medical procedures for which the nurse is not the primary provider. Guido (2001) provides an example of a surgical patient and the nurse's responsibility for postoperative teaching that is begun before surgery. The best approach is for the nurse to wait until the patient's physician explains the procedure and obtains informed consent and then to begin patient teaching. Some hospitals and other types of health care organizations may prohibit nurses from obtaining written consent for specific procedures that are provided by other providers. It is important for each nurse to know about these prohibitions and to follow them. Physicians may legally delegate getting informed consent to a nurse; however, if a problem occurs the physician is still at risk. In this situation the nurse is also at risk (Guido, 2001).

■ Informed consent for human research is very important. Many nurses participate in research in a variety of settings such as hospitals, clinics, and research institutes. The key elements of consent for research include:
1. Nature, purpose, procedures, drugs, or devices involved
2. Identification of any experimental procedures
3. Potential benefits, risks, and discomforts to participant
4. Alternative treatments
5. Confidentiality of research records
6. Compensation if injury occurs
7. Persons to contact about rights, and what to do if research results in an injury
8. A statement indicating that research is voluntary and that withdrawal does not incur penalty (Karigan, 2001, p. 30)

■ **Living wills** "are directives from competent individuals to medical personnel and family members regarding the treatment they wish to receive when they can no longer make the decision for themselves" (Guido, 2001, p. 152). If a person is competent, a living will serves no purpose as the person can speak for himself. Several important points about living wills should be noted. They are usually not very specific; health care providers are not required by law to follow the living will, and there is no legal protection for the health care provider against civil or criminal liability.

■ The **durable power of attorney (medical power of attorney)** is another method that an individual can use to determine the type of care the individual wants. A competent person may appoint a surrogate (often several are identified in priority order) to make health care decisions for that person when the person is not able to do so. This solves some of the issues with the living will as there is a person who is actually making the decisions for the patient. Typically, individuals select someone that they trust will carry out their wishes, which are discussed while the individual is competent to do so. The surrogate does not have to be a family member although it is highly advisable that persons inform their family about these documents and decisions prior to needing them. Recent research indicates that despite having advance directives surrogates tend to make decisions of overtreatment (Ditto et al., 2001). In another study nurses looked at the stress that family members experience when they make decisions about withdrawing treatment (Tilden et al., 2001). All experienced stress; however, those who had advance directives, either oral or written, experienced less stress.

- The Patient Self-Determination Act of 1990 was initiated due to the need to resolve issues around these documents (Guido, 2001). Patients must now be asked by health care providers if they have living wills and durable powers of attorney or advance directives. The goal of this law is to make individuals more aware of their rights and the importance of making informed decisions that give some consideration to costs of care. Nurses must follow their organization's policies and procedures related to any of these issues.

- A **do-not-resuscitate (DNR) directive** is another form of advance directive that patients may request when they are receiving care (Guido, 2001). The physician may be implementing advance directives when writing a DNR order, but DNR orders can be written without an advance directive (Staten, 2000). Family members should also be consulted to prevent increasing family stress and possible legal actions. Health care organizations have policies and procedures to follow when patients request DNR, which should be followed. Usually there must be some discussion between the physician and patient, when the patient is able, about the decision, and there are specific intervals for reevaluation. With all of these issues related to treatment it is critical that nurses contribute by assessing the patient and communicating effectively with the patient, family, and physician. End-of-life decisions are not easy to discuss. The nurse is often in a position to discuss these critical issues; however, the physician should also be involved in the process. What happens if a patient's preferences are disregarded (Habel, 2001)? The nurse should contact the organization's ethics committee, which many health care organizations have. In doing this, the nurse acts as the patient's advocate. The nurse, of course, needs to be aware of state laws and requirements related to these serious decisions.

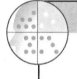

YOUR OPINION COUNTS

Find out what others think about this topic. Post your response and check out other opinions.

- Assisted suicide is another patient rights issue that has become more important; however, this one is much more complex. States typically have laws related to this popular topic in the media. The American Nurses Association opposes any nursing participation in assisted suicide, as this would violate the ANA *Code for Nurses* (2001) (ANA, 1994a, 1994b). Any concerns about potential assisted suicide should be reported to management staff and to the organization's ethics committee.

In conclusion, "nurses have an ethical and legal obligation to provide safe patient care, to maintain competency, and to identify those situations where the provision of safe care is jeopardized. Without a doubt, malpractice is a preventable problem" (Morris, 2002, p. 16). How can lawsuits be prevented, as many occur even when quality care was provided? Why do patients sue health care providers (Mock, 2001)? Many patients who sue are angry with one or more of their health care providers, perhaps about not being told what they needed to learn, lack of respect, or they may feel that they received substandard care. It is very important to understand the patient's perception as this helps explain why a lawsuit has been filed. Beckman et al. (1994) conducted a study of depositions, which are the statements that are made by witnesses (e.g., patient, family, expert witnesses, those being sued or the defendants, and so on) under oath before a case goes to trial. In 71% of the cases there were "problematic relationship issues." How can this be prevented? Since patients feel that caring was missing, providing care with a caring attitude goes a long way in preventing lawsuits. Effective communication must be part of the relationship. Effective leadership is also critical—understanding and applying legal principles while providing care and guiding others as they provide care such as UAPs and LPNs or other team members. Keys to success are connecting with the patient, appreciating the patient's situation, responding to the patient's needs, and empowering the patient (Mock, 2001).

Patient privacy: The law expands

"It has been foundational, at least since Hipporcrates, that patients have a right to have personal medical information kept private. . . . The chief public-policy rationale is that patients are unlikely to disclose intimate details that are necessary for their proper medical care to their physicians unless they trust their physicians to keep that information secret" (Annas, 2003, p. 1486). Regulations about patient privacy were added to HIPAA and went into effect in April, 2003. This established the first comprehensive federal standards for medical privacy related to the medical record or any identifiable information about the patient (Pear, 2002, August, p. A1).

Each nurse needs to be aware of and follow the policies and procedures related to oral, written, or electronic patient identifiable data set up by the health care organization regarding issues where the nurse practices; however, there are some key areas that are affected by these new privacy regulations.

- Patients must be informed of their privacy rights.
- Patients must be informed as to who will see their records and for what purpose.
- Patients have the right to inspect and obtain a copy of their medical records. (There are some exceptions to this that each organization should make clear to staff.)
- Valid authorization to release health information must contain certain information, such as a copy of the signed authorization given to the patient, in understandable language, and how the patient may revoke authorization.
- Although information may be used for research purposes to assess outbreak of a disease, all individual identifiable data must be removed.
- Personal data may not be used for marketing (for example, pharmacies may not share this information with others for this purpose).

These privacy standards are complex and require health care organizations to make changes in how they manage information. It also requires that staff are trained and updated about the changes. The standards give patients more control while at the same time make providers more accountable for keeping information private. This is federal law, but if a state has more rigorous privacy requirements then the state requirements would have to be followed.

BENCHMARKS

Now let's take a moment to test your knowledge of the concepts you have studied in this section.

Ethics: Impact on Decision Making, Planning, and Practice

Ethics is interwoven throughout health care policy development, implementation, and legal issues that arise during the delivery of health care. Nurses cannot avoid ethical issues and need to understand ethical decision making. Leadership competencies are related to ethics; for example, decision making often includes ethical issues. Implementing health policies may require consideration of ethics.

Ethical decision making

"An ethical dilemma is a difficult moral problem that involves two or more mutually exclusive, morally correct courses of action. Health care organizations are frequently confronted with two

FIGURE 10-5   Ethical decision making.

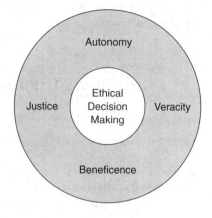

Source: Author.

key questions: "What is fair?" and "What is the right and just thing to do?" (Koloroutis & Thorstenson, 1999, p. 13). These are not easy questions to answer, and each situation is different. Organizations need to integrate an ethical framework into their daily operations and require leaders to lead by example. It is important to recognize that "articulated values have no meaning or use if they are not demonstrated in the lives of organizational members" (Koloroutis & Thorstenson, 1999, p. 16). Individual nurses and other health care providers must also deal with these critical questions when confronted with ethical issues.

Four primary principles, as described in Figure 10-5, are used to make ethical decisions: autonomy, beneficence, justice, and veracity (Chally & Loriz, 1998).

1. **Autonomy** is a principle that has always been important to nurses. Patients have the right to determine their own rights.
2. The second ethical principle is **beneficence**, or doing something good. Nurses are to inflict no harm and to safeguard the patient.
3. Patients should also be treated fairly or with **justice**. This, of course, is a problem when decisions are made as to which patients will receive treatment.
4. The fourth primary principle is **veracity**. Truth telling is critical for effective patient communication and developing trust with the patient. Informed consent is one example of a potential ethical problem that may be affected by veracity. If incomplete information is not shared with a patient, then veracity has not been met.

Koloroutis and Thorstenson (1999), however, suggest that the traditional guiding ethical principles of autonomy, beneficence, justice, and veracity probably will not be as helpful in the new health care environment that is so strongly affected by managed care. For example, autonomy is applicable with middle class Caucasian values but not with African Americans who rely more on family collective decision making. Multicultural issues are important, and they may limit the application of the four major ethical principles. Caring, advocacy, stewardship or management of finite resources, respect, honesty, and confidentiality are more relevant to this new ethical framework and require an appreciation of the impact of diversity. In the new health care environment, most of the ethical dilemmas fall into three categories: clinical, managed care or reimbursement, and general or organizational. Some examples of these dilemmas include:

- **Clinical.** Dehumanization of care due to resource constraints, end-of-life decisions, lack of informed consent and shared decision making, lack of coherent treatment plan, and lack of privacy and confidentiality in the provider–patient relationship.
- **Managed care (reimbursement).** Financial incentives, undefined role of the consumer, provider reimbursement strategies to encourage providers to provide less-than-optimum care, member confidentiality, and lack of consistency regarding coverage of investigational treatments.

■ **General organizational.** Discontinuation of services due to inadequate reimbursement, business transactions that lead to internal conflicts, and failure of management to communicate and discuss important decisions (Koloroutis & Thorstenson, 1999, p. 13).

Knowing what is right and then doing what is right can be very difficult, as sometimes it is even difficult to determine what is right (American Nurses Association, 1994a; Erlen & Mellors, 1995). When a nurse is faced with an ethical dilemma related to a clinical or a management problem, the critical questions that need to be considered during decision making are:

■ Who are the people involved? Are they directly or indirectly involved? What are their histories and involvement in the situation?
■ Who should decide and why?
■ What are the causes and consequences?
■ For whom is the decision being made?
■ What degree and type of patient consent is required?
■ What is the problem?
■ How does the problem relate to personal and professional ethical codes?
■ What are the alternative solutions?
■ What are the costs and benefits of each possible solution?
■ Who will receive the benefits? Who will pay the costs? (Costs can be more than financial.)
■ What are the probable implications or consequences of the chosen decision (Aroskar, 1980, p. 660)?

Each of these questions requires thought and data. Discussing them with peers or team members can be very helpful, which provides additional information and support and facilitates more effective decision making.

As has been discussed, professional organizations play an important role in policy making and legislation at the local, state, and federal levels, but they are also important in defining professional standards and ethics, such as the guidelines found in Box 10-2. The ANA's *Code for Nurses with Interpretive Statements* (2001) is the primary resource for nursing ethical guidance. "Individuals who become nurses are expected not only to adhere to the ideals and moral norms of the profession but also to embrace them as part of what it means to be a nurse. The ethical tradition of nursing is self-reflective, enduring, and distinctive. A code of ethics makes explicit the primary goals, values, and obligations of the profession" (American Nurses Association, 2001, p. 5). The *Code* is described in Box 10-5.

The appropriate allocation of scarce resources while reducing costs is a complex problem that is repeated every day in health care organizations. Bantz, Wieske, and Horowitz (1999) conducted a survey of nurse executives representing 100 hospitals across the United States to identify nurse executives' beliefs about ethical–economic issues that they or their staff encounter or may encounter. This sample of nurse executives did not think that there had been an overall reduction in nurse staff positions or increased risk of complications for patients. This result is surprising since more recent data indicates that these problems did exist in 1999 and today; however, "the responses may reflect an increase in the number of extra hours other nurses are working over their contracted hours to ensure patients receive the care they need" (Bantz, Wieske, & Horowitz, 1999, p. 87). These hours do have an effect on the nursing positions that were eliminated. Staff nurses, however, who had been surveyed prior to the nurse executive survey felt that patients were at greater risk. This result may reflect the different perspectives of nurses who provide direct care and those who do not. It is a major concern if nurse executives do not recognize a problem that staff nurses believe exists. This differing of views can lead to low morale or potential exacerbation of a morale problem. If nurses do not believe that their leaders recognize staff problems, this is a major problem for the profession because nurse executives represent the nursing staff in the administrative decision-making process.

Other ethical questions that were addressed in the nurse executive survey related to the care of the medically indigent. Nurse executives felt that this care should be provided; however, they were not willing to pay more taxes to cover this care, although some did indicate that they would

BOX 10-5   Code of ethics for nurses.

Provision 1

The nurse, in all professional relationships, practices with compassion and respect for the inherent dignity, worth, and uniqueness of every individual, unrestricted by considerations of social or economic status, personal attributes, or the nature of health problems.

- Respect for human dignity
- Relationships to patients
- The nature of health problems
- The right to self-determination
- Relationships with colleagues and others

Provision 2

The nurse's primary commitment is to the patient, whether an individual, family, group, or community.

- Primacy of the patient's interests
- Conflict of interest for nurses
- Collaboration
- Professional boundaries

Provision 3

The nurse promotes, advocates for, and strives to protect the health, safety, and rights of the patient.

- Privacy
- Confidentiality
- Protection of participants in research
- Standards and review mechanism
- Acting on questionable practice
- Addressing impaired practice

Provision 4

The nurse is responsible and accountable for individual nursing practice and determines the appropriate delegation of tasks consistent with the nurse's obligation to provide optimum patient care.

- Acceptance of accountability and responsibility
- Accountability for nursing judgment and action
- Responsibility for nursing judgment and action
- Delegation of nursing activities

Provision 5

The nurse owes the same duties to self as to others, including the responsibility to preserve integrity and safety, to maintain competence, and to continue personal and professional growth.

- Moral self-respect
- Professional growth and maintenance of competence
- Wholeness of character
- Preservation of integrity

Provision 6

The nurse participates in establishing, maintaining, and improving health care environments and conditions of employment conducive to the provision of quality health care and consistent with the values of the profession through individual and collective action.

- Influence of the environment on moral virtues and values
- Influence of the environment on ethical obligations
- Responsibility for the health care environment

BOX 10-5 Code of ethics for nurses. *(continued)*

Provision 7

The nurse participates in the advancement of the profession through contributions to practice, education, administration, and knowledge development.

- Advancing the profession through active involvement in nursing and in health care policy
- Advancing the profession by developing, maintaining, and implementing professional standards in clinical, administrative, and educational practice
- Advancing the profession through knowledge development, dissemination, and application to practice

---

Provision 8

The nurse collaborates with other health professionals and the public in promoting community, national, and international efforts to meet health needs.

- Health needs and concerns
- Responsibilities to the public

Provision 9

The profession of nursing, as represented by associations and their members, is responsible for articulating nursing values, for maintaining the integrity of the profession and its practice, and for shaping social policy.

- Assertion of values
- The profession carries out its collective responsibility through professional associations
- Intraprofessional integrity
- Social reform

Source: American Nurses Association. (2001). *Code for Nurses* with interpretive statements; quote 9 provisions with no interpretive statement. Washington, DC: American Nurses Publishing. Reprinted with permission.

---

donate time to provide some of this care. When asked about equality in health care, the nurse executives agreed that there should be equality, but when asked to apply this to specific case examples (e.g., age, condition, compliance), they did not agree on equal allocation of health care resources. The results of this survey are troubling because they indicate major differences in how nurse executives and nursing staff view the health care environment and its problems regarding ethical responsibility. To be effective as patient advocates and to participate in health care policy development in a difficult ethical period, nurses need to have greater agreement about the needs and problems than this survey supports.

Professional ethics

Professional ethics applies to both nursing management and clinical issues. Several nursing studies have been conducted about nursing ethics, including the one previously described. Another study that was conducted in 1994, but is still relevant today, asked nurse administrators to identify decisions that had represented ethical dilemmas for them. The following were considered important in rank order, with the first decision occurring most frequently:

1. Staffing levels and mix situations
2. Developing/maintaining standards of care
3. Allocating/rationing of scarce resources
4. Incompetent physicians
5. Demotion/termination of employees
6. Employee relations
7. Incompetent nurses
8. Selection/hiring of employees
9. Treatment versus non-treatment

10. Promotion of employees
11. Diversification of services
12. Downsizing services
13. Access to care for the indigent
14. Marketing/advertising services
15. Labor negotiations with nurses (Borawski, 1995, p. 61)

These issues indicate that nurses struggle with many situations that place them in an ethical dilemma (e.g., what to do and how to do it right). Today, these issues continue to present ethical dilemmas for nurses as practitioners and leaders.

At the 1996 American Nurses Association (ANA) convention, another survey was completed that included 1,137 nurses from all over the country (Scanlon, 1996–1997). In the survey, 37% of the nurses said they confronted ethical issues weekly, and 32% reported them daily. These are high percentages and further indicate that ethical dilemmas have been routine problems for nurses. More than half of the nurses worked in organizations that had interdisciplinary ethics committees. The five issues that they encountered the most were:

1. Cost-containment issues that jeopardized patient welfare
2. End-of-life decisions
3. Informed consent
4. Incompetent, unethical, or illegal practices of colleagues
5. Access to health care

Nurses continued to confront ethical dilemmas in all practice settings and a wide variety of locations, and they felt unprepared to cope with ethical dilemmas. Among nurses, 76% felt that the ability of nurses to act as the patient's advocate had been limited, while 64% felt that financial incentives created conflicts of interest that negatively impacted patient care. These last two findings are very troubling and indicate a changing health care environment that constrains professional roles and responsibilities, leaving health care professionals feeling powerless. What avenues of response to major ethical issues are available to nurses?

Making complaints to the board of nursing

Each state board of nursing has the responsibility to protect the public health in its state. Nurses who are licensed in a state can and should make complaints to the board when they are concerned about patient health and safety. In the late 1980s and early 1990s, Texas experienced major psychiatric health care fraud and abuse problems in some for-profit psychiatric hospitals, which is discussed in more detail later in this section. Some psychiatric nurses said they contacted their board and did not receive assistance (Mohr, 1996, 1997). Boards of nursing must be responsive, or they will find that nurses will not bother to contact them.

Leadership is required of all nurses, even those on boards of nursing. A leader is able to confront difficult issues and take risks, which is what the nurses did who reported problems. All nurses should be knowledgeable about their state's practice act and use this law and its related rules and regulations as a guide in making decisions about issues and complaints to the board (ANA, 1994a). If nurses have any concerns about legal issues and personal professional liability, consulting an attorney is also suggested. Boards of nursing have a specific process for reviewing complaints. During the investigation period, boards do not reveal the source of a complaint. Nurses can obtain information about complaint procedures from their board of nursing. The ANA's *Guidelines on Reporting Incompetent, Unethical, or Illegal Practice* (1994a) assists nurses when they confront these issues and was described in Box 10-1.

Managed care organizations and ethics

The medical industry struggles with medical and business ethical issues daily, and nurses are also confronting more and more ethical dilemmas due to these struggles. Managed care has had a major impact on health care delivery, with health care organizations and providers facing conflicts between MCO financial incentives and the MCO mission (or potential ethical duty) to provide appropriate care. Managed care organizations now play a significant role in the medical industry.

The truth of the matter is that MCOs are businesses. It is recognized that some MCOs are "good" ones, and this must imply that some type of standard has been used to compare one with the other to arrive at this conclusion. Are there standards? Can conflicts between business ethics and medical ethics within the same organization be resolved? Health care professionals want to apply medical ethics to MCOs or third-party payers and the reimbursement process because MCOs deliver medical care, which is viewed by many as being somewhat different from other business "products." Do the same ethical obligations that apply to health care professionals also apply to MCOs? Business ethics that promote fair competition—people are free to make voluntary choices to buy or sell goods or services—do not fully apply to the managed care business. Patients are not always free to choose their insurance or their provider or they may have limits placed on these decisions (Mariner, 1995). Investor-owned (for-profit) MCOs have a very important relationship with their stockholders, who expect a financial return on their investment in the MCO, and the same is true of investor-owned health care provider organizations (e.g., hospitals, clinics, home care agencies, long-term care facilities). These organizations will always experience conflicts between their business needs to control costs to meet their budgetary requirements and their contractual obligations to provide health care services to the purchasers of their services, typically the employer and their stockholders.

The relationship between the MCO and the patient/enrollee is a contractual one. The MCO is responsible only for meeting the requirements of the health plan contract, and there is no requirement that all contracts must be the same. Inequality in contracts and benefits is present in managed care, and this is not considered to be an ethical problem. Lack of choice is a common complaint about managed care; however, the very nature of managed care denies choice. "If care is managed, then, by definition, the patient is not free to choose what care he or she gets. . . . The purpose of managing care is to eliminate choices that are wasteful, harmful, or too expensive" (Mariner, 1995, p. 236). Choice comes into play in the patient/enrollee's decision to join a health plan, and even that is limited by the employer's selection of plans. Patients rarely have complete information about the plan when they join, and many do not really become interested in these details until they need services. The ideal would be the patient/enrollee who reviews each health plan option, including all of the details related to benefits, providers, outcome data, and the like, and decides on the best plan based on the individual's and his or her dependents' health status and needs. Choice is more operable in this scenario, but this rarely occurs.

If one could identify ethical standards for MCOs, these standards would include MCO accountability for the scope and quality of the patient care delivered, fairness, honesty, truthfulness, respect for persons, and justice. These standards, however, may be difficult to meet. For example, allocation of resources may conflict with many of these standards. If an MCO must ensure that all of its enrollees receive care, there will be decisions to make that will be unfair or unjust for some enrollees, but fair and just for others. Patient satisfaction is directly affected by decisions that the MCO makes, and sometimes MCOs make decisions that dissatisfy enrollees but meet the MCO's financial goals. The MCO makes a choice and decides what will bring it the most benefit; however, this is a delicate decision because patient satisfaction is also very important to MCO survival. Too much patient dissatisfaction can lead to the loss of employer health contracts.

YOUR OPINION COUNTS

Find out what others think about this topic. Post your response and check out other opinions.

Health care rationing

Health care rationing has become a topic of considerable interest (Wielawski, 1998). This is not to say that the health care system has not experienced rationing of health care resources in the past because rationing has been used. Actually, there was a time when rationing was more the norm, but the patient played a critical role. Prior to the days of insurance, patients rationed their own care and served as their own gatekeepers. As patients were financially responsible for their own care, they rationed services for themselves and their families, aided by a physician with whom they shared strong community, and often personal, ties. These physicians realized that any care provided beyond the financial means of the patient was, and would probably remain, uncompensated care (Randall, 1994). An example of rationing today is organ donation programs that allocate organs to patients based on identified criteria. Another example was Oregon's rationing system for Medicaid patients. This system prioritized diagnoses that would receive reimbursement; however, the system experienced problems. "The state has abandoned its promise of universal care. Doctors routinely find ways to get around the rationing. And conflicts with federal Medicaid regulators have impeded efforts to deny more treatments" (Kilborn, 1999, January 3, A1). Due to the problems that Oregon has encountered with its system over the 5 years of implementation, Oregon is reevaluating it. No other state has developed a rationing system similar to Oregon's.

Resource allocation is a more acceptable term for rationing. Resource allocation is necessary and inevitable in some form due to excessive health care costs and limited resources. The key question is how it should be done. Bedside rationing occurs when the individual physician declines to administer beneficial treatments because of costs that will be incurred by the insurer or services the insurer will not cover (Hall & Berenson, 1998). Is this preferable to having a rationing or resource allocation system that is centralized and bureaucratic with many rules? Is this more equitable, impartial, visible, and predictable? These are difficult questions for which there is no perfect answer. When this is applied to MCOs the view changes because managed care reimbursement focuses on the needs of the population, which is different than the traditional fee-for-service insurance plans; however, the population is only the MCO members. MCOs are generally not concerned with the greater good of the entire community, but only with decisions that affect their members. This is a major ethical dilemma that will continue to be present in the health care system.

Health care fraud and abuse

Over the past two decades health care has experienced major problems with fraud and abuse, and these have implications for nursing. Nurses have been involved in them, and it is important that nurses are aware of these situations and their outcomes, and that they consider implications for individual nurses and the profession as a whole.

Whistleblowing

The False Claims Act (FCA), was passed during the Civil War to award citizens who exposed fraud against the government; however, it became a more useful law after it was amended in 1982. How does this law relate to nursing (Canavan, 1997; Shepherd, 1998)? This is the federal law that protects whistle blowers—those who expose federal fraud. Health care fraud, as is true of most fraud, is very difficult to prove. Having people on the inside of the organization who are willing to share information is often critical to successfully prove fraud. If a nurse decides to file a suit and report fraud and the government decides to intervene in the nurse's case, the nurse is entitled to 15 to 20% of the government's ultimate recovery. If the government does not intervene with the nurse's case, and the nurse continues with the case, the nurse is entitled to 25 to 30% of the monies recovered (Polston, 1999; Shepherd, 1998). Needless to say, this is quite an incentive; however, it is not easy to report an employer. Employees have concerns about retaliation, and there is no doubt that this is a highly stressful, long, drawn-out process. Nurses have done it, though, and the FCA does provide some protections for federal cases (Canavan, 1997). If the nurse is fired, demoted, or discriminated against for these actions, he or she can bring a claim against the employer for unlawful retaliation. The nurse would be entitled to both job reinstatement and twice the amount of lost back pay. The FCA, however, applies only to federal cases, and therefore many nursing organizations and states are trying to obtain similar protective legislation for exposure of fraud within a state. When a nurse reports fraud, the nurse must be the original source of the knowledge. A nurse cannot obtain the information from a publicly disclosed source, such as a newspaper or government report, and then report it.

False claims filings in health care are increasing. In 1987, only 33 False Claims Act cases were filed nationwide by whistleblowers. The numbers have increased every year since then, reaching 221 filings in 1994 and 274 in 1995. Recoveries by the government in these cases have exploded. In 1987, the government recovered $200,000 as a result of whistleblower actions. The figure increased to $379 million in 1994, and slid back to $243 million in 1995 (Shepherd, 1998). Today it is believed that at least 10% of all government health care expenditures are procured by fraud (Hyman, 2002). This is a large percentage, representing a large amount of money wasted on unnecessary health care payments. To get an understanding of the amount of money involved, the U.S. government antifraud efforts collected $1.3 billion related to Medicare health care fraud (Department of Health and Human Services & Department of Justice, 2002). There has been much more success in recovering funds that were obtained through fraud. "From 1997 to 2000, recovery in civil fraud cases grew by more than 50 percent" (Steinhauer, 2001, p. A1). It is easy to see that there has been great growth in efforts to return funds and to charge those who have committed health care fraud.

The fraud and abuse initiative, however, has caused considerable problems for many health care organizations (Kelley, 1998). Not all who are accused of fraud and abuse are guilty. The complex, ever-changing regulations make it very difficult for organizations and their staff to keep current; consequently, it is easy to make an honest error. Calling this fraud can be a serious problem. A fraud accusation affects an organization's and its providers' reputation, and it is often difficult to erase this when an honest error is finally recognized. The number of cases has increased in the last few years, and much of this increase is due to greater efforts to discover fraud and abuse, with Congress allocating more funds to combat health care fraud and abuse.

Corporate health care fraud

"The transformation of our health care system is having several perverse effects. It is producing corporate conglomerates with billions of dollars in assets that compensate their executives as grandly as basketball players. These conglomerates are battling to control physicians in many locations and because they have cash and monopolistic power, they often succeed" (Kassirer, 1995, p. 50). At a U.S. Congressional committee meeting in 1994, the health care fraud problem was described in the following manner: "An effective antifraud program will be crucial to curing the health care crisis. Fraud is a cancer, spreading rapidly throughout our health care system. We will never, never get health care costs under control unless we do something about fraud, and waste, and abuse. The General Accounting Office estimates that 10% of our total health care expenditures, both public and private, are lost to fraud and abuse. When you consider that health care is a $1 trillion a year industry, 10% translates into $100 billion of health care fraud annually. If we could save that money, we could provide $2,500 in annual health insurance to each of the 35 million Americans who have no insurance at all" (U.S. House of Representatives, 1994, p. 1). Health care fraud has been defined by the National Health Care Anti-Fraud Association (NHCAA) as "the intentional deception or misrepresentation that an individual or entity makes when the misrepresentation could result in some unauthorized benefit to the individual, or the entity or to some other third party" (Coppola, 1997, p. 46). Health care fraud and abuse have been particularly problematic in psychiatric care, large health care corporations, and more recently in long-term care and home care.

Example: Health care fraud and abuse in psychiatric hospitals

There is no doubt that corporate health care fraud has been increasing in the last 15 years. The psychiatric health care fraud and abuse of the 1980s and 1990s provides a view of what can happen when a system confronts the care versus the bottom-line dilemma and chooses the bottom line (Mohr, 1996, 1997). During this time period, health care corporations, particularly investor-owned chains that provided psychiatric services, increased throughout the country. New hospitals were built, and hospitals were rapidly bought and sold. What happened in these hospitals? Patients were charged for care they did not receive. Patient records indicated that inappropriate care was provided, such as a large number of medications that could not have been administered in 1 day without causing detrimental effects, which indicated that the medications had not actually been administered. Patients, however, were charged for these multiple doses that never were administered. Fraudulent submissions of insurance claims were common. Patient abuse occurred when:

- Patients were admitted when they did not need to be hospitalized.
- Parents were told that their children were seriously ill when they were not.
- Patients were given medications that they did not need.
- Teenagers were abducted and admitted to the hospital.
- Patients were restrained unnecessarily and for long periods of time.
- Patients were denied their rights.
- Patients experienced verbal abuse.

These examples are only a few of the many abuses and examples of fraud from this scandal. The Federal Bureau of Investigation (FBI) conducted raids on hospitals to confiscate records and shut down computers to prevent purging of records (Rundle, 1993).

After reviewing congressional testimony, it is easy to wonder if the examples are from the late 19th century rather than the end of the 20th century (U.S. House of Representatives, 1992, 1993; U.S. Senate, 1992). Texas State Senator Michael J. Moncrief stated in one of these meetings, "In Texas, we have uncovered some of the most elaborate, aggressive, creative, deceptive, immoral, and illegal schemes being used to fill empty hospital beds with insured and paying patients" (U.S. House of Representatives, 1992, p. 7). Clearly, these health care organizations were focusing on business, using questionable business ethics, and had little concern for health care professional ethics such as the *Code for Nurses* and physician ethics.

What happened to health care professionals in these hospitals? Some staff spoke out, including nurses and physicians, but it was not uncommon for them to be threatened with job loss or to actually lose their jobs. There were threats of blacklisting and reports of false claims against employees such as use of illegal drugs to licensing boards; verbal abuse and ostracization; and other types of threats to prevent employees from reporting fraud and abuse (Mohr, 1996, 1997). Why would someone continue to work in this environment? In some cases, reporting problems to the board of nursing or state agencies did not get timely responses. Others experienced extreme stress, fear, and emotional and physical problems. In other situations, nurses felt that if they stayed and worked in the situation they might be able to help the patients who were abused, even though this typically did not happen. There were some nurses who did speak out but found it extremely stressful and painful. This example of psychiatric fraud and abuse demonstrates how easy it is for some health care organizations and individual professionals to cross the line and ignore ethical behavior. This is certainly not a positive example of what can happen when ethics are left behind, but much can be learned from it.

Example: Operation restore trust

Since the psychiatric fraud and abuse, other major health care corporations, such as Columbia/HCA, have experienced major fraud and abuse problems (Eichenwald, 1997, 1998). Federal investigations found widespread fraud, overcharges, and substandard care. The elderly are a vulnerable group in the United States, as are those with mental illness. Naturally, the vulnerable are most prone to experience the impact of fraud and abuse. When Medicare fraud and abuse occurs, the federal government can become involved because Medicare is a federal program. The psychiatric problems were exposed when patients who received Civilian Health and Medical Program of the Uniform Services (CHAMPUS) coverage, the federal program for military dependents, were abused or experienced fraud. The federal government could then become involved and use all of its related agencies such as the FBI and the General Accounting Office in the investigation. The home care Medicare fraud led to the development of a program to monitor and correct these problems called Operation Restore Trust. This program has been a burden for many home care agencies, particularly for those who have not committed fraud but made honest mistakes; however, the government is determined to correct health care fraud and abuse.

Organizational ethics

"Today, more than 500 companies have created official guardians of corporate rectitude—up from 200 just six years ago—with a mission of keeping employee conduct more upright than the law requires, if not necessarily as pure as the golden rule commands" (Kelley, 1998, p. BU1). Why all this interest in corporate ethics? Certainly, one could cite the increasing examples of health care fraud as one reason, but probably even more important was the creation of new federal sentencing guidelines in 1991. Fines were reduced for white-collar crimes if a business could demonstrate that it has a comprehensive ethics program. The Centers for Medicare and Medicaid Services established conditions of participation for providers who provide services to Medicare and Medicaid beneficiaries. The Office of Inspector General (OIG) of the Department of Health and Human Services is responsible for enforcing these rules. "In 1999, the OIG issued a model corporate compliance program for hospitals (Bartis & Sullivan, 2002, p. 67).

Since few if any hospitals do not receive these government reimbursements, most hospitals must comply. Due to these changes, health care corporate compliance committees are now more common. The quality and commitment of compliance ethics programs must, however, be monitored. Monitoring can easily be another paper process that might look good in theory but does not truly reflect the organization's culture and the behavior of its employees. Organizations must ensure that behaviors change. Some of these organizations also have ethics officers. What is their authority and how can they really effect change? These are critical questions that should be asked by organizations. It is not easy to change organizational culture, and it takes time. Is there a true commitment to improve, or is this being done to put the organization in a better legal position in case there are problems? What are some of the activities of these compliance programs?

Bartis and Sullivan (2002) describe the nursing corporate compliance program that was developed at Hartford Hospital in Connecticut, which identified five steps that needed to be taken in the program:

1. Identification of high-risk areas
2. Development of plans and tools that support the process for monitoring and measuring compliance with the high-risk areas
3. Implementation of the program
4. Education
5. Compliance related to auditing and monitoring (Bartis & Sullivan, 2002, p. 68)

The high-risk areas that this organization identified, which would vary from one organization to another, were: licensure and credentialing with current and appropriate licensure, scope of practice that is consistent with the state nurse practice act, compliance with hospital policies and procedures, and documentation.

Employee education is one im_____its outcomes. Topics that might be covered_____of conduct, compliance plan, roles and re_____ith laws and regulations, conflicts of int_____abuse, professional standards and codes of_____anization information, physician relatio_____d anti-trust issues. Some of these topics a_____ff need an understanding of financial an_____ow the procedure for reporting their conc_____e program as another "change" that will_____f behaviors. This staff attitude needs to be_____ge the organizational culture and comm_____izational leaders must be role models for a_____wrong and then do the right thing. It is n_____al issues at one time, all of which affect d_____

Koloroutis and Thorst_____organizational change that was developed_____ta. The Allina

Health System recognized that managed care was attempting to change the approach of health care to one of population-based disease and illness prevention and wellness provided within a seamless care system, which as a goal is certainly a positive one. To accomplish this, costs had to be reduced. Reducing costs led to a need to change the traditional view of ethics in the health care system. Physicians and nurses had long been patient advocates, but they found themselves in positions of being asked to control costs and access and in situations that can cause conflict. They were often caught in the middle. To address this conflict, the health care system reviewed its ethical framework and changed its focus to caring. The caring framework calls for a philosophy of moral commitment of protecting and preserving human dignity rather than reducing a person to the status of an object (Watson, 1990). This framework requires critical thinking, clinical competence, compassion, respect, listening, and acceptance. Collaboration is a key to success today, and it is compatible with the caring framework.

Nurses coping with ethical dilemmas

Nurses have responsibilities related to ethics, including maintaining knowledge of the professional *Code for Nurses*, recognition of personal values, understanding of the decision-making process and its application to nursing practice, recognition and understanding of the importance of policy and legal issues, and the ability to be assertive (Wocial, 1996). As nurses confront ethical dilemmas, there are decision-making traps that need to be avoided.

■ Prematurely reaching a decision
■ Overconfidence in your own judgment
■ Failing to follow a system
■ Inability to recognize the effect of your own personal value system
■ Inability to recognize the conflict between what is best for the patient and what is best for the organization (p. 155)

CURRENT ISSUES

Learn about events around the globe that relate to the chapter content.

Curtin (1995) advocates "putting decisions through the 'stink test'. If it smells, rethink your priorities" (p. 101). This is not a bad test because it recognizes the importance of each individual's perspective on decisions; however, it is also important to understand and recognize opposite viewpoints.

The goal is to reach a balance between the extremes, and this is not easy to accomplish. Decision making in the health care environment requires a recognition of different viewpoints and compromises. This is also true for all ethical dilemmas. Wallace and Pekel (2001) developed an ethical checklist for staff to use as they assess an ethical situation—questions to ask oneself. These questions included the following.

■ **Relevant information test.** Have I/we obtained as much information as possible to make an informed decision and action plan for this situation?
■ **Involvement test.** Have I/we involved all who have a right to have input and/or to be involved in making this decision and action plan?
■ **Consequence test.** Have I/we anticipated and attempted to accommodate for the consequences of this decision and action plan on any who are significantly affected by it?
■ **Fairness test.** If I/we were assigned to take the place of any one of the stakeholders in this situation, would I/we perceive this decision and action plan to be essentially fair, given all of the circumstances?
■ **Enduring values test.** Does this decision and action plan uphold my/our priority enduring values that are relevant to this situation?

■ **Universality test.** Would I/we want this decision and action plan to become a universal law applicable to all similar situations, even to myself/ourselves (p. 29)?

Strategies that are used by some health care organizations to cope with ethical dilemmas are ethics committees and nursing ethics groups. Ethics committees provide opportunities for interdisciplinary staff to discuss ethical dilemmas that staff experience in the organization. The committee is advisory. As is true with all discussions of ethics, there is no perfect answer. These committees are "invaluable tools for educating staff, providing a non-judicial mechanism for cases of ethical conflict, and developing organizational policies regarding ethics" (Moss, 1995, p. 283). Typical issues that are discussed by these committees are: do-not-resuscitate policies, patient self-determination, brain-death protocols, informed consent, euthanasia, and patient competency. Issues related to managed care and reimbursement and clinical decision making will also become more common topics. Ethical dilemmas such as these can lead to staff frustration and do affect the delivery of patient care.

Nursing ethics groups provide forums for discussion about nursing ethics (Moss, 1995). One problem that occurs is nurses are not always comfortable discussing their ethical dilemmas in institutional ethics committees (IECs) (Otto, 2000). Nurses, however, who participate in nursing ethics committees gain knowledge and skills that are required for ethical decision making. These nurses are then better prepared to participate in interdisciplinary ethics committees and to make their own ethical decisions.

"A political ethical conflict occurs when what one is told to do (either covertly or overtly) by those having more power in the organization or what one feels compelled to do by the organization is in conflict with one's ethical belief structure" (Brosnan & Roper, 1997, p. 42). This is demonstrated daily today in health care as nurse managers and other staff confront conflicts between financial issues and care. What is best for patients and what is best for the organization are not always the same. These can be tough choices. A health care organization is a political one, and as has been discussed in earlier chapters, leaders need to be aware of the political environment. Nurse managers and staff must consider beneficence, which is "the obligation to benefit one's institution and those it serves" (Brosnan & Roper, 1997, p. 42). However, should the team agree with the institution without thought of what this agreement means and the ethics involved? Nurses must consider nonmalfeasance and do no harm to the institution or those it serves. This obligation also relates to the employees. Respect for persons, another key principle, is also important when staff make decisions that affect patients but also when managers make decisions that affect staff. Managers have to ensure that procedures are followed; however, when this is done, it needs to be done respectfully (for example, when staff are told that mistakes have been made). Justice, or treating others fairly and impartially, is a frequent dilemma for managers. Staff need to be approached in an impartial manner with fairness. Truth telling is the obligation to be truthful or honest in decisions and approaches to others. Utility is also important, and this focuses on "maximizing the greatest good when decisions are made" (Brosnan & Roper, 1997, p. 43). Staff confront ethical issues daily; however, "The leader's actions may be 'the single most important factor in fostering corporate behavior of a high ethical standard,' but surveys rank an ethics policy as very important, too" (Dessler, 2002, p. 50).

BENCHMARKS

Now let's take a moment to test your knowledge of the concepts you have studied in this section.

Chapter Wrap-Up

Now that you've reached the end of the chapter, you may wish to explore the concepts you've been reading about in greater detail, or test yourself to see how well you've comprehended the material.

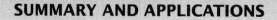

SUMMARY AND APPLICATIONS

- Summary
- Practice Quiz
- Key Terms
- Tying It All Together

- Experiential Exercises
- Case
- Links

REFERENCES

American Nurses Association. (1994a). *Guidelines on reporting incompetent, unethical, or illegal practice.* Washington, DC: Author.

American Nurses Association. (1994b). *Position statement on assisted suicide.* Washington, DC: Author.

American Nurses Association. (1998, January–February). Mass. nurses, docs spark health care revolution. *American Nurse, 30*(1), 6.

American Nurses Association. (2001). *Code for nurses with interpretive statements.* Washington, DC: American Nurses Publishing.

Annas, G. (2003). HIPAA regulations—A new era of medical-record privacy? *The New England Journal of Medicine, 348*(15), 1486–1490.

Aroskar, M. (1980). Anatomy of an ethical dilemma: The theory. *American Journal of Nursing, 80*(4), 658–663.

Bantz, D., Wieske, A., & Horowitz, J. (1999). Perspectives of nursing executives regarding ethical–economic issues. *Nursing Economics, 17*(2), 85–90.

Bartis, J., & Sullivan, T. (2002). Developing a nursing corporate compliance program. *JONA's Healthcare Law, Ethics, and Regulation, 4*(3), 67–77.

Beckman, H. et al. (1994). The doctor-patient relationship and malpractice. *Archives Internal Medicine, 154*(12), 1365.

Bodenheimer, T., & Grumbach, K. (1998). *Understanding health policy: A clinical approach* (2nd ed.). Stamford, CT: Appleton & Lange.

Borawski, D. (1995). Ethical dilemmas for nurse administrators. *Journal of Nursing Administration, 25*(7/8), 60–62.

Broder, P. (1997, October 26). Health care: The problems persist. *Washington Post,* p. A1.

Brosnan, J., & Roper, J. (1997). The reality of political ethical conflicts: Nurse manager dilemmas. *Journal of Nursing Administration, 27*(9), 42–46.

Canavan, K. (1997, May–June). Nurses confront whistle-blower retaliations. *The American Nurse,* (5), 12–13.

Center for Studying Health System Change. (1998). *A year in the life of the health care system, 1998 annual report.* Washington, DC: Author.

Chally, P., & Loriz, L. (1998). Decision making in practice: A practical model for resolving the types of ethical dilemmas you face daily. *American Journal of Nursing, 98*(6), 17–20.

Coffey, J. (2001). Universal coverage. *American Journal of Nursing, 101*(2), 11.

Coppola, M. (1997, March–April). Identifying and reducing health care fraud in managed care. *Group Practice Journal* (3), 46.

Curtin, L. (1995). Ethics in management: Creating an ethical organization. *Nursing Management, 26*(9), 96–101.

Department of Health and Human Services & Department of Justice. (2002, April). *Health care fraud and abuse control program. Annual report for FY 2001.* Retrieved April 5, 2002, from http://www.usdoj.gov/pubdoc/hipaa01fe19.ltm#c.

Dessler, G. (2002). *Management.* Upper Saddle River, NJ: Prentice Hall.

Ditto, P. et al. (2001). Advanced directives as acts of communication: A randomized controlled trial. *Archives of Internal Medicine, 161*(3), 431–440.

Eichenwald, K. (1997, November 4). Reshaping the culture at Columbia/HCA. *New York Times,* C2.

Eichenwald, K. (1998, February 14). Columbia/HCA fraud case may be widened, U.S. says. *New York Times,* B2.

Erlen, J., & Mellors, M. (1995). Managed care and the nurse's ethical obligations to patients. *Orthopaedic Nursing, 14*(6), 42–45.

Ferguson, S. (2001). An activist looks at nursing's role in health policy development. *JOGNN, 30*(5), 546–551.

Gross, L., & Reed, S. (1999). ANA calls for medicine reform. *American Journal of Nursing, 99*(11), 50, 52.

Guido, G. (2001). *Legal and ethical issues in nursing* (3rd ed.). Upper Saddle River, NJ: Prentice Hall.

Habel, M. (2001). Advance directives. *Nurse Week Great Lakes, 1*(9), 17–19.

Hadley, E. (1996). Nursing in the political and economic marketplace: Challenges for the 21st century. *Nursing Outlook, 128*(5), 396–402.

Hall, M., & Berenson, R. (1998). Ethical practice in managed care: A dose of realism. *Annals of Internal Medicine, 128*(5), 396–402.

Himmelstein, D., & Lown, B. (1997). For our patients, not for profits: A call to action. *Journal of the American Medical Association, 278*(21), 1737–1740.

Hyman, D. (2002). HIPAA and health care fraud: An empirical perspective. *Cato Journal, 22*(1), 151–178.

Institute of Medicine. (2000). To err is human: Building a safer health system. Washington, DC: National Academy Press.

Institute of Medicine. (2002). Unequal treatment: Confronting racial and ethnic disparities in health care.Washington, DC: National Academy Press.

Jones, K., Jennings, B., Moritz, P., & Moss, M. (1997). Policy issues associated with analyzing outcomes of care. *Image: Journal of Nursing Scholarship, 29*(3), 261–267.

Karigan, M. (2001). Ethics in clinical research. *American Journal of Nursing, 101*(9), 26–31.

Kassirer, J. (1995). Managed care and the morality of the marketplace. *New England Journal of Medicine, 333*(1), 50–52.

Kelley, T. (1998, February 8). Charting a course to ethical profits. *New York Times*, pp. BU1, BU12.

Kilborn, P. (1998, March 22). Looking back at Jackson Hole. *New York Times*, pp. A1, A5.

Kilborn, P. (1999, January 3). Oregon falters on a new path to health care. *New York Times*, A1, A16.

Knight, W. (1998). *Managed care: What it is and how it works.* Gaithersburg, MD: Aspen Publishers, Inc.

Koloroutis, M., & Thorstenson, T. (1999). An ethics framework for organizational change. *Nursing Administration Quarterly, 23*(2), 9–18.

Longest, B. (2002). *Health policymaking in the United States* (3rd ed.). Chicago: Health Administration Press.

Mariner, W. (1995). Business vs. medical ethics: Conflicting standards for managed care. *Journal of Law, Medicine and Ethics, 23*(3), 236–246.

McIntosh, M. (2002). The cost of health care to Americans. *JONA's Healthcare Law, Ethics, and Regulation, 4*(3), 79–89.

Mock, K. (2001). Keep lawsuits at bay with compassionate care. *RN, 64*(5), 83–84, 86.

Mohr, W. (1996). Dirty hands: The underside of marketplace health care. *Advances in Nursing Science, 19*(1), 28–37.

Mohr, W. (1997). Outcomes of corporate greed. *Image: Journal of Nursing Scholarship, 29*(1), 39–45.

Morris, K. (2002, September). Issues and answers. *Ohio Nurses Review, 77*(9), 16.

Moss, M (1995). Principles, values, and ethics set the stage for managed care nursing. *Nursing Economics, 13*(5), 276–284, 294.

Nokleby, E., et al. (1998). Managed care: The value you bring. *American Journal of Nursing, 98*(6), 34–39.

Ohlman, K. (1998). Employers can abuse info on worker's health. *Cincinnati Business Courier, 15*(3), 45.

Otto, S. (2000). A nurses's lifeline. A nursing ethics committee offers the chance to review and learn from ethical dilemmas. *American Journal of Nursing, 100*(12), 57–59.

Pear, R. (2002, August 10). Bush rolls back rules on privacy of medical data. *New York Times*, A1, A8.

Polston, M. (1999). Whistleblowing: Does the law protect you? *American Journal of Nursing, 99*(1), 26–30.

Purdum, T. (1999). California to set level of staffing for nursing care. *New York Times*, A1, A21.

Randall, V. (1994). Impact of managed care on ethic answers and underserved populations. *Journal of Health Care Poor Underserved, 5*(3), 224–236.

Reinhardt, E. (1994). Managed competition in health care reform: Just another American dream or the perfect solution. *Journal of Law, Medicine and Ethics, 22*(2), 106–120.

Robert Wood Johnson Foundation. (1997). *State health care reform: Looking back toward the future.* Princeton: NJ: Author.

Rundle, R. (1993, August 27). National medical facilities raided by U.S. agents. *Wall Street Journal*, A1, A4.

Scanlon, C. (1996–1997). Impact of cost containment on patient welfare concerns nurses. *American Nurses Association Center for Ethics and Human Rights Communique, 5*(2), 1–4.

Shepherd, S. (1998). Whistleblowing: Exposing fraud against the government. *Journal of Legal Nurse Consultants, 9*(2), 10–11.

Staten, P. (2000). Ins and outs of advance directives. *Nursing Management, 31*(3), 16, 18.

Steinhauer, J. (2001, January 10). Rebellion in white: Doctors pulling out of HMO systems. *New York Times*, pp. A1, A20.

Strunk, B., & Ginsberg, P. (2003). Tracking health care costs: Trends stabilize but remain high in 2002. *Health Affairs*, Jan–June suppl Web Exclusive W3-26674.

Tilden, V. et al. (2001). Family decision making to withdraw life-sustaining treatments from hospitalized patients. *Nursing Research, 50*(2), 105.

Toner, R. (1999, June 16). Drug coverage dominates fight brewing on Medicare. *New York Times*, pp. A1, A22.

U.S. Census Bureau. Retrieved May 7, 2004, from http://www.census.gov.

U.S. House of Representatives. (1992, April 28). *The profits of misery: How inpatient psychiatric treatment bilks the system and betrays our trust. Hearing before the Select Committee on Children, Youth and Families, One Hundred Second Congress, Second Session.* Washington, DC: U.S. Government Printing Office.

U.S. House of Representatives. (1993, February 3 & May 27). *Health care fraud: Hearings before the Subcommittee on Crime and Criminal Justice of the Committee on the Judiciary House of Representatives, One Hundred and Third Congress, First Session.* Washington, DC: U.S. Government Printing Office.

U.S. House of Representatives. (1994, July 19). *Deceit that sickens America: Health care fraud and its innocent victims. Hearings before the Subcommittee on Crime and Criminal Justice of the Committee on the Judiciary House of Representatives, One Hundred and Third Congress, Second Session.* Washington, DC: U.S. Government Printing Office.

U.S. Senate. (1992, July 28). *Hearing before the Committee on the Judiciary United States Senate, Senate Bill 2652, One Hundred Second Congress, Second Session.* Washington, DC: U.S. Government Printing Office.

Wallace, D., & Pekel, J. (2001). *Complete guide to ethics management: An ethics booklet for managers.* McNamara, CO: Fulcrum Group.

Watson, J. (1990). Transposed caring: A transcendent view of the person, health, and healing. In M. Parker (ed.), *Nursing theories in practice* (pp. 23–34). New York: National League for Nursing.

Wielawski, I. (1998). The growing gulf between what's medically available and what's affordable. *Advances,* Supplement(4).

Wocial, L. (1996). Achieving collaboration in ethical decision making: Strategies for nurses in clinical practice. *Dimensions of Critical Care Nursing, 15*(3), 150–158.

Zatkin, S. (1997). A health plan's view of government regulation. *Health Affairs, 16*(6), 33–35.

ADDITIONAL READINGS

Ahern, M. (1996). Nurses' and other experts' views of health care fraud and abuse. *Nursing Economics, 14*(1), 40–48.

Aiken, L., Gwyther, M., & Whelan, E. (1996). Federal support of graduate nursing education. Rational policy options. *Nursing Outlook, 44*(1), 10–17.

American Nurses Association. (1995). *Nursing's social policy statement.* Washington, DC: American Nurses Publishing.

American Nurses Association. (1998). *Legal aspects of standards and guidelines for clinical nursing practice.* Washington, DC: American Publishing, Inc.

Annas, G. (1998). A national bill of patients' rights. *New England Journal of Medicine, 338*(10), 695–699.

Cooper, R., Frank, G., Gouty, G., & Hansen, M. (2003). Ethical helps and challenges faced by nursing leaders in the health care industry. *Journal of Nursing Administration, 33*(1), 17–23.

Crawford, L. (2001). Regulation of registered nursing. *Reflections on Nursing Leadership,* (Fourth Quarter), 28–30, 34, 51.

Curtin, L. (1996a). The ethics of managed care—Part 1: Proposing a new ethos? *Managed Care, 27*(8), 18–19.

Curtin, L. (1996b). The ethics of managed care—Part 2: The world as it is. . . . *Managed Care, 27*(9), 53–55.

Curtin, L. (1996c). The ethics of managed care—Part 3: Toward a common vision. *Managed Care, 27*(10), 71–74.

David, B. (1999). Nurses' conflicting values in competitively managed health care. *Image: Journal of Nursing Scholarship, 31*(2), 188–189.

Erlen, J. (2001). The nursing shortage, patient care, and ethics. *Orthopedic Nursing, 20*(6), 61–65.

Ginzberg, E. (1999). The uncertain future of managed care. *New England Journal of Medicine, 340*(2), 144–148.

Goode, E. (2001, August, 27). Disparities seen in mental care for minorities. *New York Times,* A12.

Goold, S. (1998). Money and trust: Relationships between patients, physicians, and health plans. *Journal Health Political Policy Law, 23*(4), 687–695.

Gulzar, L. (1999). Access to health care. *Image: Journal of Nursing Scholarship, 31*(1), 13–19.

Harrison, J. (1999). Influence of managed care on professional nursing practice. *Image: Journal of Nursing Scholarship, 31*(2), 161–166.

Health Insurance Association. (1998). *Managed care: Integrating the delivery and financing of health care. Part A and Part B.* Washington, DC: Author.

Hoskins, J. (1999). Planning health care facilities and managing the development process. In L. Wolper (ed.). *Health care administration* (pp. 237–259). Gaithersburg, MD: Aspen Publishers, Inc.

Kerschner, S., & Cohen, J. (2004). Legislative decision making and health policy: A phenomenological study of state legislators and individual decision making. *Policy, Politics, & Nursing Practice, 3*(2), 118–128.

Kovner, C. (2000). State regulation of RN-to-patient ratios. *American Journal of Nursing, 100*(11), 61–63.

Kuttner, R. (1999a). The American health care system—Health insurance coverage. *New England Journal of Medicine, 340*(2), 163–167.

Kuttner, R. (1999b). The American health care system: Wall Street and health care. *New England Journal of Medicine, 340*(8), 664–668.

LaDuke, S. (2000). Nurses and the attorney-client relationship. *JONA's Healthcare Law, Ethics, and Regulation, 2*(4), 117–123.

Mariner, W. (1996). State regulation of managed care and the Employee Retirement Income Security Act. *New England Journal of Medicine, 335*(26), 1986–1990.

Mason, D. (2002). The politics of patient care. *American Journal of Nursing, 102*(4), 7.

Milholland, K. (1994). Privacy and confidentiality of patient information. *Journal of Nursing Administration, 24*(2), 19–24.

Milio, N. (2001). Health care reform: What went wrong? *American Journal of Nursing, 101*(12), 69–71.

Mohr, W. (1996). Ethics, nursing, and health care in the age of "reform." *N & HC: Perspectives on Community, 17*(1), 16–21.

President's Advisory Commission on Consumer Protection and Quality in the Health Care Industry. (1999). *Quality first: Better health care for all Americans.* Washington, DC: U.S. Government Printing Office.

Price, J. (2000, March). Beyond the law. One nurse's reflections on conflicts and consequences in mandated reporting. *AWHONN Lifelines, 3*(3), 41–45.

Rambur, B. (1998). Ethics, economics, and the erosion of physician authority: A leadership role for nurses. *Advances in Nursing Science, 20*(4), 62–71.

Reres, M. (1996). *Managed care. Managing the process.* Glencoe, MD: National Professional Education Institute.

Rognehaugh, R. (1998). *The managed care dictionary.* Gaithersburg, MD: Aspen Publishers, Inc.

Sabin, J. (1997). What confidentiality standards should we advocate for in mental health care, and how should we do it? *Psychiatric Services, 48*(1), 35–36, 41.

Sullivan, G. (2001). Reduce your risk in the managed care jungle. *RN, 64*(3), 71–72, 74.

The Patient Self-Determination Act. (1990, November) Sections 4206 and 4751 of the *Omnibus Reconciliation Act of 1990,* Public Law 101–508.

Wood, B. (2001). Legal and ethical considerations of patient/provider communications. *Journal of Legal Nurse Consulting, 12*(2), 10–13.

Wysoker, A. (2000). Informed consent: The ultimate right. *Journal of the American Psychiatric Association, 6*(3), 100–102.

Consumers and Nurses

MediaLink
www.prenhall.com/finkelman

The Interactive Exercises for this chapter can be found in the OneKey course at www.prenhall.com/finkelman. Click on Chapter 11 to select from the following activities: Test Your Understanding, Benchmarks, Current Issues, Your Opinion Counts, Think Critically, and Summary and Applications.

What's Ahead

The consumer's role has changed as health care has undergone major changes and managed care has become the dominant approach to health care reimbursement and delivery. This chapter addresses the role of the consumer or the patient in the health care delivery system. By its very nature the nursing process places both the patient and the patient's family in a major role. Patients as consumers of health care services have been gaining strength as they speak out about their health care; they are concerned about the quality of care and its cost. Nurses have had a role in this as well, as patient advocacy is an important component of nursing care.

There is no doubt that the patient is paying more for care as employers pay less. Premiums are higher, as are co-payments and deductibles. Recognition of consumer priorities and understanding the criteria that consumers use as they evaluate their health care services are critical to maintaining a positive relationship between the employer and the employee, especially with the increasing financial responsibility that is carried by the employee (Reif & Martin, 1996). This requires that employers, who select the plans that are offered to their employees, and third-party payers listen to their employees and enrollees and increase consumer involvement in decision making. Health care delivery organizations also need to know more about consumer issues: What does the patient want? Is the outcome what the patient wanted? Nurses also need to understand what is important to health care consumers. Consumer rights and protection are front page news as health care legislation on the state and federal levels escalates. Legislation, however, may lead to more problems, and thus must be considered carefully. A balance must exist between meeting the needs of all consumers, patients/enrollees/employees, employers, the government, providers, and insurers. Patients are turning more to nurses and asking questions about their health care and health delivery, so nurses need to be prepared to answer their questions or know how to help patients seek the answers about health care. Customer-centered health care means the nurse must be more aware of customer/patient needs. This chapter discusses consumerism, the role of the consumer or patient in health care policy, health care information and consumers, patient evaluation of health care, and the nurse as patient advocate.

OBJECTIVES

Before you begin, take a moment to familiarize yourself with the key objectives of this chapter.

- Define consumer.

- Describe the history of health care consumerism.

- Explain the relationship between public policy and the health care consumer.

- Compare and contrast the consumer implications of *The Pew Report* and *Healthy People 2010*.

- Discuss how health care information is available to the health care consumer.

- Discuss the relationship between patient education and health care consumerism.

- Describe how consumers are involved in evaluating the quality of care.

- Discuss the nurse's role as patient advocate in the health care environment.

TEST YOUR UNDERSTANDING

Before we begin our exploration of this chapter, take a short "warm-up" test to see what you know about this topic.

The Consumer and Health Care

Who is the consumer?

Consumers can be described in a variety of ways. A **macroconsumer** is a large purchaser of health care services (e.g., employers, government). The macroconsumer may also be called the customer. Clearly, this type of consumer has a major voice in health care decisions due to its size and acts as a liaison between the insurers/managed care organizations (MCOs) and employees. A **microconsumer** is the employee, the employee's family, and people who buy insurance as individuals rather than through an employer. They are the users of the health care services. All consumers, whether macro or micro, make decisions about the purchase of health care coverage, but the microconsumer is involved in more decisions about health care services that directly affect them. Choice is an important aspect of health care, and some consumers feel that their choices have diminished (e.g., choice of health plan has decreased as employers offer fewer plans and more tightly control the types of plans; the choice of provider and when the provider can be consulted have been affected; and in some cases the choice of using specialty care has diminished).

As health care reimbursement has changed, choice has become an important health care consumer issue and one that is integral in many consumer complaints and their health care.

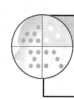

YOUR OPINION COUNTS

Find out what others think about this topic. Post your response and check out other opinions.

History of health care consumerism

Consumerism and its issues

Consumerism has been evolving over many years. With the development of managed care, consumerism has become even more important. In the 1970s, consumers were informed and assertive about their active participation in health care (Armer, 1998). During that time, the focus was on patient satisfaction and utilization of health care services. A 1971 study found that 75% of the families sampled believed that there was a crisis in health care, but only 10% said they were dissatisfied with the quality of their care (Andersen, Kravits, & Anderson, 1971). This is a confusing result; despite the fact that a high percentage felt that the health care system was in a crisis, few were critical of that care's quality. Patient satisfaction is a very complex issue, and it is not always easy to know what a patient is responding to during a satisfaction survey. Quality is also difficult to define. In the 1980s, the focus of consumer concern and provider concerns changed to the cost of health care (Boston, 1990; Preziosi, 1989; Sovie, 1990). In addition, access became an important issue for those in rural areas, the poor, the elderly, and minorities. Quality and access to services have been important issues throughout the health care consumer movement, and these issues are even more important today.

Impact of managed care on consumerism

As managed care became the dominant player in the health care system in the 1990s, a change developed regarding health care consumerism. Consumers were not as active in the early 1990s as they became at the end of the decade. Managed care developed on the West Coast and then moved to the East Coast. After that managed care slowly moved across the country, with some areas not feeling its effect until the mid-1990s. As this was occurring, managed care did not affect enough consumers to cause them to organize and protest against it. The media were not as cognizant of the changes, so it was not a front-page news item. However, as more consumers were affected by managed care, it became stronger and made a major impact on health care delivery. Consumers finally became concerned when the problems affected their personal care. Consumers, however, have reached the point of saying, "Enough!" This cry is coming from the soon-to-be-seniors generation. The Baby Boomers, in contrast, are not new to protesting and being assertive. They are now using these skills to address their concerns about health care delivery.

There is no doubt that as consumers experience problems with health care, they often criticize health care and have demanded changes in managed care. There are, however, positive aspects of managed care, such as its increased emphasis on preventive care, health promotion, and continuity. Nonetheless, it is easy to lose sight of the positive aspects of managed care. Emotions sometimes undermine rational policy changes and criticism. If the goal is to control costs, provide quality care, and increase care delivery to those who cannot afford care, it is critical to find a balance and identify the strengths and limitations of managed care, while building on its strengths.

Health care providers and third-party payers/MCOs recognize the need to listen more to consumer criticisms and are more willing to make some changes that address these criticisms. Today, patient-centered or customer-centered health care is a frequently heard term, although it does not always significantly affect health care in practical changes. More effort has been made to provide the consumer with information. The Picker Institute defined patient-centered care as "making consumers an ongoing part of quality improvement efforts by using their feedback and participation to build better health care systems" (Graham, 1996, p. 49).

Nurses have long supported this approach, but why would health care organizations and MCOs be interested? Health care organizations are increasingly aware of the need to develop satisfied consumers who participate in their care. This does affect costs in that MCOs want to hear that their enrollees are satisfied with the health care they receive. Certainly, the need to obtain contracts from employers is one driving force. MCOs also want consumers to have more understanding about their health care needs in order to be informed purchasers of care and informed users of health care services. They believe that an informed health care consumer will reduce health care costs. At the same time, consumers are turning more to government and legislation to influence health care policy making and get their needs met.

Public policy and the health care consumer

"Only through better understanding of the consumers' perceptions of the current system and their expectations for future health care delivery can policy makers and health care providers develop responsive health care programs that will meet local and national health care needs and be acceptable to consumers in the decades ahead" (Armer, 1998, p. 515). Nurses need to advocate for public policy that promotes and protects the health of the public (O'Neil & the Pew Health Professions Commission, 1998). Nursing organizations have a responsibility to advocate for the consumer and partner with consumer groups, and they frequently do this because collaboration can result in a win-win outcome. More, however, could be done. "It means we must take public stands on quality care issues and educate the public on 'public interest' issues, even when it puts us at odds with our nurse executive colleagues. It means we should support strong whistle-blowing legislation in our states, and it means we should form a circle of support for those who dare to stand up to exploitive systems on behalf of the patient. It is dangerous to continue to be silent. The American public does not take kindly to health care professionals who appear to protect the status quo, especially when the status quo is shown to be harmful" (Krauss, 1996, p. 327). The examples of health care fraud and abuse found in Chapter 10 indicate that nurses do get involved in situations when the consumer needs strong nurses who will take risks for them. This can be very difficult for nurses, but situations like these can demonstrate nurses' leadership skills.

The consumer must also become involved in the development of health care public policy. This is usually done through organizations such as the American Diabetes Association, National Alliance for the Mentally Ill, the American Association of Retired Persons, the Arthritis Foundation, and other organizations that advocate for specific policies while representing their membership. Frequently, these organizations also have health care professional members who participate in policy advocacy. Individual consumers also go directly to their legislators, on both the state and federal levels, to have a voice in policy decision making. Television, the Internet, and newspapers keep the public informed on health care policy issues and are good resources for identifying current policy issues. Nurses can be supportive of consumer involvement by ensuring that consumers get accurate information by acting as consultants, through serving as experts while writing letters to editors, and keeping up with media content. Typically, the media turns to physicians for comments about health care, but nurses are also good resources for this information. This means that nurses have to let the media know that they are competent and available to do this. Nursing organizations usually let the media know that they have representatives who are willing to be interviewed.

Consumer rights

YOUR OPINION COUNTS

Find out what others think about this topic. Post your response and check out other opinions.

Consumer rights have slowly become a major issue in health care policy, particularly due to dissatisfaction with managed care. States are active in establishing requirements related to information that the insurer must supply to the consumer and to identify grievance and appeal requirements.

The Patient Self-Determination Act of 1990 is a law that applies to all health care organizations that participate in Medicare or Medicaid by receiving reimbursement from these government sources (Shi & Singh, 1998). What does this law require? All of these facilities must provide their patients with information about patients' rights, which are typically referred to as a Bill of Patient's Rights. Some of the rights that organizations typically develop are: (a) confidentiality, (b) consent, (c) right to make medical decisions, (d) right to be informed about diagnosis and treatment, (e) right to refuse treatment, and (f) use of advance directives.

The end of the 1990s brought major efforts to pass additional federal legislation to establish a greater patient or consumer protection bill of rights. There have been many proposals in Congress, and in the fall of 1999, the Senate and the House passed two very different bills, requiring compromises on their parts; however, no patient's rights legislation has been passed as of the summer of 2005.

The consumer rights issue is highly controversial. If too many consumer rights are recognized, how will this affect the ability of MCOs to meet their goals of reducing health care costs? Reducing costs is a concern for all, not just the MCOs. What effect will it have on health care provider organizations? For example, the changes in patient privacy protection are costly to implement and yet they represent a consumer issue. Consumers also want costs lowered; however, the critical factor is what must be given up to reach this goal. Health care organizations such as hospitals, clinics, long-term care facilities, and home care agencies must consider how particular patient's rights might impact care and costs.

All of this activity indicates how the late 1980s and the 1990s were an active time for patient consumerism. Although probably initiated by dissatisfaction with managed care, many of the changes had little to do directly with managed care and really focused more on health care in general.

THINK CRITICALLY

Try this exercise to apply what you have learned about this topic.

Special reports: Do they have implications for the consumer?

Two reports about health care, one issued by a nongovernmental organization and another by the federal government, have influenced health care professionals and their services. *The Pew Report* and *Healthy People 2010* reports are very important for the consumer.

1. **The Pew Report**

In 1998 the Pew Health Professions Commission published a new edition of its *Pew Report, Recreating Health Professional Practice for a New Century* (O'Neil & the Pew Health Professions Commission, 1998). The 21 competencies identified for health care professionals for the 21st century, identified in Chapter 2, are highly relevant to the care that patients receive in all types of settings. The report emphasizes the need for changes in educational programs in order to meet the demands of the new health care environment. New values, techniques, and skill sets are necessary for the health care professional to practice in this new environment, and consumers are also requesting these changes. This report describes a shifting health care landscape for professional practice toward the need to balance the interests of the individual and society. "One of the most valuable aspects of the American health care system is its long-standing orientation to serving the needs of individual patients. . . . Much of the excellence of America's style of health care can be traced to the importance of the one-on-one relationship of the caregiver to the patient" (O'Neil & the Pew Health Professions Commission, 1998, pp. 34–35). Consumers recognize that they may be losing this special relationship, and at the same time they are concerned about the quality of care and costs. However, consumers are most concerned about changes that interfere with quality and their health care choices. Health care professional and insurer accountability is very important to consumers. As a result of greater consumer pressure, MCOs have been forced to focus more on the evaluation of care and the reimbursement process. Improvement of care, expanding access, and enhancing health are goals that have become more important in how the health care delivery system responds to problems and criticisms. These goals are also affected by the health care reimbursement system.

2. *Healthy People 2010* Objectives

Healthy People is a national prevention initiative that identifies opportunities to improve the health of all Americans by identifying goals and objectives that are used by the U.S. Department of Health and Human Services (DHHS), as well as many health care organizations and institutions, to promote health and disease and illness prevention (U.S. Department of Health and Human Services, 1998). The DHHS identified the first objectives in 1979, then additional sets in 1990, 2000, and most recently, the 2010 set, which includes two broad goals:

1. Increase quality and years of healthy life, which focuses on life expectancy, quality of life, and achieving a longer and healthier life.
2. Eliminate health disparities, which focuses on a variety of factors that have an impact on health disparities such as gender, race and ethnicity, income and education, disability, geographic location, and sexual orientation to achieve equity.

There are over 467 objectives in 28 focus areas identified to meet these broad goals. These goals and objectives for the Healthy People initiative, implemented in 2000, were created after an extensive period of input from professionals, organizations, businesses, and consumers. *Healthy People 2010* goals and objectives build on previous goals and objectives, but there were some differences, particularly due to the "broadened prevention science base; improved surveillance and data systems; a heightened awareness and demand for preventive health services and quality health care; and changes in demographics, science, technology, and disease spread that will affect the public's health in the 21st century" (U.S. Department of Health and Human Services, 1998). Figure 11-1 provides a view of *Healthy People 2010*, highlighting its major focus areas.

FIGURE 11-1 Healthy people in healthy communities.

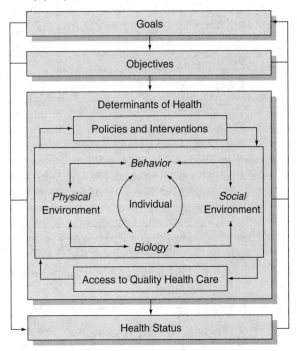

Source: U.S. Department of Health and Human Services. (2000). *Healthy People 2010* (2nd ed.). Washington, DC: U.S. Government Printing Office. http://www.healthypeople.gov, U.S. Government.

The first goal for *Healthy People 2010*—increasing quality and years of healthy life—not only focuses on longevity but also on the quality of that life. There are two views of a healthy life—that of the individual and that of the nation. Individuals want to live their lives with a full range of functional capacity during each stage of their lives. Likewise, the nation wants and needs citizens who can contribute and be productive, as illness is expensive for businesses and the government. Objectives related to this goal include:

- Decrease the total death rate to no more than 454 per 100,000 by 2010 (baseline: 503.9 age-adjusted death rate per 100,000 in 1995).
- Reduce the death rate for adolescents and young adults (15 to 24 years) to no more than 81 per 100,000 by 2010 (baseline: 95.3 per 100,000 in 1995).
- Reduce the death rate for adults (25 to 64 years) to no more than 358 per 100,000 by 2010 (baseline: 397.3 per 100,000 in 1995).
- Increase life expectancy to 77.3 years by 2010 (baseline: 75.8 years in 1995).
- Decrease years of potential life lost before age 75 to no more than 7,315 per 100,000 by 2010 (baseline: 8,128.2 age-adjusted years of potential life lost before age 75 per 100,000 in 1995).
- Increase the percentage of persons reporting good, very good, or excellent general health to at least 90% by 2010 (baseline: 86.2% of adults in 1993–1996).
- Increase healthy days to at least 26 days during the past 30 days by 2010 (baseline: 24.7 days in 1993–1996).
- Increase recent days able to do usual activities due to good physical or mental health to at least 28.7 days during the past 30 days by 2010 (baseline: 28.3 days in 1993–1996).
- Increase years of healthy life to at least 66 years (baseline: 63.9 years in 1995).
- Increase years of healthy life for persons 65 and older to 14 years (baseline: 12.0 years in 1995).

Another goal of the Healthy People national initiative is to eliminate health disparities. This is a difficult goal to meet, as it requires improved access to care for all persons as well as new knowledge about the determinants of disease and effective interventions. With the large number of uninsured in the United States, this will be a challenge. Socioeconomic disparities, demographic changes, education-related differences, race, and ethnicity are significant barriers to the success of this goal. Barriers to care will affect the implementation of *Healthy People 2010* and its results. These barriers need to be overcome to improve Healthy People results. *Healthy People 2010* also recognizes that the United States does not exist in isolation and that global forces affect any efforts to improve health (e.g., food supplies, infectious diseases, environmental interdependence, and risk of bioterrorism). This initiative is also the United States' contribution to the World Health Organization's "Health For All" strategy.

Why does the Healthy People initiative have relevance to this chapter's content? Healthy People is an example of health policy, and it provides methods to improve the health status of individual consumers and communities. One of its major overall goals is to improve the quality of health-related decisions through effective communication. Interwoven into its other goals and their objectives is the need for consumer education, advocacy, and self-management of illness via health promotion and disease and illness prevention.

CURRENT ISSUES

Learn about events around the globe that relate to the chapter content.

Information resources

Technology has revolutionized consumer access to information. For example, in 1997 there were "more than five million pages of medically related text on-line, delivered by more than 7,000 indexed Web sites" (Kleinke, 1998, p. 67). There is no doubt that this number has increased today. Interactive technology has certainly changed the availability of information, particularly electronic mail, websites, intranets, and interactive voice response systems. These new technologies offer additional ways to communicate with current customers and to collect, manage, and utilize health care information. Who uses this technology and for what reasons? Interactive audiences can be categorized into five groups:

1. Members (consumers) seeking self-care or wellness information
2. Members (consumers) seeking medical advice and treatment options
3. Consumers seeking wellness or general health information
4. Employers and employees seeking benefit or plan information
5. Providers and health professionals seeking plan or member information (Fell, 1998, p. 12)

A 1997 survey indicated that the audience for these new communication methods was still uneducated and unfocused about the new technologies. The survey results indicated that 32% of the hospitals used the Internet for some of their marketing. Although still low, however, a definite increase was seen in the past 2 years, with 46% using the Internet for 1 to 2 years and 48% for 1 year or less (Fell, 1998). This is a very new area for health care providers and insurers. As providers and insurers develop their websites, a major concern is whether the information provided will be appealing to customers. However, there are other concerns, for example:

- Accurate and useful general health/wellness information
- Provider directory/referral service with searching and sorting capabilities
- The most current health/medical/community news
- Member update/order features; for example, ordering new identification cards, e-mail access to member service representatives, frequently asked questions (FAQ) section
- Individual benefits information; for example, after identification, the member is able to access individual information, claims forms, change of address, and the like
- Access to health care professionals 24 hours a day
- Personalized health information customized to meet personal needs (Fell, 1998, pp. 17–18)

Technology opens up new roles for the nurse in health care organizations. Nurses may play an active role in the development and maintenance of these sites for providers and for insurers/MCOs who want to make them available to members. Content needs to be accurate and useful, and nurses have the clinical expertise and ability to develop this content for consumers. Health care provider organizations need to use more nurses in the development of their websites. This is something that nursing management needs to be assertive about to gain more nursing input. Nurses who participate in these projects need to understand the basics of reimbursement, clinical needs, educational principles, and the use of technology to provide information. They must also be creative. Computer expertise is a plus, but in most cases, it is not required. Most providers and insurers who are developing sites have computer experts to assist in this aspect of the project. Many consumer Internet sites provide information for consumers, and these are identified in Box 11-1.

National organizations and the government often provide the best information. *Healthy People 2010* addresses the issue of communication and emphasizes the need for appropriate communication at individual and community levels. Information and education play vital roles in promoting health; preventing, managing, and coping with disease; and supporting appropriate decisions across the spectrum of health care. For individuals, effective health communication can help raise awareness of health risks, provide motivation and skills to reduce them, bring helpful connections to others in similar situations, and offer information about difficult choices, such as health plans and providers, treatments, and long-term care. For the wider community, health communication can set the public and social agenda, advocate for healthy policies and programs, promote positive changes in the socioeconomic environment and health infrastructure, and encourage social norms that benefit health and quality of life (U.S. Department of Health and Human Services, 1998). Box 11-2 describes typical health communication activities, and Box 11-3 identifies attributes of effective health communication as identified in *Healthy People 2010*.

BOX 11-1   Consumer Internet information.

1. Consumer information is found on many Internet sites. The following are examples of sites: http://www.healthfinder.gov, http://familydoctor.org. Who sponsors the site? What information does each site provide? Is it helpful for the consumer? Is the information easy to access? Can you search for specific information? Is the information accurate? As a health care professional, how might you use the site? Can you find any information related to managed care, reimbursement, health care delivery, quality care, or patient rights? Why is the site's content related to this chapter's content?
2. http://www.ahcpr.gov. Visit this site and click on "Consumer Health." What information is available for consumers as they choose their health plans? What information is available for consumers as they use their health plans? Use the checklist to determine the health plan that is best for you.
3. http://www.graypanthers.org. What is the sponsoring organization? What are its position statements on issues such as Medicare, Social Security, and reimbursement?
4. http://www.ncqa.org. Visit this site and click on "Health Care Organization." What is CAHPS? Does it provide helpful information? How might an MCO use this information? How might a health care professional or organization use this information?

Source: Author.

BOX 11-2   Communication activities.

Telehealth

The application of telecommunications and computer technologies to the broad spectrum of public health and medicine

Interactive health communication

The interaction of an individual—consumer, patient, care-giver, or professional—with an electronic device or communication technology to access or transmit health information or to receive guidance on a health-related issue

Consumer health informatics

Interactive health communication focusing on consumers

Telemedicine

The application of telecommunications and computer technologies specifically for clinical care

Source: U.S. Department of Health and Human Services. (1998). *Healthy People 2010.* Washington, DC: U.S. Government Printing Office.

Examples of current consumer issues

The health care delivery system is complex, and consumers must cope with its complexity and barriers. Many consumers concerns also have an impact on nurses and nursing care, including four key areas of issues: (a) self-managing care, (b) use of primary care physicians and specialists, (c) medications, and (d) hospitalization. Patient education and patient advocacy, two key nursing roles that require many leadership competencies such as effective communication, coordination, collaboration, decision making, and so on, are important strategies to help patients gain strength as consumers.

1. Self-managing care

    Consumers manage their own care—even if they choose not to receive health care, they have made a decision about the importance of their health and what they want to do about it. The best way to prevent problems and reduce health care costs is to practice self-care, health promotion, and disease and illness prevention. Collaborating with health care providers to understand treatment

BOX 11-3   Attributes of effective health communication.

Availability

The content (whether targeted message or other information) must be delivered or placed where the audience can access it. This varies according to audience and purpose, from billboards and mass transit signs to prime time TV or radio, public kiosks (print or electronic), and the Internet.

Repetition

The delivery of/access to the content must be continued or repeated over time, both to reinforce the impact with a given audience and to reach new generations.

Accuracy

The content must be valid and presented accurately.

Reliability

The source of the content must be credible, and the content itself must be up-to-date and regularly updated.

Reach

The content must get to, or be available to, the largest possible number of people in the target population.

Consistency

The content must remain consistent and also should be consistent with information from other sources (the latter is a problem when other widely available content is not accurate or appropriate).

Timeliness

The content is provided or available when the audience is most receptive to, or in need of, specific information.

Balance

Where appropriate, the content presents the benefits and risks of potential actions or recognizes different but valid perspectives on the issue.

Culturally sensitive

The design or implementation process addresses special issues for specific population groups (ethnic and racial, linguistic) and also educational levels and disability.

Understandability

The reading or language level and format (including multimedia) are appropriate for the specific audience.

Evidence-based

The content and strategies are based on formative or previous evaluation with the intended audience and on applicable findings from previous communication research.

Multidimensionality

Research shows that a variety of communication activities, integrated with non-communication activities, such as programs, policies, and services, will be most successful. This implies that interagency or public-private partnerships can not only leverage resources but may also strengthen the impact. Such collaboration can have the added benefits of reducing message clutter and targeting issues that cannot be fully addressed by public resources or market incentives alone.

Source: U.S. Department of Health and Human Services. (1998). *Healthy People 2010 objectives*. Washington, DC: U.S. Government Printing Office.

choices, understand patient and health care provider responsibilities, and follow the treatment selected are critical to positive health care outcomes. If patients as health care consumers are involved in their health care decisions, they will be more satisfied with their health care. Seeking information to increase understanding is very important. In addition, enrollees need to collaborate with not only their health care providers but also with their insurers, who also play a major role in their health care decisions.

"Managed care is a structured relationship between the physician, subscriber (enrollee/member), and health plan. Things are done more formally. Records are kept on both the medical and the administrative events that occur. Authorization is part of that structure" (Cafferky, 1997, p. 80). Authorization is the approval by the insurer or MCO agreeing to pay for a health care service. As patients manage their own care, it is important to understand why authorization is done and how it is done. When patients cannot get the care that they believe is needed, it can be very frustrating and stressful for patients, their families, and staff. There are 10 reasons why an insurer uses authorization.

1. Verification of eligibility for the service coverage
2. Certification that the enrollee receives the benefits in the contract
3. Payment of claims to contracted providers
4. Validation of the medical necessity and appropriateness of care
5. Screening for procedures that require a second opinion
6. Screening for medications that are not in the plan formulary (list of drugs the health plan will cover)
7. Screening for the appropriate treatment setting
8. Provision of information for case management
9. Tracking utilization patterns
10. Controlling costs and financial management (Cafferky, 1997, pp. 80–81)

Who authorizes care? A wide variation can exist among plans as to who must authorize care, which can be very complicated. The primary care provider, as gatekeeper, may authorize treatment, or an interdisciplinary team within the health plan or an outside organization referred to as a utilization management/review organization may authorize treatment. Some MCOs use their own staff (who are often nurses) to authorize care. Another approach is to identify treatments and services that have automatic authorization (for example, Pap smears, hernia repair, vaccinations, and mammograms). The common services requiring authorization are hospital admission, emergency care, continued stay in the hospital, transfer to another facility, access to alternative care settings, experimental procedures, expensive diagnostic procedures, nuclear diagnostic procedures, treadmill stress tests, invasive diagnostic and therapeutic procedures, inpatient surgery, same day surgery, and any high-cost service. The health plan should identify what services require authorization. What happens if the patient misses an appointment for an authorized service? Some plans may require that the service be reauthorized.

2. Primary care physicians and specialists

Managed care has made the term *provider* important and uses this term for a variety of providers of care. For example, physicians, nurse practitioners, nurse-midwives, hospitals, home health agencies, and long-term care facilities are all providers. One of the most critical providers is the primary care provider (PCP), which is a model used by many plans (but not all). Usually, a physician, who is often referred to as the gatekeeper, is responsible for overseeing and coordinating the patient's care. Some plans require that the PCP approve the use of specialists before specialty care will be reimbursed. Can any physician be a PCP? Certain types of physicians are recognized as PCPs by the MCO/insurer. Typically, these are general practitioners, family practice physicians, internal medicine physicians, pediatricians, and obstetricians/gynecologists. Some plans now accept nurse practitioners and nurse-midwives as PCPs. Because most medical decisions are made by the primary care provider (e.g., medications, laboratory testing, frequency of exams, hospitalization, home care), the PCP is very important. The PCP manages the patient's needs throughout the continuum of care with the patient to ensure that needs are met. Typical services that are provided are:

- Health promotion and education
- Disease and illness prevention
- Urgent/immediate care
- Routine ambulatory care
- Diagnosis or treatment by ancillary services (e.g., physical therapy, respiratory therapy, occupational therapy)
- Acute inpatient care
- Intensive care
- Subacute skilled nursing care
- Home care nursing
- Assisted living
- Long-term care
- Hospice care

The physician does not work alone. Other professionals who often work with physicians are nurses, advanced practice nurses, nurse-midwives, physician assistants, certified registered nurse-anesthetists, and many other health care professionals. Physicians who are selected for the plan's panel of approved providers must meet criteria established by the plan. These criteria usually include board certification, which indicates that the physician has met specific standards and passed an exam. This is in addition to the physician's medical board exams. The insurer is also interested in whether or not the physician has been involved in a malpractice suit and the results of the suit. Professional references are required. Many plans also assess the physician's practice and services. At these times, plans evaluate specific practice or performance issues, such as hospitalization rates, prescription history, laboratory testing, complications, medical record review results, compliance with standards, and patient satisfaction. In order to renew a contract, physicians and other providers are evaluated carefully, and sometimes contracts are not renewed with specific providers if the health plan does not agree with the provider's decisions. In fact, some experts believe that physicians are now better evaluated than they were in the fee-for-service system or indemnity; however, this does affect patients as they may have to change providers if the health plan no longer covers services provided by a specific provider.

Referral to specialty care has been changed by many health plans as they move to managed care models and strategies. In the past, patients might have consulted with their physician about the need for a specialist or might even have decided for themselves that the problem required a specialist. The insurer did not usually tell enrollees if they could see specialists. Now, some insurers or MCOs may tell enrollees when and what provider to see or even determine if enrollees really need specialty care. Some plans require approval for every visit to a specialist and may require approval of all of the specialist's medical decisions, such as medication, laboratory testing, and hospitalization. Consumers, however, have not been pleased with this lack of choice, and now many health plans are changing their approach to allow patients more choices about their providers.

Some MCOs have also been encouraging the use of intensivists or hospitalists in hospitals; hospitals are also seeing the value in using this type of provider. (See Chapter 6 for more information about this new role.) Why would the managed care plan want to use intensivists or hospitalists? The plan may consider them to be better prepared to care for the hospitalized patient. Today, more and more care is provided outside the hospital, leaving hospital care for the most critical problems. Because these physicians are more prepared to care for hospitalized patients they may be considered to be more efficient, and thus costs may be contained while quality care is provided. This means that the physician who cares for the patient in the hospital may be a stranger who will have contact with a patient's ambulatory care physician or PCP, but will make all decisions about the patient's hospital care.

3. Medications

If a patient takes medications regularly, the patient will want to inquire about his or her health plan's formulary, hospital formularies, and policies about generic substitution and therapeutic substitution. The health plan formulary identifies the prescription drugs that the plan reimburses for its enrollees. The plan considers medication safety, effectiveness, cost, and the cost-effectiveness of the drugs it selects for its formulary. The plan may also consider how medications affect quality of life or the ability to carry on normal activities. Providers are informed about the formulary and encouraged to follow it. Some health plans track the prescription of formulary drugs versus non-formulary drugs. An important question is whether the formulary is open, closed, or incentive.

- An open formulary means that the patient can be reimbursed for nonformulary medications or medications not listed in the plan's formulary.
- If a plan uses a closed formulary, it does not reimburse for medications that are not included in its formulary.
- Incentive formularies require that the patient pay an additional co-payment if medications are used that are not in the formulary.

Medications are a very important treatment intervention today, and more and more new medications are coming on the market. Many will be very effective but also expensive. This will undoubtedly increase the importance of health plan formularies. If the plan allows generic substitution, the provider may prescribe medications that are a replacement for another medication containing the same active ingredient in the same amount and dosage form. These are sold by different pharmaceutical companies and usually are cheaper.

Therapeutic substitution may also occur. Some plans and hospitals allow pharmacists to substitute medications that are different from those prescribed by the patient's physician. The substituted medications must be in the same pharmacological or therapeutic class. The substitutions are usually in the hospital or plan formulary. How is this different from generic substitution? These drugs may have different side effects, biological effects, and interactions. In addition, the physician may not even know the substitution has been made. The plan may not only manage the enrollee's prescriptions, but it may also designate which pharmacy may fill the prescriptions. Consumers need to be concerned as the pharmacy may not be convenient or easy to access due to its hours and so on. This affects overall treatment accessibility and is very important to all consumers.

4. Hospitalization

The health plans also select the hospitals that plan enrollees may use. Some plans have several hospitals that they have approved for reimbursement, whereas others have only one. This clearly affects patient/consumer choices. Prior to a health plan's contracting with a hospital so that their enrollees will be able to use a hospital, the plan evaluates the hospital and its services. Competition among hospitals for these contracts is intense.

Patient satisfaction and quality

Patient satisfaction and quality have become more important in today's highly competitive health care delivery environment (Stumpf, 2001). Health care providers and insurers/MCOs compete for patients and enrollees. This text discusses many aspects of leadership and management, and yet sometimes it is difficult to see how this all relates to patient care. Does the health care environment and culture, work satisfaction, staff retention, and type of organizational structure matter to patients? Do they just go through the system untouched by it? Patient satisfaction outcomes seem to indicate that patients are affected by all of these factors (Hinshaw & Atwood, 1982; McDonald & Patrick, 1992; Stumpf, 2001; Weisman & Nathanson, 1985). Patients do report greater satisfaction with their care in shared governance organizations, which tend to have greater staff retention and work satisfaction (Stumpf, 2001). So the context in which staff work and patients receive their care are interrelated and affect patients' views of their care.

However, some problems do exist with patient satisfaction. "The customer satisfaction bandwagon, rampant in the business world throughout the 1990s, has now been joined by health care. Fortunately the days when health care personnel could have an attitude of 'just be grateful that we are here' are gone. In the search to improve both humanistic caring and profitability, however, many have allowed the pendulum to swing too far. They have adopted a misguided *excessive* and *exclusive* focus on customer satisfaction as the measurement of quality patient care. Making customer satisfaction the supreme goal has major inherent flaws, particularly when used in the health care arena for 'patient' customers" (Zimmermann, 2001, p. 255). Several myths related to patient satisfaction have been identified.

1. Customer satisfaction is objective and straightforward. This is not true. Surveys are difficult to develop, and they are often poorly designed (Sherman, 1998).
2. Customer satisfaction is easily measured. Satisfaction is complex and not easily measured. Patient expectations play a major role in the process, and there are many factors that can affect patient responses.
3. Customer satisfaction is accurately and precisely measured. This is not possible at this time. Attitudes are being measured.
4. Customer satisfaction is quickly and easily changed. This does not occur. In fact, "The best care may actually be accomplished by *preventing* the customer patients' return" (Zimmermann, 2001, p. 256).
5. It is obvious who the customer is. The tendency is to classify all customers as patients when there are many different customers related to a health care organization; for example, MCOs, physicians, and internal customers. (Staff within the organization become customers to other staff; e.g., laboratory provides services to the units and thus staff on the units are the laboratory's customers.) All groups of customers need to be considered when customer satisfaction is assessed (Zimmermann, 2001, pp. 255–256).

Besides these issues with the process of determining satisfaction, other issues should be considered. One issue that comes up is whether the patient, as a health care consumer, can judge what is good care. This question tends to generate strong feelings on both sides. Solovy (1998) reports that "consumers over-whelmingly state that they think quality information is useful about health care plans (87%), doctors (86%), and hospitals (83%). But only about a third actually use that information to make a decision in choosing a health care plan (34%), a doctor (35%), or a hospital (30%)" (as cited in Zimmermann, 2001, p. 258). How does the patient's illness affect the patient's impression of the treatment and how does the patient express the evaluation? Along with this issue, Zimmermann (2001) also notes that the patients who complete surveys are patients who are able to do this—alert, typically English-speaking, and often younger. This eliminates many other patients. As is true for many problems that may be identified in the evaluation process, staff tend to trivialize complaints by saying the patient was annoying or a constant complainer. This is a way of avoiding complaints and not working on improvement.

"Despite extensive research on defining and measuring quality of care, less attention has been given to consumers' views" (Oermann, Dillon, & Templin, 2000, p. 9). A study conducted on indicators of quality of care in clinics recognized that both providers and consumers are interested in assessing quality of care, but they have different views of quality (Oermann, Dillon, & Templin, 2000). What indicators are important in determining the quality of health care and nursing care? This study included a sample of 119 clinic patients in an urban ambulatory care facility. The results indicated that the most important quality indicators for health care were:

- Getting better
- Getting care and services when needed
- Having diagnoses and treatment options

Nursing care indicators were different and included:

- Communicating with the nurse
- Being treated with respect
- Being cared for by nurses who were up-to-date
- Teaching by the nurse
- Not being rushed through the visit

The indicators for nursing care appear to be more specific than those of health care quality, although clearly they are all interrelated. "Patient satisfaction studies have consistently demonstrated the importance of patients' communication with the clinician and education during hospitalization and in ambulatory care.... People with chronic illnesses also valued instruction by the nurse more than did other patients" (Oermann, Dillon, & Templin, 2000, p. 11). What is important to note here is the recognition of education, communication, and interpersonal relationships. At the same time that these are identified as key factors to patient satisfaction and patients' views of quality care, health care organizations and nurses are experiencing less time to provide care, which limits their time for communication and education with patients. This is a grave concern with staffing shortages and increased workplace stress.

Acute care is also no exception when comparing provider and consumer viewpoints. Shannon, Mitchell, and Cain (2002) conducted a study to compare patient, nurse, and physician assessments of quality of care and patient satisfaction in selected critical care units. The sample included 25 units in 14 hospitals, 489 patients, 518 nurses, and 515 physicians. Standardized instruments were used to collect the data. The results indicated that physicians rated quality of care higher than either the patients or the nurses and tended to overestimate patient satisfaction. Nurses and patients had similar ratings for quality of care. There was, however, great variation within and between units for all three groups. The study concluded that physicians, nurses, and patients view patient satisfaction and quality of care differently, and it supports the need to avoid assuming that if health care professionals have positive views of quality of care and patient satisfaction that the patient will agree. The views of all three groups need to be considered.

How do acute care patients and ambulatory care patients compare when patient satisfaction and quality of care are discussed? "Patients in hospitals have views of quality of care that are different from those of consumers in ambulatory facilities. Hospitalized patients describe high-quality care in terms of hospital staff respect for patients' values and needs, coordination of care, communication and education, physical comfort and pain management, emotional support, involvement of family, and continuity in the transition to home (Edgman-Levitan & Cleary, 1996; Ketefian, Redman, Nash, & Bogue, 1997). Although ambulatory patients are concerned with many of the same dimensions, they have other needs that are different from those of inpatients, such as access to care, length of time to get an appointment, waiting times, assistance from office staff, and follow-up care and information (Healy, Govoni, & Smolker, 1995; Krueckeberg & Hubbert, 1995; Chung et al., 1999, as cited in Oermann, Dillon, & Templin, 2000, p. 5).

The Kaiser Family Foundation (KFF) and the Harvard School of Public Health conducted a survey from 1997 to 2001 to determine public attitudes toward patients' rights and managed care (Kaiser Family Foundation, 2001) that included 1,000 adults ages 18 and older. Some of the questions addressed included:

- In general, do you think managed care health plans are doing a good job or a bad job in serving health care consumers? The data indicate that more considered that health plans are doing a bad job, although there was some change indicating plans were improving.
- What percent of Americans say they or someone they know has had problems with health plans during the past few years? The data indicated that problems decreased from 1998 to 2001.
- Do you think that ranking this issue (specific ones cited) is very important to the President and the Congress to deal with, somewhat important, not too important, or not at all important? The data indicated that all were considered important; the participants were then asked to rank them.
- Do you favor or oppose a law that would provide a Patients' Bill of Rights? Eighty-five percent were in favor of such a law.
- In relationship to the Patients' Bill of Rights, respondents were asked if they would still support it if it would mean an increase in the cost of health insurance premiums (60% still supported it), and if it meant that some businesses would stop providing health care coverage due to concerns of being sued (41% still supported it).

Patient satisfaction data are also an important component of report cards. As more is learned about the type of data that are really helpful, the report cards should become more useful and reliable for the patient, employer, all types of providers, and MCOs. It is important to recognize that the variables of satisfaction need to be identified by the patient, not the health care professional. This presents a problem. "Health care professionals tend to define the elements of patient satisfaction as mainly service components such as waiting time, courtesy, and food quality. The movement by both macroconsumers and microconsumers, however, is toward a far more complete and sophisticated inventory of both process and outcome measures that concern the quality of care along with the styles of care delivery. It is now widely recognized, if not happily embraced by providers and insurers, that care cannot be high quality unless the consumer recognizes it as satisfactory" (Sullivan, 1998, p. 573). Patient satisfaction is a core element of quality of care.

The nurse as patient advocate

CURRENT ISSUES

Learn about events around the globe that relate to the chapter content.

The nursing role

Advocacy has always been a major aspect of the nursing role with the consumer and requires leadership skills. Nursing standards that are developed by the American Nurses Association (ANA), nursing specialty organizations, and health care institutions, as well as those developed by accrediting organizations and other health care professional organizations, support many of the critical aspects of advocacy and consumerism. Patient education, patient satisfaction and complaint process, quality improvement, patient participation in health care decision making, and all components of advocacy and consumerism are found in these standards. The ANA states that the "*Standards of Clinical Nursing Practice* delineates the professional responsibilities of all registered nurses engaged in clinical practice regardless of setting" (American Nurses Association, 1998, p. 5). The *Standards of Clinical Nursing Practice* (1998) and other nursing practice guidelines serve as a basis for the following:

- Quality improvement systems
- Databases
- Regulatory systems
- Health care reimbursement and financing methodologies
- Development and evaluation of nursing service delivery systems and organizational structures
- Certification activities
- Job descriptions and performance appraisals
- Agency policies, procedures, and protocols
- Educational offerings (American Nurses Association, 1998, pp. 5–6)

There are two important components of advocacy: providing information that is useful to the patient and supporting the patient's decision, which may not be the decision the nurse desired but that—once made—must be supported. The nurse provides care while working with the patient in a collaborative relationship and advocates for the patient. The American Nurses Association has defined *collaboration* as "a true partnership, in which the power on both sides is valued by both, with recognition and acceptance of separate and combined spheres of activity and responsibility, mutual safeguarding of the legitimate interests of each party, and a commonality of goals that is recognized by both parties" (American Nurses Association, 1980, p. 3). To be an advocate, the nurse needs to be persuasive with the patient and with others with whom the nurse may interact on behalf of the patient. Advocacy does not mean that the nurse takes over for the patient, but rather the nurse helps the patient to be as independent as possible.

Managed care, however, has affected the nurse's role as an advocate. "Under managed care or other cost-containment models of health care compensation, patient advocacy by professionals is increasingly compromised" (Sullivan, 1998, p. 578). This has certainly also affected many physician–patient relationships as the physician may be involved in making decisions based on financial issues rather than as an advocate for the patient's needs. How has it affected the nurse's role as advocate? Nurses working in hospitals and home care frequently face issues with patients about reimbursement, decisions that limit the care patients receive. Nurses then feel frustrated when there is nothing they can do to assist the patient. Advanced practice nurses are experiencing many of the same conflicts as physicians.

What can the nurse do to assist the patient and advocate for the patient (Reif & Martin, 1996)? Ensuring that the nursing process is complete and includes active patient and family/significant other participation is the critical first step. Built into the process are individualized care, patient rights, respect for the patient, and patient education. The nurse also needs to empower the patient with information and support the patient and the family as health care choices are made. Accessing care, which includes services, supplies, and medical equipment, is not always easy today. Doing this today in a health care environment in which patients have shortened lengths-of-stay or do not come in for care early enough is very difficult. Patient education takes time. More and more of this load is shifting to the community. It takes commitment on the part of the nurses to ensure that it happens and that the patient education is appropriate to meet the needs of the patient. Nurses will have to be more creative in meeting the needs, probably by turning more to technology. Care does need to be taken to ensure that individual needs and human contact are still present. The nurse can help the patient understand the complex health care system and reimbursement issues related to the system in order to receive care when it is needed. Prevention is important in today's health care environment, and helping the patient understand the need for prevention and how it can benefit the individual patient is part of the nurse–patient relationship.

THINK CRITICALLY

Try this exercise to apply what you have learned about this topic.

THINK CRITICALLY

Try this exercise to apply what you have learned about this topic.

BENCHMARKS

Now let's take a moment to test your knowledge of the concepts you have studied in this section.

Chapter Wrap-Up

Now that you've reached the end of the chapter, you may wish to explore the concepts you've been reading about in greater detail, or test yourself to see how well you've comprehended the material.

SUMMARY AND APPLICATIONS

- ■ Summary
- ■ Practice Quiz
- ■ Key Terms
- ■ Tying It All Together

- ■ Experiential Exercises
- ■ Case
- ■ Links

REFERENCES

American Nurses Association. (1980). *Nursing: A social policy statement*. Washington, DC: American Nurses Publishing.

American Nurses Association. (1998). *Standards of clinical nursing practice*. Washington, DC: American Nurses Publishing.

Andersen, R., Kravits, J., & Anderson, O. (1971). The public's view of the crisis in medical care: An impetus for changing delivery systems? *Economic and Business Bulletin, 24*, 44–52.

Armer, J. (1998). Consumers as allies or partners in care. In T. Sullivan (Ed.), *Collaboration: A health care imperative* (pp. 515–533). New York: McGraw-Hill.

Boston, C. (1990). Healthcare reform. *Journal of Nursing Administration, 20*(7/8), 8–9.

Cafferky, M. (1997). *Managed care and you*. Los Angeles: Health Information Press.

Chung, K., et al. (1999). Predictors of patient satisfaction in an outpatient plastic surgery clinic. *Annals of Plastic Surgery, 42*(1), 56–60.

Edgman-Levitan, S., & Cleary, P. (1996). What information do consumers want and need? *Health Affairs, 15*(4), 42–56.

Fell, D. (1998). Customer centered health care: Why managed care organizations must capitalize on new technology to build brands and customer loyalty. *Managed Care Quarterly, 6*(2), 9–20.

Graham, J. (1996). The rise of the health care consumer. *Business and Health* (Suppl. State of Health Care in America), 49–53.

Healy, J., Govoni, L., & Smolker, E. (1995). Patient reports about ambulatory care. *Quality Management in Healthcare, 4*(1), 71–81.

Hinshaw, A., & Atwood, J. (1982). A patient satisfaction instrument: Precision by replication: A pilot study. *Nursing Research, 31*(3), 170–175.

Kaiser Family Foundation, retrieved on April 2, 2001, from http:www.kff.org.

Ketefian, S., Redman, R., Nash, M., & Bogue, E. (1997). Inpatient and ambulatory patient satisfaction with nursing care. *Quality Management in Healthcare, 5*(4), 66–75.

Kleinke, J. (1998). *Bleeding edge: The business of health care in the new century*. Gaithersburg, MD: Aspen Publishers, Inc.

Krauss, J. (1996). Advocating advocacy. *Archives of Psychiatric Nursing, 10*(6), 327.

Krueckeberg, H., & Hubbert, A. (1995). Attribute correlates of hospital outpatient satisfaction. *Journal of Ambulatory Care Marketing, 6*(1), 11–43.

McDonald, C., & Patrick, T. (1992). Leadership, nurses, and patient satisfaction: A pilot study. *Nursing Administration Quarterly, 16*(3), 72–74.

O'Neil, E. H., and the Pew Health Professions Commission. (1998). *Recreating health professional practice for a new century*. San Francisco: Pew Health Professions Commission.

Oermann, M., Dillon, S., & Templin, T. (2000). Indicators of quality care in clinics: Patient's perspectives. *Journal of Health Care Quality, 22*(6), 9–11.

Preziosi, P. (1989). *Developing a national health plan. Why now? Why nurses?* New York: National League for Nursing.

Reif, L., & Martin, K. (1996). *Nurses and consumers: Partners in assuring quality care in the home*. Washington, DC: American Nurses Publishing.

Shannon, S., Mitchell, P., & Cain, K. (2002). Patients, nurses, and physicians have differing views of quality of critical care. *Journal of Nursing Scholarship*, second quarter, 173–179.

Sherman, B. (1998). How non-profits can benefit from marketing research. *Association Forum, 28*(2), 22–23.

Shi, L., & Singh, D. (1998). *Delivering health care in America*. Gaithersburg, MD: Aspen Publishers, Inc.

Solovy, A. (1998). Trendspotting. *Hospitals and Health Networks, 72*(6), 60.

Sovie, M. (1990). Redesigning our future: Whose responsibility is it? *Nursing Economics, 8*(1), 21–26.

Stumpf, L. (2001). A comparison of governance types and patient satisfaction outcomes. *Journal of Nursing Administration, 31*(4), 196–202.

Sullivan, T. (1998). Consumers in health care, part II: Expert viewpoints. In T. Sullivan (Ed.), *Collaboration: A health care imperative* (pp. 561–590). New York: McGraw-Hill.

U.S. Department of Health and Human Services. (1998). *Healthy People 2010.* Washington, DC: U.S. Government Printing Office.

Weisman, C., & Nathanson, C. (1985). Professional satisfaction and client outcomes. *Medical Care, 23,* 1179–1192.

Zimmermann, P. (2001). The problems with health care customer satisfaction surveys. In J. Dochterman & H. Grace (Eds.), *Current issues in nursing* (6th ed., pp. 255–260). St. Louis: Mosby, Inc.

ADDITIONAL READINGS

American Nurses Association. (2000). High public esteem for nurses. *American Journal of Nursing, 100*(1), 21.

Appleby, C. (1995). The middle no more. *Hospitals and Health Network, 69*(11), 96, 98.

Bartlett, D. (1997). Preparing for the coming consumer revolution in health care. *Journal of Health Care Finance, 23*(4), 33–39.

Bournes, D. (2000). A commitment to honoring people's choices. *Nursing Science Quarterly, 13*(1), 18–23.

Byerly, R., Carpenter, J., & Davis, J. (2001). Managed care and the evolution of patient rights. *JONA's Healthcare Law, Ethics, and Regulation, 3*(2), 58–67.

Cooper-Patrick, L., et al. (1999). Race, gender, and partnership in the patient-physician relationship. *Journal of American Medical Association, 282*(6), 583–589.

Dansky, K., Yant, B., Jenkins, D., & Dellasega, C. (2003). Professional issues qualitative analysis of telehomecare nursing activities. *The Journal of Nursing Administration, 33*(7/8), 372–375.

Finocchio, L., Dower, C., Blick, N., Gragnola, C., & The Taskforce on Health Care Workforce Regulation. (1998). *Strengthening consumer protection: Priorities for health care workforce regulation.* San Francisco: Pew Health Professions Commission.

Gebbie, K. (2001). Privacy: The patient's right. *American Journal of Nursing, 101*(6), 69, 71, 73.

Government Accounting Office. (1996). *Consumer health informatics. Emerging issues.* Publication no. GAO/AIMD-96-86. Washington, DC: Author.

Harris, L. (Ed.). (1995). *Health and the new media. Technologies transforming personal and public health.* Mahwah, NJ: Lawrence Erlbaum Associates.

Hendricks, M. (1996). Marketing on the Internet. *Health Care Marketing Report, 14*(10), 8–10.

Hewitt, J. (2002). A critical review of the arguments debating the role of the nurse advocate. *Journal of Advanced Nursing, 37*(5), 439–445.

Hibbard, J., Slovic, P., & Jewett, J. (1998). Informing consumer decisions in health care: Implications from decision-making research. *Milbank Quarterly, 75*(3), 395–414.

Isaacs, S. (1996). Consumers' information needs: Results of a national survey. *Health Affairs, 15*(4), 39.

Jeffries, R., & Sells, P. (2000). Customer satisfaction measurement instruments. In health care does one size fit none? *Quality Progress, 33*(2), 118–123.

Jones, K. (1997). Consumer satisfaction: A key to financial success in the managed care environment. *Journal of Health Care Finance, 23*(4), 21–32.

Krauss, J. (1999). Advocacy and managed care. *Archives of Psychiatric Nursing, 13*(2), 65–66.

Longo, D., et al. (1997). Consumer reports in health care: Do they make a difference in patient care? *Journal of the American Medical Association, 278*(19), 1570–1584.

Lynn, M., & McMillen, B. (1999). Do nurses know what patients think is important in nursing care? *Journal of Nursing Quality, 13*(5), 65–74.

Mallik, M., & Rafferty, A. (2000). Diffusion of the concept of patient advocacy. *Journal of Nursing Scholarship,* fourth quarter, 399–404.

Mayer, T., Cates, R., Masorovich, M., & Royalty, D. (1998). Emergency department patient satisfaction: Customer service training improves patient satisfaction and rating in physician and nurse skill. *Journal of Health Care Management, 43,* 427–441.

Mayer, T., & Zimmerman, P. (1999). ED customer satisfaction survival skills. One hospital's experience. *Journal of Emergency Nursing, 25*(3), 187–191.

Oermann, M. (1999). Consumers' descriptions of quality health care. *Journal of Nursing Care Quality, 14*(1), 47–55.

Oermann, M. (2000). Indicators of quality of care in clinics: Patients' perspectives. *Journal of Healthcare Quality, 22*(6), 9–11.

Oermann, M., & Huber, D. (1999). Ignorance is bliss but not in health care: Teaching consumers about quality care. *Outcomes Management for Nursing Practice, 3*(2), 47–49.

Oermann, M., & Templin, T. (2000). Important attributes of quality health care: Consumer perspectives. *Journal of Nursing Scholarship, 32*(2), 167–172.

Office of Technology Assessment. (1995). *Bringing health care online. The role of information technologies.* Publication no. OTA-ITC-624. Washington, DC: U.S. Government Printing Office.

Perla, L. (2002). Patient compliance and satisfaction with nursing care during delivery and recovery. *Journal of Nursing Care Quality, 16*(2), 60–66.

Robinson, K. (1997). Family caregiving: Who provides the care, and at what cost? *Nursing Economics, 15*(5), 243–247.

Rosenberg, J. (1996). Five myths of customer satisfaction. *Quality Progress, 29*(12), 57–60.

Sigma Theta Tau International. (1999). New poll shows public concern about health care. *Reflections, 31*(2), 39.

Spitzer, R. (2002). Information as power. *Seminars for Nurse Managers, 10*(2), 75.

Sutton, S., Balch, G., & Lefebvre, R. (1995). Strategic questions for consumer-based health communications. *Public Health Reports, 10*(6), 725–733.

Tu, H., & Hargraves, J. (2003, March). Seeking health care information: Most consumers still on the sidelines. *Issue Brief. Findings from Health System Change,* No. 61, 1–4.

Vavra, T. (1997). Is your satisfaction survey creating dissatisfied customers? *Customer Progress, 30*(12), 51–56.

Wakefield, M. (1997). Protecting health care consumers: A bill of rights and responsibilities. *Nursing Economics, 15*(6), 315–317.

Williams, S., & Swanson, M. (2001). The effect of reading ability and response format on patients' abilities to respond to a patient's satisfaction scale. *Journal of Continuing Education in Nursing, 32*(2), 60–67.

RECRUITMENT/ RETENTION

Building on work in other domains, professional opportunities will be enhanced to attract and sustain excellent nurses for long, rewarding careers.

Desired Future Statement (Vision)

Nursing is comprised of a diverse body of individuals committed to promoting and sustaining the profession through addressing diversity, image, education, funding, practice models and environments, and professional development.

Five strategies were identified to achieve the vision and one of these was identified as the primary or driving strategy. They are:

Professional/career development opportunities across the career span. (Primary Strategy)

Funding is secured for creative educational initiatives that support nurses across the career span.

Nursing is seen as a highly desirable and appealing career choice.

Nurses develop professional practice models and work environments that ensure career satisfaction.

Comprehensive recruitment and retention strategies demonstrate nursing's strong public image and appeal to a diverse population.

Objectives to Support Primary Strategy

Establish national, professional development models for mentoring, leadership, and diversity for nurses across their career trajectory.

Address diversity issues by: obtaining funding to support an increase in minority enrollment, identifying a specific mobility track for nurses of diverse cultures throughout their careers, and creating a specific curriculum to address diversity.

Develop and distribute promotional and recruitment materials that attract individuals of diverse backgrounds into the variety of nursing career opportunities.

Recruit retired nurses to form the foundation of a professional mentoring corps.

Advocate for standardized internships and residencies through partnerships between schools of nursing, professional organizations, and practice sites. Graduates will participate in an individualized mentoring program to socialize them into the profession and enhance their knowledge of clinical practice.

Negotiate professional development opportunities with employers that are supported through a variety of resources such as: paid time off, education days, cost reimbursement, or as part of the scheduled workday.

Create a website for leadership development activities and templates, and make it available for use by hospitals and nursing organizations.

SOURCE: American Nurses Association. (2002). *Nursing's agenda for the future. A call to the nation*. Washington, DC: Author. Reprinted with permission.

CHAPTER 12

Recruitment and Retention: Meeting Staffing Requirements

CHAPTER OUTLINE

What's Ahead
Objectives
Test Your Understanding
Recruitment
   Human resources
   What is recruitment?
   The employment process
Think Critically
Think Critically
Benchmarks
Retention: Why Is It Important?
   Turnover: Costs, reasons, prevention
Current Issues
   Staff role
   Orientation: Its role in retention and
      prevention of reality shock
Think Critically
   Losing staff
Benchmarks
Performance Appraisal
Your Opinion Counts

Performance standards and position
   descriptions
Competency-based performance appraisal
Legal and regulatory issues
Performance appraisal/evaluation process
Problems with employees
Think Critically
Benchmarks
Staffing: The Critical Issue Today
Your Opinion Counts
Current Issues
   Staffing basics
   The nursing shortage
   Strategies to resolve the problems: Some
      are successful and some are not
Current Issues
Benchmarks
Chapter Wrap-Up
Summary and Applications
References
Additional Readings

 MediaLink
www.prenhall.com/finkelman

The Interactive Exercises for this chapter can be found in the OneKey course at www.prenhall.com/finkelman. Click on Chapter 12 to select from the following activities: Test Your Understanding, Benchmarks, Current Issues, Your Opinion Counts, Think Critically, and Summary and Applications.

What's Ahead

The link between recruitment and retention is clear—recruiting the right staff for the right job is the first step in retention of staff. The work environment and many other factors also affect retention, as well as the ability to recruit. Recruitment and retention may be seen as functions of human

336

resources; however, it is a wise nurse leader who recognizes that nursing staff need to be involved in this process. Staff need to help identify factors that drive recruitment and retention. Nurse managers, and in many cases staff, need to be involved in the interview and selection process of staff. Word of mouth can be a critical factor in the community—nurses let other nurses know the best places to work. Nurses in the community know which health care organizations have problems hiring and retaining staff. Organizational culture has a strong effect on recruitment and retention. Many times the factors that drive recruitment and retention problems can be identified by nurses in the community, but health care organizations do not always ask for this feedback. This chapter speaks to two perspectives: the health care organization's recruitment and retention efforts from the employer and the candidate/employee perspectives and to the critical problem of the nursing shortage, which affects recruitment and retention. Recruitment and retention also have an impact on the shortage. Consider the following data about employment in general:

- More than 90% of all hiring decisions are based on the interview.
- Interviewing is only 14% accurate in predicting performance.
- Most selection decisions are made in less than 1 hour.
- Turnover cost can be as high as 100% of annual salary.
- Many organizations do not track actual turnover cost.
- Thirty million people secured employment by lying on their resumes (Plotkin, 1997, p. 8).

Given these facts, effective recruitment and retention of competent staff are critical to meet staffing needs. The potential employee also should be aware of the critical facts and issues about recruitment and retention. With the increasing shortage of nursing staff, recruitment, retention, and related staffing activities have become critical functions within health care organizations.

OBJECTIVES

Before you begin, take a moment to familiarize yourself with the key objectives of this chapter.

- Describe how the human resources department assists the health care organization and employees.
- Describe staff recruitment.
- Explain how a position description is developed.
- Describe the employment process.
- Identify critical guidelines that a nurse should consider when applying for a position.
- Explain why it is important for nursing staff to be involved in recruitment and how they might do this.
- Discuss the importance of retention.
- Discuss the purpose of performance appraisal.
- Describe the performance appraisal process.
- Identify strategies that can be used to prevent or decrease stress and passive-aggressive behavior in the work setting.
- Discuss reasons for the nursing shortage.

TEST YOUR UNDERSTANDING

Before we begin our exploration of this chapter, take a short "warm-up" test to see what you know about this topic.

Recruitment

Recruitment focuses on finding the right staff. Issues that are included in this discussion are the department of human resources' responsibilities, policies and procedures, employment legal issues, job analysis, and the employment process. Nurses are involved in all of these issues as managers, team leaders, staff nurses, potential employees, or new employees.

Human resources

The **human resources (HR) department** in a health care organization is responsible for ensuring that staff are recruited, hired, promoted and transferred, retained, and terminated according to the organization's policies, procedures, and relevant laws. The goal is to hire and retain the best staff possible to meet the mission and goals of the organization and its components.

Functions and activities

The Joint Commission on Accreditation of Healthcare Organizations (JCAHO), the primary organization for accreditation of health care organizations, includes management of human resources in its standards. The following are the key standard focus areas:

- Human resources planning
- Orienting, training, and educating staff
- Assessing competence
- Managing staff requests (Joint Commission on Accreditation of Healthcare Organizations, 2004, p. 235)

These hospital standards identify the major goal of human resources: "to identify and provide the right number of competent staff to meet the needs of patients served by the hospital" (Joint Commission on Accreditation of Healthcare Organizations, 2004, p. 231). Meeting this goal requires planning by leaders to identify guidelines related to qualifications, competencies, and staffing. Competent staff must be provided to ensure that goals are met. Staff competencies need to be assessed, maintained, and improved, which should be an ongoing process. A culture needs to be established in which self-development and learning are supported. When the JCAHO standards are reviewed, it is clear that human resources does not work in isolation, but rather, the organization's leaders or management set the tone and guide human resources. It takes a coordinated and collaborative effort to ensure that recruitment and retention processes are functioning and effective, and this requires clear communication about the functions and activities to be carried out by human resources and management. "Recruitment is a complex process, and when it is not working, facts are required to improve it. Often it becomes an emotional area with one group blaming the other" (Finkelman, 1996, p. 2-1.2). Effective human resources departments have strong positive relationships with management, and staff feel that human resources is a support service for them, not a department that acts against them.

Human resources policies and procedures

Human resources, in collaboration with management, develops policies and procedures related to employment and staffing. Issues that are typically considered include hiring, promotion, transfers, termination, staffing and scheduling, benefits and staff requests, and other related issues. Procedures to ensure effective communication related to these policies and procedures are a critical concern as communication is a typical problem area. For example, staff may not be informed about a change in policy about work schedules, or a manager may not be informed about the hiring process. Required employment documentation needs to be clearly identified and implemented because this can have serious consequences on staff performance. Monitoring the implementation of policies and procedures is used to determine if standards are met. Health care organizations with labor unions must factor this into the management of their human resources. Labor contracts affect policies and procedures, documentation, monitoring, human resources decision making, and staff involvement.

Legal issues

Employment is heavily affected by laws, both federal and state, that protect employers and employees. It is important for both the HR staff and management to understand these laws and their implications to the hiring, promotion, and termination processes. It is equally important for employees to understand the implications of these laws, many of which are not explained during orientation. The following descriptions highlight the major laws and how they affect employers and employees.

Americans with Disabilities Act (ADA)

The Americans with Disabilities Act of 1990 prohibits discrimination in hiring and job assignments based on disability (Pell, 2000). Reasonable accommodation must be made (for example, equipment for the hearing challenged, ramps for wheelchairs, allowing employees to work in an area of the building that is easier to get to, allowing reasonable time for medical appointments, and so on). Substance abuse is classified as a disability, as is mental illness. A past history of problems in these areas cannot be used to disqualify a qualified person for employment. If, however, the employee is unable to do the job due to absences or errors, or if the employee has a history of this work behavior in a previous position, the employee can be terminated for poor work habits. However, the employee may not be terminated for a disability. The employer can refuse to hire the candidate based on poor work habits, but not a history of substance abuse or mental illness.

Employment Equal Opportunity Commission (EEOC)

The Employment Equal Opportunity Commission is the federal agency that administers the Civil Rights Act/EEO, the Age Discrimination in Employment Act, and the Americans with Disabilities Act. The EEOC is the agency that receives complaints when these laws may be violated. It conducts the investigation, makes the decisions as to fault, and designates the penalties. The EEOC can make an employer keep an employee or hire a candidate, require an employer to pay back pay, and even require that employee/candidate's legal fees are covered by the employer. The EEOC does not have to inform an employer that they are coming to investigate a complaint; however, records should not be turned over without presentation of a subpoena or a search warrant nor should staff be interviewed without legal counsel. Methods for avoiding EEOC problems include: use of routine and appropriate management education about the laws and implications, implementation of policies and procedures that comply with the laws, recruitment that does not discriminate, development of standardized interviewing process, use of application forms that meet legal requirements, and maintenance of accurate notes regarding application and hiring, promotions, and terminations.

Civil Rights Act of 1964

The Civil Rights Act of 1964 and its amendments have had a major effect on the workplace. This law prohibits discrimination in employment on the basis of race, color, sex, religion, or national origin. There is one section of this law, Title VII, that is particularly relevant, and it is referred to as the Equal Employment Opportunity (EEO) law (Pell, 2000). What does this law mean? All businesses with 15 or more employees cannot discriminate on the basis of race, color, or nationality. Questions on applications and during interviews cannot address these factors. Employment tests must be designed so as not to discriminate in these areas. The law also addresses discrimination based on religion, as businesses must now make reasonable accommodation for religious practice (for example, wearing of religious clothing and days off for religious holidays). Allowing for the latter does not mean that the business cannot make the employee use personal leave days for these days off nor are they required to pay them on these days. If meeting this requirement is an undue hardship for the business, then pay does not have to be provided. Businesses, however, can prohibit proselytizing in the workplace. This law also protects against discrimination on the basis of gender. Businesses can identify gender-specific positions; however, they must be clearly defined. Pregnancy cannot be used to discredit a woman for a position.

Affirmative action

Despite the fact that the Civil Rights Act of 1964 clearly states an employer cannot discriminate based on race, religion, national origin, or sex, giving preference to special groups continues to be a concern and is a highly controversial issue. Several presidential executive orders, beginning with those issued by President Johnson, require affirmative action for protected classes (African Americans, Hispanics, Asians or Pacific Islanders, Native Americans or Alaskan Natives, and women), which applies to all federal contractors and subcontractors that have contracts of more than $50,000 and have 50 or more employees (Pell, 2000). Executive orders are not laws and only apply to government agencies and organizations that do business with the government. Most health care organizations do business with the federal government, so many must meet these requirements. This business occurs when health care organizations accept Medicare and Medicaid payments for health care services that they provide. What does this mean to the employer? They must hire members from these protected classes "in proportion to the population of people in each class in their community" (Pell, 2000, p. 65). Employers must actively seek candidates from these minority groups. Over the years this effort has also led to accusations of reverse discrimination. In these cases, the complaint is that in giving members of the protected classes preference this denies or discriminates against someone who does not belong to one of the classes but is qualified for the position.

Family and Medical Leave Law (FMLA)

The Family and Medical Leave Law of 1996 applies to employers of 50 or more employees who work within a 75-mile radius. What does it cover? For employees who are eligible (and not all are eligible), it covers 12 weeks of unpaid leave during a 12-month period for medical reasons, which may include the birth or adoption of a child as well as care of a spouse, child, or parent who has a serious medical problem (Danaher, 2001). The medical problem may be mental or emotional illness. This law is complex, and when applied, it requires careful review. The employer may require that the employee submit medical certification of the claimed medical condition. If the employer has concerns about the validity of the certification, the employer can ask for a second medical opinion and even a third, but the employer is responsible for these costs. The employer may select the provider who will give additional medical opinions; however, this health care provider cannot be an employee of the employer (for example, a physician who works in the employer's hospital or clinic). Until all of the opinions are complete, the employee should receive FMLA benefits. For long-term or chronic conditions, the employer can request recertification but not second and third opinions.

Sexual harassment (EEOC)

Recent data from a national survey conducted from October, 2001, through March, 2002, of 7,600 nurses indicates that 19% of them had experienced sexual harassment or a hostile work environment related to other staff, and 19% had experienced harassment from physicians (*NurseWeek*, 2002). What is sexual harassment? First, it is a form of sex discrimination and a violation of the Civil Rights Act of 1964. In 1980, the Equal Employment Opportunity Commission (EEOC) further defined sexual harassment as "(1) unwelcomed sexual advances, (2) requests for sexual favors, (3) verbal conduct of a sexual nature, or (4) physical conduct of a sexual nature. These advances, requests, and types of conduct were considered sexual harassment when they (1) acted as a term or condition of employment, (2) were a criterion for employment decisions, (3) interfered with the victim's job performance, or (4) created a hostile, intimidating, or offensive work environment" (Aiken, 2001, p. 576). When a complaint is brought by an employee, the employee must prove that there is a causal connection between the harassment and the job benefit in question or a quid pro quo (Aiken, 2001). This is one type of harassment. A second type is a hostile work environment that interferes with the employee's ability to perform the job. The EEOC decides whether or not the situation qualifies as a hostile environment. Some factors that are considered are: (a) type of conduct (verbal, physical), (b) frequency of conduct, (c) whether offensive or hostile, (d) offender category such as supervisor or co-worker, (e) how many employees experienced the conduct, and (f) consistency of victim's conduct (Aiken, 2001). Other types of harassment are verbal, harassment of men, and harassment of homosexuals. Organizations should have a sexual harassment policy that describes how complaints are made. The EEOC has specific guidelines that need to be followed when complaints are filed with the EEOC (for example, there are time limits for filing complaints related to the alleged discriminatory act). Sexual harassment is a very emotional issue. Power over others plays a major role in this type of discrimination. There is abuse of authority, which is frightening. Harassers can be found at all levels and types of staff, in all types of organizations, and can be of either gender. Sexual harassment is extremely serious. "The employer can be held liable if the employer knew or should have known of the harassment and failed to take appropriate and immediate action to correct it" (Aiken, 2001, p. 579).

Age Discrimination and Employment Act (ADEA)

The Age Discrimination and Employment Act of 1967 and its amendments focus on age by prohibiting discrimination against anyone 40 years or older (Pell, 2000). In addition to this federal law, some states have their own laws protecting persons 18 years and older. This law covers businesses with 20 or more employees. As long as the person meets the requirements of the position, persons who fall in this age range cannot be denied the job. Many applications no longer include birth date or age, and most people do not include birth date on their resumes. How do some businesses try to get around this law? They say that the candidate is overqualified, the candidate made more money in his or her last position held than this position offers, or this is a trainee position. Businesses cannot say they will not cover older employees because their benefits will not cover them, because the law requires that all employees are covered by the benefit plan if it is offered. This was established by the Older Workers Benefits Protection Act of 1990 (Pell, 2000).

Federal Drug-Free Workplace Act

The Federal Drug-Free Workplace Act of 1988, which covers certain federal contractors and grantees and federal agencies, does not make screening for alcohol and drug use a requirement for employment; however, it does not make these tests illegal. This screening may be done as part of the pre-employment physical exam or at other times. Urine tests are usually used first, and then, if a problem is identified, blood tests may follow. The law does require that all federal contractors with contracts of more than $25,000: (a) Notify all employees in writing of the drug-free policy related to manufacturing, distributing, and using controlled substances, which are prohibited in the workplace. (b) Provide a drug-free awareness and education program for employees. (c) Provide employees with the policy statement, which employees must agree to follow. (d) Violation of the policy must be punished, and employees must participate in rehabilitation, and (e) Establish as a condition of employment that employees must report, within 5 days, any criminal arrest and convictions for drug-related activity in the workplace (Pell, 2000).

Workers' compensation

Workers' compensation is a very expensive type of insurance for employers, and its costs increased in the 1980s and early 1990s (Fox, 1998). This insurance is an important part of the national health care delivery system. Workers' compensation provides medical benefits and replacement of lost wages that result from injuries or illnesses that arise from the workplace. When an employee receives these benefits, the employee cannot then sue the employer for the injury. Typically, employees are provided workers' compensation coverage, as mandated by state law, employee medical benefits, and often disability benefits. Workers' compensation is not equivalent to employee medical benefits. Actually, workers' compensation was the first form of social insurance used in the United States. It is a social contract in that it is a form of mutual protection for the employee and the employer and is required by a federal law and delegated to states. The employer must follow state requirements related to benefits and limits. The financial status of the employer is not a factor in determining the type of plan it offers. The state's workers' compensation commission is the authority that supervises these health care services. States, however, do vary in the benefits they require.

Disability costs are an important part of workers' compensation costs. Workers' compensation is not, strictly speaking, health coverage. Most employers offer short-term disability that usually provides up to 60% of a worker's pay for up to 3 to 6 months after an incapacitating accident or illness. These policies may cover pregnancy and maternity leaves, usually for 10 weeks. Long-term disability becomes effective when short-term disability insurance coverage is exhausted (Gottlieb, 1998). Why is this insurance important? "For people between the ages of thirty-five and sixty-five, the odds of a disability lasting more than three months are three times greater than the chances of dying" (Gottlieb, 1998, p. 45). Paying for this care without any insurance can be a major financial crisis for most employees. Disability management is critical for most employers because it is used to control costs. Many workers who experience a disability feel a sense of entitlement of the benefit, and some experience a secondary gain from receiving this coverage. The entitlement or the worker's feeling that this benefit is "a right" can lead to workers demanding excessive medical care, and this in turn delays their return to work. As a result, employer costs also increase. Secondary gain comes from the wages the employee receives during the disability period without working.

Keeping workers' compensation separate from the traditional health care delivery system has not always proven to be the most cost-effective method of providing medical care for work-related injuries and illnesses. Workers' compensation is regulated under state laws. States vary in benefit levels, medical reimbursement schedules, and the amount of control that the employer has over employee medical choices. Occupational health nurses play an important role in the prevention of work-related injuries and illnesses as well as providing on-site treatment and follow-up.

Wagner Act of 1935 and the Taft-Hartley Act of 1948

The Wagner Act of 1935 and the Taft-Hartley Act of 1948, which amended the original law of 1935, cover issues related to employer-union relations (Pell, 2000). These laws prohibit discrimination based on union membership. Employers may not ask candidates if they are members of a union. Employers are no longer required to hire union members, but union contracts may specify that nonunion employees must join the union within a specific time period after they are hired. This is called "union shop." This issue has been taken over by some state laws, known as "right to work" laws, which prohibit "union shop" or fair-employment laws. This is an area that requires careful review of specific state law in addition to federal law.

Equal Pay Act of 1963

The Equal Pay Act of 1963 prohibits the determination of pay based on gender (Pell, 2000), referred to as "equal pay for equal work." The person must be legally able to work in the United States. Comparable worth is more than equal pay for equal work, and it is more than just addressing appropriate values to the employer. This is complicated and includes job analysis with points assigned to jobs so that even jobs that seem completely different may be of comparable worth based on such factors as education, training, responsibility, and so on.

Immigration Reform and Control Act of 1986

The Immigration Reform and Control Act of 1986 prohibits the denial of employment due to nationality. However, there are key responsibilities that must be met when hiring immigrants, such as examining required documentation to prove identity and citizenship, or documents authorizing employment of noncitizens.

What is recruitment?

Recruitment is a planned and coordinated effort to ensure that competent and appropriate staff are available to meet the goals and provide the organization's services. The recruitment process includes five steps, which are described in Figure 12-1.

After this process is completed and a candidate accepts employment, then the final steps of admitting the candidate to employment and orientation take place. There is no doubt that recruitment is critical for any organization as without competent staff organizations will not be effective and will not survive. The goal is to hire the right person in the right job at the right time.

How do human resources and management get the right person in the right job at the right time? The first step is to have a clear understanding of the job or position and then develop a position description that meets the needs. Hiring criteria need to be developed to identify the attributes of successful employees, and these can then be used to help make hiring decisions (Hutchison, 2001a). The goal is to hire staff who have a chance of succeeding in order to decrease turnover and of course better ensure high-performance employees. This is not easy to accomplish as sometimes criteria do not effectively address critical characteristics. Hutchison (2001a) notes that "Passion never should be overlooked because it is the single most universal trait of success" (p. 53). How can this attribute be evaluated? Interviewers can ask candidates about examples of when they made an extra effort to get something done and were enthusiastic

FIGURE 12-1   The recruitment process.

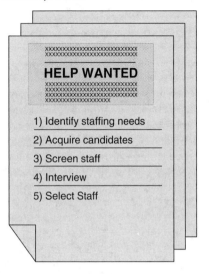

Source: Author.

about something at work. What examples can be described that indicate a drive toward success, leadership, and a pattern of growth? Other issues to consider in hiring criteria are: (a) education and work experience, (b) problem-solving skills, (c) personal values, (d) specific clinical skills, and (e) cultural fit. Cultural fit with the organization is very important as staff tend to stay in organizations where they feel there is a match between their values and the organization's values—staff will be happier when this occurs. Since change is ever present today, asking candidates to describe their experiences with change can be helpful in identifying the right employee for the job by assessing their coping styles when change occurs.

Job analysis and position descriptions

Job analysis includes a clear description of responsibilities and skills for a specific job. How does HR arrive at this description? Various methods such as observation of performance, interviews of staff who hold the position, interviews of supervisors/managers, and discussions with team members, and how other organizations describe a similar position, are used to gather data about jobs/positions. The result should be the position description, which lays out the job expectations to be used for hiring and performance evaluation. The typical parts of a job or position description include the following:

- **Education**—the type and level required to meet the job requirements (for example, a BSN degree)
- **Skills**—the skills the new employee requires to meet the job requirements (for example, EKG analysis for a cardiac care unit position)
- **Work experience**—what past experiences and duration are related to present job requirements (for example, 2 years as staff nurse in a medical-surgical unit for a home health position)
- **Physical strength or stamina**—what is required to meet the job requirements (for example, heavy lifting)
- **Intelligence**—specific requirements for the job, which may be measured by standardized tests, which is not frequently identified in health care position descriptions
- **Communication skills**—should be specified (for example, ability to lead groups for a position in a mental health clinic)
- **Accuracy of work**—jobs requiring detail and those that must be done right the first time (for example, data entry)
- **Stress level**—what is the level and need for coping skills (for example, ability to handle rapid patient turnover for a position in an Emergency Department)

■ Special factors—might include fluency in a foreign language, willingness to travel, willingness to work on weekends, or to be on call (Pell, 2000, pp. 24–25)

Each of these specifications must meet any relevant legal requirements.

The employment process

The employment process is long and complex. It, of course, begins with recruitment of candidates. Typical methods used to attract job candidates include: (a) print advertising (newspapers, professional journals), (b) Internet, (c) job fairs, and (d) use of nurse recruiters. Word-of-mouth is also an important method. The latter is what has driven the use of incentives that some health care organizations have used to encourage their staff to refer job candidates. Many employers are now meeting with nursing students in schools of nursing to attract them. After receiving resumes, these candidates then need to be screened.

During **screening,** applications are reviewed in more detail, and selections are made for interviews. Preparation for interviews takes time. After the interviews, another selection is made to determine if additional interviews are required, additional candidates should be sought, or who will be offered the position. The offer is then made, and negotiation may take place. It is important to frequently evaluate the process, which is highly dependent on communication that can easily fail.

It is very important to remember that the very first initial contact in the employment process is a potential employee's first impression of the employer. Many potential employees are lost when they are unimpressed with the process and associate this with the organization. When telephone calls go unanswered; staff do not respond when they say that they will; applications are lost; or staff are rude on the telephone, potential employees may look elsewhere for employment.

Screening

The goal of screening is to identify those candidates who should be evaluated further. Screening actually can take place more than once. The first time may be when potential candidates call or e-mail for further information. A second opportunity for screening is after candidates submit resumes and in some cases applications to determine which candidates will be interviewed. The third screening is directly involved in the final decision when choices are made about additional interviews, or a candidate is selected for the position. Sources of data that are used in screening are via telephone and e-mail, application, references, resume, licensure, certification status, and in-person interview contact.

Pros and cons of application formats

Applications are important. A candidate may send a resume and then indicate on application, "See resume." Candidates, however, should be required to complete the organization's application. First, this protects the organization legally—the organization is meeting the requirements of employment laws. Applications also provide a standard record of information about candidates that can be used when recruitment is evaluated; when consistent types of data from the applications are needed; and it also provides one consistent source of information about employees. When candidates are compared, then the application is the best source for comparison data.

Despite the fact that applications provide a consistent format for information about candidates, it is important to approach application review with some flexibility. This requires, first, a clear understanding of the position and need. If the position description says the candidate must have 5 years of experience but the candidate only has 3 years, this should be considered with an open mind. In some cases, a candidate may not have the required experience but has some characteristics that indicate the candidate could quickly adapt and learn to meet the job requirements. Reviewing the application form with a rigid eye may lead to missing out on an important candidate. Another problem that can occur is reviewing candidates too quickly because positions need to be filled. When there is a shortage in nursing, it is easy to think any nurse is better than none. In this case, little or no consideration may be given to the job requirements and matching them with the best candidate. This can lead to serious performance problems.

Resume

In reviewing **resumes,** the format or style does make a difference. The chronological style, the most commonly seen resume, is an easy style to review and provides an overall picture of the candidate with a listing of jobs by dates of employment. The functional style is organized around functions that the candidate performed in previous jobs (for example, direct care, management, and patient education functions). This style may not provide as much detailed information and also may not describe duration of employment, but it does build up experience. Red flags that require further investigation are: (a) gaps in dates, (b) more information supplied on earlier positions than more current ones, (c) overemphasis on education and non-job factors, and (d) poor grammar and spelling. (See Chapter 13 for further information about developing resumes.)

References

References are typically requested at some time during the hiring process. Human resources staff contact references via telephone or request written information. Candidates supply names, telephone numbers, and addresses for their references.

Licensure

Licensure is very important to many positions in the health care setting such as registered nurses. Some time during the application process, employers will ask for the nurse's professional license number, renewal date, and the state that issued the license. Typically after the position is accepted, the candidate must show the license and/or submit a copy of it. This is required by state licensure boards to ensure that appropriate staff such as registered nurses are licensed. Checking licensure of a nurse candidate with the state board of nursing may lead to information about professional misconduct. However, the reporting of misconduct and disciplinary action process is not perfect. "Understanding how nurses can be disciplined may help us change our minds about giving these sometimes marginalized colleagues another chance. The employment interview process offers a rich opportunity for exploring the circumstances that led to the discipline, assessing what the nurse has learned from the experience, and analyzing his or her potential to contribute to the organization" (LaDuke, 2001, p. 410). It is the employer who needs to make the decision about offering employment, but only licensed professionals can hold positions that require licensure.

Certification status

Certification is also important for some positions. Probably, the certification that covers many who work in health care is cardiopulmonary resuscitation certification. Candidates may be asked if certified and when hired to show documentation. Other certifications that may be relevant are nursing certifications for specific clinical practice.

The interview

The interview is a critical step in the hiring process; in fact, it is the most important method used in selecting staff. It is costly and time-consuming, and so must be done with thought, from the selection of the candidates to interview, preparation for the interviews, the interview itself, and then analysis of the interview results so that the best possible decisions can be made.

Interviewer: Planning for the interview

The interview step begins as soon as candidates are selected for interviews, which will affect the number and types of interviews as well as when they will take place. Interview appointments must be made, frequently requiring coordination of schedules between many people. The candidate needs to be told who will be doing the interviews and their positions, locations, time frames, and any other pertinent information such as parking and information to bring to the interview. All staff who will be involved in the interviews need to be sent a copy of the candidate's resume and, if available, an application as well as being informed about the time, place, and so on, for the interview. Prior to the interview, those who are interviewing the candidate need to review the candidate's resume and application, if the application has been completed prior to the appointment. Time should be spent in developing questions that will be asked during the interview.

Although both the interviewer and interviewee are interviewing one another, the interviewer should be in control of the process. Preparing ahead will better ensure that this control is maintained. There may be more than one interview so, after the first interview, a decision must be made to ask the candidate to return for a second interview. All of this requires planning with multiple people and receipt of their feedback. The interviewee/candidate should be told what will happen after the interview (for example, when decisions will be made and how the candidate will be informed).

Interviewing guidelines

Effective skills

An interview is a formal discussion, although many approach it more casually. An effective result requires some thought and homework. It is, however, not helpful to have an overly structured interview in which the interviewer does not allow for some flexibility as topics arise. Follow-up is critical during the interview. Effective interviewers are cognizant of the relevant laws and how they impact questions asked in the interview and on the process itself.

Restrictions on language

Language during the interview is also affected by employment laws—what can be said or not said. Another concern is actually saying too much about the position to the candidate before the candidate is given the opportunity to share information. If this is done, the candidate has more opportunity to formulate responses that match the position requirements, which may or may not be an accurate reflection of the candidate or candidate's experiences.

Barriers to effective skills

It is easy for many interviewers to quickly jump to a conclusion about a candidate soon after the interview begins or even in initial telephone conversations. Biases—what is seen or heard—can lead to positive or negative responses to the candidate. This can also work in the reverse, in that the candidate can have biases about the employer and also jump to conclusions before all the facts are known. "It is good to realize that most people are not at their best during an interview. It takes 20 minutes for most candidates to become less tense and open up for the talented interviewee to let down her guard" (Hutchison, 2001a, p. 54).

Evaluation criteria

Evaluation and selection of candidates involves reviewing all the material available on the candidates. All staff who were involved in the process need to share their feedback in a timely fashion, whether this is written or verbal. Then the hiring criteria are used to make a final determination. The person or persons who will make the final decision should be clear to all involved in the process.

An effective job interview: Hiring staff and getting the job

There are structured and unstructured interviews; however, there needs to be some structure in every interview for it to be effective. This is where planning becomes important—considering what needs to be asked and why. There may be a list of standard questions that are routinely asked and then supplemented with more job-specific and individual candidate questions. Having a list of questions better ensures that all questions are asked. Some organizations use group interviews with a group of key staff sitting in on the same interview. In this case, the group should work out procedures about asking questions and follow-up. Again, this is done to ensure that everything is covered. If the interview appears disorganized, the job candidate may then conclude that the staff are disorganized. Candidates should be told if there will be a group of interviewers.

The interview should begin with establishing rapport. Privacy, of course, is important during the entire process. Introductions of all staff present should be done with some brief statement about their roles. After a few introductory comments to put the candidate at ease, the interview should begin. Most of the questions should be open ended. Box 12-1 provides some sample questions and content to consider.

BOX 12-1   Sample job interview questions and content.

These questions and content areas might be used in a job interview. Candidates for positions should give these some thought prior to interviewing.

Clinical Experience

- Discuss your most recent nursing experience.
- Describe your experiences with nursing procedures.
- What are your strengths in nursing skills?
- Discuss the documentation system with which you are most familiar.
- Describe what you feel is an appropriate work schedule.

Nursing Skills

- How would you organize care for a patient? What needs take priority?
- Describe the nursing care you give.
- Describe how you feel about and use nursing care plans.
- Tell me about your best example of patient teaching.
- Describe what skills you have that would benefit this unit.

Leadership

- Discuss your concept of "team building" skills.
- If you had your choice, would you choose primary care, total patient care, functional care with a medication nurse, or team nursing? Why do you prefer this model?
- Tell me how you would conduct a patient care conference.
- Discuss a situation in which you approached a physician concerning a problem with a patient.
- If you were a team leader, how would you handle a problem with a team member's care?

Self-Assessment and Motivation

- Describe a major accomplishment during your last experience (college, work).
- Discuss how you plan to continue to grow personally and professionally. What are your short-term and long-term goals?
- Explain how this position fits into your career goals 3 to 5 years from now.
- What factors do you wish to avoid in nursing positions?

Human Relations and Responsibility

- Describe the working relationship between the RN, LPN, and UAP. Provide some examples from your own experience.
- What is your management style? What do you assess in supervising others?
- What factors in your college career were most and least challenging?

Source: Author.

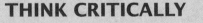

THINK CRITICALLY

Try this exercise to apply what you have learned about this topic.

The interviewer should allow the interviewee/candidate time to respond and not feed the interviewee answers or cut the interviewee off. The interview should stay on task and not wander off. As the interview progresses, information found in the candidate's resume and application should be explored. One technique that is useful is the nondirective approach, which encourages the candidate to expand on ideas (Pell, 2000). This might include: "Tell me more about. . . ." Nodding the head and using other methods to indicate interest will lead the candidate on to say more. Health care organizations are using more situational questions by asking nurse candidates what they would do for specific problems or by discussing hypothetical situations. Using real examples instead of hypothetical ones can be more helpful as "people tend to repeat actions" (Hutchison, 2001a, p. 55). When candidates discuss their own experiences this can provide information about how they might handle similar problems. This allows the interviewer to gauge the interviewee's critical thinking and ability to handle multiple problems. Of course, the interviewer must be knowledgeable about the situation proposed in order to assess the response and ask follow-up questions. Another technique is to end with summarizing questions by asking the candidate to summarize some aspect of the discussion. The candidate might also be asked about examples of when the candidate was resourceful, received criticism, worked under supervision, and worked with others. He or she may also be asked to describe him/herself. At the end of the interview, the candidate needs to be given the opportunity to ask additional questions and told about the next steps in the process. During the interview, the interviewer should take notes to ensure that information is not forgotten.

Interviewers can make serious mistakes during the interview that may lead to obtaining inadequate information and to poor decision making. Talking too much can be deadly as it limits time for the candidate to respond. Cutting the candidate off by jumping in too soon with another question or comment is not helpful, either. The interview does need to be in the control of the interviewer; if the interviewer is clear about the position, knows the interview questions that need to be asked, and is aware of the content of the candidate's resume and application, this will put the interviewer in more control. Interviewers need to listen and follow-up on questions, or important information may be ignored. Throughout the interview the interviewer's body language and communication techniques are important. The candidate will be watching for cues and interest. For example, if the interviewer communicates through body language that there is limited interest in the candidate even though this may not be the case (the interviewer may just be tired), the candidate may decide that this is not the organization where he/she wants to work. If there are doubts about the candidate and the particular position or fit with the organization, then the interviewer should comment on this and allow the candidate to respond (Carroll, 2001). This might open up the discussion, allowing the candidate to further expand on experiences and skills, and help in the selection process.

At some point in the application process, it is important to offer the candidate the opportunity to visit units or other worksites. This allows the candidate to see the work environment and staff. As this is time-consuming and costly, since it does take staff time, this visit should be planned with staff accompanying the candidate and should not disturb work or interfere with patient care. With the increasing concern and legal requirements about patient privacy and confidentiality, consideration needs to be given as to the private information about patients the candidate might view during tours. Staff who escort the candidate need to be briefed as to their role and should be willing to do this, or it will not provide the most positive view of the organization. However, this should not be a staged experience with the staff member told what to say or not to say to the candidate. The candidate will notice this, and it will not be a positive experience for the candidate. After the tour the staff member can share information with HR or a manager about questions the candidate asked, concerns expressed by the candidate, and the candidate's communication skills.

The job candidate and the interview

The job candidate should arrive at least 10 to 15 minutes early to allow time to unwind and collect his or her thoughts before the interview. Parking information and directions should be clarified before going to the interview to avoid getting lost and being late. When entering the room for the interview, it is best to first see if the interviewer offers direction to a specific seat; if this does not occur, the best seat is one that is directly opposite the interviewer. During the interview, sharing of personal information should be limited. It is important to be aware of and avoid behaviors that indicate nervousness such as swinging legs, clinching hands, pencil tapping, knuckle cracking, and chewing gum. Dress should be business attire.

Before the interview, the interviewee should consider personal career goals and experiences. If the job candidate is a new graduate, the candidate should think about clinical experiences from courses taken. These may serve as examples during the interview. Coming to the interview with prepared questions that address critical issues demonstrates an understanding of the position sought. Finding out about the organization, its nursing services, and nursing staff prior to the interview is helpful. It also communicates interest.

THINK CRITICALLY

Try this exercise to apply what you have learned about this topic.

The type of position sought is also a consideration that affects questions that might be asked (for example, questions about responsibilities and types of patients and patient problems). Other issues that might be considered are the organization's culture, mission and vision, communication within nursing, interdisciplinary and organization-wide policies, scheduling, staff development and career advancement, differential for education and certification, and ability to change positions and receive promotions. It is important for the job candidate to listen to the interviewer and to clarify questions that might be confusing before answering them. As the candidate goes through the process, the candidate should consider if this is the place he/she wants to work. The American Nurses Association (2001) developed a Bill of Rights for Registered Nurses, which can be used as a guide to assist in the evaluation of the workplace, as described in Box 12-2.

Interviewing provides experience in how to evaluate organizations and positions. Even an interview for a position that might be of limited interest can give nurses more experience about the process. Some nurses even work for temporary agencies so that they can get into an organization and learn more about it before pursuing a long-term position in the organization.

Post-interview and selection

References

References should be checked carefully, although responses are frequently vague. When this occurs, the person who calls for references should push for more information. There is only so

BOX 12-2   Bill of rights for registered nurses.

1. Nurses have the right to practice in a manner that fulfills their obligations to society and to those who receive nursing care.
2. Nurses have the right to practice in environments that allow them to act in accordance with professional standards and legally authorized scopes of practice.
3. Nurses have the right to a work environment that supports and facilitates ethical practice, in accordance with the *Code for Nurses* and its interpretive statements.
4. Nurses have the right to freely and openly advocate for themselves and their patients, without fear of retribution.
5. Nurses have the right to fair compensation for their work, consistent with their knowledge, experience, and professional responsibilities.
6. Nurses have the right to a work environment that is safe for themselves and their patients.
7. Nurses have the right to negotiate the conditions of their employment, either as individuals or collectively, in all practice settings.

Source: American Nurses Association. (2001, September/October). *The American Nurse*, p. 20. Reprinted with permission.

much that can be done to encourage a past employer to reveal information, as many organizations have been advised by attorneys not to reveal information (Pell, 2000). This does not, however, mean that attempts to obtain this information from references should not be made.

Background checks

Federal regulations require **background checks** for some health care providers who apply for clinical privileges, such as physicians and dentists (Fiesta, 1999). This information is checked in the National Practitioner Data Bank every 2 years. Long-term care employers are often required by state laws to check their employees, including nursing staff. Some acute care hospitals now do background checks. Initial registered nurse licensure now requires fingerprinting to be used for a background check. Of particular interest in criminal background checks are patient abuse and neglect, rape, and child abuse.

Personnel testing

Personnel testing is done for some positions, but it is not as common for nursing positions.

Pre-employment physical

Alcohol and drug screening may be included in the physical, but it must meet the requirements of the Federal Drug-Free Workplace Act of 1988. The candidate cannot be discriminated against based on disability.

Selection of candidates

Selection of candidates for positions must be done thoughtfully. This decision needs to include all staff who had a formal role in the process and all relevant information (the resume, application, information from interviews, and reference information). Many organizations have forms that are used to evaluate candidates based on specific criteria.

Making the offer or not

The staff member who is responsible for making the job offer should be clearly identified, and typically, this is someone in HR. This staff member needs to know what is negotiable and what is not before contacting the candidate. If negotiation is then done, the staff person needs to know who in the organization needs to be consulted about the negotiation with the candidate and kept informed of the progress.

The candidate is involved in the negotiation of the salary, but what should the candidate consider? The first step is a self-assessment of worth. This is also important when a nurse wants an increase in salary. The self-assessment should consider factors such as education, experience, certification, cost of coverage by a temporary agency nurse or outsourcing compared with the employee, and contributions that the nurse has made in previous positions (or in the present position if seeking a promotion rather than a new position). Arguments for the salary need to be clearly made, discussed, and then at the end of the meeting there should be a summarization of the critical reasons used to support the salary change. After the position is accepted, then the candidate is informed about the next steps to take and what the employer will do. If the candidate rejects the position, it is helpful to know the reason as this information may assist in understanding recruitment problems.

When is the job the right job?

The benefit package is the description of services or additional pay that the employer offers employees, and benefits are important factors when accepting a position. These benefits may be covered by the employer, or the employee and employer may share the costs for them, often at a reduced rate for the employee. The benefits that are offered vary from employer to employer. Benefits are not required, but they go a long way to attract potential competent employees to accept positions. Labor unions affect the types of benefits offered, as this is part of the negotiated labor contracts; however, not all health care organizations are unionized. Benefits should be evaluated carefully by potential employees. It is important to understand individual needs, and then evaluate the benefit package based on this information. If information is not clear or there are questions, candidates for positions, new employees, and long-term employees should address these with the organization's human resources staff. During new employee orientation, benefits are typically discussed. If a nurse changes positions, there could be an effect on benefits, so this needs to be addressed. What are some of the benefits that might be offered in a benefit package?

- Insurance: health, life, disability, dental, vision
- Vacation and/or personal leave
- Sick days
- Maternity/paternity leave
- Holidays
- Shift differential
- Charge nurse differential
- Differential for nurses with advanced degrees
- "On Call" pay
- Credit union
- Recruitment bonus
- Relocation assistance
- Housing assistance
- Uniform allowance
- Flexible scheduling/job sharing
- Orientation, refresher courses, internship, preceptorship
- Career ladder
- Education assistance
- Reduced fee for gym facilities
- Discounted or free meals in facility cafeteria
- Free or discounted parking (Burke & Whited, 1997, pp. 15–16)

Most nurses in their career will work in a variety of settings and hold several different types of positions. Some of this will be due to changes in educational levels, but it is also due to changes in interest and personal requirements such as scheduling and level of responsibility. An advantage of nursing as a profession is there are so many different ways that a nurse can practice and places where that practice can take place. With the variety of positions available, there are a number of job-related factors that the nurse needs to consider when evaluating a new position.

- The nurse applicant will want to decide whether or not the level of work required meets the nurse's personal needs and career goals. This would include: (a) working part time or full time, or (b) shifts (day, evening, night, 12-hour shifts, or short shifts, which are used to cover busy times and when there are short staff periods).
- The type of health care organization may make a difference on whether or not the nurse is able to meet individual needs, goals, and skill level. Examples of organizations are: (a) community, (b) acute care, (c) long-term care, (d) university medical centers, (e) smaller community hospitals, (f) schools, (g) home care, and (h) other types of organizations.
- A critical question should be whether or not the position focuses on direct or indirect care. Making this decision will eliminate or clarify which positions to pursue.
- As positions are evaluated, the nursing delivery model that is used may be important. Is primary nursing or a form of team nursing used?
- How are team leaders chosen and how will this affect the applicant's interests.
- If the applicant has no interest in being a team leader at the time and team leadership is rotated among team members, then this may not be the position for the nurse.
- Another area of concern that each nurse should assess is the nurse's strengths and weaknesses. Weaknesses can be changed with education and/or additional experience, but to do this they need to first be acknowledged. The areas that need consideration when identifying strengths

and weaknesses are: (a) technical skills, (b) interpersonal relationship skills, (c) communication, (d) leadership, and (e) management skills. It is not expected that a nurse be at a high level of functioning in all these areas, but an honest appraisal is helpful. Certain positions require more of some skills than others. Mental health nurses clearly need to be more skillful in interpersonal relationships and communication although they still need some basic technical skills. A nurse who works in the community needs to have strong skills in interpersonal relationships, communication, epidemiology, leadership, and management, but if the nurse is working in the community as a home health nurse, technical skills will be a critical part of the position competencies.

■ The last consideration is specialty area, something that also may change over time. Specialty positions are also affected by education and certification. Some specialty decisions may be driven by required experience level before employment in that specialty area. Some organizations offer internships to further prepare nurses for work in the specialty, such as in intensive care or the operating room.

What is happening when a lot of effort is made to find a new position, but no offers are coming in (Cardillo, 2002)? If a nurse is getting interviews, but still no offers, it is important to do an assessment of the interviews. Issues to consider are communication, how one is coming across, strengths that are emphasized, and responses to interviewer questions. Clearly, this is not easy to do as it requires stepping back and taking an objective viewpoint. Obtaining some assistance with interviewing can be helpful. Following-up with an interviewer who did not offer a job and asking for feedback with the goal of improvement might be helpful. If a nurse is not getting calls for interviews, then the resume and cover letter may need to be reviewed. Asking others to review the resume and cover letter can provide helpful, objective feedback. It could be that the positions that are sought are just not appropriate to the nurse's education or experience. Networking can be helpful, as can using mentors to help identify possible positions that might be a better fit. (See Chapter 13 for further information about mentoring.) Self-assessment is never easy, particularly when there seems to be little success; however, if done well and with as much objectivity as possible, it can lead to some changes that may result in more positive results.

BENCHMARKS

Now let's take a moment to test your knowledge of the concepts you have studied in this section.

Retention: Why Is It Important?

Organizations that ignore staff **retention** soon experience problems with quality of care and costs. Staff retention keeps the organization going and meeting its mission and goals. Staff are needed to meet these goals. "The nursing philosophy, standards, rules that determine the working conditions, perception of peer cohesion, administrative support, autonomy, task orientation, work pressure, clarity, control, and innovation all help to develop the organization culture and maintain it" (Finkelman, 1996, p. 2-1:2). When staff do not mesh with the culture, problems occur such as staff frustration, unsatisfactory job performance, and decreased quality of care. (See Chapter 17 for further discussion about an organization's culture.) These all affect staff negatively and can lead to loss of staff. Problems with retention are extremely costly for health care organizations. Every organization has to make a concerted effort to create an environment that helps to retain staff, particularly nursing staff. "The purpose of recruitment is to hire the staff necessary for your agency to provide quality care. Retention is the tool that will allow your recruitment program to meet these goals. If you cannot retain your staff, you will never be able to recruit sufficient staff" (Hutchison, 2001b, p. 15).

Turnover: Costs, reasons, prevention

CURRENT ISSUES

Learn about events around the globe that relate to the chapter content.

Turnover problems are related to retention. The costs of turnover are great, most notably in the costs that went into hiring the staff member, orientation, and maintaining the staff member, such as human resources records, staff development provided, and so on. In addition, turnover causes great strain on work teams. When new staff must be oriented and become part of the team, this affects a unit's or a team's productivity, decreasing productivity time, which is costly. If the turnover becomes a more extensive problem, the organization as a whole suffers, leading to stress and frustration as more and more staff try to cope with empty positions, orient new staff, and adjust to new team members or temporary staff. Work teams eventually develop communication and methods of working together, but all of this takes time. When this is disturbed, work is disturbed. When there is a variance that disturbs the productivity, turnover rates need to be monitored and analyzed. It is important to identify the reasons for the turnover.

Clearly, there are reasons for turnover that are related to natural life events, such as births, ill family members, spouse job changes and required relocation, a need to stay home with younger children, and a return to school. If a move is required and the health care organization is a state or national organization, encouraging staff to stay in the system can be helpful for the health care system. An example is a nurse who works for the VA system able to transfer to another VA hospital in the system. Employers need to monitor the reasons staff are leaving their jobs because some of the reasons can be addressed through prevention methods (for example, by providing child care, encouraging nurses to work part time while in school, and supporting them with educational benefits). Other reasons are of more concern and more complex, and these include:

- Lack of staff empowerment, autonomy, and respect
- Inadequate staff (interdisciplinary and within nursing staff) communication
- Inadequate staff-management communication
- Inadequate compensation
- Scheduling issues
- Inability to work with immediate supervisor
- Interdisciplinary staff communication problems
- Inadequate staff development and little support for further education
- Lack of opportunities for advancement
- Increased number of non-nursing tasks done by nursing staff
- Lack of nursing leadership (Finkelman, 1996, p. 2-1:5-1:6)

Shader et al. (2001) investigated factors that influence satisfaction and anticipated turnover for nurses in an academic medical center. The study particularly examined the relationships between work satisfaction, stress, age, cohesion, work schedule, and anticipated turnover. A survey was used to obtain data from 12 units in a 908-bed university hospital. The results indicated the following.

1. Increased job stress led to lower group cohesion, lower work satisfaction, and higher anticipated turnover.
2. Higher work satisfaction led to higher group cohesion and lower anticipated turnover.

3. The more stable the work schedule, the less work-related stress, the lower the anticipated turnover, the higher the group cohesion, and the higher the work satisfaction.
4. Job stress, work satisfaction, group cohesion, and weekend overtime were all predictors of anticipated turnover for different age groups.

Staff view reasons for turnover differently as their personal perspective comes into play. One of the simplest interventions that can be used to help prevent retention problems is to let staff know they are appreciated—recognition and "thank you" is one place to start when addressing retention problems. It is also important for organizations to ask: What is good about the organization? What does it offer its staff? What is unique about it? Where does it need to improve? Answers to these questions can help an organization develop an action plan to retain staff. Organizations want to retain their best people, but this takes effort.

When management assumes that staff must be satisfied when they are good at their jobs, this may lead to a false sense of security. "But although competence can certainly help a person get hired, its effect is generally short lived. People who are good at their jobs aren't necessarily engaged by them" (Butler & Waldroop, 1999, p. 147). Job sculpting can and should be used by managers to help retain the best. "Job sculpting is the art of matching people to jobs that allow their deeply embedded life interests to be expressed. It is the art of forging a customized career path in order to increase the chance of retaining talented people" (Butler & Waldroop, 1999, p. 146). If this process is turned over to human resources, it will not be effective because it needs to come from management. Listening to staff is the place to begin. What excites a staff member? Using performance review time to discuss those things that make the staff member excited about work can be very useful and involves the staff member in the sculpting. Job sculpting must be done from a realistic stance. What can be done to help the staff member improve? What can be changed in the workplace to assist the staff member in becoming involved in activities that really drive the staff member forward and stimulate interest? It has to be remembered that "when job sculpting requires taking away parts of a job an employee dislikes, it also means finding someone new to take them on. If staffing levels are sufficient, that won't be a problem—an uninteresting part of one person's job may be perfect for someone else" (Butler & Waldroop, 1999, p. 152). However, there are many times when there is no one else who can do the parts of the job that the staff member does not like to do. Managers must be careful about promising too much as this can lead to even greater staff frustration and retention problems. Strategies for retaining staff should focus on providing "a safe and caring work environment, offer a good orientation, create pride, have a forum for open communication, be honest in the expectations of the position, and be competitive in salary and benefits" (Hutchison, 2001b, p. 16).

Staff role

Staff play a major role in retention of other staff. How staff work together can make an important difference in whether or not staff feel comfortable in the work environment. Motivation especially has a major impact. What motivates staff to work? Motivation is complex and very individual. It helps to explain why one staff member works differently or better than another and has a direct effect on performance. The typical factors that affect motivation are: (a) job design, (b) organizational structure, (c) autonomy and empowerment, (d) staff participation in decision making, (e) communication, (f) leadership style, (g) organizational culture, (h) ethics, and (i) mutual trust between management and staff (Finkelman, 1996). Some assume that job satisfaction and motivation are the same, but they are not, although they are related. "Job satisfaction is a consequence of rewards and punishment related to past performance. Job dissatisfaction leads to decreasing morale, increasing absenteeism, and turnover" (Finkelman, 1996, p. 2-1:7). Nurse managers and their actions have an impact on staff motivation. Actions such as providing positive feedback, recognizing work effort, some degree of flexibility, asking staff to take part in decision making, providing resources staff need to do their jobs, and trying to find the best staff to fill empty positions and retain staff who improve the level of productivity all demonstrate that management is concerned about staff.

Another important factor in staff retention is the efforts that are made in career advancement. (See Chapter 13 for further information on this topic.) Identifying staff with skills and expertise for promotion is an important management responsibility. The "Peter Principle" or promoting past one's ability is not what should be done, but rather staff who can succeed should be the ones promoted. Organizations must also provide support, training, and opportunities for further education to staff (Peter & Hull, 1969). This can be very effective in retaining staff. Staff then feel recognized and more motivated to remain.

Orientation: Its role in retention and prevention of reality shock

Orientation is a key tool for getting staff ready to do the job they were hired to do and in the retention of staff. A work contract is established during orientation as new staff gain a greater understanding of the organization and its expectations. Spirit and respect are critical during the orientation process. New staff should get the sense of respect given to staff and the importance of staff input. Commitment to a job tends to decrease if staff:

- Do not feel safe and secure
- Consider their pay or benefits inadequate
- Believe their position is not what was presented in the interview and hiring process
- See their managers as non-responsive
- Perceive administration as non-responsive (Hutchison, 2001b, p. 16)

Along with orientation, staff development and continuing education are important tools in retention as well as recruitment. A strong program that ensures staff competency will be noticed by candidates for positions and will go a long way to retaining staff.

THINK CRITICALLY

Try this exercise to apply what you have learned about this topic.

Retention efforts need to be proactive. Building better relationships between physicians and nurses is extremely helpful in improving retention. Improving technology to reduce paperwork also affects retention. Recent data from a national survey of 7,600 nurses conducted by *Nurse Week* (2002) and the American Organization of Nurse Executives from October, 2001, through March, 2002, indicated that 43% of those in the sample planned on leaving their current position in the next 3 years. Reasons given for leaving were:

- 57% to take a new position
- 21% to pursue a job in another profession
- 14% to return to school
- 14% to take time out for family reasons
- 14% to retire

This same sample described their satisfaction level with being a nurse: 37% were very satisfied, 40% were satisfied, and 23% were dissatisfied. However, 40% indicated that they would not advise a high school or college student to pursue a nursing career. When nurses were asked what would be a critical factor to make them reconsider plans to leave their present position, 58% indicated higher salary or benefits, 50% cited more respect from management, and 48% noted better staffing. Salary is not always the most important factor, particularly when the working conditions are unpleasant and non-supportive (Trossman, 2002). What implications do these data have? For example, a quarter of the nurses (a large percentage) were dissatisfied, and another large percentage would not recommend nursing as a profession. Reflecting a negative view of the profession by those who practice nursing is a serious problem, and these attitudes do have an effect on how new nurses are greeted and oriented.

What is an effective orientation program? First, it must be organized, and orientee feedback needs to be used to evaluate orientation to appropriate changes. Orientation should include up-to-date general information about the organization. Typical content includes the organization's vision, mission, goals, structure, human resources or personnel policies and procedures, benefits, communication, labor union (if applicable), and staff education or development. Specific orientation is given about the worksite or unit including its relevant goals, structure, communication, policies and procedures, and (if applicable) shared governance and career advancement. Preceptors should be assigned to orientees to assist with their orientation. The best preceptors are those who volunteer and can be available to the new staff. Preceptors help new staff, particularly recent graduates, develop the following:

- Increased confidence and competence in the clinical setting
- In-depth understanding of the nurse's role
- Increased ability to problem-solve through critical thinking
- Feelings of belonging and professional nurturance (Diehl-Oplinger & Kaminski, 2000, p. 46)

When new positions are considered, nurses should ask about preceptors and their use in orientation.

Orientation can be dull at times, and programs that try to make it a more interactive experience, allowing new employees time to get to know one another as well as the other staff, are more effective. Orientation should provide new employees with the information and tools that they need to begin a new position in the organization. Orientation is also important for employees who are changing positions, from one area to another or through a promotion, but this orientation is often neglected. Potential employees should ask what is provided to staff who change positions or are promoted within the organization in these circumstances, as this will demonstrate how the organization values career advancement and change.

Losing staff

Losing staff should be an organizational concern. Analyzing the reasons for staff resignations is the place to begin and then, whenever possible, these causes need to be resolved.

Termination

Terminating staff is never easy. It needs to be done thoughtfully with a clear understanding about the reasons for the **termination.** Staff often are given the opportunity to resign. A manager may use the time to counsel the staff member, particularly if the manager feels that the position or type of nursing are not the best fit for the staff member. Most staff, however, are usually quite upset and have difficulty hearing this advice. How terminations are handled and why staff are terminated has a tremendous effect on staff morale. Although termination is initiated by the organization and not the employee, this does not mean that the organization should ignore the reasons for the terminations (for example, staff who have been terminated due to an inability to fulfill job requirements). Causes for this should be analyzed. Staff may not be clear about expectations, not know how to do the job, lack continuing education on the job responsibilities, and so on.

Resignation

Resignation should be carried out in a positive manner even when negative feelings are felt (Cardillo, 2002). The first resource a nurse should consult is the employee policies and procedures, which should describe what is expected of employees at the time of resignation. It is also important that the immediate supervisor be informed before gossip gets to the supervisor about the resignation, which can come from an internal or external source. After verbal notice is given, a written letter of resignation is provided addressed to the immediate supervisor. Copies are sent to the department director and human resources. This letter needs to be clear, well-written, and typed on good but plain stationary. It is not appropriate to use the letter as a vent for negative feedback. The letter will be kept in personnel files and thus will be referred to if references are sought. How a nurse leaves a position can make a difference in obtaining future positions. Following the appropriate process is important "because you never know when you'll need references or a recommendation from your employer or supervisor. And you never know when you'll encounter someone from that facility when you apply for work at another one later on" (Cardillo, 2002, p. 11).

Exit interview

The exit interview is an important tool for gathering information about the work environment and retention. Health care organizations need to consider the reasons staff are leaving. The following questions are important to ask in exit interviews.

- Why did you choose not to stay?
- What did you like most about your position?
- What did you like least?
- What did you like most about the agency/organization? The least?
- What could we have done differently to make your position more fulfilling (Hutchison, 2001b, p. 16)?

The interviewer should not be defensive when hearing negative comments about the organization or the job. The goal is to collect information and to try to arrive at a more positive departure viewpoint. It is important to remember that ex-employees will talk about past employers in the community, which is a public relations concern. Ex-employees who feel efforts have been made to listen to them, even though it may be late in the process, may feel more positive about the organization.

BENCHMARKS

Now let's take a moment to test your knowledge of the concepts you have studied in this section.

Performance Appraisal

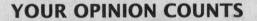

YOUR OPINION COUNTS

Find out what others think about this topic. Post your response and check out other opinions.

Performance appraisal is part of retention. During the process, management decides if staff are fulfilling job requirements and determine how to improve staff performance; by doing this, they provide guidance that will help to retain staff.

All employers have some type of performance appraisal, but performance appraisal may be called by many other terms, such as performance review, performance evaluation, performance assessment, and performance rating. Accreditation organizations require that health care organizations implement a performance evaluation process although there can be great variation in the type and effectiveness of the process. The traditional view of performance appraisal focuses on job competence and areas that need improvement; however, there are other important reasons for conducting a performance appraisal.

- It is an opportunity to provide feedback, direction, and leadership.
- It is a time to show support and encouragement.
- It is a time to initiate a discussion about areas that need improvement.
- It is an opportunity to evaluate accomplishments and to set goals (Milgram, Spector, & Treger, 1999, p. 195).

Other reasons for performance evaluation are:

- Building team cohesion
- Preventing discrimination problems
- Ensuring compliance with relevant laws
- Assisting with promotion

It is also an opportunity to reinforce the organization's vision, mission, and goals and to draw the employee into the organization's culture. The formal performance appraisal should not be the only time that the supervisor has a discussion with an employee or shares positive feedback. If this is the case, there are 364 days of lost opportunities to ensure staff improvement and growth. Staff will feel disconnected from the organization, and this affects performance, quality of care, safe care, staff dissatisfaction, and workplace stress and burnout. The ultimate result may be loss of staff and major problems with retention and recruitment as the word gets out that the organization or a unit or service is not concerned about its staff.

The idea of doing and participating in performance appraisal, despite its positive attributes, is rarely seen as a positive experience, and many dread it. Managers put off preparing appraisals and see it as an unpleasant task that often they do not feel competent to perform. The process is then conducted quickly with less thought. Employees sense this dissatisfaction with the process, and this then becomes something that just must be done. Feeling inadequate in conducting a performance appraisal is a major problem. Another potential problem is inadequate position descriptions that do not set clear performance standards for employees or for the person conducting the appraisal. If there are inadequate rewards, staff may not see the process as a positive one. Recruitment also plays a role. If staff are hired just to fill positions, then down the road there will be problems with performance appraisal when staff cannot meet the standards of the position, although this does not necessarily mean that the staff member will lose the position. There will be more of a struggle for the appraiser to find reasons to keep the staff member, especially when there are staff shortages. This, in the long run, dilutes the performance appraisal process and its results and has a direct impact on productivity, quality of care, and costs.

The major tool that is usually used for appraisal is the appraisal interview; however, before the interview can take place there are other concerns. The goal is to implement an effective performance appraisal that provides honest feedback to the employee and includes the employee in the process to better ensure quality of care, as well as improve staff performance and the organization's goals. What are issues or factors that need to be considered?

Performance standards and position descriptions

Health care organizations establish performance standards in their position descriptions. The human resources department plays a major role in all personnel issues, including performance appraisal. This department ensures that the process is maintained, keeps records, assists with development and review of standards and position descriptions, and consults with supervisory staff about performance issues and disciplinary concerns. There should be a positive relationship and effective communication between human resources and management. When this is lacking, there are major problems for all concerned.

The position description provides both the appraiser and the employee the standards or competencies that need to be met. This information needs to be given to all employees as they begin a new position. If changes are made in the description, then employees should be informed in writing. Organizations typically use a standard format for their position descriptions. Position descriptions are very important documents, and each staff member should have a copy of the description of their position. Typically, the position includes: job title, department (if applicable), status of the job (for example, full time, part time, or temporary), reporting relationship or to whom the employee reports (not a specific person but position; e.g., nurse manager), job summary, essential functions of the job or duties, qualifications, any physical requirements, and the date the description was approved. Position descriptions are also important for staff who are supervising other staff. They need to know what staff can do in their positions. For example, a team leader needs to have an understanding of the job that a UAP is expected to perform.

Competency-based performance appraisal

Competence is a frequently used term today. The National Council of State Boards of Nursing (NCSBN) defines competency as "the application of knowledge and the interpersonal, decision-making, and psychomotor skills expected for the nurse's practice role, within the context of public health, welfare, and safety" (National Council of State Boards of Nursing, 1996; as cited in Mustard, 2002, p. 37). The goal of inservice education within health care organizations is to maintain nursing competency throughout employment. (See Chapter 13 for further information on education.) Maintaining competency requires evaluation of competency, but this is not easy to accomplish. There needs to be "active reporting and corrective action without establishing a punitive environment" (Mustard, 2002, p. 41). The best approach is a proactive one that helps staff improve and prepare for changes and thus better ensure competency. The Pew 21 Competencies for the 21st Century discussed in Chapter 2 supports the need to ensure the continuing competence of regulated health care professionals. Nursing organizations also emphasize the need to develop and maintain competencies, as does the JCAHO.

Who is responsible for staff competency?

- The employer clearly has a responsibility to ensure that patients receive safe, quality care. Performance evaluation is one method that is used to ensure this.
- Regulatory boards such as the state boards of nursing also play a role when they establish the state practice act and scope of practice and monitor licensure because they are entrusted with protecting the health and safety of the public.
- Professional organizations are also involved by developing standards of practice that are used by regulatory boards, employers, and nurses to guide decisions and evaluation. These organizations are now more involved due to their participation in the certification of specialty nurses.
- Colleagues or other nurses have a role to play in peer evaluation and support of one another. The individual nurse has a major responsibility as a professional to meet state licensure requirements, maintain continuing education, participate in ongoing self-evaluation, participate in the employer-employee evaluation process, and assist colleagues through peer evaluation. The *Code for Nurses* (American Nurses Association, 2001) indicates that a nurse is responsible for professional growth and maintenance of competence. "Competence affects one's self-respect, professional status, and the meaningfulness of work. In all nursing roles, evaluation of one's own performance, coupled with peer review, is a means by which nursing practice can be held to the highest standards" (American Nurses Association, 2001, p. 18).

How competency is demonstrated continues to be a problematic issue. The Institute of Medicine report (2001) on quality care indicates that retooling practicing clinicians is critical today, and assessing this is part of performance appraisal. Should nurses be required to take only one exam in a lifetime career to demonstrate competency? How does attendance at continuing education programs demonstrate competency? Certification has been used as one method to demonstrate competency; however, it too has limitations. After the exam is taken for certification, if there are no other exams and only continuing education requirements, is competency demonstrated over time? Should this be left in the hands of professional organizations? There is no universal definition of continuing competence (Whitaker, Carson, & Sawlanski; 2000). This is a highly controversial, complex issue that has yet to be resolved. An ANA expert panel, appointed in 1999, addressed the issue of professional competence. The panel formulated several definitions.

- Continuing competence is ongoing professional nursing competence according to level of expertise, responsibility, and domains of practice.
- Professional nursing competence is behavior based on beliefs, attitudes, and knowledge matched to and in the context of a set of expected outcomes as defined by nursing scope of practice, policy, *Code for Nurses*, standards, guidelines, and benchmarks that assure safe performance of professional activities.
- Continuing professional nursing competence is determined according to level of expertise, responsibility, and domains of practice as evidenced by behavior based on beliefs, attitudes,

and knowledge matched to and in the context of a set of expected outcomes as defined by nursing scope of practice, policy, *Code of Ethics,* standards, guidelines, and benchmarks that assure safe performance of professional activities (American Nurses Association, 2001).

The panel recommended that individual nurses develop professional nurse portfolios to document ongoing behaviors that are important in promoting competent practice (Whitaker, Carson, & Sawlanski, 2000). This process should include self-reflection and peer feedback. Chapter 13 discusses portfolios in more detail as some health care organizations are using them to document staff activities and competencies for promotion or other recognition of performance.

It is important for employees to understand how the competency-based performance appraisal process is used in their organization. Part of this understanding needs to include:

- Who does the evaluation?
- Does that person understand the job that is being evaluated?
- How were the standards identified, and what occurs when they are changed?
- What methods are used to obtain data for evaluations?
- What are the performance evaluation documentation requirements?

Components of a performance management program have been changing, and there are now several new approaches that can be used. Some of these approaches are a greater emphasis on self-appraisal, continuous feedback, peer appraisal, and 360-degree appraisal.

- Self-appraisal should be part of every performance management program. Staff need to assess themselves and to include this information in their performance appraisal. How do they view their own performance? What are its strengths and limitations? What would staff recommend for improvement strategies? It is not easy to do self-evaluation, but it is an important skill to learn. Every nurse should be evaluating his/her performance daily and strive for improvement.

- Continuous feedback lets staff know as soon as they do something positive or need performance improvement. Staff need to receive clear recognition when their performance goes beyond expectations, improves, and also routinely, if their performance warrants it. Documenting this performance in the personnel file is important. This form of evaluation also helps to clarify expectations on a regular basis and offers more direct contact with staff. Timing of giving feedback is very important. During a stressful incidence, it is best to give feedback when the situation is calmer. Feedback should be given in private although it is important to provide public recognition when a staff member accomplishes something special or when a team or group of staff perform effectively. When appointments are made with staff, it is best to state the purpose of the meeting or staff may become concerned and spend time wondering about its purpose—maybe building it out of proportion.

- Peer appraisal is used in some organizations, with peers giving feedback to peers about job performance. This can be a very sensitive process that requires trust in peers to provide the constructive feedback objectively. All staff need to understand what needs to be done and how to do it. This feedback should not be the only method used in the evaluation process, but it can be helpful to know how peers respond to a staff member's performance.

- Another newer method of evaluation is 360-degree evaluation, which includes a variety of people in the feedback loop, thus forming a complete circle. This evaluation includes constructive feedback from supervisors, peers, other subordinates, self, and could include patients, family members, and other customers. All staff need to understand this method, why it is being used, and how it will be done. The staff member may choose who will do the evaluation, with a specified number identified. This feedback should be anonymous. Then feedback needs to be summarized. It is critical that those involved understand the criteria and that the focus is on performance, not personality issues. This type of evaluation should be used for development, not to make critical decisions such as salary increases.

Legal and regulatory issues

Some of the laws that were discussed earlier in this chapter are relevant to the performance appraisal process (for example, Civil Rights Act, Age Discrimination in Employment Act, Americans with Disabilities Act, and Fair Labor Standards Act). Performance appraisal must focus on performance and not individual characteristics such as gender, age, race, or sexual orientation. If any of these are used to determine a performance appraisal decision or a decision about salary, promotion, or any other job-related decision, then there is great risk of discrimination and non-compliance with required legal regulations. During the evaluation there needs to be a conscious effort to avoid generalizations, labels, personality issues, gender-based comments, and subjective language. The focus on job performance and clear examples should be provided to the staff member to support comments.

Performance appraisal/evaluation process

Appraiser's role

The appraiser is expected to provide an honest, thorough evaluation of an employee. This should not be viewed as a competition among staff but an evaluation of each staff member's performance. Objectivity is critical throughout the process. If the supervisor does not understand or feel competent to evaluate a staff member, then that supervisor is obligated to get direction and assistance with the process. Staff need to view the process as important and feel respected during the entire process.

Data or information needs to be collected in order to prepare for performance appraisal. Methods that might be used are observation, maintenance of a log of observations, or anecdotal notes. The information should be collected throughout the year. These observations take place as the staff member is providing care, in meetings, during interactions with other staff, during interactions with patients and families, or whenever the job requires. Checklists, particularly for tasks, can be used to structure observation and to keep a record. Rating scales can also be used. Documentation can be reviewed to better ensure accuracy and quality. Quality improvement data may provide helpful data. If information is collected and reviewed throughout the year, the task of the annual performance appraisal should not be viewed as such a heavy burden. After data are collected and reviewed, then the required performance appraisal forms must be completed and should provide clear information about the employee's performance.

Implementation of the following year's performance appraisal process actually begins as the current year's performance appraisal process ends. Goals are established for the next year. Throughout the coming year feedback should be provided before the formal, annual review takes place. Employees do need notice when the annual performance review is due so that they can prepare for it, and they need to know what is expected from them during the appraisal process.

The appraisal interview

The purpose of the interview can be categorized in the following ways.

1. **Probationary**—to determine if the employee has met the job's requirements; typically used for orientation to determine if the new employee meets the competency requirements for the position.
2. **Annual**—to determine the current competency of the employee, provide feedback, and plan for professional goals for the coming year as past year goals are reviewed.
3. **Ongoing–continuous**—performance appraisal should not just occur once a year but should be ongoing. Feedback needs to be given when the employee demonstrates competence or when the employee needs guidance to improve.
4. **Transfer**—if an employee is transferring to another area within the organization or receiving a promotion, a performance appraisal should take place before changing position and after orientation to a new position.
5. **Exit**—if an employee is leaving an organization, a terminal performance appraisal should be done, and as is true with all evaluations, the results should be documented in the employee's personnel file.

The supervisor (e.g., nurse manager) contacts the employee to arrange a time and place for the performance interview. There should be sufficient time for the meeting with no interruptions. Privacy, of course, should be maintained. Both parties should come to the interview prepared to discuss performance. The general format of the interview includes initial comments and greetings, review of expectations, review of previous year's goals, performance data and discussion with input from employee, and establishment of goals for the coming year. It is easy to conduct the interview by telling the employee what is wrong or right about the employee's performance with limited mutual communication and self-evaluation by the employee; however, this is an ineffective approach. It is important for the employee to be able to use self-evaluation as this is a skill that the employee needs throughout the year. Staff may also be more defensive if the approach is to tell staff what is wrong without allowing staff the opportunity to comment, or to only focus on the negative. Bias based on personal feelings should be avoided during the evaluation process and the interview. This can be difficult sometimes as there are personalities that just do not do well together; however, this needs to be recognized so the parties can work toward a more positive viewpoint. Beginning the interview with positive comments with a clear focus on job performance can get the interview off to a productive start. The interviewer needs to avoid patronizing, doing all the talking, focusing too much on negative feedback, not listening to the employee, answering own questions, and allowing interruptions to occur. Beginning with an open-ended question will draw the staff member into the process quickly, setting the standard of a dialogue instead of a lecture.

Organizations typically use a standard form during the process, and it is reviewed with the employee during the appraisal interview. Forms indicate that the organization has thought about what should be included in the evaluation process, provide some consistency, and should reflect the organization's philosophy. Regulatory requirements need to be demonstrated in the form's content. Use of a form helps the interviewer remember what should be covered. The form guides the interview; however, the supervisor needs to be flexible, encouraging the employee to participate in all aspects of the interview. If the approach is one of problem solving, identifying problems or issues and then working together to figure out the best strategy for improvement, this will stimulate more staff development. It is important that both the supervisor and the employee provide examples to support comments, and these should be specific. The focus should be on behavior and facts, and while doing this, encouraging the employee to contribute comments. Both the supervisor and employee should sign the form, which only indicates that the employee has read the form but may not necessarily mean that the employee agrees with its content. Some forms have space for employees to make their own comments about the evaluation.

All appraisal interviews must be documented with records kept in the employee's personnel file. The employee should be given a copy of the completed performance appraisal form. The supervisor may keep notes along with data about the employee. A copy of future goals should also be kept.

Employee's role

The employee plays an active role in performance appraisal. JCAHO requires that employees participate. Preparing for performance appraisal is key for the employee just as it is for the supervisor. It begins with self-evaluation. The employee should review position requirements, past year's goals, last year's evaluation, and ask colleagues for feedback. A portfolio may be developed or updated for the evaluation. This all requires time and should be a thoughtful process, not a hurried one. The idea is to have a positive experience that focuses on improvement and recognizes accomplishments, not to emphasize failures. The performance evaluation may be a time to discuss or negotiate a salary increase, change in positions, promotion, and other job-related matters. Since mutually established goals should be agreed upon in the interview, the employee should develop goals for the coming year in preparation for the performance appraisal interview. These goals need to be clear and specific and relate to the position and professional growth. Examples of content for goals are: (a) to improve documentation by describing problems more clearly, (b) to attend one conference in a specialty area, (c) to organize work better so that the employee can leave work at a scheduled time, (d) to develop more specific patient education plans, and so on. Some topics are not appropriate for the performance interview. "It's best not to cloud a discussion of your performance with issues relating to coworkers, systems that don't work, or general gossip. Let the focus be on you and your performance" (Bradley, 2001, p. 74).

Problems with employees

As with any relationships, the employer-employee relationship can experience problems. How these problems are handled can affect retention and staffing. Problems may occur during the performance appraisal or throughout the year.

During performance appraisal process

Employees and supervisors may encounter problems with one another. As managers and team leaders supervise staff they may wonder why staff are not doing what is expected of them. Some of the reasons for the inability to meet expectations may be because staff:

- Do not know what they are supposed to do.
- Do not know how to do it.
- Think the way they are told to do something will not be most effective.
- Think their way of doing a job is better.
- Think something else is more important.
- Anticipate future negative consequences.
- Have personal problems.
- Have personal limits.
- Encounter obstacles beyond their control (Fournies, 1999, p. 131).

It is important to try to understand the causes of these problems. After the job or work begins, staff may think that they are doing what they are supposed to do. They may not recognize any positive consequences for doing their job. Obstacles beyond their control may get in the way of doing the work. It may be that staff think there are more important tasks that they should be doing. Sometimes staff do not do what they are asked to do because they are punished for doing it or they may be rewarded for not doing it. If staff do not see any negative consequences for poor performance, they may not feel the need to do the job well or to improve. Personal problems, of course, can interfere with job performance at any time. The goal is to prevent these barriers from occurring so the work gets done effectively. Prevention strategies include:

- Be clear about what needs to be done (expectations).
- Find out if staff know how to do what needs to be done.
- Explain why something needs to be done.
- Listen to staff input on how to do the job and evaluate if it is a better way—if not, explain this to staff.
- Openly discuss concerns about negative consequences to clarify fact and fiction.
- When possible, ensure that personal problems will not interfere with work requirements.
- Remove all barriers to getting the job done if at all possible (Fournies, 1999).

These strategies should also be used while the work is being done so that the work can be completed effectively. Just providing negative feedback bluntly can crush employees and does little for including the employee in the process of identifying a positive strategy to resolve the problem and improve performance.

Not all evaluation interviews go smoothly. The interviewer may know before the evaluation interview that there may be problems during the interview. This is particularly true if the employee's performance has been less than expected. In this case, the appraiser needs to be very careful about preparing for the interview and spend time thinking through the evaluation and how to discuss it. The interviewer should not become defensive but stay on the subject of performance and expectations. Certainly, some positive, honest feedback should be given if at all possible. The employee may express emotion, from happiness, to frustration, to anger. Happiness is not so difficult, but frustration and anger will be stressful for both persons. Giving the staff member some time to get control is important. It allows the interviewer to also gain some composure and not respond with emotion. If the staff member cannot control emotions at the time, the interview may need to be rescheduled, although this is not preferable. If there is any threat of aggression, then the interview should be terminated. Safety is a priority. Workplace violence should never be tolerated. The supervisor may recommend that the employee seek assistance from the Employee Assistance Program (EAP), if one is available. This program provides counseling for emotional problems and substance abuse problems, and many organizations offer this service to their staff. If there is concern before the evaluation interview that the employee might respond with aggression, then the interview should not be conducted alone. Employees who are not meeting expectations need to be treated with respect. The interview should allow time to discuss performance objectively and to work on an improvement plan that includes deadlines and a clear description of what is required to improve performance. The employee needs to understand the plan and feel that it represents a joint effort.

THINK CRITICALLY

Try this exercise to apply what you have learned about this topic.

Stress on the job

Job stress is defined by the National Institute for Occupational Safety and Health Administration (NIOSH) as "the harmful physical and emotional responses that occur when the requirements of the job do not match the capabilities, resources, or needs of the worker" (National Institute for Occupational Safety and Health, 1999). The National Mental Health Association reported that workplace stress causes about 1 million employees to miss work each day (National Mental Health Association, 2005). The health care work environment is no different. Staff are experiencing much change and frustration with staff shortages and reengineering of organizations. Nurses often identify the following as reasons for their stress:

- Staff shortage
- Increasing responsibility with less time
- Excessive and/or redundant paperwork
- Interdisciplinary issues
- Job dissatisfaction
- Working different shifts
- Fatigue and overwork
- Mandatory overtime
- Decreasing quality personal time
- Poor communication
- Ineffective management

Some nurses have described themselves as experiencing chronic guilt from their inability to meet patient needs effectively as staff shortages increase while patient acuity continues to be high (Hemmila, 2002). This type of stress is destructive and can lead to major personal and performance problems. These nurses need to learn how to balance what can be done and what are unrealistic expectations. What are realistic goals? Are there staff or managers who communicate expectations that are too high? Colleagues need to support one another both by pitching in and helping to give someone a break and also by providing emotional support—communicating that we are a team that helps one another. Employers need to be aware of these feelings and assist staff who are experiencing them because in the long run such stress affects retention.

In some organizations there also seems to be a "disconnect" between staff and managers. Signs and symptoms of this "disconnect" include:

- High frustration levels reported from both staff RNs and their managers.
- A sense among staff of not being valued (for example, low self-esteem).
- Few RNs who seek a managerial career track.
- Adverse incidents that involve patients and staff.
- Ongoing misunderstanding between both groups that hurts interdisciplinary communication, cooperation, and patient care.
- An "us against them" mentality that pervades the workplace.
- Nurses telling their own patients they are overworked and understaffed.
- Poor nurse retention across the board or in particular departments.
- Labor unrest.
- High vacancy rates resulting in excessive overtime, routine use of agency nurses, or bed closure (Forman, 2001, p. 24MW).

This disconnect is related to stress within the organization.

Since it seems that stress in health care is inevitable, two key questions are what can individual nurses do to decrease their own stress and what can the organization do to decrease staff stress? Individual nurses need to first recognize what causes their own stress and how they respond to stress-producing situations. This personal self-assessment should provide valuable information that can then be used to work out a prevention plan. Strategies that can help a nurse prevent or decrease stress are:

- Set reasonable priorities.
- Ask for help and do not see this as a weakness.
- Do one task at a time.
- Take a few minutes to slow down several times during the day.
- Get sufficient sleep, eat a healthy diet, and exercise.
- Focus on what is happening rather than worrying about what could happen.
- Use appropriate self-assertion.
- View problems as challenges and opportunities.
- Laugh and take time for self.

Another strategy that can be used to learn how to better prevent or decrease stress is to better understand what occurs within oneself that can affect stress (Vernarec, 2001). For example, when a person feels overwhelmed by stress, time should be taken to write down what another person said or did that might have influenced the person's reaction. Faulty beliefs are often behind these responses. Employers can also help staff with stress. One strategy is to work with staff to develop self-care contracts (Ellis, 2000). These contracts are used to help staff identify how they will care for themselves with a focus on wellness. The contract might contain content about responsibility for self, physical fitness, nutritional awareness, stress reduction, creative activities, and appreciation for the arts. Nurse managers can recommend that the staff develop these contracts.

New graduates are particularly vulnerable to stress as they learn their new professional role. Reality shock, which has been defined as "the shock-like reaction that occurs when an individual who has been reared and educated in that subculture of nursing that is promulgated by schools of nursing suddenly discovers that nursing as practiced in the world of work is not the same—it does not operate on the same principles" (Kramer, 1985, p. 291). New graduates need an organized orientation and preceptors who take an interest in them to assist them with transition from the classroom to practice (Godinez, Schweiger, Gruver, & Ryan, 1999). Staff on the unit can make a difference in how well a new graduate adjusts. It is important for nurses to feel an obligation to assist new nurses in the profession. Reaching out is critical as many new nurses do not feel comfortable reaching out themselves. Patient assignments need to be done with care as new nurses further develop their skills and learn their way around. They need supervision and guidance with "frequent and regular opportunities for 'debriefing' with more experienced or expert nurses (Nayak, 1991, p. 66). This provides a time for the new nurse to talk through an experience and use critical thinking in a safe environment—one that does not focus on punishment but rather growth. Self-confidence builds slowly; however, when there is a staff shortage, experienced nurses often expect new nurses to gain experience quickly, although this is an unrealistic expectation. The pressure and stress that experienced nurses feel increases their impatience with colleagues. Taking time to help new nurses with the transition and supporting them will go a long way to decrease problems of rapid turnover of this vulnerable staff group, who may change jobs thinking it will get better, or eventually leave the nursing profession.

Coping with passive-aggressive behavior

Passive-aggressive behavior can be difficult to cope with in the work environment, and sadly it is something that all staff will undoubtedly experience with colleagues. When staff use passive-aggressive behavior they usually exhibit at least four of the following:

- Passively resist fulfilling routine social and occupational tasks.
- Complain of being misunderstood and unappreciated by others.
- Appear sullen and argumentative.
- Unreasonably criticize and scorn authority.
- Express resentment toward those perceived as more fortunate.
- Voice exaggerated and persistent complaints of personal misfortune.
- Alternate between hostile defiance and contrition (Whitaker, Carson, & Sawlanski, 2000, p. 82).

When coping with a staff member who exhibits this type of behavior, it is important to clarify expectations, particularly those related to assignments. The overall expectation should be that the work will be done. Apologies and excuses will not be enough. When complaints are made, it is important to consider the facts and avoid defensiveness. Seeking the truth and expecting facts will drive performance. This does not mean that a staff member cannot be understanding, but this should not interfere with performance expectations.

BENCHMARKS

Now let's take a moment to test your knowledge of the concepts you have studied in this section.

Staffing: The Critical Issue Today

YOUR OPINION COUNTS

Find out what others think about this topic. Post your response and check out other opinions.

Staffing is a critical concern in all health care organizations as "60 to 80 percent of your budget goes to staffing" (McConnell, 2000, p. 52). With the increasing costs of health care, this is an expense that must be considered daily. It is also important to remember that "staffing is both a process and an outcome. It's inextricably linked to leaders' accountability to stay within budget and control costs, regulatory and legal mandates, staff competency, quality of care, and the versatility of staffing levels and assignments based on census and acuity" (Beyers, 1999, p. 56). This discussion provides some general information about staffing basics and the nursing shortage. Each nurse needs to become familiar with the staffing policies and procedures that are used in the nurse's organization and specific unit or service. During the recruitment process it is important for the nurse candidate to ask about staffing levels, skill mix, and scheduling. All of these issues directly affect all staff, including new staff.

CURRENT ISSUES

Learn about events around the globe that relate to the chapter content.

Staffing basics

Staffing is the method used to ensure that the appropriate staff—qualifications and quantity—are available to provide the care that is needed for patients to meet their needs and thus provide quality, safe care. This is not easy to accomplish with patients changing and the ever unstable nursing workforce. Factors that must be considered in staffing are:

- Types of patients and care required.
- Number of patients.
- Workload patterns such as when patients are admitted and discharged.
- Times of procedures, and other treatment.
- Average daily census.
- Hours of work (for example, an inpatient unit is operational 24 hours a day, 7 days a week, whereas a clinic may just be operational 5 days a week but may have variable and evening hours).
- Types of nursing staff used (for example, RNs, LPNs, and UAPs).
- The use of support staff such as a unit secretary and staff to transfer patients to exams and procedures can make a big difference, as does the communication system (e.g., use of pagers, cellular phones, and handheld computers). The documentation system also is a critical factor, with computerized systems typically providing effective documentation and effective use of time.

What are some of the key terms and issues that nurses need to know to understand scheduling and staffing needs?

- A **full-time equivalent (FTE)** is the term used to designate a position, which is equal to 40 hours of work per week for 52 weeks or 2,080 hours per year. As scheduling is considered, one FTE can be filled by one person or several, with hours divided.
- Another term is nursing care hours, or the number of hours of patient care provided per unit of time.
- Staffing mix is also important, which is the type of staff that are needed to provide the care (for example, RNs and UAPs). To determine the staff mix it is important to identify the type of care that is required and who is qualified to provide that care. Staff mix also includes an assessment of staff competency to fulfill the care needs. This becomes important, for example, when staff are transferred from their usual work environment into a new one, even if temporarily; they must nonetheless be competent to carry on the assigned tasks.
- Nurse practice acts and other state regulations must always be met when staffing decisions are made. For example, if the patient requires more activities of daily living care such as would be found in a long-term care facility, then UAPs should be included in the staff mix with RNs providing supervision, assessment, and other procedures that require RN competency.
- Distribution of staff is another important factor that focuses on when staff are needed (for example, if a surgical unit gets most of its admissions on Sunday evening for Monday surgeries or if a unit has medical procedures that are done in the morning, then these factors need to be considered in the schedule).
- Shift hours have changed over the years with 8-, 10-, and 12-hour shifts used. Twelve-hour shifts have become more common; however, a recent Institute of Medicine report indicates that when shift durations exceed 12 hours, errors increase (Page, 2004). It is not yet clear what effect this conclusion will have on practice. Split shifts are also used to provide extra staff for busy times (for example, 7:00 A.M. to 11:00 A.M. or 3:00 P.M. to 7:00 P.M.). These various shifts, when used in combination, tend to meet patient needs during high workload times, satisfy staff more, and maximize the use of nurses (Sullivan & Decker, 2001).

Scheduling can be a challenge for the scheduler and for staff who want their schedule needs met. Getting a schedule established that is acceptable to management and staff is the goal, and then it can become cyclical. There will always be times when adjustments need to be made because of staff illness, vacation, and other factors. Some organizations have moved to self-scheduling, which is discussed later in this section. Supplemental staff issues have become of concern with the shortage. Extra staff hours are also needed to cover vacations, illness, and other such situations; cover vacancies; and cover when patient acuity demands it. What do organizations do? Some have their own internal pools of staff who float as needed. Others use agency nurses who are hired per shift. Use of travelers has also become a more frequent intervention. These are nurses who are hired by travel nurse agencies and then contract to work for specific hospitals and positions for specific time periods through the agency. These nurses move from one community to another. Use of agency nurses and travelers is expensive for health care organizations.

The nursing shortage

The nursing shortage is the number one topic in nursing and probably also in health care delivery in general. The shortage is compounded by the fact that it is only getting worse due to aging baby boomers, patients who will need more health care, and the fact that many practicing nurses are due to retire over the next few years. There is also a shortage of nursing faculty, which has a major impact on the ability of schools of nursing to expand enrollment. Again, this group will also be hit with larger numbers of retiring nurses. Job burnout and dissatisfaction are causing retention problems, with nurses leaving the profession or taking extended time off from work. This leads to high turnover rates, which affects costs, health care quality and safety, and the image of nursing, leading to problems with attracting people into the profession.

The present, complex shortage is primarily one of lack of supply (not enough nurses) (Nevidjon & Erickson, 2001). It is believed that past strategies, such as sign-on bonuses and premium packages, only redistribute nurses from employer to employer, rather than increase the number of nurses. In addition to not having enough nurses under usual circumstances, researchers and professional organizations have identified multiple interrelated factors that affect the demand for nurses that still need to be considered. These factors are:

- Cost-containment pressures within health care organizations resulting from managed care and an increasingly competitive health care environment.
- Hospital consolidation, downsizing, and reengineering.
- Reductions in inpatient hospitalization rates.
- Increased acuity of hospital patients.
- A shift of outpatient care from hospitals to ambulatory and community-based settings (Peterson, 2001, p. 1).

The media has been helpful in making the public more aware of the shortage, but this also makes the potential nurses more aware of how difficult it is to be a nurse today. Two media campaigns have put nursing in the forefront. "Nurses for a Healthier Tomorrow," which was initiated by 40 nursing and health care organizations, focused on 6- to 15-year-old children to try and instill the idea of nursing as important. In 2002, Johnson & Johnson initiated their "Campaign for Nursing's Future," a multimedia campaign to promote nursing careers. These ads were seen on television and were effective in sending the message that nursing is a proactive profession. These are expensive campaigns, and thus having partners to conduct them is critical.

What are the data that indicate there is a shortage? The U.S. Department of Health and Human Services and several other governmental agencies (2002, July) provided information about the shortage. This 2002 report indicated that "in 2000, the national supply of FTE registered nurses was estimated at 1.89 million while the demand was estimated at 2 million, a shortage of 110,000 or 6 percent. Based on what is known about trends in the supply of RNs and their anticipated demand, the shortage is expected to grow relatively slowly until 2010, by which time it will have reached 12 percent. At that point demand will begin to exceed supply at an acceler-

BOX 12-3 Websites: Updates on the nursing shortage.

- American Nurses Association http://www.nursingworld.org
- American Association of College of Nursing http://www.aacn.nche.edu
- Bureau of Labor Statistics http://www.bls.gov
- Department of Health and Human Services http://www.dhhs.gov
- National League of Nursing http://www.nln.org
- American Hospital Association http://www.aha.org
- American Organization of Nurse Executives http://www.aone.org
- Health Resources Services Agency http://www.hrsa.gov

Source: Author.

ated rate and by 2015 the shortage, a relatively modest 6 percent in the year 2000, will have almost quadrupled to 20 percent. If not addressed, and if current trends continue, the shortage is projected to grow to 29 percent by 2020" (U.S. Department of Health and other governmental agencies, 2002, p. 2). Box 12-3 identifies a website that provides current data.

All areas of nursing are experiencing some shortages, including hospitals, home care, and long-term care. For example, 90% of long-term care facilities lack sufficient staff for basic care, and some home health agencies must refuse admissions (Joint Commission on Accreditation of Healthcare Organizations, 2002). Specialty care units have been particularly hard hit (for example, intensive care units and operating rooms). These are areas that usually attract younger nurses; however, with nearly 60% of the current workforce over 40 years of age and those younger than 30 decreasing, these factors have affected these specialties (Buerhaus, Staiger, & Auerbach, 2000). These nurses require intensive, costly training. Replacing them is not easy and requires time for new staff to be able to fully function. Emergency departments are also experiencing serious problems due to the staffing shortages throughout the hospital system, and this has led to diversions in many communities that are limiting emergency services to those who need them. Hospitals have had to close beds due to the shortage, and elective surgeries have had to be postponed. In addition to these very serious problems, data are also indicating that new nurses are beginning their careers with higher levels of job satisfaction; however, this good news is very quickly replaced with a larger number who are leaving nursing earlier in their careers (Sochalski, 2002). These conclusions come from the National Sample Survey of Registered Nurses conducted by the DHHS in 1992, 1996, and 2000.

Managed care has had an effect on the nursing shortage problem. Certainly, the reengineering and redesigning of health care organizations that were initiated to respond to many of the requirements made by MCOs have had a major impact. Buiser (2000) identifies specific managed care trends and how they have affected nurse job satisfaction, which is a critical element in the shortage. Case management has led to increased workload due to the decreasing length-of-stay and greater acuity. There is simply less time to provide the care. Critical pathways and protocols may have made care more routine, making nursing a less interesting job. Redesigning the workforce increased job stress while downsizing led to fear, uncertainty, and increased workload. Technology, although very helpful, may have led to feelings of loss of control over one's work. Salary and compensation continue to be issues. Alternative employment has been sought by many nurses in response to decreased satisfaction with their jobs. These are all factors that may have had an effect on retaining nurses and attracting people to nursing.

Staff turnover is extremely costly to health care organizations. The first thought when considering turnover costs is it is simple, but it is not. The following are all part of turnover costs:

- Advertising for new staff
- Interviewing job candidates (Nursing and human resources departments are involved.)
- Administrative time in human resources (job posting, position control, referencing, and investigation)

- Union requirements
- Terminal pay-outs
- Lost productivity and intellectual property
- Pre-employment physicals and drug screens
- Increased use of per diems and travelers
- Bed and unit closures
- Orientation and training costs
- Preceptor time
- Employment agencies
- Increased overtime
- Increased call-outs
- Elevated weekend rotations
- Elevated shift and floating rotations
- Impact on morale and additional turnover effects
- Increased stress that can lead to medical problems and increased use of health benefits (Colosi, 2002, p. 53)

The ANA developed nurse staffing principles that can be found in Box 12-4. The *Principles for Nurse Staffing* (ANA, 1999) describes a matrix for staffing decision making. It is composed of patients, intensity of unit and care, context, and expertise, and is described in Box 12-5.

The key elements related to patients are specific patient characteristics and number of patients for whom care is to be provided. Intensity includes "patient intensity; across the unit intensity (taking into account the heterogeneity of settings); variability of care; admissions,

BOX 12-4   ANA principles for nurse staffing.

I. Patient Care Unit Related
  A. Appropriate staffing levels for a patient care unit reflect analysis for individual and aggregate patient needs.
  B. There is a critical need to either retire or seriously question the usefulness of the concept of nursing hours per patient day (HPPD).
  C. Unit functions necessary to support delivery of quality patient care must also be considered in determining staffing levels.

II. Staff Related
  A. The specific needs of various patient populations should determine the appropriate clinical competencies required of the nurse practicing in that area.
  B. Registered nurse must have nursing management support and representation at both the operational level and the executive level.
  C. Clinical support from experienced RNs should be readily available to those RNs with less proficiency.

III. Institution/Organization Related
  A. Organizational policy should reflect an organizational climate that values registered nurses and other employees as strategic assets and exhibit a true commitment to filling budgeted positions in a timely manner.
  B. All institutions should have documented competencies for nursing staff, including agency or supplemental and traveling RNs, for those activities that they have been authorized to perform.
  C. Organizational policies should recognize the myriad needs of both patients and nursing staff.

Source: American Nurses Association. (1999). *Principles for nurse staffing.* Washington, DC: Author. Reprinted with permission.

BOX 12-5   Matrix for staffing decision making.

The American Nurses Association identified four key factors that are part of a matrix for staffing decision making in its publication *Principles for Staffing* (1999).

Patients	Intensity of Unit and Care
Context	Expertise

Source: Author (Figure).

---

discharges, and transfers; volume" (American Nurses Association, 1999, p. 3). Context incorporates some other critical elements such as architecture and layout of individual patient rooms and arrangement of the entire patient care unit(s); technology that is used such as beepers, cellular phones, and computers; and same unit or cluster of patients. The fourth element is expertise of the staff, which includes staff consistency, continuity and cohesion, use of cross-training, control of practice, involvement in quality improvement, and professional expectations. All these elements affect staffing needs and should be reviewed when staffing schedules are developed.

Strategies to resolve the problems: Some are successful and some are not

In the fall of 2002, Congress passed and funded the Nurse Reinvestment Act. This legislation addresses the issue of the nursing shortage, both of nursing staff and nursing faculty, and includes the following:

- Provides nurses for shortage areas through a National Nurse Corps
- Encourages program development and education of staff to care for the elderly
- Provides opportunities for nurses to solve their own problems
- Funds demonstration projects to enhance communication, to mentor young nurses, and to create methods for staffing and workforce deployment
- Identifies the need to prepare nurses for community-based practice and care of the vulnerable
- Highlights the need for nursing accountability (Donley et al., 2002)

Another aspect to consider when staffing problems are addressed are the trends that affect all work environments today, not just health care settings. Current trends that have been identified are:

- **Time over money**—Employees are seeking jobs that offer more personal time rather than higher pay.
- **Professional versus personal role**—Employees want to be active in both, not just in one part of their lives.
- **Rising superclass of employees**—With more employees choosing less stressful work for more personal time, some employees are carrying the heavier load.
- **Integration of home and work**—More employers are offering services that address employee stress such as child and elder care, dry cleaning, housecleaning, on-site full banking, and so on.
- **Gen X Entrepreneurs**—Employees in their twenties and thirties want greater autonomy and less bureaucracy. They are "loyal" to work rather than to their employer. Some will move to freelancing. (See Chapter 17 for more on generational issues.) There are more nurses in this age group preferring to work for agencies and travel nurse agencies.
- **Collaborative management**—There is greater interest in organizations that use teamwork and creativity with flattened hierarchies. (Hymowitz, 2000; Lancaster, 1999; Nevidjon & Erickson, 2001; Shellenbarger, 1999).

Prior to the Nurse Reinvestment Act, a federal law, California adopted a major policy related to nurse-to-patient ratios in general acute care hospitals, acute psychiatric hospitals, and special hospitals by passing a law in 1999 about this issue. The state's health services department was mandated to develop regulations that require nursing staff to be based on:

- Severity of illness
- Need for specialized equipment and technology
- Complexity of the clinical judgment needed to develop, implement, and evaluate patient care
- Ability of patients to provide self-care
- Licensure of the professional

The law also prohibits assigning nursing functions to UAPs, and it requires that certain functions can only be assigned to UAPs with supervision. This law was strongly supported by nurses and included major nursing input in California. Since then many states are moving in the same direction. It should be noted that the law itself does not state what the nurse-to-patient ratio must be but rather directs the health services department in the state to develop these regulations based on the criteria identified in the new state law. The ratios that were developed by the state took effect in July of 2003. Based on the new ratios, few of the California health care facilities would be in compliance when the ratios were implemented (Steinbrook, 2002). This is a law to improve staffing, but this still does not get to the problem of not enough staff to fill positions.

In 1997, prior to this law, the California Nursing Outcomes Coalition was established to collect prospective data, which became very important when the state tried to determine the staffing ratios (Bolton et al., 2001). This is a very complex problem—determining whether or not and how hours of care and skill mix are linked to patient care indicators of safety and quality. This Coalition bases its work on the ANA Report Card Indicators (American Nurses Association, 1995). (See Chapter 17 for more on this topic.) The indicators that the Coalition focused on were: (a) nursing staff mix and hours of care, (b) patient falls, and (c) pressure ulcer prevalence. "An understanding of the association between use of resources for patient care, their characteristics and processes (direct nursing interventions), and the effect on patients (nurse-sensitive patient care outcomes) must be prerequisite to determining the appropriate number and skill level of nurses and other direct patient care staff to provide safe, high quality patient care" (Bolton et al., 2001, p. 183).

The Nurse Reinvestment legislation is a very important step forward and supports strategies to solve the problems of the nursing shortage. In addition, in 2003 the ANA was successful in getting additional federal legislation introduced in the U.S. Senate, the Registered Nurse Safe Staffing Act of 2003 (S.991) (Federal safe staffing bill introduced, 2003). The act amends the conditions of participation in the Medicare program, which any health care organization that accepts Medicare reimbursement must meet, to establish a requirement for minimum staffing ratios. As with the California legislation, it does not specify numeric ratios but rather sets criteria for the staffing system, which must:

- Be created with input from direct-care RNs or their exclusive representative
- Be based on the number of patients and level and intensity of care to be provided, with consideration given to the admissions, discharges, and transfers that nurses must handle each shift
- Account for the architecture and geography of the environment and available technology
- Reflect the level of preparation and experience of those providing care
- Reflect staffing levels recommended by specialty nursing organizations
- Provide the requirement that an RN not be assigned to work in a particular unit without first having established the ability to provide professional care in such unit (federal safe staffing bill introduced, 2003, pp. 1, 5)

Box 12-6 highlights proposed 2003 legislation indicating that the strategy of legislating changes to respond to the shortage is an active one.

What are some other strategies that have been tried or could be tried to address the staffing problems? It is clear that there needs to be a multistrategy or multisolution approach. The following represent some strategies that are used or might be used. Some are more successful than others, but most depend upon the environment in which they are used and the support that is given to the strategy.

- Use of self-scheduling is an approach that some organizations are using (Hung, 2002). It is well known that scheduling can be an operational nightmare. In this approach nurses in a unit col-

BOX 12-6   Proposed 2003 legislation: A strategy to address nursing shortage.

- VA Medical Workforce Enhancement Act of 2003 (Introduced in House) [H.R.1951.IH]
- Nurse Loan Forgiveness Act of 2003 (Introduced in House) [H.R.501.IH]
- Recruitment and Diversity in Nursing Act of 2003 (Introduced in House) [H.R.920.IH]
- Safe Nursing and Patient Care Act of 2003 (Introduced in House) [H.R.745.IH]
- Registered Nurse Safe Staffing Act of 2003 (Introduced in Senate) [S.991.IS]
- Safe Nursing and Patient Care Act of 2003 (Introduced in Senate) [S.373.IS]
- Medicaid Nursing Incentive Act of 2003 (Introduced in House) [H.R.2295.IH]
- Teacher and Nurse Support Act of 2003 (Introduced in House) [H.R.934.IH]

Source: Author.

laborate and coordinate their schedules rather than having the nurse manager do it. Staff have a time period in which to sign up for a schedule, and at the end of the period the nurse manager or a staff designatee reviews the schedule to see if all needs are met. This type of scheduling has many benefits. It saves on management time, improves morale and professionalism, and reduces costs related to staff turnover. Nurses must take on participation, accountability, creativity, and responsibility to make this work. It is, however, not recommended that units with no scheduling problems change to this method just to do it (Hoffart & Wildermood, 1997).

- Communities are coming together to form task forces to look at the problems with representatives from health care providers and nursing education. For example, a Nursing Workforce Initiative was formed in the Greater Cincinnati (Ohio) area with the health council, nursing executives, and deans and directors of schools of nursing examining recruitment, retention, and staffing shortages. (Looking for solutions to nursing shortage, 2001). In addition to small communities forming coalitions, a large effort has been administered by the American Association of Colleges of Nursing (AACN) called the Colleagues for Caring Program. The Robert Wood Johnson Foundation established this collaboration in 1996 to "address regional nursing work force issues" (White & Rice, 2001, p. 63). The focus areas of the project are data collection and analysis, education, practice, and sustainability. Regional task forces identify common issues and possible strategies to resolve them. This collaboration includes nursing education, practice, and consumers.

- Many hospitals and other large health care organizations are using nurse retention specialists to help with recruitment and retention. The difference between a recruiter and the retention specialist is the focus not only on hiring good staff but also keeping them—retention and recruitment.

- Education and training is a critical strategy that is used in many types of situations. Using creative cross-training to allow staff from medical or surgical units to work in intensive care units (ICU) is one approach (Gilbert & Counsell, 2000; Snyder & Nethersole-Chong, 1999). The benefits from this approach are increased availability of staff who have the skills that are needed in short-term specialty care; provides opportunity for professional development; and some of the staff may wish to eventually transfer to ICU staff, which then decreases the cost of recruitment and training.

- Another staff approach might be to decrease the per diem pool and create a resource pool that is eligible to receive benefits (Beyers, 1999). The goal is to reduce overtime and use of supplementary staff. In addition, standardizing skill requirements and competencies in these groups will help make them more flexible and more acceptable to staff as they can carry expected responsibilities. This same institution also used SWAT teams or teams of staff that could be called to areas that needed extra assistance for a short time (for example, for 2 hours). These teams might assist with assessments, admissions, procedures, and so on.

- The use of unlicensed assistive personnel has been discussed in this text. This strategy for coping with RN shortages has caused much conflict. Health care organizations have supported it as a strategy to reduce costs, but this must be analyzed carefully in each situation to determine if costs will actually be reduced (Murphy, 1995). It is easy to assume that unlicensed means unskilled or uneducated, but this is not a fair assumption. UAPs can be skilled with the right education, training, and supervision; however, short training periods and lack of follow-up will lead to problems with quality and safety and require even more RN supervisory time—time that is rarely available.

■ Teaching staff how to cope with inadequate staffing is a strategy that can be incorporated in any health care organization. There are few, if any, who do not experience shortages. Filipovich (1999) recommends the following. Safety comes first and because of this nurses should: (a) assess the situation and define the implications for nursing care, (b) notify the supervisor and describe the specific problem in terms of the standards that cannot be met and the type of assistance that is needed, and (c) document staffing objectives and keep them on file. Nurses also need to conduct research to provide more data about quality indicators.

■ Use of float staff is a strategy that is used to respond to staff shortages. One of the major concerns with this strategy is whether or not the nurse is qualified and competent to practice in the clinical area where the nurse is asked to work. Nurses have the right to refuse to go but then should request training and orientation. If, however, this training and orientation is offered and the nurse refuses to attend and then refuses to float, the nurse may be terminated (Gobis, 2001). The nurse needs to know what the state's practice laws and regulations say about performing care for which one is not qualified to do.

■ The image of nursing is a critical factor that needs to be addressed. Nurses need to be the drivers of the effort to improve this image. This topic is important in much of this text's content. The ANA and other health care organizations have been working on the image of the health care system. Nursing has tried running television and radio ads as well as using print media. It is important that collaborative efforts are made with other groups to work on the image. Consumers need to know what is a nurse and what a nurse can do. Image also affects recruitment and interest of young people in the profession. Some communities have nurses and nursing students go to high schools to talk about nursing. Recruitment fairs have also become very common. Box 12-7 describes content from the ANA's *Nursing's Agenda for the Future* that describes the importance of public relations, which has a direct impact on recruitment and retention.

■ Use of mandatory overtime has become a common strategy for handling the staffing shortage, and one that has serious consequences—affecting ability to work, health of staff, retention, quality, and safety. It is a short gap or crisis approach that will not solve the problem long-term. Many states are passing legislation to limit the use of mandatory overtime, and the ANA has pushed for federal legislation in its staffing act. The Fair Labor Standards Act offers some protection. First, it does not mandate that employers provide lunch or rest breaks and does not comment on health care employee mandatory overtime (Overtime pay, 2002). It does, however, require employers to pay overtime wages for assigned hours worked over 40, of which it has knowledge, or of which it should have knowledge. Nurses need to know what their rights are in relation to overtime pay and should inquire about it. This does not, however, resolve the problems of mandatory overtime when nurses have no choice about staying at work after their scheduled time or, if they refuse, risk losing their jobs.

■ **Patient classification systems (PCS)** can be used to help identify and quantify patient needs (McConnell, 2000; Seago, 2002). The systems are used to "objectively determine workload requirements and staffing needs" (Sullivan & Decker, 2001, p. 285). There is much in the nursing literature about PCS usage. Factors that are important to consider when using a PCS, factors that can affect the PCS rating and decisions that might be made about scheduling, consider the following: "(1) the patient's preferences and medical condition, including co-morbidities, (2) time-consuming non-clinical facets such as patient turnover, (3) complex clinical decisions and the intricate interaction of health care's physical, social, ethical, emotional, and financial aspects, (4) nurses' unpredictable multitasking, and (5) caregivers' varying knowledge levels, experience, and clinical and critical thinking skills" (McConnell, 2000, p. 52). There have been criticisms of these systems, particularly the earlier systems. As technology has developed, it is now expected that newer PCS will be more effective in matching caregiver profiles with patient care needs, and caregiver-patient interactions can be tracked and monitored (Malloch & Conovaloff, 1999; Sullivan & Decker, 2001).

BOX 12-7   Public relations/communication.

Nursing's pivotal role in health care will be demonstrated on a regular basis to various publics outside of the profession.

Desired Future Statement (Vision)

- Nursing is recognized as an influential, highly rewarded profession valued for its unique knowledge and expertise. It is widely known that nurses make a difference in people's lives.
- Four strategies were identified to achieve the vision and one of these was identified as the primary or driving strategy. They are:
- **Effectively communicate nurses' impact on the quality of care and health outcomes. (Primary Strategy)**
  - Advance a valued, respected image of nursing.
  - Convey nursing's influence in health care delivery and public policy making.
  - Portray nursing as a top career choice.

Objectives to Support Primary Strategy

- Development of position statements by nursing organizations that demonstrate the positive impact of nursing on quality care. Distribute statements to nurses and the general public.
- Use Nurses for a Healthier Tomorrow (NHT) as the primary source/repository for data/information/position statements from nursing organizations regarding nursing's positive impact on quality care.
- Develop and distribute a one-sentence key message for internal and external constituents of nursing organizations about the positive impact that each nursing focus/specialty has on quality care.
- Coordinate a multiorganizational media training activity for nursing organization leaders.

Source: American Nurses Association. (2002). *Nursing's agenda for the future. A call to the nation.* Washington, DC: Author. Reprinted with permission.

- Skill mix is an important aspect of staffing. Nursing skill mix is "the proportion of RNs to the total complement of nursing staff" (Mark, Salyer, & Wan, 2000, p. 552). It is a topic that has been the focus of many research studies.

- Magnet recognition is another strategy that has been used to improve recruitment, retention, and staffing during staff shortages. These hospitals, as discussed in Chapter 6, meet certain standards that tend to support staff recruitment and retention.

- Increased compensation will not be enough to solve the problem although it does help some and should not be ignored.

- Job sharing, which has been used in a variety of work settings, is now also used in some health care organizations. It is an innovative approach, but it will not work for all positions. "An alliance of two nurses in a job-sharing role is one option for successfully meeting the challenges of today's health care, while promoting job satisfaction and personal endeavors" (Gliss, 2000, p. 40). Some key issues are selecting the job that can be done by two people and finding the right staff matches. It requires partnership and sharing. This strategy can attract nurses who want to work part-time and still make a contribution.

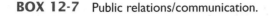

CURRENT ISSUES

Learn about events around the globe that relate to the chapter content.

- Employers need to change their view of staff—moving away from viewing staff as an expense but rather as an asset. Strategies to value staff need to be used (Nevidjon & Erikson, 2001).

■ Providing clinical practice opportunities and responsibility that match the nurse's knowledge and skill can help to retain nurses.

■ The *Code for Nurses* (American Nurses Association, 2001) requires that nurses should participate in the development of workplaces so that they are environments in which quality care can be provided. Nurses must advocate for their patients. This type of workplace should help to retain nurses and also to attract nurses—decreasing job dissatisfaction.

■ When hospitals and other health care organizations identify areas or services that are particularly short on staff, such as critical care and operating rooms, they need to develop training programs for staff to attract them to these areas.

■ Nurses need more assistance with developing delegation skills because delegation is required more and more with the increased use of non-RN caregivers. "Nurses must know what tasks are appropriate to 'give away,' how to manage the workload and be accountable for outcomes, and how to provide for the growth and development of non-RN caregivers and other support staff. Nurses sometimes feel less valued when they must delegate tasks to a non-nurse. However, nursing can consider delegation, along with shared governance, as another form of empowerment" (Andreoli, 1992; as cited in Nevidjon & Erickson, 2001, p. 10).

■ The decreasing number of nursing faculty is a serious problem. Attracting more nurses into teaching is critical. There is now more funding available for graduate education. Schools of nursing need to develop programs to educate future faculty.

■ Nursing curricula need to be current. Graduates must be prepared to practice. If they are not, there is a risk of losing the new nurse early in the career track.

■ Greater attention needs to be given to orientation, preceptorships, internships and residencies, and other creative methods to assist in helping new graduates adjust to the workplace and retain them.

■ The recruitment of foreign nurses, a strategy that has been used in past nursing shortages, is increasing again. These nurses need to be able to pass the NCLEX exam, speak English, and provide assistance with culture adjustment. Some ethical issues with this strategy should be considered. Many countries are experiencing shortages, so the United States is taking nurses from some countries who need them, too (Pearson & Peels, 2001; Steefel, 2001). The International Council of Nurses (ICN) "condemns the practice of recruitment of nurses to countries where governments and other relevant authorities have failed to address deficiencies known to cause nurses to leave the profession" (Steefel, 2001, p. 36). The Rural and Urban Health Care Act of 2001 proposed an expansion of the H-1C category to allow all hospitals to hire nurses on temporary visas and allow them to stay in the United States for up to 6 years. The goal was to reduce barriers in getting these nurses to come to the United States. Addressing the nursing shortage with this approach will not have a long-term impact on the problem.

■ As hospitals begin to realize that they must figure out how to deliver quality care more effectively despite the shortage, they have arrived at a number of staffing strategies. One strategy looks at the delivery system. "The delivery system determines the way that nursing care will be delivered" (Manthey, 2001, p. 424). One of these is a core incremental staffing plan (Manthey, 2001). This plan has two major components: (a) experienced, full-time staff who manage and/or deliver care and (b) part-time, short-term, transitional regular employees and supplemental staff (agency and travelers), who deliver most of the daily care activities. The first level of staff is the senior staff. This level would include the appropriate skill mix for the patient acuity level. The staffing plan is part of the system as is the care delivery model (for example, team nursing, primary care nursing, and so on). The risk with this approach is creating a class system by communicating that one level of staff is better than the other. The real focus should be that some RNs have chosen different lifestyles and career interests (e.g., travelers and agency nurses) and want the flexibility. The core staff are responsible for continuity of care.

■ Regulatory and policy issues may be a factor affecting the shortage (Nevidjon & Erickson, 2001). One particular area is documentation that is often affected by regulations. Documentation is complex and time-consuming. It can be very repetitive, and staff may not see the value in the documentation. Documentation needs to be streamlined, standardized, and must take advantage of computers. In addition, state boards of nursing should review their policies and procedures and determine what is contemporary or out-of-date as these policies and procedures may not be helpful in retaining nurses.

■ Organizations need to explore how staff spend their time and if there are better ways of doing things to decrease activities that could be better done by someone else. Nurses spend more time than they need to on non-nursing tasks. Over the years these tasks have only increased. Effective management requires that work be allocated according to who is the best person to do the work. As this problem area is explored, it is important to consider trends such as patient population, staffing patterns, workload, and care practices (Hader & Clandio, 2002). All of this should be directed at effective staff utilization and allocation of limited resources.

■ Some health care organizations are using their own staff to increase the pool of RNs. They are identifying nonprofessional staff who might be interested and have the ability to pursue nursing education (Fox & Brooks, 2000). This is an excellent example of an organization supporting career advancement. In addition, many organizations are supporting RN efforts to obtain a BSN degree. Support can be in the form of tuition reimbursement, scheduling flexibility, and other types of services to make it easier to go back to school. Some organizations have partnered with nursing schools to conduct courses onsite or to develop online programs. These efforts indicate that the organizations really do want to help staff develop themselves.

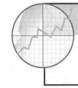

BENCHMARKS

Now let's take a moment to test your knowledge of the concepts you have studied in this section.

Chapter Wrap-Up

Now that you've reached the end of the chapter, you may wish to explore the concepts you've been reading about in greater detail, or test yourself to see how well you've comprehended the material.

SUMMARY AND APPLICATIONS

■ Summary   ■ Experiential Exercises
■ Practice Quiz   ■ Case
■ Key Terms   ■ Links
■ Tying It All Together

REFERENCES

Aiken, T. (2001). Sexual harassment. In J. Dochterman & H. Grace (Eds.), *Current issues in nursing* (6th ed., pp. 576–582). St. Louis, MO: Mosby, Inc.

American Hospital Association. (2002). *In our hands*. Oakbrook Terrace, IL: Author.

American Nurses Association. (1995). *Nursing report card for acute care settings*. Washington, DC: Author.

American Nurses Association. (1999). *Principles for nurse staffing*. Washington, DC: Author.

American Nurses Association. (2001). *Code for nurses with interpretive statements*. Washington, DC: Nursing Publishing, Inc.

American Organization of Nurse Executives. (1999). *Nurse staffing survey: February 23, 1999*. Chicago, IL: American Hospital Association.

Andreoli, K. (1992). Primary nursing for the 1990s and beyond. *Journal of Professional Nursing* 8(4), 24.

Beyers, M. (1999). About how to reduce overtime and use of per diem staff. *Nursing Management, 30*(12), 56.

Bolton, L. et al. (2001). A response to California's mandated nursing ratios. *Journal of Nursing Scholarship* (second quarter), 179–184.

Bradley, C. (2001). A response to California's mandated nursing ratios. *Journal of Nursing Scholarship* (second quarter), 179–184.

Buerhaus, P., Staiger, D., & Auerbach, D. (2000). Why are shortages of hospital RNs concentrated in specialty care units? *Nursing Economics, 18*(3), 111–116.

Buiser, M. (2000). Surviving managed care: The effect of job satisfaction in hospital-based nursing. *MEDSURG Nursing, 9*(3), 129–134.

Burke, S., & Whited, M. (1997). *How to find your perfect job in nursing.* Freeman, SD: Pine Hill Press, Inc.

Butler, T., & Waldroop, J. (1999). Job sculpting: The art of retaining your best people. *Harvard Business Review, 87*(September–October), 143–152.

Cardillo, D. (2002). How to resign in style. *Nursing Spectrum Metro Edition, 3*(2), 11.

Carroll, P. (2001). Questions to avoid when conducting interviews. Retrieved on April 28, 2001, from http://www.nurses.com/content. . . 12-11D5-A770-D0B7694F32}&Bucket=Columns.

Colosi, M. (2002). Rules of engagement for the nursing shortage. *JONA Healthcare Law, Ethics, and Regulation, 4*(3), 50–54.

Danaher, M. (2001). Medical leave under the family and medical leave act: Understanding the impact of the act's interpretive guidance. *Journal of Legal Nurse Consultants, 12*(3), 3–6.

Diehl-Oplinger, L., & Kaminski, M. (2000). Need critical care nurses? Inquire within. Use preceptors to orient your facility's nurses to critical care. *Nursing Management, 31*(3), 44, 46.

Donley, R., et al. (2002). What does the Nurse Reinvestment Act mean to you? *Online Journal of Issues in Nursing, 8*(1). Retrieved on May 7 from http://www.nursingworld.org/ojin_on.

Ellis, L. (2000, March). Have you and your staff signed self-care contracts? *Nursing Management,* 47–48.

Federal safe staffing bill introduced. (2003). *The American Nurse, 35*(3), 1, 5.

Fiesta, J. (1999). Greater need for background checks. *Nursing management, 30*(11), 26.

Filipovich, C. (1999). Teach nurses effective ways to deal with inadequate staffing. *Nursing Management, 30*(12), 38.

Finkelman, A. (1996). *Psychiatric nursing administration manual.* Gaithersburg, MD: Aspen Publishers.

Forman, H. (2001). Diagnosis: Disconnect. *Nursing Spectrum Midwest Region, 2*(9), 24–25MW.

Fournies, F. (1999). *Why employees don't do what they're supposed to do.* New York: McGraw-Hill.

Fox, D., & Brooks, M. (2000). The professional nurse education program. A work force development model. *Journal of Nursing Administration, 30*(10), 490–496.

Fox, K. (1998). Workers' compensation and managed care. NCSL LegisBrief. *National Conference of State Legislatures, 6*(31), 1–2.

Gilbert, M., & Counsell, C. (2000). Intensive care unit cross training: Saving dollars while retraining staff. *Journal of Nursing Administration, 30*(6), 308, 324.

Gliss, R. (2000). Job sharing: An option for professional nurses. *Nursing Economics, 18*(1), 40–41.

Gobis, L. (2001). The perils of floating. *American Journal of Nursing, 101*(9), 78.

Godinez, G., Schweiger, J., Gruver, J., & Ryan, P. (1999, May–June). Role transition from graduate to staff nurse: A qualitative analysis. *Journal for Nurses in Staff Development, 15*(3), 97–110.

Gottlieb, M. (1998). *The confused consumer's guide to choosing a health care plan.* New York: Hyperion.

Hader, R., & Clandio, T. (2002). Seven methods to effectively manage patient care labor resources. *Journal of Nursing Administration, 32*(2), 66–68.

Hemmila, D. (2002). When helping hurts. *Nurse Week. Great Lakes Region, 2*(2), 7.

Hoffart, N., & Wildermood, S. (1997). Self-scheduling in five med/surg units. *Nursing Management, 28*(4), 42–45.

Hung, R. (2002). A note on nurse self-scheduling. *Nursing Economics, 20*(1), 37–39.

Hutchison, P. (2001a). Strategies for recruiting and retaining health care professionals. Part 1. *Home Care Provider, 6*(2), 53–55.

Hutchison, P. (2001b). Strategies for recruiting and retaining health care professionals. Part 2: The right candidate. *Home Care Provider, 6*(4), 14–17.

Hymowitz, C. (2000, January 4). How can a manager encourage employees to take bold risks? *Wall Street Journal,* B1.

Institute of Medicine. (2001). *Crossing the quality chasm.* Washington, DC: National Academy Press.

Joint Commission on Accreditation of Healthcare Organizations. (2002). *Health care at the crossroads. Strategies for addressing the evolving nursing crisis.* Oakbrook Terrace, IL: Author. Retrieved January 5, 2003, from http://www.jcaho.org.

Joint Commission on Accreditation of Healthcare Organizations. (2004). *Hospital accreditation standards.* Oakbrook Terrace, IL: Author.

Kramer, M. (1985). Why does reality shock continue? In J. McCloskey & H. Grace (Eds.), *Current issues in nursing* (pp. 891–903). Boston, MA: Blackwell Scientific Publication.

LaDuke, S. (2001). Professional misconduct: Issues related to hiring and firing. *Journal of Nursing Administration, 31*(9), 408–410.

Lancaster, H. (1999, December 21). A father goes to work and finds new ways to make sense. *Wall Street Journal*, B1.

Looking for solutions to nursing shortage. (2001, May). *M.D. News*, 15.

Malloch, K., & Conovaloff, A. (1999). Patient classification systems, Part 1: The third generation. *Journal of Nursing Administration, 29*(7/8), 49–56.

Manthey, M. (2001). A core incremental staffing plan. *Journal of Nursing Administration, 31*(9), 424–425.

Mark, B., Salyer, J., & Wan, T. (2000). Market, hospital, and nursing unit characteristics as predictors of nursing unit skill mix. *Journal of Nursing Administration, 30*(11), 552–560.

McConnell, E. (2000). Staffing and scheduling at your fingertips. *Nursing Management, 31*(3), 52–53.

Milgram, L., Spector, A., & Treger, M. (1999). *Managing smart*. Houston, TX: Gulf Publishing Company.

Murphy, E. (1995). Unsubstantiated assumptions about unlicensed assistive personnel obscure the challenge of delivering quality care. *AORN, 62*(7), 8, 10.

Mustard, L. (2002). Caring and competence. *JONA's Healthcare Law, Ethics, and Regulation, 4*(2), 36–43.

National Council of State Boards of Nursing. (1996). *Definition of competence and standards for competence*. Chicago: Author.

National Institute for Occupational Safety and Health. (1999) *Stress at work*. Washington, DC: Department of Health and Human Services.

National Mental Health Association. Promoting mental health in the workplace. Retrieved from http://www.nmha.org. on March 10, 2005.

Nayak, S. (1991, March/April). Strategies to support the new nurse in practice. *Journal of Nursing Staff Development*, 64–66.

Nevidjon, B., & Erickson, J. (2001). The nursing shortage: Solutions for the short and long term. *Online Journal of Issues in Nursing, 6*(1). Retrieved June 6, 2001, from http://www.nursingworld.org/ojin.

Nurse Reinvestment Act, H.R.3487ENR, 107th Congress. (2002). Retrieved on December 8, 2002, from http://www.access.gpo.gov/nara/publaw/107publ.html.

NurseWeek & American Organization of Nurse Executives. (2002). Registered nurses survey. Retrieved on April 17, 2002, from http://www.nurseweek.com/survey/fullresults2.asp.

Overtime pay. (2002). *Ohio Nurses Review*, July 6.

Page, A. (Ed.). (2004). *Keeping patients safe: Transforming the work environment of nurses*. Washington, DC: Institute of Medicine of the National Academies Press.

Pearson, A., & Peels, S. (2001). A global view of nursing in the new millennium—2: The nursing workforce. *International Journal of Nursing Practice, 7*(S5–S10), 55–59.

Pell, A. (2000). *The complete idiot's guide to recruiting the right stuff*. Indianapolis, IN: Alpha Books.

Peter, L., & Hull, R. (1969). *The Peter Principle: Why things go wrong*. New York: William Morrow.

Peterson, C. (2001). Nursing shortage: Not a simple problem—no easy answers. *Online Journal of Issues in Nursing, 6*(1). Retrieved June 6, 2001, from http://www.nursingworld.org/ojin.

Plotkin, H. (1997). *Building a winning team*. Los Angeles: Griffin Publishers.

Seago, J. (2002). A comparison of two patient classification instruments in an acute care hospital. *Journal of Nursing Administration, 32*(5), 243–249.

Shader, K., et al. (2001). Factors influencing satisfaction and anticipated turnover for nurses in an academic medical center. *Journal of Nursing Administration, 31*(4), 250–263.

Shellenbarger, S. (1999, December 29). For harried workers in the 21st century: Six trends to watch. *Wall Street Journal*, B1.

Snyder, J., & Nethersole-Chong, D. (1999). Is cross-training medical/surgical RNs to ICU the answer? *Nursing Management, 30*(2), 58–60.

Sochalski, J. (2002). Nursing shortage redux: Turning the turnover on as an enduring problem. *Health Affairs, 21* (4), 157–164.

Steefel, L. (2001, May). Hands from abroad shore up nursing shortages. *Nursing Spectrum Metro Edition*, 35–36.

Steinbrook, R. (2002). Nursing in the crossfire. *New England Journal of Medicine, 346*(22), 1757–1766.

Sullivan, E., & Decker, P. (2001). *Effective leadership and management in nursing*. Upper Saddle River, NJ: Prentice Hall.

Trossman, S. (2002). Satisfaction guaranteed? A sampling of strategies to keep experienced nurses on the job. *The American Nurse, 102*(5), 1, 12, 14.

U.S. Department of Health and Human Services, Health Resources and Services Administration, Bureau of Health Professions, & National Center for Health Workforce Analysis. (2002, July). *Projected supply, demand, and shortages of registered nurses: 2000–2020*. Washington, DC: Authors. Retrieved on July 8, 2003, from http://www.hrsa.gov.

Vernarec, E. (2001). How to cope with job stress. *RN, 64*(3), 244–246.

Whitaker, C., Carson, D. & Sawlanski, J. (2000). Dealing with difficult behavior. *Nursing 2000, 30*(6), 81–82.

White, N., & Rice, R. (2001). Collaboration to nurture the nursing work environment. The Colleagues in Caring practice task force. *Journal of Nursing Administration, 31*(2), 63–66.

ADDITIONAL READINGS

Abelson, R. (2002, May 6). With nurses in short supply, patient load becomes a big issue. *New York Times*, A14.

American Association of Colleges of Nursing. Colleagues for Caring Project. Retrieved from http://aacn.nche.edu/CaringProject.

Benner, P. (2001). *From novice to expert. Excellence and power in clinical nursing practice* (Commemorative Edition). Upper Saddle River, NJ: Prentice Hall.

Bradley, C. (2001). Your role in your annual performance evaluation. *AJN, 101*(7), 71, 73.

Cardillo, D. (2001). Job hunting challenges take some troubleshooting. *Nursing Spectrum Metro Edition, 2*(8), 25.

Carroll, P. (2001). Questions to avoid when conducting interviews. Retrieved on April 28, 2001, from http://www.nurses.com/content. . . 12-11D5-A770-D0B7694F32}&Bucket=Columns.

Crimlisk, J., McNaulty, M., & Francione, D. (2002). New graduate RNs in a float pool. *Journal of Nursing Administration, 32*(4), 211–217.

Dellefield, M. (2000, June). The relationship between nurse staffing in nursing homes and quality indicators. *Journal of Gerontological Nursing,* 15–28.

Donley, R., et al. (2002). What does the Nurse Reinvestment Act mean to you? *Online Journal of Issues in Nursing, 8*(1). Retrieved on May 7 from http://www.nursingworld.org/ojin.

Fosbinder, D., Everson-Bates, S., & Hendrix, L. (2000). Using an interview guide to identify effective nurse managers: Phase II, outcomes. *Nursing Administration Quarterly, 24*(2), 72–82.

Furlow, L. (2000). Job profiling: Building a winning team using behavioral assessments. *Journal of Nursing Administration, 30*(3), 107–111.

Garrett, D., & McDaniel, A. (2001). A new look at nurse burnout. *Journal of Nursing Administration, 31*(2), 91–96.

Goode, C., & Williams, C. (2004). Post-baccalaureate nurse residency program. *Journal of Nursing Administration, 34*(2), 71–77.

Hartigan, C. (2000). The synergy model in practice. Establishing criteria for 1:1 staffing ratios. *Critical Care Nurse, 20*(2), 112, 114–116.

Ingersoll, G., et al. (2002). Nurses' job satisfaction, organizational commitment, and career intent. *Journal of Nursing Administration, 32*(5), 250–263.

Institute of Medicine. (2001). *Health professions education. A bridge to quality.* Washington, DC: National Academy Press.

Jacobsen, C., et al. (2002). Surviving the perfect storm: Staff perceptions of mandatory overtime. *JONA's Healthcare Law, Ethics, and Regulation, 4*(3), 57–66.

Keeling, B. (1999). How to allocate the right staff mix across shifts, Part 1. *Nursing Management, 30*(9), 16–17.

Kovner, C., & Harrington, C. (2000). Counting nurses. Data show many nursing homes to be short staffed. *American Journal of Nursing, 100*(9), 53.

Legislative Network for Nurses. (2002). *The nurse staffing shortage Part 2: The crisis continues.* Silver Spring, MD: Business Publishers, Inc.

Mark, B. (2002). What explains nurses' perceptions of staffing adequacy? *Journal of Nursing Administration, 32*(5), 234–241.

McGillis, L., Pink, G., Johnson, L., & Schraa, E. (2000). Development of a nursing management practice atlas. Part 2, variation in use of nursing and financial resources. *Journal of Nursing Administration, 30*(9), 440–448.

O'Connor, M. (2002). Nurse leader: Heal thyself. *Nursing Administration Quarterly, 26*(2), 69–79.

O'Neil, E., & the Pew Health Professions. (1998). *Recreating health professional practice for a new century.* San Francisco, CA: Pew Health Professions Commission.

Price, C. (2000). A national uprising. United actions push mandatory overtime, inadequate staffing to forefront. *American Journal of Nursing, 100*(12), 75–76.

Shullanberger, G. (2000). Nurse staffing decisions: An integrative review of the literature. *Nursing Economics, 18*(3), 124–132, 146–148.

Trossman, S. (2004a). Move over eBay? A potential trend involving bidding for shifts online. *The American Nurse, 36*(3), 1, 8, 12.

Trossman, S. (2004b). New overtime regulations may harm RNs. *The American Nurse, 36*(3), 1, 3.

Vernarec, E. (2000). Just say 'no' to mandatory overtime? *RN, 63*(12), 69–70, 72, 74, 76.

Worthington, K. (2001a). Stress and overwork top nurses' concerns. *American Journal of Nursing, 101*(12), 96.

Worthington, K. (2001b). The health risks of mandatory overtime. *American Journal of Nursing, 101*(5), 96.

NURSING/PROFESSIONAL CULTURE

Asserting nursing's high standards of professional practice, education, leadership, and collaboration will enhance professionalism, image, and career satisfaction.

Desired Future Statement (Vision)

All nurses believe they are, and all nurses are viewed to be, critical strategic health care assets valued by the public, policy makers, employers, and health care colleagues as equal partners in health care. Nurses embrace their professional responsibility and accountability, including: collaborating, mentoring, promoting diversity, and adhering to standards and ethical codes of professional practice.

Five strategies were identified to achieve the vision and one of these was identified as the primary or driving strategy. They are:

Professionalism is supported by infrastructures for education and leadership development. (Primary Strategy)

Nurses promote a health environment of respect and caring for one another.

Nurses believe, articulate, and demonstrate the value of nursing.

Collaboration is a professional imperative.

Nurses achieve substantial external influence and recognition for their value to society.

Objectives to Support Primary Strategy

Promote membership, participation, and connection with professional nursing organizations; demonstrate the relevance and image of such organizations.

Establish certification as a professional benchmark. Through innovations and new models, increase the number of certification programs available for all nursing roles (especially all identified specialties) and increase the number of certified nurses.

Provide ongoing leadership development by bringing together widely diverse groups of nurses to discuss and advance professional nursing culture.

Expand nurse managers' leadership skills to champion professional culture in their workplace.

SOURCE: American Nurses Association. (2002). *Nursing's agenda for the future. A call to the nation.* Washington, DC: Author. Reprinted with permission.

Keys to Professional Success

CHAPTER OUTLINE

MediaLink
www.prenhall.com/finkelman

The Interactive Exercises for this chapter can be found in the OneKey course at www.prenhall.com/finkelman. Click on Chapter 13 to select from the following activities: Test Your Understanding, Benchmarks, Current Issues, Your Opinion Counts, Think Critically, and Summary and Applications.

What's Ahead

Nursing professionalism begins when students enter nursing programs and continues throughout their careers. This chapter discusses some critical keys for professional nursing success. Career development is a theme throughout one's career and includes strategies such as mentoring, coaching, and precepting to get the needed guidance. Lifelong learning, including career development, is an individual nursing responsibility as well as important to health care providers and the profession as a whole. Time management is also key to successful practice and to decreasing stress, both of which affect retention.

OBJECTIVES

Before you begin, take a moment to familiarize yourself with the key objectives of this chapter.

- Describe the critical elements of a career plan.
- Develop a resume.
- Discuss how networking, coaching, and mentoring might be beneficial to a new nurse.
- Discuss the implications of lifelong learning.
- Collect time data and analyze how time is used.
- Identify time management improvement strategies.

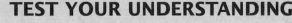

TEST YOUR UNDERSTANDING

Before we begin our exploration of this chapter, take a short "warm-up" test to see what you know about this topic.

Career Development

Career development is a lifelong professional activity. At various stages in a nursing career it is more important (for example, on entering the profession and at junctures when decisions are made about position changes or promotions). The first step is the first job. Here is where the new nurse confronts the most difficult situations. Duchscher (2001) has identified some of the problems new nurses find in the real world. Dependency on others is a critical issue. New nurses want to be a contributing team member but do not yet feel ready to do so. Many view "not knowing" as a weakness rather than seeing it as something that new nurses would be expected to experience (Duchscher, 2001). A struggle takes place between wanting to be independent and not yet being ready for it. Recognizing this to be the case is critical. Asking for help is never easy, but it is a sign of a professional nurse. New nurses may not consider career development, but it begins to happen automatically when the first job is taken and situations are confronted that create questions and a need to develop additional skills to cope with workplace issues and problems. If the nurse does not actively plan for it, success may be problematic.

First job: Early issues

For many new nurses, a problem area that is confronted early on is fear of physicians. Much of this comes from the fact that most student nurses have little contact with physicians and certainly little with medical students. The recent Institute of Medicine reports on quality of care highlight the need for more interdisciplinary learning, as this is the type of care that needs to be provided and it requires collaboration and communication. Asking experienced nurses for help with nurse-physician communication is very important. What to say, how to say it, and when to say it are skills that can be learned. The key to this approach is remembering that the patient is the focus, and care must be safe and reach required outcomes. This can be a problem as many new graduates are self-absorbed. They have "a tendency to focus on themselves rather than on their patients; there was a strong propensity to visualize patient outcomes in terms of their effect on the new nurse rather than on the patient" (Duchscher, 2001, p. 428). This happens even though nursing education emphasizes patient outcomes, not nursing outcomes. As new graduates "leave the nest" of their schools they encounter a world that requires flexibility and innovation and clearly expects nurses to take on responsibility. Along with this they assume that experienced nurses are always right, only to find out this is not always the case. This causes frustration and stress. New graduates want to be accepted, not criticized, which may certainly occur. Many new graduates already see this happening as students when they experience nurturing from nurses, but sometimes they experience or observe negativity. How does the new nurse typically respond? The nurse turns the focus to doing—getting tasks done efficiently. Few nurses have not had the experience early on in their careers of going home wondering what damage they may have done—the fear can be very stressful and is one reason why finding role models who can help and provide support is so critical at this stage of one's career.

Several months down the road, Duchscher (2001) notes that many new nurses begin to find the meaning of nursing. At this time, the nurse views oneself less as student and more as a practicing nurse. The nurse is more realistic, accepts limitations better, and tries to find some stability in the workplace. Nurses become "resigned themselves to their own fallibility, recognizing that they needed to learn to understand that some degree of uncertainty is always in the job" (Duchscher, 2001, p. 430). They begin to trust themselves as independent nurses and gain more self-awareness. Care then becomes more patient-centered. This is a critical transition, and new nurses reach it at different times.

Throughout the adjustment phase of entering a new career, change, stress, and lack of self-confidence are critical factors that can motivate or limit a new nurse. Using orientation to learn as much as possible about the organization and the job, finding support in a preceptor, attending education opportunities in the workplace, allowing oneself to make errors without punishing oneself but then learn from the errors, gaining assertiveness and communication skills, learning to manage time, and finding time for personal self are all critical to success—lifelong career success.

Career Plan: A Professional Growth Action Plan

To meet career goals it is important to first plan for them or to develop a map to reach them. This is called a career plan. Just as is done for all planning in organizations, individuals need to be aware of changes that might affect a career now or possibly in the future. The professional **portfolio** is a method to demonstrate competency. The overall purpose of the portfolio is to "provide a repository for the historical information about one's career" (Bell, 2001, p. 69). As the portfolio is developed, emphasis should be placed on outcome achievement. New graduates will begin this process when they apply for their first job as a nurse. Some health care organizations are now requiring nursing staff to submit portfolios if the nurses participate in a career ladder program. The portfolio is used in the evaluation process to determine which level in the career ladder is appropriate for an individual nurse. The components of a career plan include the following:

- **Biosketch:** This is a short summary paragraph describing critical elements about oneself. A biosketch should be changed based on its purpose. Examples to model can be found in author biosketches, in marketing material for a continuing education program, and so on.
- **Resume:** This is a 1- to 2-page review of the nurse's career which is kept fairly current and includes core information. Information that is typically included is demographic data, education, credentials, goals and objectives, and relevant experience. As is true for all of the information, it needs to be updated annually. It is this format that is typically used by new graduates who have a shorter employer and professional history.
- **Curriculum Vitae (CV):** This document is much more detailed than a resume and includes all of the information about the nurse's professional career. Other additional information that is included in a CV, as opposed to a resume, is: (a) continuing education, (b) committees, (c) presentations, (d) publications, (e) honors and awards, (f) community activities, and (g) grants. This type of format is more difficult for nurses to use who have a shorter employer and professional history.

The purpose of the resume is to identify key professional experiences and education. Most employers, with exception of academic ones, want to see a resume rather than a curriculum vitae (CV), even when they ask for a CV. The resume focuses on selected information. Key current experience should be listed. When considering whether or not to add such information as publications, only relevant ones should be included on a resume. Box 13-1 provides some tips to developing a resume and Boxes 13-2, 13-3, and 13-4 provide examples of resumes.

What credentials and format should be used? There are four typical types of credentials: degrees (BSN, MSN, PhD), licensure (RN, LPN/LVN), certification (APN, APRN, NP, CNS),

BOX 13-1 Tips for developing a resume.

Three types of resumes

1. Chronological: describes positions held in reverse order
2. Functional: highlights skills with less emphasis on position titles
3. Combination: provides information in both styles

- Before writing a resume, a thorough review and collection of information about work history is required. Getting all the information together will help to make the process more efficient. This is the time to get out the career plan and use it as a guide.
- Resumes should be no longer than 1 to 2 pages (curriculum vitae are longer and more detailed).
- Educational background goes at the end of a resume unless a new graduate, and this information is stronger than work experience. If a recent graduate, grade point average (GPA) can be included.
- Nurses do not need to include their license number as this will be asked for later during the application process.
- An objective should be identified. If the applicant is not sure about what area of nursing, the best approach is to say a position in the nursing profession.
- Personal data should not be included.
- Resumes should include positive qualities.
- Information about relevant work experience, paid and unpaid, are included.
- Using clear writing style with action verbs demonstrates a positive approach to the employer.

The final product

Quality paper should be used in white or ivory.

It is best to use a simple, clear font such as Times Roman or Helvetica. Fancy script styles should not be used.

Proofreading cannot be overdone. Having another person review the resume can be very helpful.

Electronic resumes are now accepted by some organizations, but inquire before sending one. It is important to make sure that the correct e-mail address is used. Formatting may not be maintained, but sending it as an attachment ensures a better chance that the document will arrive as written.

Chronological resume

1. Name, address, telephone, e-mail address.
2. Objective—brief and current.
3. Profile—a summary of skills, personality traits, and achievements related to objective.
4. Education (can be put at the end of the resume)—degree, school, graduation date, certified, state licensure—state(s) and type of licensure (do not need to include number).
5. Professional experience or related experience—dates positions started and ended, organization (name, city, and state), description of the job, achievements at the job. Provide information from most recent to least recent.

Functional resume

1. Name, address, telephone, e-mail address.
2. Objective—brief and current.
3. Profile—a summary of skills, personality traits, and achievements related to objective.
4. Education (can be put at the end of the resume)—degree, school, graduation date, certified, state licensure—state(s) and type of licensure (do not need to include number).
5. Professional experience or related experience—instead of a chronological list the focus is on what was done in positions. Begin descriptions with action verbs.
6. Employment history—dates positions started and ended, organization (name, city, and state), description of the job, achievements at the job. Provide information from most recent to least recent.

Guidelines for interview process

- Doing research before the interview can pay off. What is the job? Look beyond the title as titles do not give the full picture of a position.
- Prepare a list of references so that when employers ask for this information it is easily retrievable. References need to be contacted before their names are given out. Include name, title, organization, and contact information in the list. Some references may be more appropriate for some jobs than others so you may want to have a number of names for different types of jobs.
- When setting up appointments, clarify the time, place, who will be met, directions, and parking arragements. If distance travel is involved, it is important to give the employer contact information such as hotel number or cell phone in case changes need to be made.
- A thank you note should be sent soon after the interview. This should be a personalized note.

Source: Author.

BOX 13-2 Example of a chronological resume.

Cathleen T. McClellan
00 Boyd Road
Toledo, OH 45011
513.872.0000

OBJECTIVE: Staff nurse medical unit

EDUCATION/LICENSE: BSN, to be awarded, May, 2004
                          XYZ University, Indianapolis, IN

                          Certified to sit for boards, State of Ohio

EXPERIENCE:

2003–Present   **Patient Care Assistant**
                          Medical Unit
                          Good Hope Hospital
                          Indianapolis, IN

Summer, 2003   **Patient Care Assistant**
                          Long Term Care Unit
                          The Rehab Hospital
                          Cincinnati, OH

Summer, 2002   **Registration Assistant**
                          Physicians' Clinic
                          Cincinnati, OH

1999–2001   **Sales, part-time**
                          Boxer Department Store
                          Cincinnati, OH

AFFILIATIONS:

                          • Sigma Theta Tau, 2004–
                          • National Student Nurses Association, 2002–President of chapter
                          • Dean's List, 2002–2004

Source: Author. Fictitious resume.

---

and awards or honors (Fellow of the American Academy of Nursing-FAAN) (Smolenski, 2002). The only credentials that are required legally (for example, on medical documentation) are those that state law requires for practice in the state (for example, RN). Other credentials would not be required on medical documentation unless state law requires it. Then the question comes up as to the order for designating credentials. The rule is to start with the credential that has the least chance of being taken away, which is the academic degree (Smolenski, 2002). This is followed by licensure and then the most recently earned certification, followed by honors and awards. An example would be: Jane Jones, MSN, RN, CNS.

A cover letter should be sent with the resume. It should be short (no longer than one page is a good gauge). The first paragraph should catch the reader's attention and explain why the resume is being sent. The second paragraph needs to convince the reader that this position would best be filled by the author of the letter. The third paragraph can expand on reasons and skills. The last paragraph should request an interview, state when and how follow-up will be done, and provide contact information. There should also be some expression of thanking the reader for taking the time to review the material. This cover letter should be customized for specific positions and organizations. Developing the letter requires some research about the organization and

BOX 13-3 Example of a functional resume.

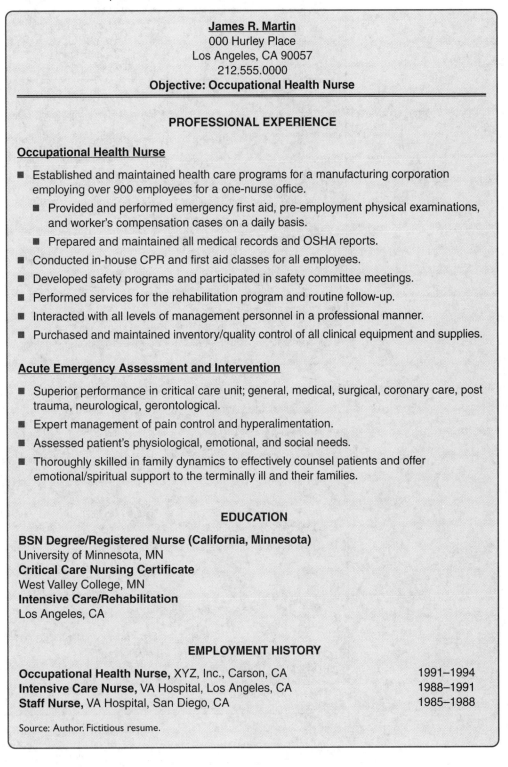

James R. Martin
000 Hurley Place
Los Angeles, CA 90057
212.555.0000
Objective: Occupational Health Nurse

PROFESSIONAL EXPERIENCE

Occupational Health Nurse

- Established and maintained health care programs for a manufacturing corporation employing over 900 employees for a one-nurse office.
  - Provided and performed emergency first aid, pre-employment physical examinations, and worker's compensation cases on a daily basis.
  - Prepared and maintained all medical records and OSHA reports.
- Conducted in-house CPR and first aid classes for all employees.
- Developed safety programs and participated in safety committee meetings.
- Performed services for the rehabilitation program and routine follow-up.
- Interacted with all levels of management personnel in a professional manner.
- Purchased and maintained inventory/quality control of all clinical equipment and supplies.

Acute Emergency Assessment and Intervention

- Superior performance in critical care unit; general, medical, surgical, coronary care, post trauma, neurological, gerontological.
- Expert management of pain control and hyperalimentation.
- Assessed patient's physiological, emotional, and social needs.
- Thoroughly skilled in family dynamics to effectively counsel patients and offer emotional/spiritual support to the terminally ill and their families.

EDUCATION

BSN Degree/Registered Nurse (California, Minnesota)
University of Minnesota, MN
Critical Care Nursing Certificate
West Valley College, MN
Intensive Care/Rehabilitation
Los Angeles, CA

EMPLOYMENT HISTORY

Occupational Health Nurse, XYZ, Inc., Carson, CA	1991–1994
Intensive Care Nurse, VA Hospital, Los Angeles, CA	1988–1991
Staff Nurse, VA Hospital, San Diego, CA	1985–1988

Source: Author. Fictitious resume.

position, which will also be helpful for the job interview. The Internet is one source, as well as reviewing published material, networking to find others who may know something about the organization, and so on.

- **The portfolio:** This is a detailed collection of data about the nurse that focuses on the nurse's career goals and objectives. An annual work plan or the nurse's focus for a specific year is included. For example, the plan might include the following goals: Obtain first nursing position

BOX 13-4 Example of a combination resume.

Sandra Lee Schafer
0000 Somers Drive
Philadelphia, Pennsylvania 15243
412.278.0000

OBJECTIVE
A Clinical Nurse Specialist

CURRENT PROFESSIONAL EXPERIENCE

REGISTERED NURSE   1992–present
Shadyside Hospital, Philadelphia, PA
- Provide, direct, and evaluate nursing care clients and their significant others.
- Develop health care programs.
- Participate in nursing research.
- Provide counseling, guidance, and appropriate referrals for patients, families, and all caregivers.
- Evaluate and document effectiveness of patient care plan and degree of goal attainment.
- Teach patient/family.
- Utilize approaches and techniques to accomplish stated goals and objectives while coordinating patient care with other health care professionals.
- Clinical preceptor for baccalaureate and graduate nursing students.

PROFESSIONAL PROFILE
- Advanced knowledge and technical skills in clinical area of nursing.
- Ability to perform unit-specific system-by-system patient assessment.
- Highly developed intellectual and interpersonal skills in clinical area of nursing.
- Preparation on the Master's level with didactic content, complimented by a clinical synthesis component.
- Orchestrated hospital's participation in the second annual PCSA Program sponsored by the Prostate Cancer Education Council (PCEC) and the Association of Community Cancer Centers (ACCC).
- Co-coordinated Breast Cancer Detection Awareness Program (BCDA).

EDUCATION
Master's of Nursing, 1982
University of Pittsburgh School of Nursing, Pittsburgh, PA

PREVIOUS EMPLOYMENT HISTORY
Adjunct Faculty, Roche College, Philadelphia, PA   1995–1999
Staff Nurse, Shadyville Hospital, Philadelphia, PA   1993–1995

Source: Author. Fictitious resume.

---

that meets personal requirements, complete orientation, complete a critical care internship, and feel like a member of the team. Mentors may be used to help the nurse identify the plan's focus to avoid trying to do everything. Annual performance appraisals can be placed in the portfolio. The portfolio should highlight annual successes or accomplishments (for example, a presentation to staff, patient satisfaction data, or completion of a critical care competency). All of this information should be written in the third person. Expectations of the nurse's position should be identified, as well as the year's accomplishments. All special skills and competencies are also documented and kept in a file. Positive feedback such as letters of appreciation from patients or colleagues can also be included in the portfolio. Participation in volunteer community activities and community involvement should be described. If presentations have been made, these are included, describing the topic, audience type, location, and date. Information about all publications should be updated. Committee work is also documented, including the title of the committee, position held, time of involvement, offices held, and at what level (local/state/national). Kudos need to be added when they occur. Keeping a log throughout the year is one way to ensure that information is not forgotten when the portfolio is reviewed and annually updated. New nurses should begin this log with their first nursing position.

■ **Professional career development plan:** This is the nurse's self-assessment, identification of goals and objectives, and determination of the best strategies to reach identified goals for 1 year, 2 years, and so on. The plan includes: professional goals, target time frame/timeline, strategies/activities to reach goals, and status of goals.

Self-assessment must be done as a career plan is developed. What might be considered in this self-assessment? The first phase focuses on the nurse as a person. What are the nurse's personal needs? Examples of needs are: (a) time to spend with self, (b) time to spend with family, (c) time for community volunteer work, (d) time to travel, and (e) other similar needs. Short-term goals should be developed that focus on what the nurse hopes to accomplish in non-nursing areas. The same would be done for long-term goals. The self-assessment should include aspects of self that are liked and not liked. This will help the nurse look at his or her life. From a variety of perspectives a career plan really cannot be effective if the nurse does not complete a holistic self-assessment—separating professional from personal so that conflict may be avoided. It is important to understand that when one accepts a position it will take time to adjust and to understand the implications of the position's responsibilities on one's personal life (for example, the amount of stress and the time that is required to do the job). It is always better to appreciate these factors before accepting a job, if this is possible. The second phase of the self-assessment focuses on the same questions but from a professional or career perspective. What are the nurse's career needs? Examples might be a position with low stress, a position with direct care, or a position that requires more technical skills. Short-term and long-term career goals then need to be identified with consideration given to the identified career goals, which need to be reasonable. Clarifying these goals will serve the nurse well throughout the nurse's career. After the list of goals is developed, priority goals are identified. For example, what is more important for the nurse: to develop competencies to function as a staff nurse the first year or to begin graduate courses following completion of the BSN?

THINK CRITICALLY

Try this exercise to apply what you have learned about this topic.

Getting guidance

Learning how to seek out professional guidance is a skill that helps nurses cope with professional problems and also with career development. Several methods can be used: networking, mentoring, and coaching.

Networking

Networking focuses on using any contact that might help a nurse in career advancement or in the work that the nurse is doing. This allows for informal communication with others—exchanging information, ideas, and other contacts to meet professional goals. One develops a network through contacts from school, work, professional organizations, professional meetings, and even from the nurse's personal life, as there may be someone who is met in a personal encounter who may be helpful later. While attending meetings, nurses should make an effort to meet other nurses and find someone who may be helpful in the future—someone with similar interests and goals. Keeping a list of these people and their contact information may be helpful in the future. The Internet and e-mail offer additional methods for networking, from making initial contact with someone who might be helpful to continuing networking with long-term colleagues. Many people feel more comfortable contacting someone they do not know by e-mail than calling him or her on the telephone.

What are the advantages of developing a network?

- Build support systems
- Foster self-help
- Improve productivity and work life
- Foster a sense of belonging
- Expedite the exchange of information
- Encourage the development of new ideas
- Generate other connections and develop the network
- Enhance both personal and professional development
- Liberate creativity and innovation
- Emphasize cooperation (Henderson & McGettigan, 1994, p. 286)

Networking is not a "one-way street" in that both parties need to help one another. Sharing information is one way to begin to initiate a networking relationship. This sets a positive tone. Competition does not lead to effective networking.

Mentoring

Mentoring, an important career development tool that can be used by nurses in any type of setting or specialty, can be used to develop the critical leadership skills needed by nurses. "All successful leaders have had mentors and are mentors. They had someone they could confide in, seek advice from, and get help from, and they do the same for others. Being influential and making a difference often are the result of learning leadership skills from others. The skill of gaining recognition and power and the ability to influence others often are learned from those who have recognition, power, and influence" (Bower, 2000, p. 255). These relationships help nurses grow. Seeking out a mentor is not a sign of inadequacy, but rather a sign of a professional who knows the value of support and positive criticism. "Mentors awaken our confidence in our capacity and work with us on how we view ourselves" (Klein & Dickenson-Hazard, 2000, p. 20). Mentors act as teachers by sharing knowledge and expertise, counselors by providing psychological support, intervenors by providing access to resources and protection, and sponsors by promoting the protégé as he or she facilitates development of independence, self-confidence, job satisfaction, upward mobility, decision-making skills, and problem-solving skills (Gordon, 2000). Mentoring does not just occur with new graduates; it may be sought at various points in a nurse's career (Domrose, 2002). "The conclusions drawn from the literature indicate that mentorship has some bearing on career advancement, social and political skill development, and work satisfaction" (Carey & Campbell, 1994, p. 40).

Since mentoring may have negative effects, particularly if there is not a good match between mentor and protégé, which may lead to intimidation, overmanipulation, and demands for loyalty (Gordon, 2000), it is important to explore the relationship aspect of mentoring. There are three steps in the mentoring relationship (Bower, 2000).

1. The first phase is the selection process. Does the mentor select the protégé or does the protégé select the mentor? Typically, the mentor selects the protégé; however, a protégé may approach someone and suggest a mentorship. Mentoring is not new to nurses although when stress increases (such as during times of high staff shortage) there can be less interest in mentoring. When stress is felt there is less energy available to reach out to others. The mentoring process is a socializing relationship as the mentor guides the protégé. Even though it may be more common for the mentor to select the protégé, it is perfectly acceptable for a nurse who wants career guidance to select a mentor to help guide the process. Mentoring should

be a win-win experience for the protégé and the mentor (Shaffer, Tallarica, & Walsh, 2000). Compatibility is important for a successful mentoring experience. Critical questions to consider are: (a) Does the mentor have time for the relationship? (b) Does the mentor have the skills that can assist the protégé? (c) Is the mentor willing to include the protégé in his or her professional activities? Vance (2003) identifies some of the important characteristics of the mentor and the protégé. The mentor should demonstrate generosity, competence, self-confidence, and openness to mutuality. The protégé should demonstrate initiative, career commitment, self-identity, and openness to mutuality. A mentor is not a friend or supervisor and should be well-respected. Protégés should expect mentors to challenge them and stimulate new considerations.

2. The second phase is goal-setting. The protégé develops goals detailing what he or she hopes to accomplish by having a mentor. Mentors also have goals for the relationship. They work together to ensure that goals do not conflict and are reasonable, given time and skills. Goals need to be periodically evaluated.

3. The third phase is the working phase. The relationship is developed as boundaries are established and both decide how and what type of contact they will have with one another. Then they begin to exchange feedback and resources, which may be contacts to assist the protégé in the pursuit of his or her goals. Transition during the working phase happens subtly as the protégé gradually becomes a colleague, although it is possible to be a colleague and be mentored.

One assumes that a mentor and protégé must be in the same location in order to interact; however, with today's technological communication systems this is not the case. E-mail can be used as well as the telephone. These methods may actually provide more accessibility even when the mentor and protégé live in the same location.

Coaching

Coaching is "a personal performance-focused conversation of discovery. Not only to help nurses improve performance, it can renew their commitment to self-sufficiency, organizational goals and values, continuous learning, and improved achievement" (Kinlaw, 1999; as cited in Lachman, 2000, p. 19). Helping colleagues develop self-efficacy through coaching involves four strategies:

1. Help the nurse master challenges, remembering that success breeds success.
2. Use vicarious experience to encourage action. The coach is a role model for providing customer service, portraying confidence with peers, and dealing with difficult families.
3. Use social persuasion, as self-confidence can improve with others who have confidence, such as the coach.
4. Promote self-care, as taking care of oneself improves self-efficacy (Lachman, 2000, p. 15).

When nurses have performance problems, coaching may be used to help these nurses develop solutions. Other strategies that can be used in the coaching process include:

■ **Create a positive mind-set**—shifting the focus to performance improvement rather than the problem and negative consequences.
■ **Get the facts straight**—arriving at a clear and complete assessment of the problem.
■ **Start on an up note**—when the coaching process begins it should focus on the qualities of the staff member rather than jumping right into the problem.
■ **Present the problem concisely**—from the perspective of its effect on the team, unit, division, and organization.
■ **Ask about the nurse's perspective of the problem**—using open-ended questions to involve the staff member, summarizing and repeating to get to the issues, avoiding blame placing and overemphasis on resentments that may come out, then agreeing on major causes.
■ **Search for solutions**—involve the nurse by asking what the nurse would do to solve the problem; avoid the temptation to set a strict direction for the solution even when the nurse cannot seem to identify one.

Comparison of mentors, preceptors, and coaches

Preceptors and coaches may sound very similar to mentors, but they are different. Gordon (2000) compares these three roles. A preceptor is a formalized role with a definite time period and a focus on task accomplishment. Typically, preceptors are assigned. An example of a preceptorship is what may occur in a health care setting when a new nurse is assigned to an experienced nurse for a specific time period for assistance with orientation. Characteristics of an effective preceptor include:

- Sufficient experience with confidence and competence, typically at least 2 years
- Excellent communication skills exercised with peers, medical staff, and patients
- The ability to successfully use mechanisms for coping with stress and conflicting priorities
- Excellent teaching and mentoring skills
- The ability to identify and assess alternatives for problem solving
- The willingness to share knowledge and experience
- Experience in evaluating job performance objectively
- The ability to recognize bad habits in self and others and the willingness to make efforts to correct them promptly (Jackson, 2001, p. 24C)

In comparing preceptorship with mentoring, the mentor-protégé relationship usually occurs more naturally with no designated beginning and ending time, and each agrees to enter the relationship. There is also less focus on tasks. The mentor and protégé may not even be employed by the same employer. As described earlier, a nurse who feels the need for some career guidance would select a mentor, negotiate a mentorship relationship, and continue that relationship as long as both feel it is appropriate to meet goals that were developed. A coach focuses on a specific event, and there is less emphasis on the development of an interpersonal relationship, which facilitates the meeting of the goals.

THINK CRITICALLY

Try this exercise to apply what you have learned about this topic.

Licensure

Licensure is provided through states, and examination for licensure is reciprocal in that the examination does not have to be retaken if a nurse moves to another state and still has a valid license in at least one state, although there is a required application process and licensure fee. Some states do have **continuing education** requirements for renewal. Nurses are then required to maintain records of continuing education and should know what should be included in these records. Licensure renewal occurs every 2 years, and a fee is paid at the time of application for initial licensure in a state and for each renewal. Nurses can go on inactive status, but before doing this nurses should find out what this means long-term if they should decide to become active again. Most nurses keep an up-to-date license in at least one state regardless of their employment status.

To obtain an RN license in a state, either the first RN license or when transferring from one state to another, there are specific state requirements that vary from state to state (for example, submission of transcripts, copies of all RN licenses from other states, application, demonstration of continuing education credits, and other requirements). The contact for this information is the state board of nursing, the authorized state entity with the legal authority to regulate nursing. The nurse practice act in each state typically:

- Defines the authority of the board of nursing, its composition, and powers.
- Defines nursing and the boundaries of the scope of nursing practice.

- Identifies types of licenses and titles.
- States the requirements for licensure.
- Protects titles.
- Identifies the grounds for disciplinary action (Retrieved National Council of State Boards of Nursing, Inc., May 16, 2003).

The scope of practice in nurse practice acts focuses on independent and dependent functions. The key difference is that dependent functions require direction or authorization from another health care provider who is authorized to practice in the state, such as a medication order from a physician that the nurse then administers. Independent functions do not have this requirement.

The state board of nursing also makes administrative rules and regulations that clarify and assist with implementation of the laws. Nurses and the public can make comments on the rules and regulations during a specified period of time before the rules are implemented. Mutual recognition, which is discussed in Chapter 2, is a new approach to multiple licensure to ensure that nurses can easily practice in several states.

THINK CRITICALLY

Try this exercise to apply what you have learned about this topic.

Certification

Certification is now available for most major specialty areas. The focus is on lifelong learning and improvement. This effort should improve the quality of care provided to patients. A recent study identified what some certified nurses perceive to be the benefits from certification, including:

- Recognized as an expert in the field by colleagues
- Certification recognized or publicized
- Full or partial reimbursement of costs
- Salary increases, advancement in career
- Retention in position, one-time bonus
- Eligibility for a higher-level position
- Promoted to a higher level position (Carey, 2001)

However, more than 25% of the respondents stated that they believe they receive no benefit from certification.

The American Nurses Credentialing Center (ANCC) offers 37 certification examinations. There are two levels of credentialing: (a) baccalaureate-prepared nurses and (b) advanced practice registered nurses, who can become board certified. Associate degree- and diploma-prepared nurses can also be certified. These credentials are based on education, skills, proven experience in a specialty area, and passage of a certification examination. Recertification at specific intervals is determined by demonstration of ongoing practice in a specialty area and required continuing education. Nurses can be certified in more than one area as long as they meet the requirements for that specialty. Another choice is to retake the examination after 5 years. Nurses take pride in this accomplishment, and many health care organizations recognize nurses who have achieved certification.

THINK CRITICALLY

Try this exercise to apply what you have learned about this topic.

Professional organizations: Developing a nursing career

Professionalism is part of being a registered nurse. The characteristics of professionalism include:

- Belief in self-regulation and public service
- Commitment to the profession beyond the economic incentives
- A sense of autonomy in practice
- Professional association

Most major professions have organizations that represent various professional issues, and nursing is no exception. The nursing profession's general nursing organization is the American Nurses Association (ANA), but there are also many nursing specialty organizations. There are even organizations whose membership is composed of multiple nursing organizations. An example is the Nursing Organizations Alliance, which was formed in 2001. The goal of this type of professional organization is to utilize the power of the collective membership to make a difference and make nursing more visible.

Involvement in professional organizations develops leadership skills, improves networking, provides access to mentors or the possibility to be a mentor, provides input into professional issues, expands professional education, and increases professional socialization with other members of the profession. Membership is part of professional obligation, although many nurses do not see this as important. Being a professional means belonging to or being connected to a profession, and commitment to that profession involves having a voice in what the profession is and could be. Much of this process takes place in professional organizations. For example, the ANA as well as many specialty nursing organizations develop standards that affect nursing practice.

Attending meetings and conferences provides good opportunities for networking and identifying possible mentors, which are methods for improving professional and leadership skills. Becoming active in organizations by holding office and serving as a meeting delegate are ways to enhance participation in meetings. Submitting abstracts for presentations also increases involvement and opportunities at meetings. If a nurse has not submitted abstracts before, it is helpful to seek out a mentor with experience in this area who will help with the process. Nursing needs more involvement of nurses from all types of settings and experience levels to participate in meetings and conferences. Continuing education credit usually can be obtained at meetings. When considering which conferences to attend, the conference schedule should be reviewed to determine which content is of interest, whether or not the schedule allows for attendance at the sessions of interest with limited conflicts, cost, and location. Evaluation of speakers should also be included. Out-of-town meetings require not only registration fees but also travel costs, meals, and lodging, all of which need to be factored into the cost-benefit analysis of attending a specific meeting or conference. Some of these costs may be tax-deductible depending on how an individual's taxes are calculated, so receipts should be kept. Some employers assist with conference costs, but this is not routine. It is important to inquire about this during the employment process.

Seeking promotion

At some point in everyone's career, promotion is considered. This promotion may be sought at the nurse's present employer or may mean the nurse will look at other organizations for a new position that represents a promotion. A promotion to a management position is one type of promotion although certainly not the only type. What can be expected when applying for a promotion to a management position? The following are some examples of questions that might be asked in an interview, and these questions can be applied to more than just management positions.

1. What are your strengths and skills?
2. Where will you need the most support or assistance?
3. What are the most rewarding nursing experiences that you can recall?
4. What were your least rewarding nursing experiences?
5. What new ideas have you tried out in any previous employment, in the community, or in school?

6. If you assume this position, what would be the first thing you would consider changing (Manning, 1991, p. 26)?

Characteristics that are usually important for nurses who take management positions are leadership, enthusiasm, honesty, communication skills, and personality that "fits" the unit or service. As is true with any position sought, the nurse needs information about the type of support that will be offered—education, guidance on the job, time period of orientation, and so on. If the nurse has never held a management position, it is critical to openly discuss leadership and management skills and if the organization will provide management development courses or pay for academic courses. If the organization provides this content, the nurse needs additional information about the type of content, such as who teaches it, time frame, and expectations. This is not an area in which many health care organizations have been very effective. Promotions occur, and then new nurse managers are left to deal with the process of management by themselves or with minimal support. When organizations make promotions, this is one of the most important decisions that they make. Many serious errors can be made that affect many staff. Promoting a nurse to a nurse manager position because the nurse is popular or provides excellent patient care may lead to a disaster for the unit. Promoting from within can, however, improve retention as well as recruitment when job candidates learn that promotion does occur, which provides opportunity for advancement. Organizations need to avoid the **"Peter Principle"** or promoting to the level of incompetence (Laborde & Lee, 2000). Some methods that organizations can use to increase managerial effectiveness include:

1. Dual career ladders when nurses continue to develop their technical skills and begin development of management skills (Lissy, 1993).
2. Succession planning that identifies someone who will take the place of a manager and allows time for that nurse to develop management skills (McConnell, 1996).
3. Mentoring to help potential new managers develop.

A key to successful promotion is development of criteria and competencies required for positions. These can then be used in the selection process and will also help candidates better understand the position (Laborde & Lee, 2000).

Entrepreneur/intrapreneur

Entrepreneurship and intrapreneurship are important as they provide opportunities for growth and advancement. What is the difference in an **intrapreneur** and an **entrepreneur?** Intrapreneurs are probably more common. These are nurses who are risk-takers and innovators within an organization. This nurse views change as a plus, seeks ways to respond effectively to change, and is proactive. Intrapreneurs offer change within organizations. A nurse manager may be an intrapreneur within an organization when the nurse manager steps back and views the organization's culture and change within that culture, and then steps up and offers creative ideas and approaches to problems. This nurse needs to be assertive, have high self-esteem, and be confident. To be effective as an intrapreneur the nurse needs to demonstrate negotiation skills, time management, leadership skills, and risk-taking. This nurse will come face to face with the "old guard" or those who want to keep things the way they are. The intrapreneur wants to look beyond the "way things are" and will also avoid accepting the first solution as the best one. Listening, observing, comparing ideas, questioning the status quo, using new frames of reference for solutions, networking, and planning are critical for the nurse intrapreneur.

Both intrapreneurs and entrepreneurs require risk-takers who are willing to address critical issues with innovative ideas. Nurse entrepreneurs are typically consultants or nurses who have established their own business. Legal nurse consultants are an example of a growing group of entrepreneurs. Successful consultation in any area is highly dependent on marketing and seeking out consulting projects. It is definitely risky financially, and many nurses who do this have multiple facets to their work so that they are not dependent on only one "product or service." They may also phase in consultation by having a full-time or part-time job and then gradually increase their entrepreneurial work. What are other typical areas of nurse entrepreneurship? Examples are:

■ Development of continuing education material
■ Teaching in continuing education programs

- Assisting health care organizations with management problems, clinical improvement, and so on
- Consulting with pharmaceutical and medical equipment companies on projects
- Working with medical equipment companies

These opportunities do not just happen. The nurse consultant has to be active and make them happen. The key is that there is no limit, and creativity in finding these projects is required. Some nurses like to be involved in entrepreneurship because of its flexibility and the many different opportunities that can be explored. Some nurses, however, need more structure. Entrepreneurship requires a high level of self-discipline, as much of the work is done in isolation. Entrepreneurs have to decide if they have something to offer, a product or service, and then set up a business plan and market it themselves. It can be stressful or exciting, and different personalities respond differently. Whenever this route is taken, it is important to do periodic self-assessments because it may not be the best experience and it is important to recognize this early on.

Lifelong learning: Nursing professional development

Nurses must be lifelong learners in today's changing health care environment, as new science, technology, treatments, management methods, and so on, are constantly coming into play. To remain up-to-date each nurse must meet the competency requirements for the job that needs to be done. The Institute of Medicine report (2003) that addresses health professions education notes that "health professionals are not adequately prepared—in either academic or continuing education venues—to address the nation's patient population" (p. 2). This report emphasizes the need to focus on five core competencies:

1. Provide patient-centered care
2. Work in interdisciplinary teams
3. Employ evidence-based practice
4. Apply quality improvement
5. Utilize informatics (p. 3)

Given the need to keep learning, how does a nurse meet this goal? The goal can be met in a variety of ways—participating in continuing education, fulfilling required employer education

FIGURE 13-1   Framework for nursing professional development.

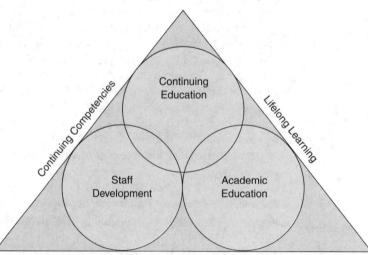

Source: American Nurses Association. (2000). *Scope and standards of practice for nursing professional development.* Washington, DC: American Nurses Publishing.

and training, participating in orientation for new positions, and pursuing formal academic programs. In addition to these approaches, nurses who are current with the literature in their area of expertise and participate in professional activities gain knowledge that can be applied to their practice. The ANA standards (2000a) describe the framework for nursing professional development, which is provided in Figure 13-1.

This framework is based on the Philosophy of Nursing Professional Development that is described in Box 13-5.

Competency-based learning

The ANA has stated that continuing competence is "ongoing professional nursing competence according to level of expertise, responsibility, and domains of practice as evidenced by behavior based on beliefs, attitudes, and knowledge matched to and in the context of a set of expected outcomes as defined by nursing scope of practice, policy, *Code for Nurses,* standards, guidelines, and benchmarks that assure safe performance of professional activities" (2000b, p. 16). Many factors affect staff education needs, and the most important one is the accountability and responsibility accepted by each nurse.

For a long time the nursing profession has been conflicted about the employer's need to pay for and also provide education. How much of this is covered by the employer is highly variable and should be discussed during the employment process. The key question throughout this discussion is who is responsible for continuing competence? The ANA standards, *Scope and Standards of Practice for Nursing Professional Development* (2000a), identifies four sources of responsibilities: (a) the individual nurse, (b) the professional association, (c) the employer, and (d) regulatory agencies.

1. Individual nurses are responsible for maintaining individual competence so that their practice is based on current knowledge and skills. To accomplish this each nurse must practice self-evaluation to regularly identify learning needs and then obtain required education. Peer review may be part of this process.
2. The professional association, which in the case of these standards is identified as the ANA and its constituencies (state and local), has the responsibility of developing standards, providing continuing education programs, monitoring health policy to determine educational needs, and supporting nursing research, which may indicate the need for additional learning needs. Other nursing organizations such as specialty organizations also participate at this level.
3. The employer is directly concerned with practice that is safe and of the highest quality. They, too, are responsible for ensuring that staff are able to do their jobs effectively and thus are concerned with ongoing competency. As change occurs in the workplace the employer must ensure that staff are able to provide the care that is required. In addition, the employer confirms that nurses have the correct academic preparation, licensure, and, when required, certification.
4. The last important source of responsibility involves regulatory agencies. State boards of nursing are required by law to ensure that the state's citizens receive safe and quality care. They do this through establishing standards and providing licensure. Some states have specific continuing education requirements that must be met when licensure renewal occurs.

YOUR OPINION COUNTS

Find out what others think about this topic. Post your response and check out other opinions.

Change, as has been noted, is clearly a major factor driving education needs. What are some of the other critical factors affecting lifelong learning? Diversity is another factor, which is found in both health care staff as well as patients and their families. Chapter 17 discusses this topic in much more detail. Another factor discussed in Chapter 17 that needs to be considered with staff

BOX 13-5   Philosophy of nursing professional development.

Beliefs

The following beliefs guided development of the *Scope and Standards of Practice for Professional Nursing Development:*

- Lifelong learning is the responsibility of the nurse and is essential to maintain and increase competence in nursing practice.
- Continuing professional nursing competence is essential to the provision of safe, quality health care to all members of society.
- The public has a right to expect continuing professional nursing competence throughout the career of the nurse.
- Assurance of continuing professional nursing competence must be shaped and guided by the nursing profession.
- Continuing professional nursing competence is definable, measurable, and can be evaluated.
- The nurse as the learner actively partners with the nurse professional development educator in the educational process and in the maintenance of the nurse's continuing professional nursing competence.
- The nursing professional development educator incorporates the roles of facilitator, change agent, consultant, leader, or researcher in the learning activities that support the nurse in developing and maintaining continuing professional nursing competence.
- Self-directed learning is an integral part of continuing education, staff development, and academic education.
- Use of adult learning principles contributes to effective professional development activities.
- A variety of educational options are necessary to meet the diverse needs of the nursing population, including, but not limited to, academic education, experiential learning, consultation, teaching others, professional reading, distance learning, research, and self-directed activities.
- The learning activity may be related to resolving the current knowledge or skill deficit of the nurse to ensure continuing professional nursing competence.
- Ongoing evaluation of educational activities is essential to maintain and enhance professional development and the quality and cost-effectiveness of health care.
- The practice of nursing professional development is guided by principles of ethics.

Influencing Factors

Professional development needs of nurses are influenced by many factors, such as:

- Nurses' acceptance of accountability and responsibility for their practice.
- Specialization in nursing, cultural backgrounds, changes in educational levels, and other demographic characteristics of nursing adult learners.
- Changes in demographic characteristics of health care consumer populations.
- Knowledgeable consumers who recognize their right to health care and demand accountability for services rendered.
- Changing health care delivery systems and financing methods.
- A rapidly evolving body of knowledge and research applications from nursing, social, physiological, and the basic sciences.
- Advances in nursing practice, health care delivery, and technology.
- Participation of nurses in intra- and interdisciplinary efforts that affect health care delivery systems.
- The numbers and variety of health personnel, health care consumer populations, and types of services provided in any given setting.
- Health care consumer, organizational, legislative, policy, regulatory, or professional development requirements.
- Increased focus on evidence-based practice outcomes.
- Political, social, economic, legislative, and regulatory factors that influence nursing and health care throughout the world.

Source: American Nurses Association. (2000). *Scope and standards of practice for nursing professional development.* Washington, DC: American Nurses Publishing. Reprinted with permission.

education is generational issues, which affect people's learning, motivation, effectiveness of learning strategies, and so on. Consumers also affect education when they demand quality, safe care. With their growing knowledge and access to important information, consumers ask more questions, thereby requiring that staff are more knowledgeable. The changing demographics such as a growing aging population requires new approaches to care and the need for knowledge and expertise about care for those with chronic diseases. The development of knowledge about science and other aspects of care (for example, genetics) requires that staff update their own knowledge. Different management approaches, reimbursement issues, and health policy changes all lead to more educational needs. The push to provide more evidence-based care means that staff need to understand this process and participate in the development of this information. Nurses who think their learning days are over when they graduate and obtain their license will soon find that this is not the case. Quality practice requires updates on current regulations. In addition, the Joint Commission on Accreditation of Healthcare Organizations (JCAHO) also requires that its accredited health care organizations address this issue by requiring that all full-time, part-time or per diem, volunteer, or agency employees be provided with "an effective, systematic approach to orientation; continuing education based on identified need; and a mechanism for competency assessment and validation" (Burke, 2000, p. 21).

Pursuit of educational activities

The ANA (2000a) has developed standards related to professional development. These standards emphasize that adult learning principles should be applied when professional development occurs, which should be "based on recognition of the adult individual's autonomy and self-direction, life experiences, readiness to learn, and problem orientation to learning" (American Nurses Association, 2000a, p. 23). Some key definitions related to professional development that sometimes can be confusing but are important in determining what type of education activity is offered include the following.

- **Orientation.** Orientation is the process of introducing nursing staff to the philosophy, goals, policies, procedures, role expectations, and other factors needed to function in a specific work setting. Orientation is provided for new employees as well as employees facing changes in their roles, responsibilities, and practice settings.
- **Inservice educational activities.** These learning experiences are provided in the work setting for the purpose of assisting staff members in performing their assigned functions in that particular agency or institution; for example, staff are taught how to use new cardiac monitoring equipment.
- **Staff development.** Development is the systematic process of assessment, development, and evaluation that enhances the performance or professional development of health care providers and their continuing competence (National Nursing Staff Development Organization, 1999).
- **Continuing education (CE).** Continuing education features systematic professional learning experiences designed to augment the knowledge, skills, and attitudes of nurses and therefore enrich the nurses' contributions to quality health care and their pursuit of professional career goals; for example, a nurse attends a session at an annual meeting about treatment of chronic illness in the community.
- **Academic education.** Courses can be taken for undergraduate or graduate credit in an institution of higher learning that may or may not lead to a degree or completion of a certificate program. This term specifically refers to courses taken after the completion of a basic nursing education program (American Nurses Association, 2000a, pp. 23–25).

What should staff expect in education programs that they participate in for continuing education credit? The program should be planned and organized, and content should include:

- Identification of needs and adult learning principles
- Identification of learners
- Identification of learner objectives
- Content which is relevant and current
- Learning environment, conducive to learning
- Teaching methods, appropriate for content and learner level
- Implementation; faculty should be qualified and able to teach the content
- Evaluation

Attendance should be checked, and attendees/learners are required to identify themselves either by social security number and/or RN licensure number. The organization that provides the program is required by their continuing education accrediting organization to keep records for a specific number of years. Evaluations are also required; once completed, they provide feedback that can be used to improve the program.

Health care organizations typically provide some educational programs for their staff in addition to orientation, and these programs should meet the same requirements as cited previously whether or not they are offered for continuing education credit. The organization's education department may be centralized, decentralized, or sometimes a mix of both. A centralized service means that education staff provide education both for the organization as a whole and also for individual unit service needs such as for the labor and delivery unit. The decentralized approach focuses all the education on the unit or department level, with few or any overall education staff. The mix combines these two approaches and is probably the more common approach today. Staff may also get involved in teaching one another, either in formal situations or informally as they help one another.

Orientation is, of course, a major issue in all organizations. It is very costly, and requires much staff time. Preceptors are used to assist new staff as they adjust to, and learn about, the organization. Orientation should focus on the overall organization, department, and job orientation information. Many health care organizations use some type of skills checklist for their staff. What are some of the typical topics included in orientation?

- Organization mission, vision, and goals
- Organization structure
- Organizational culture
- Diversity
- Types of patients
- Position descriptions (roles and responsibilities)
- Human resources policies and procedures
- Benefits
- Scheduling
- Performance improvement process and policies
- Safety
- Ethics, patient rights, and related issues
- Patient care delivery models and tools used (such as pathways)
- Communication
- Computer system and usage
- Documentation of patient care
- Specific direct care orientation (for example, to equipment, procedures, and so on)
- Admission, transfer, and discharge procedures

Documentation of professional development activities

Every nurse should develop and maintain personal education files, which should contain all copies of certificates of attendance that document continuing education credit, as well as documentation about completed academic courses. This information is needed in some states that require a specific number of CE hours at licensure renewal time, although all nurses should maintain a file for their portfolios and development of resumes. Continuing education credit is noted by contact hours, which is one contact hour per 50 minutes. Some states require that some of the CE credits include specific content (for example, content on HIV/AIDS, medication safety, or state regulations that affect nursing practice). Health care organizations may require specific content for specific positions. Nurses who hold specialty certification must also meet the specialty certification continuing education requirements, which are not identical to those required by the state board of nursing for relicensure.

Returning to school: What needs to be done?

The following quote provides a view of continuing one's education that is very positive:

> My formal education is like a wave that's propelling me into my future. I've had many new and exciting opportunities come my way in the past five years. School has prepared me to meet those challenges and given me the confidence to try new things and keep moving forward. You can't possibly appreciate what higher education will do for you until you start taking classes. It keeps you young, it makes you feel alive, and it keeps the blood coursing through your veins. It's never too late to go back to school. It's a gift you give yourself and a way to enrich your life. You'll have more to give yourself, your family, your patients, and the world around you. (Cardillo, 2001, October, p. 12)

Returning to school, whether it be for a baccalaureate, masters, or doctoral degree or to obtain certification in a different specialty, requires careful thought and a plan. Career advancement planning, as discussed earlier in this chapter, is the place to begin. What is the goal(s) for returning to school? It might be to receive a promotion, gain knowledge and skills, receive additional pay, seek a new and different position, or just for the internal need to expand oneself. There are also internal reasons that may not be as obvious—self-esteem, need to get ahead, competition with others, and so on. Going back to school alters a person's lifestyle, and this can have a major impact on family and personal life. Family members should be open about reactions and concerns and discuss the implications. This will help to prevent some of the stress that is inevitable as an adult tries to balance school, work, and a personal life. Most nurses must also consider the financial implications (for example, cost of education and how this might affect how quickly one can finish); loss of hours worked, reducing income; cost of child care for school hours; typical activities such as vacations and entertainment that might have to be limited to cover costs; costs of books, computer, e-mail access, and other learning resources; and travel time if this is required. Scholarships, grants, tuition reimbursement from employer, and loans are external sources of financial assistance.

The Nurse Reinvestment Act of 2002 (funded in 2003) is landmark nursing legislation that provides strategies to resolve some of the issues that have exacerbated the nursing shortage. This law, passed with tremendous effort and support from nurses across the country, "offers funds to project a new image of nursing in the twenty-first century. It establishes a National Nurse Corps to provide nurses for shortage areas. It finances the education of the next generation of teachers (nursing faculty). It encourages program development and education of persons to care for the nation's aged. It offers nursing the opportunity to solve one of its own problems—the culture of the workplace. It provides funds for demonstration projects to enhance communication, to mentor young nurses through internships and residences, and to create new methods for staffing and work force deployment" (Donley et al., 2002, p. 1). This legislation has implications, as described, for all nurses. Nurses need to make the most of the funds to demonstrate that the profession can lead the way in resolving nursing shortage issues that have implications for the entire health care delivery system such as quality of care and costs.

Time is always a concern with so little of it available, so it is important to assess this aspect of returning to school. Returning full time means completing a degree sooner, but it may also mean a loss of income or trying to balance work with going to school full time, leading to major stress. Part-time study is possible in some programs and might be a better approach for some nurses, but it takes longer to complete the degree. Online degree programs are a choice many nurses are making, and all three types of degrees can be obtained this way. This approach allows for greater time flexibility. Nurses also need to consider the schedule that the educational program requires. For example, are courses taught more than once a year? If not, this means a nurse might have to wait a year to get a course that is needed. The general steps a nurse goes through in the process of returning to school are described in Box 13-6.

Selecting the right school or program can be difficult. Factors that are important to consider include professional goals and personal needs, distance, cost, quality of school/program and faculty, and type of program (for example, online learning versus onground learning where courses are attended on a campus, or in some cases a mixture of both). It is helpful to assess different types of programs to compare and contrast curricula and instructional methods. Asking to review course descriptions and inquiring about specific course requirements and clinical experience are critical in selecting the right school. Potential students tend to focus on "them liking me and accepting

BOX 13-6   The process of returning to school.

1. Making the decision
2. Considering financial issues, both costs of school and impact on personal finances
3. Completing required testing
4. Selecting the schools/programs
5. Completing the application and interview process
6. Making final decision when acceptances arrive
7. Preparing to begin

Source: Author.

me" rather than seeing the importance of the potential student evaluating and interviewing the program and its faculty. What needs to be considered when a program or school is assessed (McGettigan & Henderson, 1994)? The degree that is sought and whether or not certification preparation is offered are important (for example, advanced practice with ability to sit for certification exam in family practice advanced practice nursing). Nurses who are returning to school to obtain a baccalaureate degree will want to examine the type of credit awarded for previous nursing courses and general education prerequisites courses. Transcripts and course descriptions from previous credit received are important information in this process. Nursing programs tend to have a schema of their curriculum that provides the framework for the approach used in the courses.

One should always be concerned about the quality of an educational program as there can be variability. How can this be determined? The school should be accredited. The interview is a time to inquire about student success on boards and certification exams; faculty clinical and research work (for example, publications and research); number of students in clinical groups and courses; number of faculty who are tenured or non-tenured, which means they are not permanent; number of part-time faculty; and where faculty received their degrees. If one is considering graduate school (particularly doctoral programs), it is important to learn more about faculty research and determine if their areas of research are comparable to personal professional interests. The Internet makes it easy to initiate a publication search and learn more about the work of individual faculty members. An evaluation of student services is also part of this process. Items of interest are student advisors, counseling, library, parking, health services, and Internet access and technology services. The latter is particularly important when taking online courses. Talking with students often reveals critical information about the learning environment and how students are treated by faculty and staff.

An increasing number of schools offer Web-based and other forms of distance learning academic degrees. Some only offer specific courses while others offer the entire degree online. It is important to evaluate distance learning programs before selecting them. A distance learning program is "the transmission of educational programming to geographically dispersed individuals through technology. The technology may be the World Wide Web, e-mail, video- or audiotapes, videoconferencing, fax, or snail mail" (Day, 2001, p. 23). Courses toward degrees or full degrees that are offered in this manner are BSN, RN to BSN, MSN, and PhD. Certificate programs are also turning in this direction.

Before considering a program of this type it is important to do a self-assessment that focuses on personal learning style. Factors that are important to assess are commitment and self-motivation, flexibility, self-discipline, and ability to function as an independent learner. If it is important for a nurse to have one-to-one in-person contact, then this is not the type of learning that will be successful for him or her. It also requires organization and self-discipline as there may be no specific time for class attendance. The structure must come from within. This is not to say that these programs do not have structure, as they do. They typically require much work, and in some cases, more work than traditional classroom courses. It also does not mean that students do not get to know one another or the faculty, since some of these courses provide a greater opportunity to get to know one another. These courses typically offer greater opportunities to study with students from all over the country (and, in some courses, the world). There is greater cross-learning and discovery about how others are practicing nursing and exploration about different health problems and similarities in a broad range of communities.

There is no doubt that technology plays a major role in these courses, and this may seem to be problematic for some students. The key is having the right equipment and software and learning how to use them. These programs typically build on self-directed learning, which is an essential skill in today's health care environment (O'Shea, 2003). Self-directed learning occurs "when students take the initiative for their own learning, diagnosing needs, formulating goals, identifying resources, implementing appropriate activities and evaluating outcomes" (Spencer & Jordan, 1999, p. 1281). Responsibility is placed in the hands of the learner, and this is often more apparent in programs such as online programs.

If the decision is made to explore online programs or a program that offers some of their courses online, what might be some aspects to include in the evaluation? Many of these aspects should be evaluated for any type of nursing program that is considered.

- What is the program's accreditation status? Consult with the state board of nursing regarding regulations if considering advanced practice nursing. To avoid problems with legitimacy the program should be university-based. If the goal is to seek certification (for example, for advanced nurse practitioner), will the program provide the content and required clinical hours?

- Time is a critical issue with all educational endeavors, and distance learning views time differently than traditional programs. Is the program synchronous, meaning the students have to be available at a specific time (for example, in a chat room) or asynchronous with no specific times? There are, of course, always due dates. Some of these courses no longer use the traditional time frames of semesters and quarters but rather specify a specific period such as 5 or 6 weeks for a course. This has great implications because students are doing the work or learning that would normally be done in traditional credit hours (for example, over an entire semester). Some programs limit the number of courses that can be taken at one time, which is much lower than in traditional academic programs, as they recognize that the workload is great. For courses that use videoconferencing in specific locations, students will need to consider travel time to those sites. If clinical hours are required, this time must be considered.

- Costs are, of course, always important. Sometimes there is no distinction made between in-state and out-of-state students in distance learning courses, so it is important to inquire about this. Additional costs to consider are computer and printer equipment, software required, and Internet connection costs. With the latter, it is best to get the type of connection that is not charged per time used because much time will be spent online. If travel is required to a distant site, then this cost must be factored into the student's budget. Some programs mail textbooks and material to students although students pay for the texts, material, and the postage. Typically, papers are sent via e-mail or the Web; however, if they have to be mailed or faxed, then this is an additional cost. The idea is to inquire about the hidden costs or costs that would not be typically considered in traditional programs. Of course, if no travel is required, costs will be saved in travel and parking. Those with children can save money in child care costs and time taken off from work.

- Learning and evaluation methods should be considered for any educational program; however, they seem to be even more important with distance learning. Many programs are using creative methods, and most rely much more on group projects, independent learning, faculty facilitation of learning, and critical thinking activities. Testing may also occur. This testing may be based on the honor system, and some programs may require that the student go to a testing site. Many students in these programs actually find that they have an opportunity to explore content in more depth. Discussions are often of higher quality as students have time to think about the topic and respond. Potential students should ask how courses are conducted and for information about the types of learning activities that can be expected. Sizes of classes are also important. Larger classes are difficult to manage online. Typical effective sizes range from 8 to 12 students.

- If a practicum is required, how is this arranged? Who identifies the site and preceptor, type of required communication, required hours, and so on?

- Admission requirements should not be much different than in traditional academic programs. It is important to find out about deadlines and meet them. How are the courses offered (for example, are courses offered multiple times during the year or just once)? The latter has great implications for student flexibility and the type of barriers that might exist in completing the program in a timely fashion. Admission requirements typically include licensure considerations, liability insurance, and for practicum or clinical, cardiopulmonary resuscitation, immunizations for practica, and so on.

■ Technology is critical in this type of learning environment. The program should be able to produce a very specific list of the required type of equipment and software. Many programs now offer some discounts on the computer, equipment, printer, and software when purchased through the university. Does the program offer software that can be downloaded? The type of technology support can make or break a learning experience. All will say they have 24-7 support, but asking about wait times and qualifications of tech support staff can be helpful. Contacting students in the program or who have completed the program can provide the important information about how accessible and helpful tech support has been. Each student should always have a backup plan or another computer that could be used, which might be a family member's, friends, one at work, or one at a public or local university library.

■ Resources are always important, such as student guidance and the library. How they are contacted or accessed can make a big difference. What types of resources does the library offer that can be accessed from home? Are there any fees?

■ Faculty should never be ignored. Who are the faculty and what are their qualifications? What type of experience do they have in nursing, nursing education, and, if relevant, in distance learning? How accessible are faculty, and how are they contacted? What is the faculty role in the course? Talking with students is important when trying to find out more about these issues.

There is no doubt that distance learning offers many advantages from a flexibility point-of-view. Most nurses who return to school continue to work. Trying to juggle work schedules with getting to class can be a nightmare. Distance learning can make this much easier. If taking an online course, the classroom can be open 24-7. Nurses also have personal lives and obligations that demand much from their schedules. A flexible method for obtaining further education can help decrease the stress or pull on personal lives. This is not to say that these courses are easy or require minimal work but rather that the time factor is more in the control of the individual nurse student. Naturally, these online courses are not appropriate for every nurse.

CURRENT ISSUES

Learn about events around the globe that relate to the chapter content.

Professional issues

Continuing competency: Where is the profession going?

The ANA has been exploring and developing its viewpoint about continuing competency. The following have been identified as assumptions regarding continuing competence.

1. The purpose of ensuring continuing competency is the protection of the public and advancement of the profession through the professional development of nurses.
2. The public has a right to expect competence throughout nurses' careers.
3. Any process of competency assurance must be shaped and guided by the profession of nursing.
4. Assurance of continuing competence is the shared responsibility of the profession, regulatory bodies, organizations/workplaces, and individual nurses.
5. Nurses are individually responsible for maintaining continuing competence.
6. The employer's responsibility is to provide an environment conducive to competent practice.
7. Continuing competence is definable, measurable, and can be evaluated.
8. Competence is considered in the context of level of expertise, responsibility, and domains of practice (American Nurses Association, 2000b).

In order to appreciate these assumptions it is important to understand three critical terms: continuing competence, professional nursing competence, and continuing professional nursing competence.

1. Continuing competence is an important goal for nurses, and we have not yet developed mechanisms to accomplish this.
2. Professional nursing competence looks at two factors: expected outcomes and behavior. Expected outcomes for practicing nurses (competencies) are identified by a variety of sources: nursing scope of practice, policy, *Code for Nurses,* standards, guidelines, and benchmarks. These expected outcomes need to demonstrate the nurse's behavior, which is also affected by beliefs, attitudes, and knowledge.
3. These two terms are combined to form continuing professional nursing competence. The *Nursing's Agenda for the 21st Century* (American Nurses Association, 2002) describes continuing competence as the "ongoing professional nursing competence according to level of expertise, responsibility, and domains of practice as evidenced by behavior based on beliefs, attitudes, and knowledge matched to and in the context of a set of expected outcomes as defined by nursing scope of practice, policy, *Code for Nurses,* standards, guidelines, and benchmarks that assure safe performance of professional activities" (American Nurses Association, 2000b, p. 3).

BENCHMARKS

Now let's take a moment to test your knowledge of the concepts you have studied in this section.

Time Management to Get the Work Done

Time management is included in this chapter because it has an impact on career development and is a major issue in how successful a nurse will be. This discussion provides some guidelines for understanding time management.

Making the most of your time

"We can't control the amount of time available; we can only control how we use it. Once time is passed, it's gone and cannot be replaced" (Brumm, 2002a, p. 14MW). This quote highlights the critical time management issue. It is a rare person who is successful under time pressure, and this type of pressure has severe wear and tear consequences on individual staff and the work environment. Time management includes aspects of communication, planning, prioritization, and delegation. With today's rapid change environment and overabundance of information, time management is a key to success in this hectic health care environment.

Productivity is critical to organizations, and individuals soon learn that to be effective workers, it is also important to them. What is productivity? Simply put, it is the ratio of outputs to inputs, or what resources need to be used to complete an action, service, and so on. Typically, one thinks of productivity as being associated with organization goals, staffing, and budgets; however, staff need to consider their own productivity levels. In simplest terms, nurses all experience days when they have felt, "I just didn't seem to get anything done." This relates directly to productivity. Inevitably, *time* gets to be an awful word, and time is associated with productivity. Time is a precious resource that always seems to run short. However, it is a resource that can be managed. It has become even more critical to manage time because organizations expect staff and managers to be more decisive and to focus on "now" while still considering long-term goals. As time appears to be in short supply, staff and managers then move their focus further from long-term goals and zero in on "now." In the long run, the loss of a balance between long-term and present needs is detrimental to staff, management, and the organization.

All levels of nursing staff need to practice time management. New nurses struggle with this hourly, and their co-workers and managers need to help them learn the critical skills associated with effective time management. This will benefit the organization and patient care. More importantly, when a person feels in control and recognizes time has been managed as best as it can be, less stress is experienced. Less stress means less wear and tear on oneself, improved critical thinking, better decisions, more effective communication and collaboration, and improved quality of care. How one uses time actually is a nonverbal message that is noticed by others. Effective time management also means more efficiency and effectiveness in the care delivery process. Efficiency means doing things right while effectiveness means doing the right things. This text emphasizes the importance of participatory leadership with staff playing an important role in decision making; however, it should be noted that this type of approach takes more time. It is not uncommon to hear statements such as, "It's easier if I do it myself." Why is this so? Negotiation, conflict management, communication, and group decision making take time. Improving time management "requires an understanding of strengths and limitations related to work habits, setting priorities, taking responsibility to reach goals, and developing an organized work system" (Finkelman, 1996, p. 1-6:1).

Some time management strategies may have serious ethical, legal, and emotional implications (Bowers, Lauring, & Jacobson, 2001). This happens when procedures are missed or shortened, medications are not administered when ordered, and patients are neglected or have less time with staff. In these cases time has become the controlling element in care and can seriously affect the quality of care. Time management, however, can result in different results.

- Gain more control over work
- Make the job easier
- Save time
- Determine what is important
- Accomplish what is important (Gleeson, 2000, p. 4)

To reach these outcomes a nurse may use a number of strategies.

Time analysis

Where does one begin with time management? As is true for all issues or problems, assessment is required: How is time spent? What are the person's strengths and limitations with time management? What can be realistically changed? It is very easy to say, "I spend hours doing this or that" without really having reliable data about the amount of time that is actually used or how that time is actually used. The only real way to obtain reliable data is to conduct a personal time analysis. Most shudder at the thought of doing this, as it takes more time to do it. Keeping a log or diary for a time period, and remembering that all days are not alike, can be helpful. After the log is kept for a specified time period, such as a week, an honest review of the data is required. This analysis might consider some of the questions identified in Box 13-7. Other questions can be added, although some of these may not be relevant based on the nurse's position. It is important to ensure that the analysis gets to the critical time management issues.

After the analysis, major time management problems need to be identified. Honesty is important in this process, or time management will not be corrected. Time management can be improved, but it requires effort. Correcting a time management problem does not mean it will never be a problem again. Slipping back into old habits is very easy to do, so reevaluation of time management should be part of the ongoing improvement process. What are some of the common problems that people have with time management?

- Lack of goals and inadequate setting of priorities
- Problems with delegation (not delegating when we should, inadequate directions, lack of supervision, too much supervision, inability to let go, poor communication, lack of understanding about what a delgatee can and cannot do)
- Too many interruptions
- Overworking

BOX 13-7 Time analysis questions.

- Did I spend any time organizing my day? Was this organizing done the day before or at the beginning of the day?
- Did I stick to my plan?
- How do I begin and end my day?
- Do I jump from task to task?
- Do I complete a task before undertaking a new one?
- How many telephone calls did I make, and how many of these calls were really required?
- Did I do another task while on the telephone?
- Did I spend time looking for information? For medical records? For forms? For supplies?
- How much time was spent completing forms or writing reports? When were they due?
- Did I ask support staff to do something that saved me time?
- Did I prepare for patient procedures and other activities so that I did not have to stop what I was doing to get supplies or other items I needed?
- Did I get a complete report so that I had information I needed?
- Who interrupted my work and why?
- Did I repeat actions that I did not need to repeat?
- Did I spend a lot of time getting ready to do a task?
- Was I prepared to do a procedure?
- Did I take a break and have a meal break?
- Did I prepare for meetings? For shift report?
- Did I have my appointment book/calendar with me to make appointments?
- Did I have time to talk with my patients? With family members?
- Did I return all my phone calls and e-mails?
- Did I take some time to evaluate my day? When?

Source: Author.

- Responding with frustration when need to be flexible
- Difficulty jumping in and getting started
- Attending meetings that do not go anywhere
- Difficulty knowing when to stop
- Inattentiveness and lack of concentration
- Inability to say "no"
- Wasting time on smaller tasks
- Lack of planning (individual task, shift, daily, weekly, and long term)
- Not using the most effective and efficient communication method (verbal one-to-one, group, written, telephone, e-mail)
- Focusing on a large project in total rather than breaking it down into small components
- Waiting for the "right time" to do something
- Overcommitment
- Failure to follow-up on uncompleted tasks
- Insecurity, fear of failure, and lack of confidence and self-esteem
- Treating every problem as a crisis
- Unawareness of the importance of tasks, situations, and communications
- Socializing

- Confusion over responsibilities and roles
- Inability to find information when you need it
- Inability to take a break
- Feeling incompetent to do a task
- Poor leadership that fails to set clear lines of responsibility and authority
- Inadequate information systems
- Unclear about what has to be done (Cesta, Tahan, & Fink, 1998, p. 46; Finkelman, 1996, p. 1-6:2; Milgram, Spector, & Treger, 1999, p. 154)

This is not a complete list of possible time management problems but identifies some of the common ones. Most people have more than one problem area. A critical problem area for many staff is trying to do everything or solve all problems. This can be addressed by prioritizing.

Goal setting and priorities

Identifying a list of time management problems does not mean the problems are solved. An important next step is to consider the tasks that are typically required. Rather than thinking all of this must be done on a shift, during the day, or for the week, the better approach is to identify goals and then set priorities. What factors are important to determine priorities, whether in a direct care position or a management position? Prioritizing means identifying what is important at a given time, but still recognizing that a priority list can change. Consider the following:

1. Activities that are the most necessary or critical to complete
2. Activities that are routine activities
3. Activities that are those that one would like to accomplish but could be postponed (Katz, 2001, p. 101)

The first concern is whether or not the task is urgent or has a deadline. Deadlines need to be considered carefully. Whose deadline is it, and is it reasonable? Most people feel what they do or want is important when they set a deadline. When priorities are set the individual must consider all that must be done. Clearly, the role or position of the person setting the deadline and that of the person who must meet the deadline are important. If a nurse's manager says something is due at 3 P.M., the nurse will more than likely try to get it done. However, if the nurse has a clear understanding of his/her schedule and prioritization of tasks for the day, the nurse may see that it cannot be done by the deadline. The nurse then needs to talk with the manager and explain the situation. This is part of saying "no" using a reasoned approach. Another issue related to prioritizing is the pressure that the staff member feels in getting the task done, which is often related to the importance placed on the task, who is asking that the task be done, how long the staff member has put off doing the task, and whether the staff member feels competent to do the task. Policies and procedures also affect whether or not a task is considered low or high priority. Steps that must be followed in sequence are going to have a higher priority. Tasks that are highly related to high priority goals will move to the top of the priority list. If a task is part of a high priority larger project it may be of higher priority than one that is not. Personal preference should not be ignored as it plays an important role. People like to do enjoyable things, and so these tasks creep up to the category of higher priority, even when they should not be a priority. Other questions should be considered when the list of tasks or activities is prioritized, and these are identified in Box 13-8. Using these questions to guide an analysis to prioritize tasks and activities is helpful.

If there is a large complex project to do, what is the best way to approach it? First, staff need to have a reasonable picture of what is involved in the project. This may take some research—talking with people, reviewing written directions about the project, and so on. It is important to have an idea about the amount of time the project might take, which may not necessarily correspond with the deadlines set by others. Time is not only something most people feel they are short of, but it is also something that is not so easy to estimate—how much time will it take? However, at some point staff must set up a reasonable time schedule for a project. When this is done, staff must factor in other responsibilities and the time that these responsibilities consume.

BOX 13-8   Prioritizing tasks and activities.

- Does this task have to be done now or today?
- What will happen if it is not done?
- Can someone else do it?
- Is this task worth the time required to do it?
- Could the task be divided into smaller parts?
- Could this task be done differently so that it will require less time?
- If this is a weekly, monthly, quarterly, or annual task, what is the best way to schedule its completion to meet deadlines?
- Is it necessary to consult with anyone before work can begin?
- If meetings are required, how will this requirement affect the schedule and priorities?
- If work requires a team how will this affect the work?

Source: Author.

As is true for every schedule, a perfect trajectory through the schedule will be impossible; inevitably, interruptions, crises, staff changes, or even change in the direction of the project or some of its components will occur. Schedules need to be reevaluated to make them more reasonable. It is important to recognize that tasks may take longer than expected and then to make effective adjustments as needed.

Daily planning and scheduling

To improve time management, it is important to plan; however, health care is not the most stable climate in which to work. As has been discussed in previous chapters, change is ever present, which means flexibility is required for survival. Planning the day is the place to begin. Some will do this the day before at the end of the day, some will plan out the week, and others will focus on planning at the beginning of the day. A nurse who is providing direct care will have to do this planning at the beginning of the day or shift; however, some thought can be given to required activities that occur routinely prior to the beginning of the day. Examples are typical required patient care needs, regular meetings, required reports, and other routine activities. Some of the issues that need to be reviewed as the plan is developed are: (a) daily appointments (with whom, purpose, time, and other related content information); (b) meetings, including committees, staff, and shift report (type of meeting, purpose, time, place, material, or information needed); (c) phone calls (to whom, purpose, and time frame); (d) rounds (time, with whom, purpose); (e) report or documentation preparation; (f) reading literature and reports; and (g) special activities. What element has been left off this not-all-inclusive list? Breaks and meal times, which can be overlooked. For staff who are involved in direct care, critical factors will be driven by patient needs (for example, procedures, admissions, discharges, and transfers), medications, when patients go to surgery, care that must be provided and routine schedules (for example, meal times, radiological schedule, laboratory tests, and so on), supervision of other staff such as UAPs, communication with other health care disciplines, documentation, phone calls, contact with family, assessment needs, planning care, and other related patient care activities. From this consideration will come the "To Do" list. The list needs to be focused because it is easy to keep adding to it when it is unrealistic that all the items will be accomplished within the time frame. "To Do" lists also need deadlines—when will the tasks be accomplished. If there are no deadlines or deadlines are not met, the result will be frustration and a feeling of inadequacy. Fatigue can be very detrimental to getting work done, and can be reduced through planning. The plan should always leave some time for the unexpected. "Both problems and opportunities come up when you least expect them" (Milgram, Spector, & Treger, 1999, p. 156). "If you over schedule your time and consistently run over, you will feel even more harried and hassled. Allot sufficient time between scheduled activities" (Marrelli, 1993, p. 127). Overscheduling also makes it difficult to cope with the unexpected.

Techniques to better manage time

Bowers, Lauring, and Jacobson (2001) conducted a study to determine how nurses manage time and work in long-term care. Interviews and observation were used to better understand how work conditions affect nurses' practice. The conclusion of the study indicated that "time was an extremely salient work condition for the nurses interviewed. Under conditions of too little time and many interruptions, nurses compensated by developing strategies to keep up or catch up" (Bowers, Lauring, & Jacobson, 2001, p. 484). Even though this study included a very small sample of 18 nurses in two long-term care facilities, the results may be more true than not. Three types of strategies were used by the nurses as they compensated. The first, minimizing time spent doing required tasks, meant that nurses wanted to work more efficiently. To reduce time the nurses established and maintained routines, but these routines had patient care implications. Consistent resident assignments were sought to reduce the time needed to get to know new residents and their needs. Some nurses organized their work around residents or tasks. When the resident approach was used, nurses did as much as they could for a resident in one episode of care. This allowed more time to talk with residents and decreased time "running around." If organized by task, the resident's care was focused on individual tasks (for example, doing all blood pressures for all patients). This may lead to fragmentation of care, which can be a problem. Prioritizing and reprioritizing work was also used to minimize time spent on tasks. Many factors affected prioritization such as who requested that the task be done, resident characteristics, family characteristics, and visibility of the resident's needs. The second major type of strategy used by nurses in the study was creating new time when time was short. Nurses did have their own benchmarks about time to determine when they were running short of time. The nurses might then work faster, combine tasks, change the sequence of tasks, communicate inaccessibility, convert wasted time, and negotiate "actual time" or the time available to complete the work. The third major strategy was changing work responsibilities, which was used when time could not be created. The nurse might assign the work to another shift and delegate tasks to others, often less trained staff. The strategies used by nurses in this sample are used by many nurses in a variety of health care settings.

The following are some examples of techniques that can be used to improve time management.

- **Calendar.** A calendar is essential for effective time management (Katz, 2001). The type that is used is a personal decision. A day-at-a-glance or week-at-a-glance are two typical planner types, although most who work in health care settings do need a daily calendar. This should have space for more than appointments. Goals and objectives, critical information, tasks to do, telephone calls to make, contact information, expenses, and much more can be added to these "calendars." Electronic planners have become more popular and are easy for clinical staff to carry with them. Notes can be added, information can be easily changed, and clinical resources can be added. This type of planner is, however, more expensive and takes a little time to learn how to use.
- **Handle once rule.** It is very easy to slip into the habit of going back to review written materials again when what needs to be done is make a decision the first time they are read. The same applies to mail. Get it, read it, and take action to avoid letting it pile up on the desk. This will help with the piles of work to do that can interfere with effective work habits and also losing information. Searching for information takes time.
- **Batch work.** Set aside blocks of time to work on particular tasks that make sense together. This process, called **batching work,** focuses the work and concentration.
- **Minimize routine work.** Routine work can be minimized or improved by being organized. Keep a list of "most called numbers" and an up-to-date electronic mail (e-mail) address list. When making telephone calls, jot down critical points to be made or questions to keep the calls as short as possible. Leave complete voice messages, many of which may not need call back as they are informational, and provide good times to return the call. Using e-mail to conduct work may be faster than getting involved in a telephone call or an in-person conversation. Set up specific times to do routine tasks. Periodically review routine tasks to determine if they are still required. It is easy to get stuck and continue to do tasks that are really no longer necessary.
- **Say "no."** Saying "no" graciously is a skill that is required of everyone who wants to improve his or her own time management. It is not easy to do. When does one say "no?" Consideration

needs to be given to who is asking, the task or activity, benefits or consequences of doing or not doing the task, available time, interest in the task, and other related factors. When staff have problems with saying "no," the typical results are overload, overtime, and overstress. "There is a difference between the problem of attempting to accomplish too much and the inability to say 'no.' Those who attempt too much suffer from overconfidence. The inability to say 'no' means not knowing how or not having the emotional fortitude to refuse" (Brumm, 2002b, p. 27MW).

- **Anticipate.** Anticipation helps decrease the mode of seeing everything as a crisis that must be solved immediately. Anticipating problems before they occur may help to decrease them and to solve them more effectively. "If you spend all your time putting out fires, you will not be able to gain control over your job" (Milgram, Spector, & Treger, 1999, p. 155).

- **Streamline paperwork.** Paperwork is ever present in clinical and management positions. Saving time related to paperwork is critical. The first step is to have an organized paperwork system for filing or use of some type of documentation system. Know what needs urgent action, needs to be read, needs to be answered, is needed for information only, are low priority items for action, and so on. A very good rule to follow is to see a piece of paper only once, take action on those things that can be responded to, and then move it along. Make notes on paperwork that will help clarify or expand on its content. It is also important to evaluate the existence of paperwork. Does this information help others to do their job? Does it help to do personal work? How much written information is required? Use of e-mail and the Internet has made a difference in the amount of paperwork in organizations. Many organizations are sending more and more information through these means and cutting down on hardcopy memos. However, the next step after information is sent electronically is what the receiver does with the information. Many make hard copy files so the paperwork trail is still ever present. It is important to keep information that might be needed frequently in files, so that it can be accessed easily. Similar categories, such as "correspondence," "projects," and "current data," should be used for hard copy files and computer files. This, too, will make it easier to get to the information.

- **Use the Pareto Principle.** "To help prioritize, take advantage of the **'Pareto Principle'** or the 80/20 rule. Choose the 20% of your activities that will generate 80% of your results. Then pare down or delegate the remaining 80% of your activities" (Milgram, Spector, & Treger, 1999, p. 156). This is a key time management guideline.

- **Improve reading skills.** Professionals have a responsibility to keep up with current literature, which takes time. If one can, taking a speed-reading course or some type of training to help with reading may be helpful. There are, however, other strategies that can be used. When new issues of journals are available, scan the table of contents to select what is most important. Scan headlines to determine what is important. Read only pertinent material. The Internet has opened up many opportunities to help nurses get the literature they need. Nurses subscribe to services, often at no cost, that send via e-mail summaries of current literature or relevant health news. If something is very important, then the nurse can go to the original article and read it. Joining a journal club or forming one can stimulate one to read. A journal club is a group of professionals who agree to read and present material for discussion on a scheduled basis. This can even be done on the computer with e-mail and a listserv or a chat room. This saves time in that members can do it anytime and do not have to be at a specific place.

- **Determine the best time.** Scheduling activities to do, if this timing is the individual's choice, should be based on the complexity of the task. Some people function better earlier in the morning, others mid-day, and then there are the night owls. Difficult tasks should be done when a person is operating optimally. If this is not considered, the work may be postponed as the person just does not have the energy or the work result may be ineffective. Direct care, however, provides limited flexibility in this area for staff.

- **Control social time.** It is important to have some downtime and to enjoy time with co-workers. However, as this can consume too much time at work, it is important to monitor social time. In clinical situations staff may need to push for break times, which are critical for decreasing staff stress.

- **Improve communication.** Ineffective communication can cause time-consuming problems (Brumm, 2002a, p. 14MW). Redoing tasks and projects due to poor communication is not pleasant and increases stress. Improving listening skills and asking questions leads to more effective communication. Clear directions are important for the receiver and sender. It is also important to know what information is necessary to complete a task or project. Wasting time on gathering new information, analyzing information that is not helpful, or having to redo work due to inadequate communication uses up time. Avoiding assumptions about information is also important.

- **Follow-up systems.** Setting up methods to make sure that tasks have been done needs to be part of a time management plan. Some factors to consider include knowing when something needs to be done or checked to confirm completion, or when to monitor quality. Incorporating these checks is critical, or tasks may be lost.

- **Seek help.** Ask for help when needed. Sometimes a colleague, team leader, or manager may be helpful in planning and time management. Find someone who can assist with identifying time management problems and strategies to resolve. New graduates often have problems with time management and yet may be shy about admitting that this is a problem, fearful about what their nurse manager, team leader, co-workers, or preceptor may think. The problem only gets worse this way, stress increases, and work is affected. Not only should the new graduate ask for assistance, but nurses working with new graduates should offer assistance about time management.

- **Self-discipline.** All of the planning to improve time management will be wasted if the staff member does not have self-discipline. Plans, deadlines, and use of time management strategies need to be followed. The only person who is responsible for this is the individual involved.

THINK CRITICALLY

Try this exercise to apply what you have learned about this topic.

Making rounds

Making rounds is an important tool for planning work and thus has an effect on time management. Data are collected that will affect "To Do" lists and prioritization of work based on objectives. When staff members walk through their work area they are able to assess the status of patients, the environment, other staff and their performance, family and visitors, safety issues, and a host of other factors. Rounds need to be made in a thoughtful manner with some ideas about what will be observed or assessed. Every nurse should make rounds in the patient care area, particularly focusing on the nurse's patient assignment. In the community, nurses make rounds as they drive or walk through the community. They notice community needs, improvements, possible health problems, and the environment. A home health nurse does this when a home visit is made. After rounds, the nurse uses this information to develop or alter a work plan. Team leaders use rounds to see how the team is working, make adjustments in work distribution, determine quality of care, talk with staff and with patients, provide feedback, and plan for further work needs. Box 13-9 identifies some key guidelines for making rounds for a staff nurse.

Time management implementation and barriers

Time management implementation is an ongoing process that requires adjustments as situations change. Some adjustments will be affected by barriers. What are some of these strategies that might be used to prevent or eliminate the barriers?

Information overload

There is no doubt that information piles up—papers, e-mails, voice messages, meetings, and professional literature. If information is not managed, information overload can interfere with time management. What information is really needed? What information is not necessary? It seems that as information grows, there is a sense that it is more important. Some staff fear discarding

BOX 13-9   Rounds.

Patient rounds should be done by every nurse, whether he or she is a team leader or providing care to a group of patients. The team leader makes rounds on all the patients covered by the team while an individual nurse would make rounds on the patients included in the nurse's assignment for that shift. What should be included in the rounds?

- Observe each patient and assess for needs
- Assess IVs
- Assess dressings and wounds
- Observe patient's emotional status
- Converse with the patient, include the patient in planning, ask the patient about how the patient feels, perform patient education, and so on
- If family is present, converse with them
- Observe for safety risk (bed rails, patient's ability to get out of bed, and any other safety issues related to equipment and the environment)
- Observe UAP performance and outcomes of delegated tasks
- Talk with UAPs and discuss their work, patients, and support that they may require

Source: Author.

information, as it may be needed later. Determining what's needed requires an understanding of goals and objectives, deadlines, responsibilities, and roles.

Interruptions

Interruptions drain time and energy. If staff automatically participate in the interruption without thinking about whether or not it is a reasonable interruption, then staff will find less and less time available to do the work that needs to be done. Staff also need to stop and think before interrupting others when experiencing interruptions.

- Can this be postponed?
- Can someone else do it?
- Can it be done later?
- Does it tell me something about the person who is interrupting me?
- Is it something I would rather do now?
- What are the risks if I do not get involved?
- Do I want to take it on because I do not trust someone else to do it (Finkelman, 1996, p. 1-6:3)?

Working alone in a quiet place or closing the door may be necessary in order to get something accomplished. This limits distractions and interruptions; however, interruptions are not only from external sources. The individual may think of something else to do, make a phone call, or do some other action that gets the person off track. This is related to procrastination. Interruptions may require that the person say "no" in order to prevent disruption in work. Interruptions are also a serious problem in interfering with precious break or meal times. This time should be protected as it increases efficiency and job satisfaction.

Respecting time

An important element of respecting time is respecting its importance to oneself. This means it is important to take breaks and meal times. Learning relaxation techniques that can be used in the workplace can help reduce stress when time seems to be the evil monster. Developing an exercise routine helps decrease stress. Most tend to put all those "must" and "should" do's on the "To Do" list without thought to those activities that help to support and provide energy to get the work done. Respecting time means that there is an understanding that time can drain energy, but it can be managed even though the amount of time—24 hours in a day—will never change.

Wasting time and procrastination, perfectionism, and prioritization

Most people are pretty good at wasting time so it is important to identify what the typical methods are that an individual uses to waste time. This can be highly individualized. Some examples of methods are: (a) taking a lot of time to find material, information, or supplies to do a task; (b) making phone calls that could wait; (c) expanding the "To Do" list; (d) cleaning up desk or work area; (e) beginning and stopping a work activity; (f) socializing; (g) becoming overly involved in one task when another is more important; (h) volunteering; (i) interfering with others' work; (j) daydreaming; and (k) redoing a task or activity to improve it. On the surface, many of these examples look productive and may be in some situations if they are not wasting time; however, that is why it is important to analyze their effectiveness. If they are used to waste time, they are not effective.

The three "Ps" can lead to major problems in time management and waste time (Marrelli, 1993). Procrastination and perfectionism related to prioritizing are important factors in improving time management. Procrastination occurs when a staff member habitually puts off tasks. Something always seems more important. It is a delay that only increases stress, not decreases it. Procrastination is particularly useful, although not helpful, for tasks that staff do not want to do as they may be boring, too challenging, or unpleasant. One method for coping with procrastination is to break up larger tasks or projects into smaller components. The task may then seem smaller and more manageable or less boring and routine. Lakein (1974) referred to this as the "Swiss cheese" method. It might also include working on a project or task in segments, at different intervals in the day (Smith, 2000). Another strategy that can be used to unlearn the procrastination habit is to recognize how good it feels to accomplish the task and see that it might not have been as bad as imagined. It is important to consider the "benefits (to you and others) of completing the task versus the effects of procrastination" (Katz, 2001, p. 104). Gleeson (2000) recommends the following for overcoming procrastination.

- Do it once. "Do it later" piles or files are deadly. Rarely are views changed when one goes back to a memo or document.
- Clear your mind. If one's mind is filled with a lot of little facts and thoughts this will interfere with work, result in task overload, and lead to procrastination.
- Solve problems while they are small. When the little red flag goes up that says something may be wrong, taking care of it then is much easier than it will be later.
- Reduce interruptions. When staff respond to interruptions, then work is delayed.
- Clean up backlogs. Backlogs of work increase work in the long run. Identifying them and then getting through them is important, but it is also important to identify the causes of the backlogs to prevent recurrence.
- Start operating toward the future instead of the past. A backlog focuses staff on the past, not on the future.
- Stop worrying about it. It is not great to waste time by doing things again or putting them off until later; however, what is even more detrimental is the worrying and stress that arises from procrastination (pp. 13–20).

It is important to recognize that not everything should be done "now." This is where prioritization comes into play. What is important based on goals and objectives?

"Perfectionism is known generally to mean that work is never perceived to be 'good enough'" (Marrelli, 1993, p. 120). Procrastination is a common method used by perfectionists. The task is put off because the staff member feels the final result will not be what it should be. "Any work product is better than none, and you may never have the luxury of time or other resources to accomplish a given project in the manner you believe it should be accomplished. Trying to be perfect wastes time and is an unrealistic goal" (Marrelli, 1993, p. 120).

Prioritizing, as has been discussed, is critical to time management. Information about what is required, why, when, and the amount of effort it will take must be analyzed and then decisions made based on priority. Why is this related to procrastination and perfectionism (Marrelli, 1993)? When tasks are delayed this then affects prioritization. The "To Do" list gets changed, but not because something is accomplished or because there is a rational reason for a change. Deadlines make a difference in the prioritization list, but when items are delayed due to procrastination or perfectionism, the high priority list grows and then becomes overwhelming. Perfectionism may lead the staff member to believe that it is too late to perform the task as it "should" be done. How should this be dealt with? One step that can be taken is to begin, even if the result is not the final product. Moving forward seems to make a big difference.

Working in blocks of time

Working in blocks of times is more efficient than sporadic bursts of work for short periods of time. An example is returning telephone calls. If there are many telephone calls to return and if none are urgent, then taking a block of time to return calls may be more effective. Responding to e-mail is another task that can be done in blocks of time. Some people have an e-mail notification system. This can be an interruption if one feels compelled to check the message and respond. Planning several times a day to check e-mail is more efficient.

Work expansion

It is easy to expand work. For example, if one allows 1 hour to complete a task, which actually only needs half an hour, it will take about 1 hour. Setting realistic time frames will help to prevent this.

Using delegation effectively

Chapter 8 discusses delegation extensively; however, it is important to note that delegation does play a major role in time management. Effective use of delegation can save time. The "Forest or the Trees" phenomenon can be a real problem for staff, as getting overly involved in details can lead to exhaustion. Details need to be managed and assigned to appropriate tasks and projects. Sometimes details need to be handled by others although many have trouble giving up details. Oversupervision related to delegation occurs when the delegator, team leader, or manager will not leave staff alone to do the work. This takes time for the manager and often affects the staff member trying to do the job. It appears as if the manager or the team leader does not trust that the staff member can do the job. Some refer to this as micromanaging.

Meetings

Just the use of the word *meetings* can send some staff into a state of frustration. This is because many meetings are unproductive, other than being great time wasters. Meetings are not going away, even those that clearly need to be evaluated and should go away. However, those that should be continued can often be improved. The critical question to ask is, "Is the meeting necessary?" Meetings may be informal or formal; this discussion will focus on formal meetings. The following questions can guide decisions about the meetings.

- Is the purpose of the meeting clear to everyone? Typical purposes of meetings are: sharing information or advice, issuing directions, addressing grievances or arbitrating, making or implementing decisions, generating creative ideas, arriving at consensus, and presenting a proposal for discussion and, usually, for ultimate resolution. Individual views of the purpose of the meeting are critical to the effectiveness of a meeting. If there is conflict in purposes, then the meeting will get bogged down.
- Does everyone need to attend the entire meeting? The purpose of the meeting affects who should attend.
- Is there a better way of addressing the issues than having a meeting? Other methods are e-mail, discussion boards on an Internet site, one-to-one meeting, written reports, and so on.
- Are there other people who do not usually attend the meetings who might make a useful contribution this time? Sometimes key persons do not attend, and this interferes with the work that needs to be done (Hindle, 1998, p. 8).

Committees are found in every organization. The two major types are standing committees that meet on a regular basis and have a specific responsibility given to them by some authority within the organization, and ad hoc committees that are established to focus on some specific issue and are disbanded when work is completed. Committees usually have specific operating rules, such as *Robert's Rules of Order,* and report back to some other group in the organization. For example, a nursing staff ad hoc committee (which may be called a task force) may be formed in the nursing or patient care department to assess the need for a new documentation system. This committee might report back to the nurse manager group. Committees may also be interdisciplinary, such as the pharmacy committee or medical information system committees, which would include physicians, nurses, pharmacists, technical staff, administration, and so on.

Preparing for a meeting

When preparing for a meeting, key issues to resolve upfront are to define the purpose, decide how long the meeting should last, and decide who should attend. Today, there are many options of methods that groups can use to meet. The most common method is still to physically get together in one location. Virtual communication, however, is growing (Hindle, 1998). One of these methods, videoconferencing, is particularly helpful when members want to see each other but are in different locations, do not want to travel to meet, and want to decrease costs. Videoconferencing requires equipment and uses real time audio and video links. Telephone conferencing is also used, but does not include video. People who work in different locations in the city, different states, or even different countries can meet by using these methods. Time is important since these are real time methods, so time zones need to be considered. What might be 4:00 P.M. for one person may be 7:00 P.M. for another. E-mail correspondence also plays a role in meetings. This method can be used to notify members of meetings and changes; send minutes and other documents; allow for discussion prior to meetings, which can decrease the time spent in meetings as well as preparation time; and in some cases can be done in a chat room format.

The agenda is a very important document that is typically prepared by the chair, although members should have input into the agenda. Some agendas not only list the items to be covered but also the time period for each item to control the amount of time spent on each. The usual format is approval of minutes, old business, new business, and announcements. Agendas that come out too late for members to review and consider them are not helpful when it comes time for the meeting. The meeting may then flounder as members try to figure out what is going on and what their responses might be. As the meeting is planned, all equipment, supplies, and written material should be present to reduce time spent during the meeting looking for items or copying material. If audiovisuals are to be used, they should be checked prior to beginning the meeting.

Attending a meeting

Members should also prepare for meetings. Reading the agenda, minutes of the past meeting, and other material relevant to the agenda will help move a meeting on and improve participation. Some issues may require talking to people prior to the meeting or even planning negotiation about an issue that may be conflictual.

Confidentiality may be an issue in meetings. Information may be shared in meetings that should not then be shared outside the meeting. This topic may need to be discussed in the initial meeting. It should be clear to all when information is confidential. Members should be asked to control as much as possible interruptions of pagers and cell phones, although this is very difficult to do in a health care setting. Silent options on the telephone or pager should be used during meetings.

It may be difficult for some staff to speak up in a meeting, due to their lack of confidence, lack of knowledge of the issue, or the presence of "very important people." If there is an issue that a staff member knows he or she wants to comment on, practicing what to say before the meeting may build confidence. What points should be made? Who might disagree and why? Who might agree and why? What is the best way to frame the comments? Seeking advice from those who might know about the issue may also be helpful. Listening is important for all committee members, but it is also a way to learn how to communicate in the group. Observing nonverbal communication may help because this type of communication may say more than the verbal communication. For example, someone who sits with arms folded may indicate a lack of support, a barrier, or even anger. Another person may sit in a relaxed fashion, moving arms freely to indicate interest in the topic. Nonverbal communication can be incongruent with verbal communication.

Self-evaluation of participation in meetings is important for members, particularly staff who have less experience with groups and meetings. The following are some statements that can be made in a self-assessment.

- I allow speakers to finish making their point before I speak.
- I am confident when making a point or stating my views.
- I am able to concede when I am wrong.
- I can control the tone of my voice when I feel nervous or angry.
- My body language suggests self-confidence.
- I listen carefully to what other people are saying in a meeting.
- I am thoroughly prepared for every meeting that I attend.
- I carefully review the minutes of the previous meeting.
- I research in advance the views of the other participants at a meeting.
- I know what my objectives are before I attend a meeting.
- I share a common purpose with the other participants at the meeting.
- I arrive on time for the meeting (Hindle, 1998, pp. 44–45).

These guidelines for self-appraisal also apply to shift reports. Table 13-1 identifies some critical elements related to shift reports.

Chairing a meeting

Chairpersons can be selected by a number of different methods. They may be selected by the group or an outside group, selected by someone outside the group, or selected because of the person's position or title. The challenge for the meeting's chair is leading the meeting and keeping the discussion on track. Planning ahead will help the meeting move forward. Meetings need to begin and end on time, with roles such as minute taking clearly identified prior to the meeting. Some groups require a quorum or minimum number of members for business to be conducted. If a quorum is not present, then the meeting may be cancelled or there may be no voting, which is noted in the minutes. Issues are discussed, following the agenda that is developed and shared with members prior to the meeting, and decisions are reached. The key duties of the chair are to listen to the viewpoints of others, ensure that all participants make contributions, block negative tactics, and summarize views and decisions in an objective manner (Hindle, 1998). The chair must also be very aware of nonverbal communication in order to assess the mood of the group and the roles and feelings of individual members.

The following are some examples of common nonverbals that may indicate important group member reactions.

- Posture alert: Interest
- Clenched fists: Anger
- Staring at papers or into space: No interest
- Pointing at another person: Anger, argumentative
- Eye contact: Interest
- Group laughter appropriate: Group comfortable
- Members occupied with non-meeting work during the meeting: Disinterest, questionable effective meeting

Minutes from the previous meeting need to be approved after changes are noted. Minutes for the present meeting also need to be taken. The secretary for the group or assigned secretary for the particular meeting should pass around a sign-in sheet and note those who are absent as well as those present, which will be included in the minutes. Minutes need to indicate the group name, date and time, and location of meeting. Minutes should indicate that they were approved

TABLE 13-1   Shift report.

The critical elements of the shift report are the patients, the treatment they have received, and their plan of care.

This list does not include everything that might be included in a shift report, and speciality units may have specific information that would be reported for their patients (for example, intensive care units, behavioral care units, substance treatment units, labor and delivery, and so on). New nurses should ask for assistance when giving their first reports and also listen as others give reports to get some idea of what is generally expected. Asking for feedback about a report can help to improve the process and information.

Guidelines for Giving the Report	Content of the Shift Report	How Should Staff Listen to the Report?
• The report should be concise and pertinent. • Time is always a concern so the report needs to stay on task and avoid "storytelling," which occurs when more details are told than necessary, leading one to eventually wander off the topic of the report. • The best reports are planned before they are given, which decreases rambling and inclusion of information that is not required to provide quality care. • The staff member giving the report should collect information from all relevant staff so that the report is as complete as possible. • The goal is to share important information, and if this is done, staff will listen. • Make sure that before the report begins all necessary information is available. • Shift reports must be set up so that there is still coverage of the patients while the report is given. • Privacy and confidentially must be part of the report—choose a location that provides a quiet environment. Some reports are recorded so equipment must be operable and available when needed. Just because a report is recorded does not mean the report does not take time. Staff still need time to record it, and then incoming staff need to listen to it.	• Review each patient • Significant symptoms and problems • On stat, unusual, or PRN medications; why and outcomes • Identify any change in diagnosis • Significant laboratory reports • Procedures completed and outcomes • Significant communication with physicians and other health care providers • Significant intake and output alterations • Significant discharge plan issues • Significant contact with family or significant others • Significant patient education issues • Procedures, laboratory exams, or the treatment expected in the incoming shift • Expected admissions and significant information about them (e.g., diagnosis, type of admission (transfer from another unit, ER, direct admission)) • Expected discharges during the incoming shift. Shift report also includes any critical work-related communications (e.g., staffing, incidents, policy and procedure issues, communication problems, management issues, and so on)	• Staff need to be present when the report begins. • Staff need to listen to the report. • Staff should ask relevant questions. • Staff should take notes so that information does not need to be repeated. The shift report does provide a time for the staff to work together as a team. Some time may be spent on socializing, which is important for team bonding; however, this type of interaction must be limited as it can interfere with the report process. Staff then become restless, knowing that work still needs to be done, and then listening decreases.

Following Report: Planning
• Depending on the nursing model used, the team leader or an individual staff member need to plan the work that needs to be done during the shift.
• The report provides the framework of critical elements.
• The patients' plans of care are reviewed as well as physician orders.
• Assignments are made for all staff.
• During the shift the team leader needs to follow-up to ensure that work is completed appropriately and make rounds. Individual staff will do the same.
• Planning work requires that the team leader or staff member consider what must be done and when, assessment of the patient, general routine of the unit (physician rounds, when meals are served, general lab work schedules, radiological tests scheduled, and so on), patient transportation needs to procedures, exams, and so on, delegation, discharge and admission of patients, medication schedules, level of staffing if this changes during the shift (for example, if some staff overlap a shift), staff breaks, and meal times.

Source: Author.

with or without changes, or with specific changes noted. Motions need to be described, regarding who made the motion, seconded the motion, and whether it passed or not. Motions can be amended—the minutes should note the amendment to the motion stated, discussed, and approved or not. The motion is discussed and moved on before amendments. Some more formal organizations require that there is advance notice of amendments to motions, but this is not the case for most meetings. Passing resolutions, which is the written statement of a future action, or voting on a motion is important if the group is using this formal method of decision making. Some groups indicate the actual number of votes cast in the minutes rather than just passed or failed. Minutes should follow the agenda, and sentences should be short and to the point. Typically, minutes are set up in four columns: agenda topic, summary of discussion, motion/action, and responsibility and deadline. Keeping the same format for all minutes helps organize the information and takes less time for review. At the end of the minutes the secretary notes: "Adjourned at" and "Respectfully submitted" with the secretary's name and signature. If copies are sent out to non-group members, then this should be noted at the end of the minutes, unless the organization has a standing system for distribution and it is decided that this is not required. The secretary can ask the chair to review the minutes prior to the final draft to decrease errors, although the minutes still need approval from the entire group.

The chairperson can use the following self-assessment to determine meeting effectiveness.

- Has everybody had a chance to express his or her views?
- Have the procedural rules of the organization been followed?
- Did you have a firm control of the meeting with the agenda on track?
- Did you encourage people to speak by asking them questions (Hindle, 1998, p. 34)?

Meetings are closed with the chair summarizing key points and thanking everyone for their participation and ideas.

BENCHMARKS

Now let's take a moment to test your knowledge of the concepts you have studied in this section.

Chapter Wrap-Up

Now that you've reached the end of the chapter, you may wish to explore the concepts you've been reading about in greater detail, or test yourself to see how well you've comprehended the material.

SUMMARY AND APPLICATIONS

- Summary
- Practice Quiz
- Key Terms
- Tying It All Together

- Experiential Exercises
- Case
- Links

REFERENCES

American Nurses Association. (2000a). *Scope and standards of practice for nursing professional development*. Washington, DC: American Nurses Publishing.

American Nurses Association. (2000b). *Code for Nurses with Interpretive statements*. Washington, DC: American Nurses Publishing.

American Nurses Association. (2002). *Nursing Agenda for the Future A call to Nation*. Washington, DC: Author.

Bell, S. (2001). Professional nurse's portfolio. *Nursing Administration Quarterly, 25*(2), 69–73.

Bower, F. (2000). Mentoring others. In F. Bower (Ed.), *Nurses taking the lead* (pp. 255–276). Philadelphia: W. B. Saunders Company.

Bowers, B., Lauring, C., & Jacobson, N. (2001). How nurses manage time and work in long-term care. *Journal of Advanced Nursing, 33*(4), 484–491.

Brumm, J. (2002a, March). Put time on your side, Part 1. *Nursing Spectrum Metro Edition*, 14MW–15MW.

Brumm, J. (2002b, April). Put time on your side, Part 2. *Nursing Spectrum Metro Edition*, 26MW–27MW.

Burke, A. (2000). Organization-wide competency and education. *Nursing Management, 31*(2), 21–25.

Cardillo, D. (2001). Job hunting challenges take some troubleshooting. *Nursing Spectrum Metro Edition, 2*(8), 25.

Carey, A. (2001). Certified registered nurses. *American Journal of Nursing, 101*(1), 44–52.

Carey, S., & Campbell, S. (1994). Preceptor, mentor, and sponsor roles. *Journal of Nursing Administration, 24*(12), 39–48.

Cesta, T., Tahan, H., & Fink, L. (1998). *The case manager's survival guide*. St. Louis, MO: Mosby-Year Book, Inc.

Day, G. (2001). Evaluating distance learning programs. *Journal of Legal Nurse Consultants, 12*(1), 23–24.

Domrose, C. (2002). A guiding hand. *Nurse Week Great Lakes, 2*(3), 9–10.

Donley, R., et al. (2002). What does the Nurse Reinvestment Act mean to you? *Online Journal of Issues in Nursing, 8*(1). Retrieved on May 7, 2003, from http://www.nursingworld.org/ojin.

Duchscher, J. (2001). Out in the real world. *Journal of Nursing Administration, 31*(9), 426–439.

Finkelman, A. (1996). *Psychiatric nursing administration manual*. Gaithersburg, MD: Aspen Publishers, Inc.

Gleeson, K. (2000). *The personal efficiency program* (2nd ed.). New York: John Wiley & Sons, Inc.

Gordon, P. (2000, March). The road to success with a mentor. *Journal of Vascular Nursing*, 30–33.

Henderson, F., & McGettigan, B. (1994). Influencing others and using resources. In F. Henderson & B. McGettigan (Eds.), *Managing your career in nursing* (pp. 260–304). New York: National League for Nursing.

Hindle, T. (1998). *Managing meetings*. New York: DK Publishing, Inc.

Institute of Medicine. (2003). *Health professions education*. Washington, DC: National Academy Press.

Jackson, M. (2001). A preceptor incentive program. *American Journal of Nursing, 101*(6), 24A, 24C, 24E.

Katz, J. (2001). *Keys to nursing success*. Upper Saddle River, NJ: Prentice Hall.

Kinlaw, D. (1999). Coaching for commitment. San Francisco: Jossey-Bass.

Klein, E., & Dickenson-Hazard, N. (2000). The spirit of mentoring. *Reflections on Nursing Leadership: Sigma Theta Tau International* (third quarter), 18–22.

Laborde, S., & Lee, J. (2000). Skills needed for promotion in the nursing profession. *Journal of Nursing Administration, 30*(9), 432–439.

Lachman, V. (2000). Coaching techniques. *Nursing Management, 30*(1), 15–19.

Lissy, W. (1993). Currents in compensation and benefits. *Compensation and Benefits Review, 25*(1), 8–17.

Lakein, A. (1974). *How to get control of your life*. NY: Signet

Manning, G. (1991). INVEST: A plan for developing new managers. *Nursing Management, 22*(12), 26–28.

Marrelli, T. (1993). "Effective time management and productivity." In T. Marrelli (Ed.), *The nurse manager's survival guide* (pp. 119–133). St. Louis, MO: Mosby-Year Book, Inc.

McConnell, C. (1996). Succeeding with succession planning. *Health Care Supervisor, 15*(2), 69–78.

McGettigan, B., & Henderson, F. (1994). Enriching self and revitalizing career. In F. Henderson & B. McGettigan (Eds.), *Managing your career in nursing* (pp. 304–334). New York: National League for Nursing.

Milgram, L., Spector, A., & Treger, M. (1999). *Managing smart*. Houston, TX: Gulf Publishing Company.

National Council of State Boards of Nursing, Inc. Retrieved on May 16, 2003, from http://www.ncsbn.org.

National Nursing Staff Development Organization. (1999). *Strategic plan 2000*. Pensacola, FL: National Nursing Staff Development Organization.

Nurse Reinvestment Act, H.R.3487ENR, 107th Congress (2002). Retrieved on December 8, 2002, from http://www.access.gpo.gov/nara/publaw/107publ.html.

O'Shea, E. (2003). Self-directed learning in nurse education: A review of the literature. *Journal of Advanced Nursing, 43*(1), 62–70.

Shaffer, B., Tallarica, B., & Walsh, J. (2000). Win-win mentoring. *Nursing Management, 30*(1), 32–34.

Smith, S. (2000). Time management and feelings of accomplishment are directly related! What is wrong with this statement? *INSIGHT, 23*(2), 38.

Smolenski, M. (2002). Playing the credentials game. *Nursing Spectrum Midwest Region, 3*(7), 26–27MW.

Spencer, J., & Jordan, K. (1999). Learner centered approaches in medical education. *British Medical Journal, 318,* 1280–1283.

Vance, C. (2003). Mentoring at the edge of chaos. *Nurse Leader, 1*(1), 42–43.

ADDITIONAL READINGS

Andrica, D. (2000). Managing effective committees. *Nursing Economics, 18*(2), 94.

Bagott, I., & Bagott, J. (2001). Talk the talk: Overcome your fear of public speaking. *Nursing Spectrum Midwest Edition, 2*(7), 12–13.

Benner, P. (2001). *From novice to expert. Excellence and power in clinical nursing practice* (Commemorative Edition). Upper Saddle River, NJ: Prentice Hall.

Burke, S., & Whited, M. (1997). *How to find your perfect job in nursing.* Freeman, SD: Pine Hill Press, Inc.

Cardillo, D. (2001a). Go back to school and change your life. *Nursing Spectrum Metro Edition, 2*(10), 12.

Cardillo, D. (2001b). How to get back to school. *Nursing Spectrum Metro Edition, 2*(11), 26.

Cardillo, D. (2001c). Myths about networking. *Nursing Spectrum Metro Edition, 2*(9), 28–29.

Cardillo, D. (2001d). Resume versus CV: Which is right for you? *Nursing Spectrum Metro Edition, 2*(7), 25.

Cardillo, D. (2002a). How to change specialties. *Nursing Spectrum Metro Edition, 3*(5), 12.

Cardillo, D. (2002b). How to write an effective cover letter. *Nursing Spectrum Midwest Edition, 3*(7), 12.

Cardillo, D. (2002c). Six steps to getting the most from your job. *Nursing Spectrum Midwest Region, 3*(1), 28.

Chapman, L. (2000). Distance learning for post-registered nursing: The facts. *Nursing Standards, 14*(18), 33–36.

Cragg, C., Plotnikoff, R., Hugo, K., & Casey, A. (2001). Perspective transformation in RN-to-BSN distance education. *Journal of Nursing Education, 40*(7), 317–322.

Crawford, L. (2001). Regulation of registered nursing. *Reflections on Nursing LEADERSHIP, 27*(4), 28–29, 34.

DeBourgh, G. (2001). Using web technology in a clinical nursing course. *Nursing Education, 26*(5), 227–233.

Detmer, S. (2002). Coaching your unit team for results. *Seminars for Nurse Managers, 10*(3), 189–195.

Gates, D. (2001). Stress and coping. A model for the workplace. *AAOHN Journal, 49*(8), 390–398.

Gelbert, R. (2000). Integrating web-based instruction into a graduate nursing program taught via video-conferencing. Challenges and solutions. *Computers in Nursing, 18*(1), 26–34.

Godinez, G., Schweiger, J., Gruver, J., & Ryan, P. (1999, May/June). Role transition from graduate to staff nurse: A qualitative analysis. *Journal for Nurses in Staff Development,* 97–110.

Greene, M., & Puetzer, M. (2002). The value of mentoring: A strategic approach to retention and recruitment. *Journal of Nursing Quality, 17*(1), 63–70.

Helge, D. (2001). Turning workplace anger and anxiety into peak performance. *AAOHN Journal, 49*(8), 399–408.

Herrin, D. (2001). E-learning. Directions for nurses in executive practice. *Journal of Nursing Administration, 31*(1), 5–6.

Huston, C., Shovein, J., Damazo, B., & Fox, S. (2001). The RN-BSN bridge course: Transitioning the re-entry learner. *Journal of Continuing Education Nursing, 32*(6), 250–253.

Joel, L. (2002). Education for entry into nursing practice: Revisited for the 21st century. *Online Journal of Nursing,* Retrieved May 31 from http://www.nursingworld.org/ojin.

Kjervik, D., & Leonard, D. (2001). Nurse responses to re-tooling practice, education, and management roles. *The Journal of Continuing Education, 32*(6), 254–259.

Kozlowski, D. (2002). Returning to school: An alternative to 'traditional' education. *Orthopedic Nursing, 21*(4), 41–47.

Laschinger, H., Finegan, J., Shamian, J., & Wilk, P. (2001). Impact of structural and psychological empowerment on job strain in nursing work settings. *Journal of Nursing Administration, 31*(5), 260–272.

Marino, K. (2000). *Resumes for the health care professional.* New York: John Wiley & Sons, Inc.

Mills, A., & Blaesing, S. (2000). A lesson from the last shortage. The influence of work values on career satisfaction with nursing. *Journal of Nursing Administration, 30*(6), 309–315.

Mills, N., Haun, L., & Daldrup, D. (2000). Kansas City colleagues for caring: Giving new meaning to networking. *Journal of Nursing Education, 39*(2), 54–56.

Posting resumes on-line. *American Nursing Student, 4*(3), 18–19.

Prontis-Ruotolo, D. (2001). Surviving the night shift. *American Journal of Nursing, 101*(7), 63, 65, 67–68.

Restifo, V., & Yoder, L. (2004). Partnership: Making the most of mentoring. *Nursing Spectrum/Midwestern Edition, 5*(5), 21–23.

Robinson-Walker, C. (2002a). Coaching culture. *Seminars for Nurse Managers, 10*(3), 148–149.

Robinson-Walker, C. (2002b). The role of coaching in creating cultures of engagement. *Seminars for Nurse Managers, 10*(3), 150–156.

Roe, C. (2000). The regulation of nursing practice today. *Home Care Provider, 5*(2), 25–32.

Saver, C. (2001). The forgotten specialty. *Spectrum Metro Edition, 2*(9), 5.

Shaffer, F. (2001). Career portfolio: A professional mandate for the 21st century. *Seminars for Nurse Managers, 9*(4), 233–237.

Smeltzer, C., & Truong, C. (2000). A management tool for achieving success. *Journal of Nursing Administration, 30*(12), 574–576.

Washer, P. (2001). Barriers to the use of Web-based learning in nursing education. *Nursing Education Today, 21*(6), 455–460.

Weston, M. (2001). Leading into the future: Coaching and mentoring Generation X employees. *Seminars for Nurse Managers, 9*(3), 157–160.

Whittaker, S., Carson, W., & Smolenski, M. (2000). Assuring continued competence-policy questions and approaches: How should the profession respond? *Online Journal of Nursing.* Retrieved on June 30 from http://www.nursingworld.org/ojin.

ECONOMIC VALUE

How society values nursing must change to make major strides in recruiting and retaining nurses. Educating the public about nursing's pivotal role in health care will be basic to involving nurses in health care policy formulation and in key business decisions that affect nursing's future.

Desired Future Statement (Vision)

Nurses are recognized as providers of quality, viewed as cost-effective health care, compensated for their value, and supported through public policy.

Five strategies were identified to achieve the vision and one of these was identified as the primary or driving strategy. They are:

Leadership provided to leverage economic influence. (Primary Strategy)

A united profession achieves its key economic goals.

The economic value of nursing is better understood through the use of quantified nursing data.

Innovative compensation strategies are widely implemented.

New and existing economic resources are applied to support nursing education.

Objectives to Support Primary Strategy

Create a comprehensive database/repository for evidence-based research related to quality, value, and cost of nursing services.

Design a model for reimbursement for nursing services.

Devise and/or evaluate varying models of innovative compensation packages designed to recruit and retain registered nurses.

Advocate for passage of state tax relief for registered nurses.

Develop five new educational reimbursement programs for individuals pursuing careers in nursing, working in collaboration with policy makers.

SOURCE: American Nurses Association. (2002). *Nursing's agenda for the future. A call to the nation.* Washington, DC: Author. Reprinted with permission.

Health Care Financial Issues

CHAPTER OUTLINE

MediaLink
www.prenhall.com/finkelman

The Interactive Exercises for this chapter can be found in the OneKey course at www.prenhall.com/finkelman. Click on Chapter 14 to select from the following activities: Test Your Understanding, Benchmarks, Current Issues, Your Opinion Counts, Think Critically, and Summary and Applications.

What's Ahead

Understanding health care financial issues is important for nurses as they practice in the health care environment as well as when they assume leadership roles. Financial issues can be viewed from a macro and micro perspective. The macro perspective concerns broad health care expenditures from a national view and reimbursement for health care services. The micro perspective focuses on the financial issues related to individual health care organizations (for example, budgeting). This chapter focuses more on the macro perspective because this perspective must come first, and it is the one that most directly affects budgets and all nurses, regardless of their position. This is not to say that the micro perspective is not important or will not be discussed. The basics of micro issues will be discussed; however, extensive details about budgeting and health care organization financing is content that is more appropriate to nurses who are entering management positions where these skills are absolutely critical. The critical need for new nurses is to understand who pays for health care, how this payment is made, and how reimbursement affects health care delivery, which is the macro perspective, and then some essential basics related to budgeting in health care organizations, nurses' role in the process, and how budgets impact nursing care.

OBJECTIVES

Before you begin, take a moment to familiarize yourself with the key objectives of this chapter.

- Distinguish between the macrolevel and microlevel view of health care financial issues.
- Discuss critical issues related to national health care expenditures.
- Describe the role of the third-party payer.
- Explain how health care insurance is paid for and by whom.
- Identify the importance of the diagnosis-related groups.
- Discuss the importance of the various government benefit programs.
- Define two examples of managed care models.
- Discuss how managed care has changed since it began.
- Define the service strategies used by managed care to control costs and quality.
- Define the reimbursement strategies used by managed care to control costs and quality.
- Discuss the impact of reimbursement on health care delivery.
- Define key financial management terms.
- Describe the budgetary process and its importance to nursing.
- Define productivity.
- Identify strategies that nurses can use to participate in cost containment in their practice.

TEST YOUR UNDERSTANDING

Before we begin our exploration of this chapter, take a short "warm-up" test to see what you know about this topic.

YOUR OPINION COUNTS

Find out what others think about this topic. Post your response and check out other opinions.

Health Care Financial Issues: The Macrolevel

During nursing's long history, little interest was shown in financial issues. Nurses were typically unprepared to participate in financial decision making, and health care administrators often did not encourage or support nurse managers/leaders to participate in the financial side of health care. The inclusion of content related to health economics, finance, and business management into nursing curricula evolved slowly, which became a serious limitation as it prevented active nursing involvement in health care finance. Gradually, nurse administrators have developed an increased interest in budgeting; however, they have had to contend with hospital administrators who did not feel that nurse administrators needed to be involved in the budget.

In 1978, the National League for Nursing published conference papers from a meeting of nurse executives, who represented acute care, long-term care, community health, and university settings (National League for Nursing, 1978). The conference focused on raising nurse executives' awareness of the need to be involved in budget preparation. One administrator stated, "The 1980s will find us even more concerned with belt tightening and intensifying voluntary efforts to contain health care costs. The future is in our hands" (National League for Nursing, 1978, p. 5). The belt tightening that was predicted for the 1980s does not come close to what is expected today. Nurse administrators began to realize that they needed to play an active role in budget development in order to meet their goals for nursing services and to increase their understanding of health care reimbursement. Why is it important for nurses to understand reimbursement?

- Reimbursement affects patient care delivery: types of treatment, choice of provider, length of treatment.
- Reimbursement has an impact on provider performance and patient outcomes.
- Reimbursement affects financial resources that are available for health care organizations (for example, for staffing, equipment and supplies, renovation and expansion, and so on).

This early recognition of the need for involvement, however, focused only on the nursing management level: nurse executives and nurse managers. Staff nurses were, in most cases, still out of the loop; however, nursing can no longer afford to isolate staff nurses from financial issues. All nurses need a greater understanding of how financial decisions are made, by whom, why, and how these decisions make a difference in the care a patient receives; number of staff available to provide that care; access to services, supplies, and equipment; and so on. This section of the chapter discusses these critical issues.

National health care expenditures

The health care industry is extremely large, and its financing is influenced by many factors, particularly social expectation, economic trends, technological developments, and political factors (Britt, Schraeder, & Shelton, 1998). Financial issues affect all aspects of the provision of care, settings, and services, such as inpatient care, ambulatory care, home care, primary care, long-term care, public health, pharmaceutical, medical supplies, medical transportation, medical technology, medical research, and so on. Compared with other countries, the United States has the most expensive health care system and the highest living standards and economic status. Despite this, the United States has a large number of people without insurance: 45 million people in 2004, with an increase in the number of uncovered children. The breakdown of cultural or ethnic groups was as follows:

- Non-Hispanic white   11.1%
- Hispanic   32.8%
- Black   19.5%
- Asian   18.7% (U.S. Census Bureau, 2004)
- American Indian and Alaska Native   27.5%

The actual and projected national health care expenditures for selected years from 1970 through 2007 are described in Table 14-1.

The largest portion of health care expenditures is found in the hospital industry, despite decreasing lengths-of-stay and increasing use of non-hospital services. Figure 14-1 provides another description of health care expenses: projected expenditures into 2030.

These data indicate that health care expenditures are expected to increase, just about doubling from 2010 to 2020 and again from 2020 to 2030! These estimates are based on historical data and analysis.

An understanding of health care expenditures includes an appreciation of how the nation's health dollar is spent and also who pays for health care or the health care funding sources. Typically, reported data such as national financial data are a few years behind. Figure 14-2 includes both types of data. It is also important to recognize that health care expenditures change annually.

TABLE 14-1 Actual and projected national health expenditures for selected calendar years from 1970 through 2007[*].

SPENDING CATEGORY	1970	1980	1990	1998	2007
	BILLIONS OF DOLLARS (PERCENT)				
Total national expenditures	73.2 (100.0)	247.3 (100.0)	699.5 (100.0)	1,146.8 (100.0)	2,133.3 (100.0)
Expenditures for health					
services and supplies	67.9 (92.8)	235.6 (95.3)	775.0 (96.50)	1,113.2 (97.1)	2,085.3 (97.8)
Personal health care	63.8 (87.2)	217.0 (87.8)	614.7 (87.9)	998.2 (87.0)	1,859.2 (87.2)
Hospital care	28.0 (38.2)	102.7 (41.5)	256.4 (36.7)	383.2 (33.4)	649.4 (30.4)
Physicians' services	13.6 (18.6)	45.2 (18.3)	146.3 (20.9)	221.4 (19.3)	427.3 (20.0)
Dental services	4.7 (6.4)	13.3 (5.4)	31.6 (4.5)	53.7 (4.7)	95.2 (4.5)
Other professional services	1.4 (1.9)	6.4 (2.6)	34.7 (5.0)	66.8 (5.8)	134.5 (6.3)
Home health care[†]	0.2 (0.3)	2.4 (1.0)	13.1 (1.9)	33.2 (.29)	66.1 (3.10)
Drugs and other nondurable					
medical products	8.8 (12.0)	21.6 (8.7)	59.9 (8.6)	106.1 (9.3)	223.6 (10.5)
Prescription drugs	5.5 (7.50)	12.0 (4.9)	37.7 (5.4)	74.3 (7.5)	171.1 (8.0)
Vision products and other					
durable medical products	1.6 (2.2)	3.8 (1.5)	10.5 (1.5)	14.3 (1.2)	23.3 (1.1)
Nursing home care[†]	4.2 (5.7)	17.6 (7.1)	50.9 (7.3)	87.3 (7.6)	148.3 (7.0)
Other personal health care	1.3 (1.8)	4.0 (1.6)	11.2 (1.6)	32.4 (2.8)	91.4 (4.3)
Program administration					
and net cost	2.7 (3.7)	11.9 (4.8)	40.7 (5.8)	74.1 (6.5)	151.3 (7.1)
Government public health					
activities	1.3 (1.8)	6.7 (2.7)	19.6 (2.8)	40.9 (3.6)	74.9 (3.5)
Expenditures for research					
and construction	5.3 (7.2)	11.6 (4.7)	24.5 (3.5)	33.5 (2.9)	48.0 (2.3)
Research[‡]	2.0 (2.7)	5.5 (2.2)	12.2 (1.7)	18.4 (1.6)	27.5 (1.3)
Construction	3.4 (4.6)	6.2 (2.5)	12.3 (1.8)	15.1 (1.3)	20.5 (1.0)

[*] Figures for 2007 are projections. Numbers may not add to totals because of rounding. Data are from the Health Care Financing Administration, Office of the Actuary, National Health Statistics Group.

[†] This category includes free-standing facilities only. Additional services of this type are provided in hospital-based facilities and counted as hospital care.

[‡] Research-and-development expenditures of drug companies and other manufacturers and providers of medical equipment and supplies are excluded from this category and instead are included in the category in which the product falls.

Source: U.S. Department of Health and Human Services, Health Care Financing Administration, Office of Actuary, National Health Statistics Group.

Several changes have been noted when comparing specific service categories and their expenditures, as indicated in Figure 14-2, the Nation's Health Care Dollar in 2001, to similar data from 1997. The percentage of a dollar that paid for hospital care changed from 34% or 34 cents (1997) to 32% or 32 cents per dollar (2001). At the same time, physician and clinical services increased from 19.9% or 19.9 cents (1997) to 22% or 22 cents (2001). What might be a reason for this change? Managed care reimbursement, as discussed in this chapter, affected usage of out-of-hospital care. Decreasing hospitalization has been greatly influenced by the need to decrease costs;

FIGURE 14-1 Projected national health expenditures, 2000–2030.

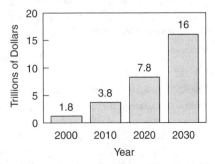

Source: U.S. Department of Health and Human Services; Health Care Financing Administration, 1995.

FIGURE 14-2   The nation's health dollar: 2001.

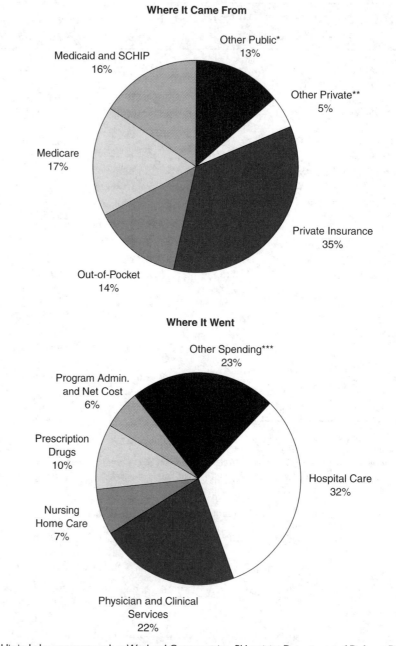

Where It Came From

Other Public*
13%

Medicaid and SCHIP
16%

Other Private**
5%

Medicare
17%

Private Insurance
35%

Out-of-Pocket
14%

Where It Went

Other Spending***
23%

Program Admin.
and Net Cost
6%

Hospital Care
32%

Prescription
Drugs
10%

Nursing
Home Care
7%

Physician and Clinical
Services
22%

* Other public includes programs such as Workers' Compensation, PH activity, Department of Defense, Department of Veteran's Affairs, Indian Health Services, and state and local hospital subsidies and school health.
** Other private individual inpatient, privately funded construction and non-patient reserves, including philanthropy.
*** Other spending includes dental services, other group services, home health care, durable medical providers, over-the-counter medications, sundries, research, and construction.

Source: DHHC, Centers for Medicare and Medicaid Services, Office of the Actuary, National Health Statistics Group. http://www.cms.hhs.gov/statistics/nhe/historical/chart.asp. August 16, 2003.

however, new advances in health care and new methods for providing health care have made it easier to lower hospitalization stays and costs. Some examples of these advances that are clearly connected to increasing and decreasing costs and have an impact on nursing care are: (a) increased use of outpatient or ambulatory care surgery, (b) early ambulation of patients, (c) rapid-acting antibiotics, (d) greater ability to provide complex services in the home, (e) increased use of skilled nursing facilities, (f) research supporting benefits of shorter hospital stays, and (g) patient classification systems that identify parameters of usual hospital stays (Reres, 1996). Prescription costs also have risen due to an increase in the cost of drugs, increased costs of many new effective drugs, and

TABLE 14-2 Hospital statistics.

	1998	1999	2000	2001	2002
Number of hospitals	5,039	4,977	4,934	4,927	4,949
Beds in thousands	842	831	825	828	823
Admissions in thousands	31,830	32,377	33,102	33,834	34,501
Average length-of-stay	6.9 days	5.9 days	5.8 days	5.8 days	5.7 days
Expenses adjusted per inpatient stay dollars	$6,387.53	$6,512.44	$6,650.68	$6,979.29	$7,353.17
Expenses adjusted per day dollars	$1,064.93	$1,101.47	$1,147.99	$1,216.04	$1,288.63

All data refer to nonfederal short-term general and other hospitals.

Source: Data summarized by Author from American Hospital Association. (2004). *Hospital statistics.* Oakbrook Terrace, IL.

broader health insurance coverage. This major concern is discussed further later in this chapter. Insurance premium costs have also risen. In 2003, the total cost for premiums for annual employer-sponsored health insurance was $2,426 for an individual and $7,035 for a family, and in 2004 it was $3,383 for individuals and $9,068 for family coverage (U.S. Census Bureau, 2004). Table 14-2 and Figures 14-3 and 14-4 provide additional data about hospital statistics and health care expenses.

Health care utilization and expenditures data are used to evaluate cost control outcomes and sometimes demonstrate that expenditures for patients increased and cost control was not very effective.

However, another perspective on health care expenditures exists that is more complex. Is spending more on medical care worth it in terms of its impact on the length and quality of life? Third-party payers must view health care expenditures from many perspectives (for example, using cost-benefit analysis as described in this study of myocardial infarction patients). Health care providers must also view expenditures from many different perspectives. To gain a better understanding of health care expenditures, nurses need a better understanding of health care reimbursement and the role of the third-party payer.

Reimbursement for health care delivery services

You enter a patient's room, and he is speaking on the telephone. You overhear him say, "I don't care how much this hospitalization is costing. My insurance pays for it." You nod and agree. This example almost seems as if it came from another world, certainly not the real one, and both the patient and you, the nurse, need to enter the real one. Is it this simple?

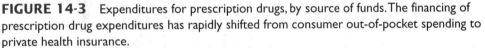

FIGURE 14-3 Expenditures for prescription drugs, by source of funds. The financing of prescription drug expenditures has rapidly shifted from consumer out-of-pocket spending to private health insurance.

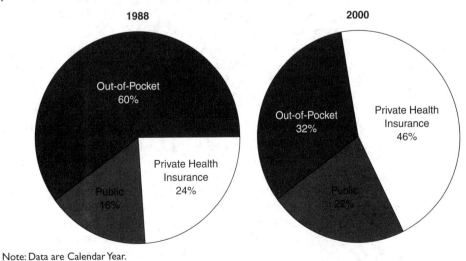

Note: Data are Calendar Year.

Source: CMS, Office of the Actuary, National Health Statistics Group. June 2002 Edition.

FIGURE 14-4   Centers for Medicare and Medicaid Services. Disbribution of funding for freestanding nursing home expenditures for all payers, CY 2000. Medicaid remains the largest single payer of nursing home care.

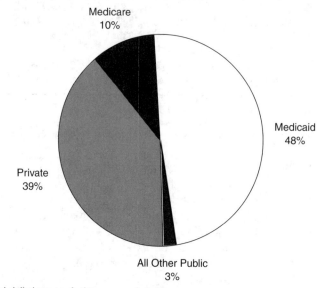

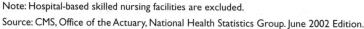

Note: Hospital-based skilled nursing facilities are excluded.

Source: CMS, Office of the Actuary, National Health Statistics Group. June 2002 Edition.

Health care reimbursement in the United States is a pluralistic payment system with multiple payers from both the public and private sectors. It is complex, with many players, motivations, and a long history of change. Insurance began in Boston in 1847. By the end of the 1860s, there were 60 health insurance companies. In 1911, Montgomery Ward and Company offered a plan that provided benefits to its employees who were unable to work due to illness or injury (Health Insurance Association of America, 1998). Employers began to offer health insurance coverage instead of increasing wages. Over time businesses offered insurance to get the tax benefit it provided to employers because employers' contributions for insurance benefits are exempt from federal and state taxes, which is a very important savings for employers.

From 1987 to 1997, health insurance premiums rose 90%, which was an incredible increase for those earning low wages (Cooper & Schone, 1997). With the increase in premiums as well as the increase in other out-of-pocket expenses, people began to make choices; for some people, these were unwise decisions, although they may have been made for legitimate financial reasons. Some decided not to sign up for health insurance and others limited their use of services to cut down on their personal costs. Employees who choose not to purchase coverage decide to take the risk and gamble that they will not need health care services.

Cost consciousness in the face of limited health care dollars has reached a level that crosses all care settings and patient populations to a much greater extent than in the past. It has created a heightened awareness of the need to provide cost-effective care in a clinically responsible manner (Britt, Schraeder, & Shelton, 1998). Today, health care purchasers, typically employers and governments, are in a very influential position, because the purchaser usually is involved in major decisions (e.g., approval of reimbursable services, provider choice, length-of-stay, length of treatment, quality). All nurses require a greater knowledge of reimbursement in order to understand how reimbursement affects care provided, denial of care, and numerous factors related to the nursing practice within all types of organizations. In the past, nurses did not discuss health care reimbursement with their patients. The business office would be called to come and talk with a patient when questions arose. This is not an inappropriate intervention when a patient has billing questions; however, it has fostered a climate of separation. Nurses provide care, and "someone" pays. Patients, however, expect that nurses have some knowledge about reimbursement. The growth of managed care has made this knowledge even more important. Nursing standards identify financial resource management as an important nursing responsibility.

FIGURE 14-5 Key players in the health care environment.

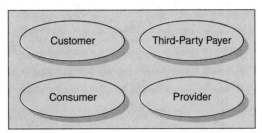

Source: A. Finkelman. (2001). *Managed care. A nursing perspective.* Upper Saddle River, NJ: Prentice Hall, p. 6. Reprinted with permission.

Key players in the reimbursement process

The key players in reimbursement strategies are the insurer (third-party payer), the customer, the consumer, and the provider. These players are identified in Figure 14-5.

1. Third-party payer/managed care organization/insurer

   With the development of managed care the insurer, **third-party payer**, or MCO no longer carries all of the financial risk for health care. Reimbursement strategies used by MCOs are primarily aimed at reducing MCO financial risk; however, these strategies are often difficult to separate from service strategies. The insurer may use any of the managed care models and may be a national or regional insurer. With the advent of managed care, the insurer has increased power to influence care and reimbursement and has been more successful in decreasing its financial risk by using reimbursement and service strategies.

2. Customer

   The **customer** is the person who contracts with the insurer. In most cases this is an employer since the U.S. reimbursement system is employer-based. The employer looks for the most cost-effective plans to meet the needs of its employees.

3. Consumer/patient/enrollee

   The patient or enrollee is a key player in the health care system. If patients did not exist, there would be no need for insurers or providers. When a person chooses a health insurance plan, the person is referred to as a plan member or enrollee.

4. Provider

   Who is the provider? Provider is a generic term. Any of the following may be considered a provider: physician, advanced practice nurse or nurse practitioner, nurse-midwife, registered nurse, physician assistant, nurse anesthetist, pharmacist, dentist, optometrist, chiropractor, podiatrist, hospital, home health agency, hospice, long-term care facility, psychiatric hospital, skilled nursing home, infusion therapy agency, and so on. In short, a provider is any person or organization that provides health care.

What is health insurance?

An insurer or third-party payer is the organization, private or public, that pays or underwrites coverage for health care for another entity, such as a business or individual. The third-party payer provides either group coverage or individual coverage. Most people who have insurance coverage receive it as an employee benefit or through membership in an organization, which is group coverage (e.g., a health care professional organization might offer health plans to its members). Most group insurers are commercial or for-profit insurers. Individual or personal insurance that is not part of employment is much more expensive for the purchaser or the enrollee. Sometimes individuals purchase personal insurance to cover gaps in their employment insurance. Others who may be self-employed may have to purchase individual coverage plans. In the insurance schema, the patient is referred to as the first party, the provider as the second party, and the third party is the payer or insurance carrier, such as a commercial insurer, managed care organization, Blue Cross and Blue Shield, and the government programs (e.g.,

Medicare, Medicaid). The third-party payer actually pays the bills; however, the process is not simple. As insurance has grown, there has been an increase in insurer financial risk. The insurer could lose the money it invests or it could miscalculate the amount of money it needs to cover all of its expenses, expected and unexpected. This could happen if too many of the health plan members require more health care than was estimated. If the insurer is a for-profit organization, it must also yield profits to pay its stockholders. Insurer administrative costs (e.g., staff, facilities, supplies, information systems, and other similar activities and functions) can also be very high.

How does the insurance process actually work to yield payment for health care services?

1. An individual experiences uncertainty about health care needs and treatment costs. Without this consumer uncertainty, there would be less need for insurance and less financial risk associated with health care. Given this uncertainty, there is a need to share the financial risk with other consumers to decrease individual risk.
2. When individuals decide to join an insurance plan, they put a specific amount of money into the pool or the insurance fund. The pool consists of the group of people that the insurer is covering for health care services.
3. The insurer takes on the role of managing or administering the pool of money. Plan members really do not want to do this for themselves.

For example, a large manufacturing company offers several health care coverage options to its employees. This company does not want to use its own resources to administer employee health care coverage, so it contracts with insurers. The insurer will be better served, as will the purchaser of the health care plan (the employer) and the enrollees, if there are a large number of members/enrollees. This decreases the financial risk and the administrative costs and usually means that there is greater diversification in the health status of members, with some healthier than others. The amount that is then paid to obtain the coverage, the premiums, is usually lower. There also will be a greater chance of a pool of members who will have different health care needs: some requiring no care, others needing limited care, and some with major medical care and long-term needs. The worst scenario for the insurer is to have a group of unhealthy members.

Prospective versus retrospective payment

Typically, when a customer considers purchasing a product, such as a car, the price is known before the purchase. The seller sets the price, and then the purchaser decides to buy or not to buy the product, usually considering need, price, quality, and the like. This is **prospective payment.** The health care industry has had a different experience with setting prices. In the past, third-party purchasers of health care services devised a **retrospective payment** system. In this system, the provider spent money while providing the care, requested payment for these expenses, and then was paid. Providers liked this because they knew they would be paid for their services when they submitted their bills. This payment method was known as fee-for-service or billed charges for health care services. The provider establishes the fee-for-service, and the patient pays, usually through a third-party payer. This was the major form of payment for health care for a long time. Fee-for-service payment typically did not put many limitations on the provider, and the insurer accepted the charges identified by the provider so the provider made most, if not all, of the treatment decisions with the patient. As a consequence, there was little incentive to be cost-effective when the provider knew that the requested charge would be paid in full. Box 14-1 describes indemnity insurance or the more traditional view of insurance coverage.

Third-party payers thought that retrospective payment using a fee-for-service method was a good approach, but after a time, this became an expensive way to do business. Then, third-party payers began to put some limits on what they would reimburse, eliminating an automatic acceptance of all charges. The federal government via its Medicare and Medicaid programs was the first purchaser or third-party payer to develop a comprehensive **prospective payment system (PPS).** The purpose of changing to this payment system was to decrease hospital costs. This sys-

BOX 14-1   Characteristics of traditional indemnity insurance.

- Fee-for-service reimbursement for providers
- Insurer assumes all financial risk
- No restrictions on choice of provider
- Limited financial incentives to be cost-effective
- No organized interest in quality measurement
- No organized interest in appropriateness of services

Source: Author.

tem is not based on actual charges but rather on estimated, predetermined prices made by the payer, not the provider. The provider knows before the care is provided what the payer will pay for a particular service. Usually, additional resources such as specialty care that may be used are not figured into this amount. In changing to prospective payment, the health care industry moved to the approach used by most sellers of products—here is the price; you either buy it or do not buy it. Now, it is quite clear that health care is a much more complex product. Just consider: Do consumers (patients) usually have a choice when they need care? Getting sick is different from deciding to buy a book, chair, dress, car, and so on.

Compensation for health services

Since the product, health care services, is not as simple as other types of products, a number of different approaches are used to pay for these services. Nurses will hear these terms, and they are related to the type of care the patient receives. They have an effect on how much money is actually received for services, which has a trickle down effect (for example, how much money is available for hiring staff, buying supplies, paying for overtime, and so on). The typical types of reimbursement methods are discounted fee-for-service, per diem rates, diagnosis-related groups, capitation, and **resource-based relative value scale.** Home health care usually is reimbursed on a per-hour or per-visit basis.

Discounted fee-for-service

In the mid-1970s, early forms of managed care began to use discounts. **Discounted fee-for-service** is a payment method that offers to pay the provider a specific percentage of the provider's usual charge or a reduced rate. The percentage can be a straight one, in which only a certain percentage is taken off the charge, or it can be a sliding scale, with the percentage changing based on specified criteria. Discounted services are part of a contractual arrangement with a third-party payer. An insurer may contract with a health care facility or any other type of provider to receive a discount for services provided. For example, an insurer's enrollees who receive care at that facility receive a 20% discount, or rather are only charged 80% of the usual charge for the services. Clearly, this is an advantage for the insurer/MCO. Sliding scales, another type of discount, are reflective of the volume of services provided. If the insurer requires a specific level of service, the fee scale will be adjusted or decreased. Most health care facilities, such as hospitals, have many contracts with insurers that have different discounts. If not all care is reimbursed at 100% of the cost, this leaves the health care provider with expenses that are not covered, which can have serious ramifications for the provider over the long term if the provider cannot cover these unpaid expenses. Providers, such as hospitals, outpatient clinics, physician practices, and home care agencies, must be very careful about the amount of care that is discounted and consider how the unpaid portion will be covered, since an insurer advantage can become a health care provider disaster. If a provider's expenses are not fully covered by reimbursement, then the provider (for example, a hospital) may have to decrease its costs (e.g., decrease staffing, postpone renovation or purchase of new equipment, decrease amount of educational programs provided to staff, and so on).

Per diem rates

A **per diem rate** is reimbursement that is fixed, based on each day in a health care facility (e.g., $600 per day). Services that may be covered, as well as expected length-of-stay and intensity of services, may be included in the agreed-upon per diem rate. This rate may also be discounted by the contract between the third-party payer and the provider. The per diem rate is an estimate of what the charges would be; however, this prospectively determined rate is all that is paid even if the actual expenses are greater. Usually, per diem rates vary for specialty areas; for example, daily rates for critical care, psychiatric care, medical care, surgical care, or obstetrical care would not be the same (e.g., critical care per diem would be higher than medical care per diem due to the staffing level, equipment, supplies, and so on). Per diem reimbursement is the negotiated rate per day times the number of days of care (e.g., $600 per day times the number of days in the hospital—3 days would equal $1,800 per diem reimbursement).

Diagnosis-related groups

Diagnosis-related groups (DRGs) is a statistical prospective payment system that classifies care or diagnoses into groups. These groups, which include inpatient care, are then used to identify payment rates. This is a per-stay reimbursement, focusing on a single episode of care related to a diagnosis and includes all predetermined expected services delivered for that episode of care. DRGs were established as the payment system for Medicare reimbursement by the Tax Equity and Fiscal Responsibility Act of 1982 (TEFRA). Over time some third-party payers also adopted it. The DRG system considers the types of patients a hospital treats or its case mix and the costs for treatment. Resources used and length-of-stay or bed days are important aspects of the incurred costs. Case-mix characteristics include severity of illness and intensity of service, as described in Box 14-2.

This system focuses not on the number of patients, but rather on the types of patients and the resources they require. The major diagnostic categories (MDCs) are based on anatomical or pathophysiological groups and/or their clinical management. Each MDC includes one to ten DRGs. The DRG rates are also affected by the:

- Location of the hospital (rural or urban)
- Wage index, which affects hospital costs
- Teaching hospital status and house staff training
- Recognition of outliers

Some patients, called outliers, will not meet the DRG requirements for a specific DRG. They are outside the expected in either length-of-stay or costs.

DRGs have had, and continue to have, an impact on nursing care. Nurses who work in acute care will hear about DRGs in their practice. Coordination of all aspects of care becomes critical in order to meet length-of-stay requirements for a specific DRG. Patients who stay longer incur more costs. Timely admissions and discharges are important components of cost-effective care.

BOX 14-2   DRG criteria: Severity and intensity.

Severity of Illness	Intensity of Illness
Clinical Findings	Physical Evaluation
Chief Complaint Working Diagnosis	
Vital Signs	Monitoring Clinical Elements
Imaging	Treatment/Medications
Diagnostic Radiology	
Ultrasound	
Nuclear Medicine Results	
Hematology, Chemistry, and Microbiology Results	Schedules Procedures
Other Clinical Parameters	

Source: A. Finkelman. (2001). *Managed care. A nursing perspective.* Upper Saddle River, NJ: Prentice Hall, p. 27. Reprinted with permission.

The nursing staff does most of the documentation, and it is this documentation that provides required information to assign the DRG to a specific patient. The DRG is assigned after the patient is discharged when it is too late to change the care or the documentation. Documentation, of course, should never be adjusted due to payment/reimbursement requirements to get more money for the care.

The DRG system takes outliers into consideration. If a patient's hospital stay is longer than expected or total costs are greater than expected for the patient's DRG, then the patient is considered to be an outlier. Additional reimbursement may be received for these patients; however, nursing staff, as well as other staff, need to analyze why outliers are occurring. Reimbursement for outliers cannot be assumed, and reimbursement may be limited or not paid at all. Changes in care and the coordination of that care may be required to decrease the number of outliers, and thus decrease financial risk for the organization and risk of additional payment denials. Hospitals are very concerned when they have outliers because they need to investigate the reasons to ensure that costs are controlled. Box 14-3 describes the case-mix index, another important component of the DRG system.

There is no doubt that Medicare and its DRG payment system have had a tremendous impact on health care. They have decreased hospital stays, but they have also increased the need for home care, long-term care facilities, and ambulatory care. Costs have been shifted to other settings, ones that are thought to be more cost-effective. There is an increased need for nurses to work in these non-hospital settings to meet the needs of patients who may still be very sick (for example, home care and long-term care). This is an example of how a reimbursement decision can have a direct impact on nursing care, such as the type of care provided and need for staff.

Capitation

The growth of managed care introduced one of the major changes in health care reimbursement—**capitation**. Capitation is a prepayment to a provider to deliver health care services to enrollees of a health plan. This is usually a monthly payment, but it can also be paid on an annual basis. The provider agrees to provide all care for the enrollee's health care needs that the provider is qualified to provide. If the enrollee requires no services in the allotted time period, the provider is still paid. If the enrollee's care incurs additional expenses, the provider receives no extra payment. The capitation method is dependent on a contract between the provider and a third-party payer. The focus is on covered lives or the number of persons who are enrolled in a health plan rather than individuals. For example, costs are typically described as inpatient days per 1,000, visits per 1,000, and cost per life. "Capitation changes the focus from how much a provider will be paid, as is the case with fee-for-service, to how much it costs to provide the care required" (Baldor, 1998). In doing this, the third-party payer no longer carries the full financial risk for the employer because much of it is shifted to the provider to keep costs down when decisions are made about care.

BOX 14-3   DRG: Case-mix index.

> Case-mix index (CMI) is the sum of all DRG-relative weights divided by the number of cases. This index is used to assign case-mix complexity to a hospital. The CMI is affected by five factors.
>
> ■ Severity of Illness
>
> ■ Prognosis
>
> ■ Treatment Difficulty
>
> ■ Need for Intervention
>
> ■ Resource Intensity
>
> Source: A. Finkelman. (2001). *Managed care. A nursing perspective.* Upper Saddle River, NJ: Prentice Hall, p. 28. Reprinted with permission.

Employee contributions to coverage

The employee pays some parts of the insurance coverage with the employer paying another part. The amount an employee pays, the premium, varies depending on the amount paid by the employer, the insurer's contract, and the amount of health care services used and how they are used. **Premium rate setting** is one of the most important decisions that a third-party payer can make, and also an important decision for consumers. Rating is pricing. The third-party payer determines the premiums (price or rate) for its products or services. Premiums are usually calculated as an amount per member per month (PMPM). If the third-party payer miscalculates, it can mean that the insurer loses money and may become financially unstable because the third-party payer will then not have enough funds to pay for the health care services that its members require and to cover administrative expenses that are needed to manage the insurance plan.

These costs continue to increase. The employee contribution to medical coverage usually includes some form of a deductible, co-payment/coinsurance, and annual limits. Insurance/MCOs plans are highly variable; these methods may not be included in all plans and can vary in how they are applied. Deductibles and co-payments/coinsurance represent the employee's out-of-pocket health care expenses and are used by the insurer to control its costs. When the insurer increases the out-of-pocket expenses, the insurer pays less and the enrollee or member pays more.

1. **Deductibles**

    A **deductible** is the amount the employee must pay before the third-party payer will begin to pay for health care services. The deductible is handled in two ways. Some plans require that the employee pay a single deductible for the employee and also for family members, which is applied to all services in the plan. The deductible for family members often is higher. The second method is the use of separate deductibles for categories of services, such as hospitalization, ambulatory care, and so on. Usually, when employers and employees pay high premiums, the employee pays a lower deductible. Deductibles are usually not used by **Health Maintenance Organizations (HMOs)**. Figure 14-6 describes the relationship of the deductible to other payments in the major medical model.

    Most major medical plans start with a deductible of $100, $250, or higher. This payment keeps the cost of the plan down because the enrollee is accepting responsibility for the most frequent charges, those under the deductible limit. After the deductible is paid, the enrollee shares the expenses by paying the co-payment or coinsurance. Typically, this is shared with the insurer on an 80/20 basis. Each dollar above the deductible is paid in this manner—insurer 80 cents and enrollee 20 cents. If the medical bill is large, 20% can still be a sizable amount. A patient example illustrating how this is implemented is found in Box 14-4.

FIGURE 14-6 Major medical model (Deductible, coinsurance, and high policy limits).

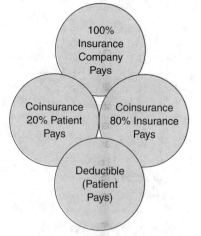

Source: A. Finkelman. (2001). *Managed care. A nursing perspective.* Upper Saddle River, NJ: Prentice Hall, p. 31. Reprinted with permission.

BOX 14-4   Deductibles and co-payments: A patient example.

Deductibles and Co-payments: A Patient Example		
Hospital Bill	$20,000	
Patient Deductible	− $ 200	
	$19,800	**Medical charges after deductible paid**
Medical Charges after Deductible Paid	$19,800	
Patient Share/Co-payment	× . 20	
	$ 3,960	**Amount of medical expenses to be paid by patient/co-payment**

Deductible must be paid before the insurer will pay its portion. Patient must pay deductible and co-payment.

Deductible	$ 200	
Co-payment	+$ 3,960	
	$ 4,160	**Total amount to be paid by patient**

Despite insurance coverage, the patient must still pay $4,160, which is not a small amount.

Source: A. Finkelman. (2001). *Managed care. A nursing perspective.* Upper Saddle River, NJ: Prentice Hall, p. 32. Reprinted with permission.

2. Co-payments/coinsurance

A **co-payment/coinsurance** is the fixed payment that the employee must pay per physician visit, procedure/treatment, or prescription. This is payment sharing between the insurer and the enrollee/patient. The payment typically is required at the time of the service and usually is an established amount, such as $5 or $10, or it can be a percentage. Co-payments may be found in all types of coverage. Box 14-5 describes an example of a patient's out-of-pocket expenses for an insurance plan.

Employers are increasing their efforts to contain their own costs; to achieve this, out-of-pocket expenses for employees typically increase. Employees then carry more of the responsibility for paying for the costs of care.

Annual limits

Annual limits are very important, particularly for employees and their families who experience major medical expenses in a year. All plans have some type of limit on the amount that the employee is required to pay annually. For example, coverage for an individual employee might have an annual limit of $1,000, and for the employee's family coverage $2,000. After

BOX 14-5   Out-of-pocket expenses: An example.

Physician's bill for office visit: Bronchitis:	$120
Insurer's reasonable and customary charge for this visit:	$100
Patient's co-payment of 30% ($100 × .30) =	$ 30
Uncovered part of bill to be paid by patient ($120 − $100) =	$ 20
Patient's total out-of-pocket expenses Co-payment ($30) + uncovered portion ($20) =	$ 50
The $50 represents 41.6% of the total charge, which was $120.	

Source: A. Finkelman. (2001). *Managed care. A nursing perspective.* Upper Saddle River, NJ: Prentice Hall, p. 32. Reprinted with permission.

this is paid, the health care services are covered 100%. In addition, some plans have lifetime limits on benefits, which means that after the employee's total expenditures for health care reach a specific amount, the plan will not pay for any more services. Plans may have a lifetime limit as high as $1 million; however, for some major illnesses, such as prematurity, major mental illness, or severe injuries with disability, this amount can quickly be spent. This may seem like an attractive benefit, but in reality it may not cover the costs. Not all plans have lifetime limits.

When an employee joins a health plan or when an individual purchases insurance, the person becomes an enrollee/member/subscriber in the plan. The enrollee's family is not usually referred to as the enrollee. They are dependents who are included in the plan's coverage, if that is an option available to the enrollee. The contract or covered services plan describes the eligibility criteria, benefits, and payments. These criteria identify when the enrollee and dependents are eligible for the services as well as when they are not eligible. For instance, a dependent child typically is not covered after a specific age or when he or she is no longer considered a dependent.

Coverage renewability is particularly important with individual health insurance policies and long-term care contracts. Until the Health Insurance Portability and Accountability Act (HIPAA) was passed in 1996, this was a major problem for enrollees or dependents with major or chronic health problems. This legislation provides guaranteed renewability, with exceptions made for fraud and nonpayment of premiums.

Covered services and enrollee benefits

The written **benefit plan** describes the benefits that are provided to the enrollee as well as the financial coverage for those benefits and is referred to as the covered services. Before covered services can be described, it is important to understand the relationship between the enrollee and eligibility for the covered services. Federal law requires that all employees eligible for a particular plan be offered enrollment, at the same price, regardless of their health status.

Benefits are a very important part of any health care plan. Important factors are the covered services, exclusions (what is not covered), and limitations. Great variability exists among plans in their benefit description and what is included or excluded. As an employee makes decisions about coverage, benefits can be a critical issue to consider, depending on the health and financial needs of the employee and the employee's family. They may or may not make the difference in coverage for treatment. In some cases, when there are major or chronic health problems, paying higher premiums to obtain maximum benefits may be the wisest choice. Plan benefits are also important to the provider because medical decisions are often based on the benefits that will be covered, which may not necessarily be what the patient needs.

Covered services are the health care services that the plan will cover or reimburse; however, the care or services must be medically necessary. What are the criteria used to determine if care is medically necessary? These criteria include consistency among diagnosis, medical documentation, and the likelihood of acceptance by medical peers that the treatment is necessary for the patient (Rognehaugh, 1998). The insurer determines medical necessity with input from the provider. Clearly, this is an area that creates conflict because the insurer becomes the major decision maker, not the health care provider. Typical benefits included in health care plans are:

- Hospital room and board
- Outpatient and inpatient surgery
- Office and inpatient physician visits
- Nursing services
- Diagnostic and radiological laboratory tests
- Ambulance services
- Medical equipment, such as might be used in the home

Some plans include more specialized care, such as home health care, extended care, hospice care, inpatient and outpatient mental health care, and alcohol and substance abuse treatment. When plans cover these services, specific descriptions are included in the covered services document or plan. Typically, home health care is used when skilled nursing care is required and usually covers supplies and equipment required for the delivery of the skilled care in the home; when hospice care is provided, it is usually covered for terminally ill patients who have 6 months or less to live. Extended care is provided for patients who need less intensive care than hospital care and require skilled nursing care, rehabilitation, and/or convalescent services. Mental health services and alcohol and substance abuse treatment services usually have more stringent limitations. The insurer identifies not only the benefits that are offered but often who may provide these services, a requirement that must be met for the insurer to cover or pay for the health care service. Table 14-2 provides information about hospital statistics.

Special health care needs are always a concern for the insurer because they increase costs. Dental and vision coverage are services that receive special attention. If an employer offers these services, it usually covers only one of them. Employers are beginning to pay a smaller portion of the premiums for these services. Some are only offering the option of dental HMOs. In addition, the use of medical technology has become an increased concern for MCOs and for consumers. The development of new medical technologies is a wonderful step forward for health care delivery, but they cost money to develop and use. Insurers must evaluate new technologies carefully before agreeing to cover these new therapies.

Health promotion and disease prevention have become more important to insurers, particularly in the managed care environment. In the past, traditional indemnity plans usually did not cover, or provided limited coverage for, these services. Examples of preventive care that might now be included are annual physical exams, childhood immunizations, and mammograms, usually within a specified age range. Health promotion examples are health education classes, wellness centers, and smoking cessation groups.

Exclusions are the services that will not be covered by a health care plan. Examples of conditions that might be excluded are:

- Conception by artificial means (Some plans cover artificial insemination and treatment for medical problems that cause infertility.)
- Reversal of voluntary sterilization (i.e., post-tubal ligation or a vasectomy)
- Contraception such as diaphragms, intrauterine devices, and some drugs (Oral contraceptive pills are usually covered.)
- Elective abortions
- Processing of blood
- Cosmetic surgery unless cause is due to injury, disease, or birth defect
- Orthodontic treatment
- Experimental or investigational treatments
- Transplants (If covered, specific types are identified.)
- Disabilities related to military service
- On-the-job injuries covered by workers' compensation
- Marriage and relationship therapy
- Mental health services ordered by the court (Korczyk & Witte, 1998, p. 48)

Prior to the passage of HIPAA, insurers used preexisting conditions to control some of their costs. Preexisting conditions are health conditions that exist prior to the date that insurance becomes effective. This was a problem for enrollees who had chronic illnesses, such as rheumatoid arthritis, diabetes, or renal disease. HIPAA requires that a group insurer may only refuse or limit coverage of a new employee with a preexisting condition treated or diagnosed in the 6-month period prior to enrollment for only 12 months. This 12-month period is reduced by the period of continuous coverage before enrollment in the new policy and is for one time only. For example, a person with renal disease who was diagnosed with the illness maintains continuous coverage for 5 months. Upon changing jobs, the person's coverage can be limited or denied for 7 months. At the conclusion of the 7-month waiting period, the person becomes eligible for the same insurance coverage offered to all employees. Having once met the 12-month waiting period, a person cannot be denied coverage when changing jobs as long as the person has had continuous

BOX 14-6 Health Care Federal Budget for FY 2004.

The following are examples of federal budget proposed health care expenditures. This does not mean that funds will actually be authorized as this is a different step in the budget approval process. These were included in the budget resolution passed by Congress.

- More than $500 billion for health programs and research

- Over the next 10 years, $500 billion has been set aside to reform Medicare, Medicaid, and help the uninsured

- About $266.5 billion will be used to fund Medicare in 2004, which is a 7.2% increase from 2003 budget

- Over the next 10 years, $400 billion has been set aside to reform Medicare and add a prescription drug benefit. (This is not expected to have a major impact on Medicare as it is expected that Medicare will have a $1.8 trillion bill for prescription drugs during this time period.)

- About $170.8 billion for Medicaid

- About $69.8 for the State Children's Health Insurance Program (SCHIP)

Source: Data retrieved on August 1, 2003, from http://Thomas.loc.gov and summarized by Author.

coverage. This can be complicated; however, it is critical for persons who have chronic illness, which is a larger and larger portion of the population who use many health care services.

Government health benefit programs

The federal government is the major player in the health care arena because it covers at a minimum 40% of the health care reimbursement in the United States (Health Insurance Association of America, 1998), which means that nursing care is directly affected by government health benefit programs. The federal government benefit plans are Medicare, Medicaid, the Federal Employees' Health Benefit Program (FEHBP), TriCare, and the Civilian Health and Medical Program of the Uniform Services (CHAMPUS). Health care is the major item in the federal budget each year. Nurses are involved in the care of all of these groups of patients, civilian and military. Box 14-6 identifies some of the key examples of health care expenditures found in the federal budget for fiscal year (FY) 2004.

Medicare

Nurses play major roles in all of the settings in which Medicare beneficiaries receive their care: inpatient, skilled nursing facilities, and home care; thus, Medicare payments, benefits, and requirements directly affect nursing care. Medicare is the federal health care insurance program that was established in 1965 by Title XVIII, Health Insurance for the Aged, an amendment to the Social Security Act of 1935. Eligibility requirements include being 65 years old or over and employed for 10 full-time equivalent work quarters or having a spouse who has met this requirement. Others who also qualify are persons with permanent kidney failure and persons receiving Social Security disability payments for 2 years, regardless of age. Medicare is the largest single payer in the United States. Over the last few years, there has been considerable concern about the growth of Medicare. The "Baby Boomers," people born between 1946 and 1964, have not yet entered the Medicare beneficiary age range, which will begin in 2010. The number of beneficiaries in May, 2004, was approximately 40 million (U.S. Census, 2004). This will greatly increase the number of Medicare beneficiaries.

In the late 1990s there was a slight decrease in Medicare costs, primarily because of the major effort to reduce hospital, home health, and provider payments. There are, however, some results that are troubling, which have had a ripple effect throughout the health care system. Home care agencies have had to make adjustments. Some home care agencies have had to avoid admitting higher-cost patients/clients to keep their costs in control (Pear, 1999). In acute care,

FIGURE 14-7 Medicare spending. Overall Medicare spending grew from $3.3 billion in 1967 to nearly $241 billion in 2001.

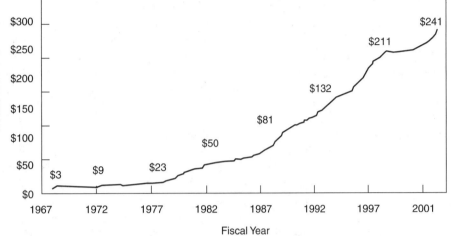

Note: Overall spending includes benefit dollars, administrative costs, and program integrity costs Figure represents federal spending only.
Source: CMS, Office of the Actuary. June 2002 Edition.

home care, and long-term care patients are sicker when they receive care, and thus need more intensive care at a time when nursing staff levels are reduced. Families are also greatly affected when they are left with the burden of caring for seriously ill family members at home with limited or no health care support. However, as can be seen in Figure 14-7, Medicare spending is on the rise, and that trend is predicted to continue.

The administrator for the Medicare program is the Centers for Medicare and Medicaid (CMS), which is part of the Department of Health and Human Services. The Medicare program is composed of two parts: A and B.

1. Medicare, Part A, is the hospital insurance plan, paying for inpatient treatment, skilled nursing facilities, and home health care. Medicare, Part B, is the supplementary medical insurance program, which includes coverage for physician services, outpatient treatment, and laboratory testing.

2. Part B, however, is voluntary and requires that the enrollee is entitled to Part A and willing to pay Part B premiums. The government pays 75% of the cost. The monthly premium is paid by the beneficiary. The Medicare beneficiary must also pay deductibles and co-payments, which are not high. If the person also qualifies for Medicaid by meeting the requirement of limited financial resources, Medicaid pays the deductibles and co-payments for the beneficiary. There is great concern that, as changes are considered in Medicare (benefits, eligibility, services, and so on), costs for beneficiaries will increase.

Medicare is funded by the Medicare Trust Fund, which includes payroll tax contributions. There has been much discussion in the last few years about fears that this fund will run out of money, particularly as the "Baby Boomers" age. Through Medicare Part A and Part B, over 39 million beneficiaries are provided with a comprehensive range of health care benefits. Because of the increasing number of individuals reaching age 65, costs are projected to grow.

THINK CRITICALLY

Try this exercise to apply what you have learned about this topic.

Medicaid

Medicaid, the health plan for low-income individuals, was established by Title XIX of the Social Security Act, enacted in 1965. This is not just a state program, but a program that is jointly funded by the federal government and the states. Each state has its own Medicaid program that provides funding for health care and long-term care or nursing home care. What is the role of the federal government? The federal government's matching funds are designed so that poorer states receive a larger percentage of the federal Medicaid funds to ensure more equity among the state programs, which must meet federal guidelines established by CMS. Each state, however, determines its own benefits, its eligibility requirements, and provider fee schedules. This is where problems and inequality occur. In May, 2004, the number of persons covered by Medicaid was 51 million (Centers for Medicare and Medicaid Services, 2004).

Despite efforts to ensure equal Medicaid programs among the states, there is still a wide difference in programs from state to state, particularly in eligibility requirements. All states, however, must include persons who qualify for Aid to Families with Dependent Children (AFDC), all needy children under the age of 21, Old-Age Assistance, Aid to the Blind, persons who are permanently and totally disabled, and the elderly over 65 years who are on welfare. When states set eligibility standards, these standards can cause major problems for many people who need these health care services and then cannot receive Medicaid reimbursement. Nurses who work in community health soon learn about the impact that Medicaid cuts have on the availability of health care services to vulnerable populations. Eligibility standards may have a major effect on providers, who may end up providing care with no reimbursement to cover their costs. Medicaid benefits cover:

- Comprehensive services for inpatient and outpatient care
- Professional services, including mental health
- Diagnostic testing, prevention, and screening for children and adolescents
- Nursing home care
- Home health care

Optional benefits that states may include are prescription medications, prosthetic devices, hearing aids, and care for people who are mentally retarded (Kaiser Commission on the Future of Medicaid, 1997).

Federal employees' health benefit program (FEHBP)

The FEHBP provides health care coverage to over 10 million federal employees, retirees, and their dependents (Knight, 1998). This coverage is mandated by law and administered by the federal government's Office of Personnel Management. Members or enrollees of the FEHBP choose from a wide variety of health care plans, including managed care plans, during the government's annual enrollment period. Minimum benefits are required for plans to contract with the FEHBP. Since the federal government's departments and agencies have facilities and offices throughout the United States, FEHBP coverage can be found outside Washington, D.C. for VA employees, CDC, EPA, FBI, and so on.

Military health care

Health care coverage for military personnel and their dependents is another major health care expenditure for the government. The military health services system (MHSS) is not only an insurer but also a provider through its health care facilities found throughout the world. Military nurses are part of many of these facilities. MHSS provides health benefits to more than 9 million active-duty military personnel, as well as retirees, dependents, and survivors through its CHAMPUS program. Almost 10% of the beneficiaries are over 65 years of age, and this proportion is expected to increase (Health Insurance Association of America, 1998). CHAMPUS was a fee-for-service insurance program for dependents; however, due to its increasing costs, the federal government began to experiment with the use of managed care. The military has been restructuring its health care system to include both military and civilian providers and facilities.

This restructuring has developed an organization that has 12 regional care areas. The goal is to provide more cost-effective care by using military health care facilities, contracts with civilian managed care organizations, quality assurance programs, and information technology (Knight, 1998). Military medicine is changing just as civilian care has changed. The Veteran's Administration medical system has also undergone recent changes (e.g., introducing primary care, regional centers and marketing, case management). This system provides ambulatory care, acute care, and, in some cases long-term care for military veterans, and is separate from the military health system.

State insurance programs

States also offer insurance to their state employees. The state government is usually a state's largest employer, and consequently largest insurer. Usually, there is some degree of choice for state employees among several plan options. State employees contribute to the payment of this coverage in the same way they would if they were employed in the private sector.

Managed care

Health care reimbursement is a complex process, which has been made even more complex by the use of managed care. Understanding how this process works and who the players are in the process helps health care providers advocate for their patients and intervene in the process to ensure that quality care is not compromised and that health care professional needs are considered. Today, reimbursement and managed care are inseparable. Nurses play active roles in the various models of managed care, and these models affect the practice of most health care professionals daily in many health care settings. As managed care grows, nurses will need to participate more actively in these organizations. Nurses are also employed by MCOs. They provide direct care, work with enrollees, determine allocation of benefits, and act as case managers. Some nurses hold management positions in MCOs, and this trend will probably increase. To remain a viable health care profession and be the patient's advocate, nurses cannot ignore managed care and its impact on health care delivery. By assuming leadership roles and participating in the changing health care environment, nursing care needs will not be ignored.

Managed care is changing due to demands from providers and consumers. What will happen in the future with the managed care approach to reimbursement is still unknown. Some believe that the traditional approach or the managed care approach that is now used will not be successful in the long term. The ideal managed care delivery system will be an organized body of health services and financial mechanisms. It will operate in an integrated and systematic fashion to manage and provide the right wellness, medical, and related services at the right place and time. The system's organizational goal will be to improve the long-term health status of the community (Wolford, Brown, & McCool, 1996).

Continuity of care, wellness and illness, long-term care, and the health status of the community will be important aspects of the future health care delivery system. This system will need to be a seamless one and will require an information system that allows for efficient sharing of information among the system's organized parts. Accountability and responsibility must be part of this system. Accountability is the acceptance of ownership for the results of an action or lack of results. Responsibility is an obligation to accomplish a task (Sullivan & Decker, 2001).

The goal of improving the community's health status, however, may be difficult to reach. Today, the system operates with self-interest as the main concern, and this is far from a community interest (Wolford, Brown, & McCool, 1996). Are communities ready to consider what health services they really need when this might mean that some providers and facilities would no longer be needed? The government would have to provide financial support so that the health needs of all citizens are met. Consideration of this approach has thus far not been successful. Change does not come easily in this environment. The insurer needs to collaborate more with the provider and vice versa. The patient needs to be more knowledgeable and assertive. Choices will vary depending on the size of the community. This vision focuses on a system whose individual parts are concerned about the success of all of the parts, because this means success for the entire system. This alone is a major challenge.

Managed care models

The HMO was the first managed care model; however, many others have been developed. Why did this happen? Consumers have not always been happy with HMOs. The problem of increasing health care costs was not resolved in the 1980s when managed care began to expand. Insurers, who were in competition with HMOs, began to develop new models for health care management, and employers were interested in these other options. Today, health care professionals and consumers experience a maze of different MCO models. Trying to compare and contrast their characteristics can be an overwhelming task; however, to appreciate the implications of managed care, this understanding is important. First, it is helpful to review a definition of managed health care, which has been described as "... a regrettably nebulous term. At the very least, managed care can be described as a system of health care delivery that tries to manage the cost of health care, the quality of that health care, and the access to that care. Common denominators seen in MCOs include a panel of contracted providers, who are mostly physicians but may include other health care professionals such as advanced practice nurses, that is less than the entire universe of available providers, some type of limitations on benefits to subscribers who use non-contracted providers (unless authorized to do so), and some type of **authorization** system" (Kongstvedt, 2001, p. 1367). The most important difference in the managed care models is the relationship between the managed care organization and the participating providers, particularly physicians. The major role of traditional indemnity insurance was to process and pay medical bills. MCOs have a more comprehensive approach that has affected how they are organized. MCOs continue to process and pay medical bills, but they have become more involved in the management of their members' health care, focusing on appropriate care, when it is needed, and illness and disease prevention. Table 14-3 summarizes the more common MCO models, including the HMO, **Preferred Provider Organization**, **Point-of-Service**, and carve-outs.

THINK CRITICALLY

Try this exercise to apply what you have learned about this topic.

The changing view of managed care

In May 1998, managed care was experiencing trying times. "Despite continued enrollment growth, the profitability of most managed care plans has declined significantly since 1994" (Taylor, 1998, p. 1). Others also predicted that national health care spending would double in the next 10 years (Ginsburg & Gabel, 1998). Expenses increased due to the increased use of prescription drugs, demand for new and improved technology, and increased payments to physicians. Consumer insistence on provider choice and use of office-based services will undoubtedly increase physician payments (Smith et al., 1998). There are, however, other reasons for expected increases in health care costs. There is now more flexibility within managed care in consumer choice because consumers demanded more, and this has and will continue to make it more difficult for managed care organizations to control costs. The growing criticism of managed care and threats of greater legal regulation have created a difficult situation for MCOs. On the one hand, there is a national move to hold health plans more accountable for their care and services. To do that, plans need to manage care more tightly. On the other hand, consumers, employers, and policy makers are pressuring health plans for greater provider choice. In addition, MCOs are confronting more powerful providers than they did in the early years of managed care. Physicians and hospitals, as well as other types of providers, are joining together to gain more negotiating power with MCOs. External forces have become more important, with increased legislation and regulation that further constrain MCO efforts to control costs. MCOs have always used various strategies to control costs and monitor provider performance. These have become even more important, and some strategies have actually had to be adjusted due to consumer and provider complaints.

TABLE 14-3 Common managed care models.

All MCOs have provider panels, which is the group of providers who are contracted to provide health care services to enrollees in the MCO. Providers are typically direct care providers (for example, physicians, advanced practice nurses, nurse-midwives, hospitals, clinics, long-term care facilities, home health agencies, laboratories, durable equipment suppliers, pharmacies, and so on). Provider panels are selected and organized in a variety of ways. Control is a major issue with MCOs, particularly control over provider decisions, which have a direct impact on costs. The following are several of the more common managed care models.

Health Maintenance Organization (HMO)	Preferred Provider Organization (PPO)	Point-of-Service (POS)	Carve-Outs
The HMO is the original model or prototype of managed care, which integrates the delivery of service with reimbursement for those services. The HMO pays the bills for its members' health services, but it also manages and provides care to its members. An enrollee in an HMO such as Group Health goes to one site to receive care, both primary and usually specialty care. Most HMOs do require that the patient/enrollee pay a small co-payment. There may be limited provider choice. The HMO develops incentives to encourage its providers to provide the lowest-cost care to the HMO members.	A PPO is a delivery network of providers, physicians, advanced practice nurses, hospitals, and other providers. The PPO does not assume any financial risk or receive premiums, but it does charge for use of its provider network. The PPO itself is not directly involved in the delivery of health care services; rather, it acts as an intermediary to negotiate and manage the managed care contracts on behalf of the individual providers. Capitation is not common with a PPO, but rather reimbursement is usually based on the fee schedule identified by the PPO. Typically, members pay lower deductibles and coinsurance when they use providers in the PPO provider panel. PPOs do not focus on utilization management and quality assurance, which is not true of other MCO models. The PPO has become the most acceptable MCO model because consumers have the most choice in providers and do not have to get a referral from a primary care provider to see a specialist.	The POS model provides more choice for the enrollee/patient, but at a price to the enrollee. The enrollee may determine at the time that a health care service is needed whether to use a provider in the MCO panel or one outside the panel. If the enrollee chooses a provider outside the panel, then the enrollee pays higher co-payments and deductibles. When the enrollee goes outside the panel, the provider is paid on a fee-for-service basis. The MCO hopes that over time the enrollee will choose not to use the POS option. A POS option may be found in a number of different MCO models.	A carve-out is another method for organizing managed care services. These are health care services that are separated or carved out of a regular health care service contract and then are contracted separately in a separate plan. Services that are carved out are ones that are high volume or high cost. Psychiatric services, substance abuse treatment, prescriptions, radiology, laboratory, vision, and dental are typical services that are often carved out. The patient may need to pay an additional premium and meet different requirements for the use of these services, particularly related to referrals. Mental health treatment and substance abuse treatment are the two most common services offered in this manner. The enrollee usually does not even realize that a carve-out exists.

Source: Author.

Managed care strategies to control cost and quality

How do MCOs cut health care expenses and yet still ensure quality care? Service and reimbursement strategies are used to manage the health care services provided and to reduce costs. It is important for all health care providers, including nurses in all types of settings, to understand the strategies that are used and their purposes. Service strategies are methods used by MCOs to manage delivery of care in all types of health care settings. The purpose of these strategies is to decrease cost and provide quality care. The MCO wants to find better, more cost-effective treatments; however, this is a strategy that has not been fully utilized. It is quite clear by now that as MCOs have been trying to decrease health care costs, provider roles, and responsibilities, provider–insurer/MCO relationships, patient needs, and societal health care needs have undergone major changes and will continue to do so. There is no doubt that health care delivery has been affected by managed care service strategies, but it is not always clear if costs have been better controlled with these strategies or if the quality of care has changed, positively or negatively.

Efficiency is a critical component of these strategies. The goal is to minimize costs and choose services with the maximum excess of benefits over costs. Just focusing cost-containment efforts on decreasing costs will not be enough in the long run. Achieving the desired outcome has become more important over the past few years, which definitely relates to achieving greater benefits over costs. Have MCOs been successful with strategies to increase efficiency? At this time, not much data are available to support linking costs with outcomes. The belief is, however, that managed care has more ability to do this than did traditional indemnity insurance. This is more likely to occur because MCOs are ". . . better equipped to measure the outcomes of care, identify quality problems, and implement strategies for improvement, such as adopting clinical guidelines to reduce unjustified variations in medical practice. Managed care plans also have a unique opportunity to intervene at the system level, and thus have the potential to overcome the fragmentation that underlies much of the inefficiency of the poorly organized fee-for-service sector" (Priester, 1997, p. 58). Table 14-4 summarizes some of the service strategies that are used, such as **primary care providers,** resource management, and **utilization management**.

Service strategies have had an impact on changing health care and costs; however, reimbursement strategies probably receive the brunt of the criticisms directed at managed care. MCOs use a variety of strategies that focus on reimbursement to control medical costs, and these strategies require an understanding of the incentives that are important to managed care and buyers of health care (employers and government primarily). The incentive for MCOs is profit, which requires reduced costs. The incentive for the buyer, who is usually the employer, is reduced costs. The situation becomes complicated when one considers that the goal of the provider, especially the physician, advanced practice nurses, hospitals, and other health care professionals, is to provide quality care. Clearly, these may be conflicting goals, and this affects the outcomes. Even the choice of reimbursement strategies has caused conflict, more so than service strategies. The following provides a brief overview of some of these strategies: provider performance, capitation, length-of-stay management, and formularies.

Provider performance

Provider performance has never been more important. Today, when MCOs contract with new providers to join their **provider panels** or renew contracts with providers, the MCOs base their provider selection on specific criteria. Why is this so important? The MCO wants providers who offer cost-effective, quality care that meets the MCO criteria. As managed care developed through the 1980s and 1990s, cost-effectiveness became more important than quality; today, quality issues are slowly becoming more important. The goal of performance-based reimbursement evaluation is to alter provider performance. How the MCO goes about reaching this goal can vary and can mean the difference in success or failure. Rewards work better than sanctions, but both have been used. The MCO may financially reward providers who meet the MCO's criteria for cost-effective care by offering bonuses or close the provider off from receiving new enrollees. The goal is to discourage the use of inappropriate and costly services. MCOs typically use continuing education, data and feedback, practice guidelines, and protocols to encourage providers to change their behavior. Examples of indicators that are used to evaluate provider performance are:

- Member satisfaction data
- Member complaint and grievance rates
- Wait time for appointments
- Utilization rates
- Immunization rates
- Complication rates
- Overall medical costs or medical costs per member per month

TABLE 14-4 Service strategies.

Changing Practice Patterns

There is no doubt that managed care has affected how physicians, registered nurses, and all other types of providers deliver their care and services today. The greatest change in practice patterns has been the gradual move from the acute care setting to the home and community. Today, many providers focus on ambulatory care. There is also an increased emphasis on primary care. Providers are now more concerned with what treatment is really necessary and how to get the job done quickly. Hospitals have changed the way that they deliver care and are more interested in shortening length-of-stay, the utilization of resources, and the development of ambulatory services (e.g., clinics, wellness centers, ambulatory surgery, home care). Changing practice patterns has been positive for nursing and will continue to offer new opportunities for nursing. For example, physicians and health care organizations are recognizing the value of using advanced practice nurses and nurse-midwives to assist them in increasing their patient volume and reallocating their time. MCOs have gained more control over physician practice. With financial incentives driving many physician decisions, can the patient trust the physician to be completely honest about treatment options, even the expensive ones? This is one reason why it is important for all health care providers, such as nurses, to understand incentives and other service and reimbursement strategies used by MCOs. These strategies affect nursing care and the nursing profession; treatment patients receive or do not receive; length-of-stay and length-of-treatment; communication with providers; and trust in all health care providers. Consumers also need to be aware of these strategies, and they will turn to nurses for guidance and information.

Primary Care

The primary care provider (PCP) plays a major role in the managed care environment. The major PCP responsibility is to coordinate comprehensive care and serve as a gatekeeper. Not all models of managed care require that every enrollee have a PCP. The managed care organization identifies the qualifications of the PCP, which may vary among MCOs. In addition, pressures from consumers and physicians have also changed how MCOs describe primary care providers. The traditional view was that the PCP should be a family practice physician. Other health care providers who may now be classified as PCPs are medical internists, pediatricians, obstetrician–gynecologists, and ophthalmologists, and some MCOs have contracted with advanced practice nurses to serve as PCPs. Another important characteristic of a PCP is the patient does not need a referral from a provider to see the PCP. The gatekeeping responsibility is used to control over-utilization of specialists and other medical costs. Patient choice is limited by this strategy. The PCP, in the role of the gatekeeper, does this for the patient. In addition, the PCP coordinates the patient's care, which should improve the outcomes. Concerns about cost and appropriate treatment utilization are not illegitimate; however, consumers have generally disliked the idea of having to go through a physician or another provider in order to see a specialist. The PCP is typically paid using the capitation method to provide the contracted services identified by the MCO. This strategy provides additional cost control. In addition, MCO performance profiles provide descriptive data on the provider's utilization of services, such as laboratory testing, referrals to specialists, use of formulary, and the like, and are used to control costs.

Specialty Care

In the managed care environment, the PCP and the authorization process have a major impact on specialty care. The rigid approach to specialty care used in the early 1990s, however, has been loosening up. This has occurred primarily because consumers dislike the lack of physician choice and have spoken out against this approach. Specialty physicians also found the rigid process associated with gatekeeping and authorization a major deterrent to practice survival. Open access, allowing for greater direct access to specialists, is provided in different ways by more MCOs today. The patient may have to pay an additional co-payment to have a choice of specialists, but some MCOs are not charging for the option of choice although still requiring authorization from the PCP. MCOs are providing more information to enrollees about the use of specialists and access to them. This information is often found on the Internet. There was concern about increased utilization and continuity of care; specialty referrals were not as tightly controlled. However, some MCOs have found that these concerns have not played out the way they expected. Usually, these MCOs have developed systems to keep PCPs informed about their specialty usage.

Resource Management

Resource management is important to any MCO. The MCO's goal is to ensure that care is cost-effective, efficient, and of the appropriate quality. To do this, resources need to be used wisely. Resource management is interconnected with utilization and authorization. In the past the system of care was characterized by an independent array of disjointed providers and purchasers. Each provided many effective services for the consumers of health care, but they failed to overcome their independent interests to focus on the values of overall effectiveness. This led, in part, to oversupply of capacity, tremendous variability of outcomes, and duplication of resources. Managed care has now made it very clear that resources must be managed better than in the past. Nursing needs to take a lead in defining how nursing resources should be managed in order to meet outcomes of cost and quality. It becomes more important to identify clear outcomes, use scientifically determined best practices to achieve outcomes, measure progress, and when required, to reinvent the processes through which care is delivered.

(continued)

TABLE 14-4   Service strategies—*continued.*

Utilization Management

Utilization management is the process of evaluating the necessity, appropriateness, and efficiency of health care services used by the enrollees/patients who receive care from a provider. Utilization data are used to assess care and by external organizations to assess the quality of the MCO's services. Authorization is the major method used in utilization management. It is the payer's approval for a health care provider to provide specific care. The MCO or payer identifies what services or benefits require authorization. To be truly effective in controlling costs, an MCO must be able to influence provider utilization behavior. For example, if an MCO cannot find a way to decrease a provider's number of hospital admissions or the number of referrals to specialists, costs will continue to be a problem. The purchaser of the plan, the employer, does not like the idea of health care costs increasing and may decide to drop the MCO and contract with another, more cost-effective MCO. Who can authorize services is a critical decision. This decision is made in several ways. Probably, the most recognized method is to have authorization done by the primary care provider/physician. If an enrollee wants to see the PCP, no authorization is required. Some MCOs require that plan staff authorize services. In this case, the physician or other type of provider calls a plan representative and describes the patient's problems and need for services. The staff representative compares this information with predetermined criteria. Often, this representative is a nurse. Nurses are finding many new roles in managed care, and this is one of them. The nurse discusses the patient's needs with the provider and determines whether authorization can be provided. If the provider does not agree with the decision, the provider is referred to a supervisor or the medical director. Some plans use a different system. They have the enrollee call the plan directly, using a nurse advice line. The enrollee does not have to go to the PCP to use a specialist but uses the advice line to gain authorization. The nurse uses predetermined criteria to assess the enrollee's needs for care and then tells the enrollee the type of provider that is required.

Health Promotion & Disease and Illness Prevention

Health promotion and disease and illness prevention are strategies that focus on encouraging the enrollee to become a partner in maintaining health. Education is a key method for accomplishing this partnership. Each time an MCO develops health promotion and disease and illness prevention services, it reassesses the costs and benefits of these services. MCOs vary in how much of this strategy is applied to its plan. The goals of health promotion are to help people modify their lifestyles and make choices to improve their health and quality of life. Health education is very important in helping enrollees/patients to accomplish this goal. After the MCO identifies the health promotion and disease and illness preventive services to offer, it must develop the services, ensure that providers provide the services, and then communicate their availability to the enrollees. MCOs use newsletters, personal letters, information provided at the worksite, and the Internet to share information with their enrollees. Models of managed care other than HMOs, such as PPOs, may cover the services or may set a dollar amount for preventive services. In the latter case, the enrollee has more choice as to how to use the money set aside for health promotion and prevention. Some plans may require co-payments and deductibles for these services.

Management of Ancillary Services

Diagnostic and therapeutic services are ancillary services, and they greatly affect the costs of medical care. Typical diagnostic services are radiology, laboratory testing, electrocardiography, invasive imaging, and cardiac testing. Examples of ancillary therapeutic services are physical therapy, occupational therapy, speech therapy, and cardiac rehabilitation. Pharmacy service is also an ancillary service. These services are different from other services in that they require an order from a provider. Patients cannot just request a specific laboratory test or the like. These services have been identified as high-cost services with potential for overutilization. Their overuse or inappropriate use has often increased health care costs. How does the MCO control the utilization of these services? Collection of utilization data is very important. These data are collected so that individual providers can be evaluated. Standards of care and protocols are developed by the MCO to educate and guide the provider when decisions are made to use ancillary services. Another method used to control usage is the authorization process and limiting who can authorize services, which provides more rigid control. Some MCOs also limit how many times the enrollee can receive the service before reauthorization is required. For example, how many physical therapy sessions can a stroke patient receive before reauthorization is required? The reauthorization typically requires reassessment of the patient's needs. This control of usage has been a problem for some patients and providers.

Source: Author

- Hospital readmission rates
- Mammography rates
- Number and typed procedures
- Length-of-stay
- Number and type of prescriptions
- Capitation

Capitation is the payment of a fixed monthly fee to provide health care. Services that are included are defined with a contractual arrangement. This is a reimbursement strategy, and one that has increased in the managed care environment.

Length-of-stay management

Hospital occupancy rates and LOS for all types of patients have been decreasing, which has been supported by managed care. This change has increased the utilization of ambulatory care services, home care, subacute services, and other types of services that replace inpatient treatment. Nursing has been concerned about the decrease as it has affected patient care and patients' needs. A 1994 study that examined LOS and hours-per-patient-day based on the GRASP®, a patient classification and workload measurement, indicated that there was a relationship between LOS and required nursing care hours (Shamian, Hagen, Hu, & Fogarty, 1994). There is increased nursing resource consumption as LOS is reduced. The first hospitalization days have higher requirements for nursing hours, particularly the first 2 days. Nurses are now encountering more acute patients on admission because patients are kept out of the hospital until it is absolutely necessary to admit them. This has increased care needs. There is also increased pressure to provide rapid patient and family education, with little time to provide it. Is money actually saved when LOS is shortened? At what point does the decreased LOS actually increase nursing costs? These are critical questions that require further research. Other studies have demonstrated that the reduction of LOS by 1 day is not necessarily equal to reduction of an average cost per day (Arndt & Skydell, 1985; Fosbinder, 1986). These are old studies; however, it is important for nursing to continue to pursue these issues.

Formularies

Advances in pharmaceuticals have helped patients live more normal lives and have decreased health care costs, but at the same time these advances have increased medical costs. This may seem contradictory; however, both have occurred. For example, new AIDS medications have decreased the number of hospital days, but these drugs are also very expensive. Antibiotics prevent patients from becoming sick or sicker; however, some antibiotics are very expensive. Careful cost-benefit analysis is required. The federal government is more concerned about the increasing costs of drugs. Senior citizens comprise less than one-fifth of the population, and yet today they account for approximately one-third of the total prescriptive drug sales (Meinhardt, 1998). In 2004, Medicare began to offer some coverage for prescriptions, although not enough to cover most of the costs.

Formularies are used to cope with these increasing pharmaceutical costs. The formulary is the MCO's list of drugs or classes of drugs that the MCO prefers that providers use. How does an MCO determine which drugs to include in its formulary? Most MCOs use safety, effectiveness, cost, and cost-effectiveness as their criteria. No MCO formulary includes all of the drugs approved by the Food and Drug Administration (FDA). The formulary typically focuses on generic drugs, because these tend to be less expensive than the brand-name products, although they are usually chemically equivalent. Many drugs are the same, but their therapeutic effect or their side effects may vary. For some patients, excluding drugs that they have found helpful may be a serious problem. This is particularly important for patients with chronic illnesses for whom a specific drug is more effective. When the MCO's formulary changes and a drug is not included, or if the patient changes third-party payers and the new MCO formulary does not include the drug, the patient suffers.

Managed care must also consider adding new drugs that are expensive, including biotechnology products. For example, biotech hemophilia therapy per patient per month may cost between $4,000 and $17,000; biotech therapy for Gaucher's disease may cost between $13,000 and $27,000 per patient per month (McCarthy, R., 1998). Clearly, an MCO must weigh the costs and benefits of using these therapies. It needs data that demonstrate significant clinical advantages, but these advantages still may not be enough to support the decision to cover their use. MCO protocols and authorization are established for these highly expensive drugs. Another complication is that most of the new biotech treatments are injectable, and typically, MCOs do not cover injectables under the category of pharmacy but rather as medical expenses. As these drugs become more common, this classification as a medical expense will require reconsideration. The pharmacy coverage may be different from other benefits—often more limited—and thus there may be some advantage in reclassifying biotech drugs as pharmacy expenses.

Clinical trials, for example with drugs, have been a long-standing problem with MCOs, which have typically refused to cover most costs for trials; HMOs, however, have agreed to help pay the costs of care for members who enroll in clinical trials (Pear, 1999). Some MCOs have agreed to pay for experimental cancer therapy (Kolata & Eichenwald, 1999). Hopefully, this will increase the number of people willing to participate in clinical trials, which has been a problem as more Americans have joined MCOs.

Reimbursement issues: Impact on nurses and nursing care

Managed care is slowly making a major impact on nursing care. What are some ways this impact has been felt? Reorganization, reengineering, and restructuring of health care organizations are frequent today, and they have affected nursing care. As discussed in Chapter 5, managed care has caused health care organizations to evaluate their structure and processes and to make changes. The first setting in which managed care had a major impact on nursing care was the acute setting. There were then ripple-down effects to other types of health care settings. The new systems of health care have been created from restructuring and mergers. They have been "challenged to 1) manage within fixed resources; 2) decrease costs by reducing waste and inefficiencies; 3) focus on health and prevention of illness through primary care networks; 4) improve quality and outcomes; and 5) improve access to care" (Stickler, 1994, p. 49). All of these changes continue to require adaptation, and nursing must continue to play a major role with each of them.

Reimbursement does affect nurses and nursing care. Nurses are not expected to be reimbursement experts, but understanding how care is paid for is important. It is particularly important if reimbursement affects who delivers care, to whom it is delivered, where and when it is delivered, what type of care can be provided, and when care might have to end. If one does not understand reimbursement and its role in health care delivery, one might think that these decisions have nothing to do with the payment of care and are only connected to the provider and the patient. This, however, is not true. Reimbursement is another layer to the complex health care delivery process and system that cannot be ignored. How have nursing and nurses been affected by reimbursement and how can they affect reduction in costs, which is a concern of third-party payers? The following are some examples.

- Managing within fixed resources and decreasing costs by reducing waste and inefficiencies are more important to nursing today than they were in the past. Compared with other providers, nurses use the most resources, such as supplies and equipment, in the acute care setting, and through their usage they can make a difference in reducing waste and inefficiencies. The early history of nursing was one of "you don't need to know the budget or what things cost." This attitude is no longer acceptable if the organization expects to make a difference in reducing its costs.
- Nursing staff levels have also been affected by reimbursement as hospitals and other health care organizations have had to change staffing levels due to costs. This change requires that nurses assess how they deliver care and search for more efficient methods. In addition, nurses are speaking out more about staffing levels and their impact on patient care and quality and safety outcomes.
- Nursing has always been concerned with health promotion and prevention of illness and disease—important aspects of managed care. Nursing education emphasizes this content even more today. Nurses have even entered the primary care area with the increased usage of advanced practice nurses, who may serve as primary care providers.
- Quality and outcomes are not foreign to nursing, but nurses are not experts in these areas. Nurses, like other health care professionals, have yet to fully implement programs that access quality and outcomes. Much must be learned about these critical processes, and managed care seems to be driving the need for further development. Nurses could play an important role in this development. Health care professionals need to reexamine how they have assessed the quality of their care (see Chapter 16).

■ Access to care has also been a concern of nursing, but again nursing has not been any more successful in this area than any other health care profession. Nurses have the opportunity to make major contributions when access to care is discussed in planning meetings in the acute care setting, and access issues are part of an important concern in community health. Nurses must participate actively in this planning, or they will be left out of the process.

■ Nurses have been comfortable working in differentiated structures that are organized around specific diagnostic clusters (e.g., medicine, critical care, obstetrics, and support services such as nutritional or environmental services). More organizations are recognizing that this might not be the most effective way to structure the work. Greater emphasis is now placed on coordination of work across parts of the organization. "Significant cost savings have been reported by conducting joint programs, eliminating duplicative positions in entities with proximal geographic areas, clustering marketing and planning areas central to service-line rather than entity, and developing of 'centers of excellence' for specific service areas" (Stickler, 1994, p. 53). To survive the changes in the future and develop new roles, nurses need to be active participants in these new delivery systems.

The following are some issues that are particularly affected by the macrolevel of health care financial issues.

1. Cost of care is more important than charges for care. This factor drives all decisions that are made, whether they are patient-related or not. Operating costs have to be covered.
2. Understanding of managed care and reimbursement is critical, and not just by nurse leaders/ managers, but also staff nurses.
3. The continuum of care has become more important and will continue to be so. What are its components; are they easily accessible; what are the roles of nurses in helping the patient through the continuum; and the roles of nurses within each component? Getting the appropriate care in the best setting from the most appropriate provider reduces costs.
4. There is an increased emphasis on patient education, promotion, and prevention, which are aimed at improving quality but also decreasing costs.
5. Caregivers (families, significant others) have taken on major roles in the health care delivery system. Are they prepared for this? Are they available for this? How does their usage affect health care costs?
6. Provider performance evaluation is now the norm, even if it does cause stress. This includes performance data about hospitals, clinics, home care, long-term care, physicians, advanced practice nurses, and so on. Development of computer technology has helped move this along. These data are used to make reimbursement decisions.
7. The hospital discharge process has become more important. This affects the entire continuum of care and yet staff must care for sicker patients who are discharged, with less staff and less time.
8. Outcomes are constantly monitored. Paying for something that does reach expected outcomes is costly.

BENCHMARKS

Now let's take a moment to test your knowledge of the concepts you have studied in this section.

Financial Issues: Microlevel

The microlevel focuses on the financial issues of an individual health care organization. New nurses are typically not responsible for budgeting; however, a general understanding of the process as well as other related issues is important as they affect nurses and how they practice.

Prior to entering a more detailed discussion, it is helpful to review that some organizations are classified as for-profit and others as not-for-profit. It is not uncommon for staff to have only negative views of for-profit organizations. What do these two classifications really mean? In simplest terms, a for-profit organization must return some of its profits to its stockholders or owners. A not-for-profit organization does not have stockholders or owners who require returned profit; however, in this case the profit is reinvested in the organization. All organizations need to make a profit to stay in the "black" because, if this does not occur, debt will increase, the organization may be in the "red," and the organization over the long term will fail financially. This organization will be forced to reduce costs, which will impact care delivery and nurses. The key difference between these two types of organizations is what is done with the profit. Even for-profit organizations need to use some of their profit on their organization; therefore, not all of it goes to stockholders or owners.

A second critical area in microlevel financing is the idea that budgeting is a very real description of the financial status of the organization. It is not something that is just described on paper; when the **budget** is prepared, it is just an educated guess. This process requires data that are as accurate as they can be. Change has been a frequent theme in this text, and this is certainly true of budgets. Changes in many factors that affect health care delivery can mean the provider or organization must make budget adjustments. Examples of these factors are number of patients admitted, length-of-stay, decreasing amount of reimbursement, increased staffing costs or costs of staff benefits, change in the cost of supplies, need to renovate or expand space, expansion of computerized documentation, and need to purchase new medical equipment.

The third critical issue is microlevel financial issues have a direct impact on the delivery of health care and on nursing. Much more will be discussed about this issue. These finances directly affect decisions about staffing, supplies and equipment, renovation of facilities, types of services provided, quality of services, accessibility of services, employee education and training, and much more. So even if staff nurses do not prepare the budget, it directly affects them.

This section of the chapter discusses an overall review of the financial component of hospital/other types of health care organizations, key financial management terminology, the budgeting process, productivity, and cost containment. Staff nurses typically do not become directly involved in these functions, although at times they may be asked for input on the budget at the unit level, and their work affects productivity and cost containment. Nurses who go into management positions need to become more involved in budgeting, and when this occurs, they need to devote more time to learning much more about financial health care issues at the microlevel.

Financial component of hospitals and other types of health care organizations

Each health care organization has its own financial system; however, there are some common elements of these systems that are helpful for nurses to understand. They affect nursing staff and nursing care. The governing body of the organization such as the board of directors is ultimately responsible for the financial activities and stability of the organization. The board oversees the organization's budgetary process and approves the final budget.

- This budget is prepared and submitted by the organization's chief executive officer (CEO).
- The CEO may delegate the day-to-day financial operations to other staff such as a chief financial officer (CFO) or comptroller.
- The chief nurse executive (CNE) is typically responsible for the nursing budget that is submitted to the CFO and then to the CEO.

■ The key higher level management staff should collaborate in the development of the overall organizational budget. Department heads, which should include directors of nursing for services and nurse managers, participate by developing budgets for their services and units, and then these budgets are passed up the line to become part of the overall budget.

This does not mean that all of these budgets are accepted as originally submitted. As the budgets go up the line, compromises need to be made—not everyone gets what they request. The final product or organization budget is a compilation of all of these budget requests.

This process takes time. Data from past budgets are used in developing subsequent budgets. Staff may participate at the unit or service level as these managers request staff input about budgetary needs for the coming year. All through the budget process consideration should be given to the organization's vision, mission, and goals and marketing plan. For example, if an expansion of services is planned then this would need to be included in the budget planning with consideration given to additional staffing, equipment and supplies, physical plant changes, marketing expenses, staff training, the impact expansion will have on other services, and so on. This process is really the same in all types of health care organizations, but, of course, the smaller and less complex organizations may not have as many levels in the process.

Key financial management terminology

Financial management is highly complex and a specialty area in health care administration. The key goal is to obtain the funds necessary to meet the organization's goals. Nurses are not expected to be experts; however, they will hear some financial/budgetary terms and need to know what they are in order to participate as much as is possible in this process. The organization needs accurate data to do the following: (a) guide operations of the organization, (b) make effective decisions about financial issues, and (c) monitor and control operations by using variance analysis.

The following are common budget terms.

■ **Accounts receivable:** An amount owed to the health care organization (HCO) by a patient or customer for services. (As discussed earlier in this chapter, third-party payers such as MCOs, Medicare, and Medicaid are the most common payers for these services.) If these accounts are not paid in a timely manner, this does have an effect on the HCO's ability to pay its own bills.

■ **Actual figures:** The exact amount of revenue and expenses the HOC experiences; these figures are not the amounts that were estimated or proposed for the budget, but rather the real numbers.

■ **Asset:** An item owned by the HCO with value that can be identified objectively (for example, the value of equipment used in the operating room over a long period of time).

■ **Bad debt:** An amount due to the HCO that will never be collected (for example, a patient who has no coverage for care and cannot pay the bill). Too much bad debt will be a serious problem for an organization.

■ **Balance sheet:** A financial statement identifying the HCO's assets and liabilities at a specific time. Assets are always found on the left of the balance sheet and liabilities on the right.

■ **Budgeted figures:** The projected numbers the HCO expects in revenues and expenses that are identified in the budget.

■ **Cost center:** The smallest functional unit that can be identified for cost control and accountability (for example, the cardiac care unit, the emergency department, pharmacy, etc.).

■ **Cost per case:** The expense to the HCO for providing care to a specific patient from admission to discharge.

■ **Cost per unit of service or unit cost:** The cost to produce a single unit of service (for example, provide a specific laboratory test, administer medications, prepare a meal, clean a room after discharge, or make a home visit).

■ **Depreciation:** Allocation of cost of large capital assets by recognizing a portion of the cost for each year of its estimated life. If the HCO purchases an MRI machine, it would estimate how long these machines typically last and then determine how much of the cost to allocate to the budget each year. For example, if the equipment costs $10,000, and the equipment is expected to last for 5 years, the organization would allocate a certain amount of the $10,000 for each year. At the end of the 5 years the equipment would not be an asset with value.

- **Direct costs:** Costs that are incurred in giving direct care, which is not so simple to allocate as it depends on the focus. For example, direct cost for a nurse working in a neonatal unit would be costs of the nurse's time to provide an infant care or the supplies required to provide that care.
- **Expenditure:** A liability that is incurred from the acquisition of an asset (e.g., buying new equipment for the laboratory).
- **Expense:** A decrease in the HCO's equity due to operations (e.g., funds to purchase medical supplies, staff hours).
- **Fiscal year:** The identified time period for each budget cycle (July to July or January to January), which is then subdivided in a variety of ways—for example, biweekly, monthly, quarterly, semiannually.
- **Fixed costs:** The costs that do not increase or decrease as a result of changes in volume or patient days (for example, specific salary levels, minimum staffing required, electricity, depreciation, telephone, computer).
- **Income statement:** A statement of revenues and expenses for a specific time period (see Box 14-7).
- **Indirect costs:** Costs that are indirectly related to patient care; for example, supplies needed to provide care would be direct costs while the unit secretary's time to order supplies would be indirect. However, despite the distinction noted in this definition and the definition of direct costs, the salaries for all involved in the examples (nurses, supervisor, and unit secretary) would be listed under direct costs in the budget.
- **Indirect overhead:** Costs that cannot be associated with a specific patient care provided or support services. These costs are usually allocated to a department (for example, time spent completing unit data logs or ordering supplies).

BOX 14-7   Sample income statement form.

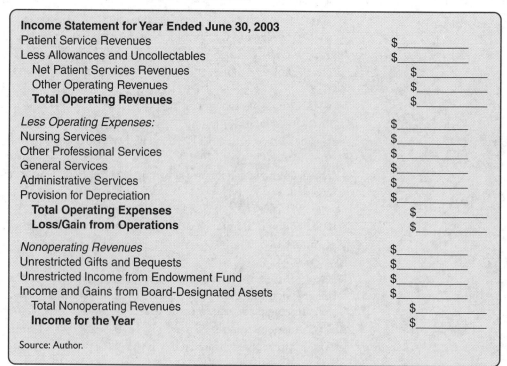

Income Statement for Year Ended June 30, 2003

Patient Service Revenues	$_____	
Less Allowances and Uncollectables	$_____	
Net Patient Services Revenues		$_____
Other Operating Revenues		$_____
Total Operating Revenues		$_____
Less Operating Expenses:	$_____	
Nursing Services	$_____	
Other Professional Services	$_____	
General Services	$_____	
Administrative Services	$_____	
Provision for Depreciation	$_____	
Total Operating Expenses		$_____
Loss/Gain from Operations		$_____
Nonoperating Revenues	$_____	
Unrestricted Gifts and Bequests	$_____	
Unrestricted Income from Endowment Fund	$_____	
Income and Gains from Board-Designated Assets	$_____	
Total Nonoperating Revenues		$_____
Income for the Year		$_____

Source: Author.

- **Liabilities:** Money an organization owes to someone.
- **Overhead:** Any cost of doing business that is not a direct cost of service and cannot easily be allocated to individual patients and even to individual units or services (e.g., utility costs).
- **PD:** Patient day.
- **Per diem reimbursement:** Payment for a day of care regardless of the specific services provided each day.
- **Prospective reimbursement:** Payment schedules established prior to providing services.
- **Retrospective reimbursement:** Payment for services after they are provided (e.g., DRGs).
- **Total costs:** The combination of fixed and variable costs.
- **Unit of services:** The specific unit of health care service that a department or unit provides to its consumers (e.g., patient day, specific treatment or procedures, meals served, patient visits to a clinic, number of home visits).
- **Variable costs:** Costs that fluctuate with census or patient days, treatments, clinic visits, home visits, and so on. Costs that might be affected are number of meals, staffing levels, linen requirements, supplies, and so on.
- **Variance report:** A report describing the difference between the budgeted and actual figures.
- **Wage index:** The factor that is used to compare wages paid to specific categories of personnel in HCOs, such as hospitals, across the country (Finkelman, 1996, pp. 1-4:2-4:3; Finkler & Korney, 2000).

The budgeting process: An overview

The budgetary process is long and cyclic. As soon as it is complete for the year, it begins again. Effective and realistic budgets require reliable data. What is a budget? It is a statement, usually annual, that describes the expected revenues or money that will be made by the organization and expected expenses that will be required to provide the services. The budget should identify financial resources, who will use them, when, and the purpose of their use. Box 14-8 provides a sample departmental budget form.

Budgets must be live documents as they will need to be adjusted. Effective budgets are consistent with critical organizational qualifiers such as the vision, mission, goals, short-term and long-term strategic plans, and marketing plan. Budgets are composed of three parts:

1. **Salary and wage budget,** which is the largest part and includes salaries and wages, earned benefits (sick time, vacation time, health benefits, and so on), premium or overtime pay, and merit raises.
2. **Operational budget,** which includes the estimate of the volume and mix of activities and services, and the resources required to provide them.
3. **Capital budget,** which is the estimate of purchases of major capital items such as equipment, building, new furniture; it typically sets a cost amount to identify which items are to be included.

Management is responsible for three major budget functions.

- The first function is planning the budget, which is ongoing.
- The second function is management of ongoing activities and services in relationship to the budgeted items.
- The third function is control of spending, which requires careful identification of variances when the budget is not met and analysis of reasons for these variances. There has to be frequent review of the proposed budget and the actual budget. If there is a variance or difference between what was proposed in the budget and what was actually spent or money received, then this needs to be analyzed. For example, if the proposed annual budget allocated an amount for staff recruitment and then the hospital finds that more staff have resigned than was expected, the hospital will need more funds for additional recruitment expenses. This may affect other aspects of the organization if there is a need to cut other expenses to cover these other important needs. Patterns are then analyzed. Critical variance questions are:
    1. What effect does the variance have?
    2. Why did the variance occur?

BOX 14-8 Department budget.

Department/Unit:_____Fiscal Year:_____

Unit of Service/Patient Days		
Unit of Service/_____ *	_____ Revenue	_____
Unit of Service/_____ *	_____ Revenue	
	_____ Revenue	
	Total Revenue	

Expenses
Productive Salaries
Nonproductive Salaries
  TOTAL SALARIES
Employee Benefits
Medical Supplies
Dietary
Minor Equipment
Equipment Rental
Audiovisual Supplies
Recreational Supplies
Copying
Printing
Books/Literature Staff
Books/Literature Patients
Maintenance
Housekeeping
Linens

Total Expenses
Profit

*Unit of service (UOS) may include more than patient days and should be identified in option categories such as UOS/procedure, group session, patient visit.
Comments:

Nurse Manager Signature:_____Date:_____

Source: Author.

3. What can be done to prevent its re-occurrence?
4. What needs to be done to make the best of the situation?

Data about variances will also be used when the next year's budget is developed to better estimate needs. Box 14-9 provides an example of a variance analysis.

Why are budgets developed? Every organization has one, and it consumes staff time to develop the annual budget and then to implement it. The major reasons for developing the budget are to:

1. Provide a financial and statistical expression of the plans for the organization
2. Identify how resources (staff, equipment, space, finances) are to be allocated
3. Provide a basis for measurement and evaluation of actual performance of the organization's plan
4. Provide periodic reports that assist in management decision making
5. Create cost awareness throughout the organization
6. Assist management in determining rates or prices

Budgets are more than just the initial financial data described; otherwise, these goals could not be met. The budget includes data about performance as the budget is applied over the year. It is this performance that organizations use to guide budgetary decisions throughout the year. Is the organization making as much money (revenues) as they thought they would? If not, what impact does this have on expenses? If more money is made than was predicted in the budget, should the organization use that money or invest it? All of these questions have an impact on nurses and nursing care.

BOX 14-9 Budget Variance Analysis and Justification Form.

BUDGET VARIANCE ANALYSIS AND JUSTIFICATION FORM
Month_____ Year_____ Unit_____

PART A:

	Budgeted	Actual	Variance		Variance%
1. Patient Days/Visits/Cases	_____	_____	_____	Days/Visits/Cases	_____
2. Staff Vacancy (full-time equivalents [FTEs])	_____	_____	_____	FTEs	_____
3. Acuity	_____	_____	_____	HPPD	_____
Other:					
4. Orientation	_____	_____	_____	hours	_____
5. Benefits	_____	_____	_____	hours	_____
6. Charge Pay	_____	_____	_____	hours	_____
7. Call Back	_____	_____	_____	hours	_____
8. Minimum Staffing	_____	_____	_____	hours	_____

PART B:

			Current Month		Year-to-date	
Salaries	Budgeted	Actual	Variance	Budgeted	Actual	Variance
Staff _____	_____	—_____	_____	_____	_____	_____
Agency _____	_____	—_____	_____	_____	_____	_____
TOTAL _____	_____	—_____	_____	_____	_____	_____

PLAN OF ACTION/FOLLOW UP: JUSTIFICATION

1. Patient Days/Visits/Cases Variance	= $_____
2. FTE Variance Hours	= $_____
Agency ×_____ Hour	= $_____
Other ×_____ Hour	= $_____
3. Acuity Variance*	= $_____
4. Orientation Variance	= $_____
5. Benefit Variance	= $_____
6. Charge Pay	= $_____
7. Call Back	= $_____
8. Minimum Staffing	= $_____
TOTAL JUSTIFIED VARIANCE	= $_____
TOTAL UNJUSTIFIED VARIANCE	= $_____

*In order to USE acuity in justification process, all acuity audits must be complete for the month and accuracy must be between 95 and 100%.

Items	Budgeted	Actual	$ Variance	Year-to-Date	$ Variance Justification	Follow-up	Plan of Action
Contract Service Fees	_____	_____	_____	_____	_____	_____	_____
General Supplies	_____	_____	_____	_____	_____	_____	_____
Food	_____	_____	_____	_____	_____	_____	_____
Medical/Surgical Supplies	_____	_____	_____	_____	_____	_____	_____
Drugs	_____	_____	_____	_____	_____	_____	_____
Copies	_____	_____	_____	_____	_____	_____	_____
Printing	_____	_____	_____	_____	_____	_____	_____
Minor Equipment	_____	_____	_____	_____	_____	_____	_____
Equipment Repairs	_____	_____	_____	_____	_____	_____	_____
Equipment Rental	_____	_____	_____	_____	_____	_____	_____
Books/Literature	_____	_____	_____	_____	_____	_____	_____
Travel	_____	_____	_____	_____	_____	_____	_____
Education	_____	_____	_____	_____	_____	_____	_____

Items that require justification and plan of action/follow-up should be checked and the information attached to this report.

TOTAL EXPENSE (includes salary plus agency)		**CURRENT MONTH**	**YEAR-TO-DATE**
	Budgeted	$_____	$_____
	Actual	$_____	$_____
	Variance	$_____	$_____
	Justified	$_____	$_____
	Unjustified	$_____	$_____

Source: Felteau, A., Budget variance analysis and justification. *Nursing Management, 23*(2), 1992 S-N Publications, Inc., Reprinted with permission.

There are several advantages to developing and implementing a budget. First, of course, budgets force the organization to plan. Just as a family that has a certain income should plan how money will be spent, saved, and invested, an organization has this responsibility. It encourages many levels of staff to participate in overall and unit/service/department planning. Cost containment is another major advantage of budgeting—forcing staff to consider how they use resources (allocation of services) and to consider how money needs to be conserved. The budgetary process provides opportunity for self-analysis, motivating staff, and the organization to improve performance.

There are also disadvantages to budgeting. There can be disagreement among management staff about the budget, and consensus can be difficult to obtain. Staff at all levels need to understand the process and its implications, which requires education or training. Many organizations do not provide this to their staff. Budgeting does require flexibility as needs change, and sometimes making these changes is difficult. Another difficulty is some managers may focus too much on the budget without consideration of other organizational issues found in the vision, mission, goals, and strategic plans. Clearly, overbudgeting can lead to major problems, as can ignoring downturns and not adjusting the budget accordingly. The latter issues can lead to problems of survival for the organization as it might slip into "the red" and then not be able to meet its financial demands.

As budgets are developed, the two main components of the budget are revenues and expenses. Revenues are projected based on past experiences and plans for the probable future. Types of data that are important to consider are number of patient days, procedures, treatments, length-of-stay, number of clinic visits, number of home visits, types of patients, and so on. If the organization plans on adding new services, then data will have to be based on more speculation based on what might be. Data about other organizations might be used to project these revenues (for example, adding a new home care service and how this service might compete with other home care agencies). Strategic plans are also reviewed to identify possible revenues and expenses that might be affected by the plan. Probable expenses are carefully analyzed, again using past data. Examples of typical expense categories are:

- Salary and wages
- Benefits
- Medical supplies and other supplies
- Depreciation
- Administration costs
- Housekeeping
- Dietary
- Professional fees and other fees the HCO may be required to pay
- Capital equipment
- Furniture and furnishings
- Maintenance
- Pharmacy
- Orientation and education
- Printing
- Information technology
- Utilities
- Landscaping
- Legal fees
- Parking and security

Some of the expenses are fixed as they do not change due to activity and service levels, and some are variable as they do change due to activity and service levels. For example, costs for orientation increase when the numbers of new staff increase; number of deliveries increases costs for the obstetrical department; and number of snow storms increases the need for parking lot snow removal.

Productivity

Productivity must be considered during the budgetary process and also when changes occur in the health care arena. **Productivity** is the ratio of output (products and services) to input (resources consumed). The goal is to increase productivity or at the minimum not to decrease it. To do this, factors that affect both input and output need to be evaluated.

■ Examples of factors affecting input are: staff characteristics (mix, qualifications, experience, stability, length of shift, mandatory overtime), patients (number, ages, acuity, diagnoses, treatments), and organization (unit configuration, size, staffing, leadership and management, equipment, services, financial status).

■ Examples of factors affecting output are: number of emergency visits, deliveries, admissions, clinic visits, meals served, radiological procedures, total number of patient days, surgical procedures, and acuity.

What methods are used to assess productivity? Some examples are a patient acuity or classification system, cost accounting, budget reports, position control, quality improvement monitoring, and full-time equivalent (FTE) analysis. An FTE is a full-time position that is equated to 40 hours of work per week, 80 hours per pay period, or 2,080 hours per year. It is not a person but a unit of time or time actually worked. Nonproductive time is included in the paid hours; productive time is actual time worked. The principal measure of input is worked hours, worked FTEs, or paid hours. However, it is also important to measure both "worked hours" productivity and paid hours productivity, which includes benefit allowances for sick time, vacation, and holidays.

Productivity = output divided by input

EXAMPLE:

Input: 24 hours of nursing care (one patient day). Inputs are predetermined budgeted nursing care hours per patient day based on the patient's acuity and required patient care activities.
Outputs: the outcomes; achieved patient goals.

Two critical issues in productivity are efficiency and effectiveness. Efficiency is doing things right while effectiveness is doing the right things. Both of these need to be assessed when productivity is analyzed. Cost containment and quality are related to productivity. Analyzing outcome variances is part of the process. Productivity is affected by staffing patterns, methods of organization, and the usage of nurse extender mechanisms such as other support staff to assist nurses (Eastnaugh, 2002).

Cost containment

Cost containment must be part of the budgetary process, or the HCO may not survive. The problem with cost containment is it has a bad name. Seeing it only as a negative experience will limit the success of the effort. Quality and cost containment should be and are definitely connected. When decisions are made to control costs, there needs to be a balance. How does the cost of care affect quality? If costs are reduced, will quality of care be affected and in what way? These are critical questions that must be asked, and nurses who are involved in budgetary decisions should speak up and ask them. As this process occurs, ethical issues may be brought up when difficult decisions are made. The typical cost-containment methods are:

■ Decrease overtime expenses
■ Decrease sick time expenses

- Prevent costly expenses for repair of equipment
- Use supplies wisely
- Decrease the inventory of supplies that are infrequently used or not used at all
- Maintain productivity standards
- Prevent employee accidents
- Use methods to improve staffing decisions (Finkelman, 1996, p. 1-4:12)

There often is a fear in organizations that cost-containment decisions are only made by financial staff. This is a legitimate concern. These decisions should be made jointly with other management staff who appreciate the clinical implications of these decisions. There is no doubt today that budget cuts do occur, and many are necessary. Staff need to understand the reason for the cuts before the rumor mill about the cuts does major damage to morale. Nursing management should seek out facts to respond to budget cuts and to plan. If nursing management approaches all budget cuts with a negative attitude, assuming that all cuts are nonproductive, nursing management will not be able to work collaboratively with the HCO's other management staff. Cost-containment efforts require an honest appraisal of the needs and approaches to resolving them. Nurse leaders need to be team players and willing to step back and objectively assess a problem. This does not mean that they do not advocate for nursing and for patient care delivery, but rather they do this in a professional manner. They need to approach communication about the problems and the cuts openly with other staff, providing explanations and support as needed. Staff too can be brought into the process as they may have some excellent ideas about how problems may be resolved. In the end, budget cuts need to be made carefully with consideration given to short-term and long-term effects. Nurse leaders must assume an active role in all phases of the process.

BENCHMARKS

Now let's take a moment to test your knowledge of the concepts you have studied in this section.

Chapter Wrap-Up

Now that you've reached the end of the chapter, you may wish to explore the concepts you've been reading about in greater detail, or test yourself to see how well you've comprehended the material.

SUMMARY AND APPLICATIONS

- Summary
- Practice Quiz
- Key Terms
- Tying It All Together

- Experiential Exercises
- Case
- Links

REFERENCES

Arndt, M., & Skydell, B. (1985). Inpatient nursing services: Productivity and cost. In E. Shaffer (Ed.), *Costing out nursing: Pricing our products.* New York: National League for Nursing.

Baldor, R. (1998). *Managed care made simple* (2nd ed.). Malden, MA: Blackwell Science.

Britt, T., Schraeder, C., & Shelton, P. (1998). *Managed care and capitation: Issues in nursing.* Washington, DC: American Nurses Publishing.

Centers for Medicare and Medicaid Services (http://www.cms.gov). Retrieved from June, 2004.

Cooper, P., & Schone, B. (1997). More offers, fewer takers for employment-based health insurance: 1987–1996. *Health Affairs, 16*(6), 142–149.

Eastnaugh, S. (2002). Hospital nurse productivity. *Journal of Health Care Finance, 29*(1), 14–22.

Finkelman, A. (1996). *Quality assurance for psychiatric nursing.* Gaithersburg, MD: Aspen Publishers, Inc.

Finkler, S., & Korney, C. (2000). *Financial management for nurse managers and executives.* Philadelphia: W. B. Saunders Company.

Fosbinder, D. (1986). Nursing costs/DRG: A patient classification system and comparative study. *Journal of Nursing Administration, 16*(11), 18–23.

Ginsburg, P., & Gabel, J. (1998). Tracking health care costs: What's new in 1997? *Health Affairs, 17*(5), 142–146.

Gottlieb, M. (1998). *The confused consumer's guide to choosing a health care plan.* New York: Hyperion.

Health Insurance Association of America. (1998). *Managed care: Integrating the delivery and financing of health care, Part A.* Washington, DC: Author.

Kaiser Commission on the Future of Medicaid. (1997). *Medicaid facts: The Medicaid program at a glance.* Washington, DC: The Kaiser Foundation.

Knight, W. (1998). *Managed care: What it is and how it works.* Gaithersburg, MD: Aspen Publishers, Inc.

Kolata, G., & Eichenwald, F. (1999, December 16). Group of insurers to pay for experimental cancer therapy. *New York Times,* C1, C10.

Kongstvedt, P. (2001), *The managed care handbook,* Gaithersburg, MD: Aspen Publishers, Inc.

Korczyk, S., & Witte, H. (1998). *The idiot's guide to managed health care.* New York: Alpha Books.

McCarthy, R. (1998). Biotech millennium: All you need is $1 million and a dream. *Drug Benefit Trends, 10*(11), 33–38.

McQueen, J., & Marwick, P. (1995). Introduction: Evolution of patient-focused care within the contractual framework of an integrated delivery system. *Journal of Health Care Finance, 51*(6), 5–9.

Meinhardt, R. (1998). Legal matters—Congress takes aim at retail pharmacy pricing. *Drug Benefit Trends, 10*(11), 21–22.

National League for Nursing. (1978). *Financial management of department of nursing services.* New York: Author.

Pear, R. (1999, May 23). Insurers ask government to extend health plans. *New York Times,* Y16.

Pear, R. (2003a, September 3). Emergency rooms get eased rules on patient care. *New York Times,* A1, A15.

Pear, R. (2003b, December 9). Medicare law's costs and benefits are elusive. *New York Times,* A1, A18.

Priester, R. (1997). Does managed care offer value to society? *Managed Care Quarterly, 5*(1), 57–63.

Reres, M. (1996). *Managed care: Managing the process.* Glencoe, MO: National Professional Education Institute.

Rognehaugh, R. (1998). *The managed health care dictionary.* Gaithersburg, MD: Aspen Publishers, Inc.

Schmidt, D. (2001). Financial management for patient care managers. In J. Dochterman & H. Grace (Eds.), *Current issues in nursing* (6th ed., pp. 420–429). St. Louis, MO: Mosby, Inc.

Seefeldt, F., Garg, M., & Grace, H. (2001). Controlling health care costs: Regulation vs. competition. In J. Dochterman & H. Grace (Eds.), *Current issues in nursing* (6th ed., pp. 377–387). St. Louis, MO: Mosby, Inc.

Shamian, J., Hagen, B., Hu, T., & Fogarty, T. (1994). The relationship between length-of-stay and required nursing care hours. *Journal of Nursing Administration, 24*(7/8), 52–58.

Smith, S., et al. (1998). The next 10 years of health spending: What does the future hold? *Health Affairs, 16*(6), 128–140.

Stickler, J. (1994). System development and integration in health care. *Journal of Nursing Administration, 24*(10), 48–53.

Sullivan, F., & Decker, P. (2001) *Effective leadership and management in nursing.* Upper Saddle River, NJ: Prentice Hall, Inc.

Taylor, R. (1998). Managed care woes: Industry trends and conflicts. *Issue Brief: Center for Studying Health System Change, 13*(May), 1–4.

U.S. Census Bureau (2004). http://www.census.gov.

Wolford, G., Brown, M., & McCool, B. (1996). Getting to go in managed care. In M. Brown (Ed.), *Integrated health care delivery* (pp. 12–24). Gaithersburg, MD: Aspen Publishers, Inc.

ADDITIONAL READINGS

American Nurses Association. (1995). *Nursing's social policy statement.* Washington, DC: American Nurses Publishing.

Boulter, C., Maben, P., & Oatway, D. (1999). *Prospective payment for long term care.* Washington, DC: American Nurses Association.

Dochterman, J., & Grace, H. (2001). Overview: A concern for costs. In J. Dochterman & H. Grace (Eds.), *Current issues in nursing* (6th ed., pp. 374–376). St. Louis, MO: Mosby, Inc.

Eastaugh, S. (2002). Hospital nurse productivity. *Journal of Health Care Finance, 29*(1), 14–22.

Grimaldi, P. (1995a). Capitation savvy a must. *Nursing Management, 26*(2), 33–34.

Grimaldi, P. (1995b). Searching for managed care savings. *Nursing Management, 26*(10), 14, 17.

Hunt, P. (2001). Speaking the language of finance. *AORN Journal, 73*(4), 774–786.

Kilborn, P. (1999, February 26). Uninsured in U.S. span many groups. *New York Times,* A1, A14.

Klemczak, J., & Dontje, K. (2001). Paradigm shift: Taking care of patients and taking care of business. In J. Dochterman & H. Grace (Eds.), *Current issues in nursing* (6th ed., pp. 405–410). St. Louis, MO: Mosby, Inc.

Kuttner, R. (1999a). The American health care system. Health insurance coverage. *New England Journal of Medicine, 340*(2), 163–168.

Kuttner, R. (1999b). The American health care system. Employer-sponsored health coverage. *New England Journal of Medicine, 340*(3), 248–252.

Lagnado, I. (1998, November 17). The uncovered: Drug costs can leave elderly a grim choice: Pills or other needs. *Wall Street Journal,* A1.

Lamb, G. (1995). Early lessons learned from a capitated community-based nursing model. *Nursing Administration Quarterly, 19*(1), 18–26.

Lee, J. (2001). Reimbursement for alternative providers. In J. Dochterman & H. Grace (Eds.), *Current issues in nursing* (6th ed., pp. 411–419). St. Louis, MO: Mosby, Inc.

Lesser, C., & Ginsburg, P. (2003). Health care cost and access: Problems intensify. *Issue Briefs,* No. 63.

Maddox, P. (2001). Managed care, prospective payment, and reimbursement trends: Impact and implications for nursing. In J. Dochterman & H. Grace (Eds.), *Current issues in nursing* (6th ed., pp. 387–400). St. Louis, MO: Mosby, Inc.

Malloch, K., & Porter-O'Grady, T. (1999). Partnership economics: Nursing's challenge in a quantum age. *Nursing Economics, 17*(6), 299–307.

Scala-Foley, M., Caruso, J., Archer, D., & Reinhard, S. (2004). Making sense of Medicare. Medicare's preventive services. *American Journal of Nursing, 104*(4), 73–75.

Scala-Foley, M., Caruso, J., Ramos, R., & Reinhard, S. (2004). Making sense of Medicare. Medicare eligibility, enrollment, and coverage. *American Journal of Nursing, 104*(2), 81–83.

WORK ENVIRONMENT

In this area so basic to nursing's future, members of the profession will work to improve nurses' work environments so that quality patient care is optimized and professional nursing staff is retained.

Desired Future Statement (Vision)

Nurses provide quality care in dynamic and satisfying environments that utilize their specialized skills and knowledge. These environments promote health and safety, appropriate staffing, shared decision making, collaboration, mentoring, and professional growth.

Six strategies were identified to achieve the vision and one of these was identified as the primary or driving strategy. They are:

Nurses have an effective voice in decision making. (Primary Strategy)

Professional development is fostered for nurses in all roles.

Sound methods are identified and utilized to assure appropriate staffing.

Collaborative work relationships are actively enhanced and promoted.

Support is demonstrated for quality of work life and safety at work.

Practices are defined and implemented that produce quality patient care.

Objectives to Support Primary Strategy

Build educational programs that result in articulate nurses who effectively participate in decision making.

Create infrastructures and practices in health care that foster nurses' participation in decision making at all levels or organizations.

Increase significantly nurses' representation and participation in health policy agencies, committees, and consumer boards.

Develop and disseminate reliable systems, based on scientific evidence, that guide staffing and resource allocation.

SOURCE: American Nurses Association. (2002). *Nursing's agenda for the future. A call to the nation*. Washington, DC: Author. Reprinted with permission.

Technology and Health Care

MediaLink
www.prenhall.com/finkelman

The Interactive Exercises for this chapter can be found in the OneKey course at www.prenhall.com/finkelman. Click on Chapter 15 to select from the following activities: Test Your Understanding, Benchmarks, Current Issues, Your Opinion Counts, Think Critically, and Summary and Applications.

What's Ahead

"A massive communications revolution (paradigm shift) is under way, one that will have profound effects upon the art and science of nursing" (Richards, 2001, p. 6). This offers important opportunities for nursing education, practice, research, and administration. Is nursing ready for this? Will nursing move too slowly to gain full benefits of the movement? "Imagine a world where no matter who you are or where you are, you get the health care you need when you need it. A world where people living in far-flung areas need not travel hundreds of miles to get specialty care that could save their lives? A world where you will be treated in an emergency room by a nurse at your side and a physician at a distant emergency department? A world where doctors and nurses in rural America can learn about new medical practices at the touch of a computer key" (U.S. Human Resources and Services Administration, 1999). For nurses to participate in the technology revolution, whether staff nurse or in a management position, they need to be knowledgeable about health care technology, appreciate the implications of its use, develop the required skills, and apply them to practice and management. This chapter discusses critical technology issues and their implications for health care practice and management.

OBJECTIVES

Before you begin, take a moment to familiarize yourself with the key objectives of this chapter.

■ Discuss the importance of information and clinical technology to nursing.

■ Describe the critical issues related to privacy and confidentiality.

■ Define telehealth.

■ Identify the implications of telehealth to nursing practice, education, administration, and research.

■ Describe how telehealth can be used for patient education.

TEST YOUR UNDERSTANDING

Before we begin our exploration of this chapter, take a short "warm-up" test to see what you know about this topic.

Importance of Information and Clinical Technology

Critical factors

The explosion of information and technology has brought the health care delivery system into a new era, which has allowed health care to expand into new areas and to improve others. Information and technology have affected clinical practice, communication, structure of organizations, consumers, workforce issues, quality care issues and outcomes, costs and reimbursement, and ethical and legal concerns. In July 2002, the American Nurses Association (ANA) sponsored an important conference, "Using Innovative Technology to Enhance Patient Care Delivery." This conference focused on the following seven issues that reflect the broad impact of technology in today's health care environment, all of which have an impact on nurses.

■ Improve patient safety and quality

■ Improve operational efficiency and effectiveness in interdisciplinary practice

■ Improve medication use processes to decrease errors

■ Improve health technologies that empower patient and enhance patient care

■ Create future care environments that improve efficiencies, clinical outcomes, and the healing experience

■ Improve practice environments through simulation

■ Improve workforce productivity through automation

There is much known and much unknown about the implications of a technologically driven environment. At the same time that technology and information are surging forward, health care is confronted with a severe nursing shortage as well as shortages of other health care providers. Can information technology help to resolve this problem (Meadows, 2002)? Many examples are described in this chapter that may make a difference or at least make health care delivery more efficient and effective. Technology may be one of these factors. "Clinical information systems can be one of those immediate actions that can help nurses feel more confident about the care they are delivering. In addition to preventing medical errors, streamlining workflow and communications, and reducing redundant data entry, these systems can have a lasting and positive effect on overall job satisfaction, providing significant influence on retaining our invaluable nursing resources" (Meadows, 2002, p. 48).

Even though there are many positive aspects of information technology (IT), some drawbacks exist that need to be considered as health care organizations incorporate more IT. "Connectivity is the buzzword of the new millennium. We are connected to the Internet, to local area networks, and to paging systems and voice mailboxes. But are we forgetting the goal of emotional connectivity" (Simpson & Keegan, 2002, p. 80)? It is particularly important for health care providers to consider the total impact of technology on practice and organizations. Emotional Intelligence leadership, which was discussed in Chapter 1, has become more important in organizations with staff tuning in more to their emotions and reactions, how these emotions and reactions affect others, and making changes in behavior to improve relationships and communications. Technology may interfere with this process. Talking through "machines" limits real observations and emotional connections. Does it increase isolation? Does it prevent honest communication? If it does, then it is important to try to figure out ways to prevent these problems. Advancement of technologies is not going away so it is important to use it effectively. Patients need providers who are connected to them, understand the emotional side of health care, and use the power of the human interaction. The goal should not be to throw out or ignore information technology but rather to be aware of potential problems and build in methods to maintain personal connection with patients. It is also important to note that this feeling of isolationism can occur with staff. Despite these concerns, "The recognition is finally here that you can't practice medicine in the 21st century without information technology support" (Landro, 2002, June 10, p. 1). IT cannot be separated from knowledge expansion—with so much increasing knowledge how can one keep up? Health care organizations now need clinical decision-support tools and information systems more than ever. This is very costly, but no organization can afford not to invest in the technology to keep up. In addition, insurers, managed care, and accrediting groups demand more and more data to demonstrate outcomes. The nursing profession needs to appreciate the importance of data and how best to use data. IT provides much data about health care including nursing, and tapping into these data to better understand both the impact of nursing care on patient outcomes and the cost of care can benefit nursing.

CURRENT ISSUES

Learn about events around the globe that relate to the chapter content.

Technical skills

Is nursing ready to play a major role in the revolution of information and technology? There has been a major deficiency in nurses' computer skills; however, the younger generations are very different because they have grown up with computers. "These new graduates will bring with them new, powerful tools for inquiry, analysis, and self-expression. They will begin to question the implicit values contained in information we have historically championed and cherished within our profession" (Richards, 2001, p. 6). This is the Net Generation, who in 1999 were between the ages of 2 and 22 (Richards, 2001). They are media-literate and expect interactivity. This group demands more and more communication, information, and interactivity. Nurses outside this group will be playing catch up, and many of these nurses are now the ones in leadership positions. If these leaders do not recognize the importance of the IT environment, miss opportunities, and reject changes, the newer nurses will be frustrated with their leadership.

Technical IQ (TIQ) focuses on knowledge of specific functioning of a technology and an understanding of relationships among technology, staff and consumers, and systems (Kerfoot, 2000). The first issue is to keep ahead and to anticipate based on technological changes that can and will affect patient care and thus require changes in education, research, and administration. Information and computers are shifting from binary units to "fuzzy logic" (Kosko, 1999). What does this mean to nursing? The clean lines that separate concepts are disappearing, if they were ever there. Kerfoot (2000) shares the example of how health care has structured the hospital into discrete units. With these units, walls have been created—barriers to intercommunication, collaboration, coordination, and effective communication. Patient-centered care is an attempt to remove these walls and move away from linear, binary thinking to systems thinking. Computer systems will help with this change. The five areas that are more than likely the top key change areas of the near future are:

1. Computing—moving toward more and more innovations that will increase the chance of developing artificial intelligence
2. Telemedicine
3. Lasers
4. Genetic engineering
5. Alternative energy sources (Stix & Lacob, 1999, as cited in Kerfoot, 2000, pp. 30–31)

Many other potential innovations probably exist that have not even been thought of at this time.

Information technology: Critical issues

As information explodes and staff try to cope with it and want it to be helpful to them, several issues become important, particularly privacy and confidentiality and the clinical information system.

Privacy and confidentiality

The 1996 Health Insurance Portability and Accountability Act (HIPAA) has had major effects on IT. First, the act mandates that there be a standardized method for insurance companies and physicians to reduce overhead and increase the payment time for patient care, but this must be done in a manner that ensures patient privacy. Privacy and confidentiality have long been issues in health care, and IT developed with little control related to privacy and confidentiality. This law, however, has had an effect on IT. Chapter 10 contains additional content about this law and recent changes. The law identifies steps that must be taken by health care providers to protect this privacy. Today health care organizations of all types are required to meet certain requirements to better ensure patient privacy and confidentiality.

Clinical information system

"The ability of health care delivery networks to effectively manage and leverage clinical information to meet strategic clinical goals is a cornerstone of their transformation and survival as integrated information-based clinical enterprises. Successful health care delivery networks will be those that can apply emerging clinical information technologies to meet strategic clinical goals" (Kissinger & Borchardt, 1996; Snyder-Halpern & Chervany, 2000, p. 591). It is difficult to find a health care organization that is not using or evaluating for use some type of clinical information system. Some systems have been more effective than others. Making decisions about these clinical information systems is a complex process requiring input from many staff throughout an organization. Selecting the right system is not easy. It is also a very costly decision. After the selection, staff require training and need time to adjust. What is needed to develop a clinical information system strategic plan?

1. A clinical vision should be developed that describes the organization's future view of itself. What does the organization believe about the role of IT in its services? This will provide guidelines for how invested the organization will be and at what cost.
2. Clinical strategy should include the general organizational activities that support the organization's vision. This needs to include external influences. How will or could IT affect this strategy?
3. Strategic clinical goals are then developed that are important for the organization and its work. What needs to be included in the goals to support IT?
4. Strategic clinical vital signs are used to evaluate whether or not goals are obtained. How can IT be used to collect data, analyze data, and perform decision making? These goals are then used in the evaluation of IT to assist in determining needed improvements (Snyder-Halpern & Chervany, 2000, pp. 585–586).

As these questions are considered, the organization needs to review such factors as the role of nurses. Will nurses be able to access the IT system for documentation, to obtain clinical resource information, e-mail, and so on? Will physician orders be covered by the system, which has an impact on nursing? Will the IT system become integral to all aspects of the organization? How will staff have input into the system? These are only a few of the considerations that have an impact on health care IT systems.

BENCHMARKS

Now let's take a moment to test your knowledge of the concepts you have studied in this section.

Technology: Implications on Health Care Delivery

Technology is more than just IT, as it also includes technology that can be applied to clinical care, education, and research. The following discussion provides some information about the impact that technology has had and will continue to have on various aspects of health care delivery.

Telehealth

Telehealth is the use of telecommunications equipment and communications networks for transferring health care information between participants at different locations. This technology offers opportunities to provide care when face-to-face interaction is impossible. Telehealth applies telecommunication and computer technologies to the broad spectrum of public health and medicine (U.S. Department of Health and Human Services 1998). In addition, it provides many opportunities for consumer health informatics (see Chapter 11). Using technology in health care was even addressed in bioterrorism legislation, which included funding for telemedicine network expansion (Wiley, 2002). The hope is that there would be greater use of this technology to expand emergency public health response to bioterrorism and other public health emergencies. The future holds more opportunity for telehealth with the following changes occurring in telehealth.

■ A shift from a predominately rural focus to the provision of home care and school-based health care in the inner city

■ The movement from a preoccupation with acquisition and transport of information to an emphasis on the quality of the information being transmitted

■ A switch from a practitioner-based health care system to a patient-empowered and preventive health care system, and in turn, from a patient-based system to a consumer-oriented system (Dakins, 2002, p. 14)

See Box 15-1 for descriptions of key telehealth terms, such as **Telenursing**, Telemedicine, **Telepresence**, and **videoconferencing**.

"The most successful telehealth systems employ a variety of telecommunication modalities including two-way interactive video consultations, teleradiology, and telepathology that link primary care providers in rural areas or inner city clinics to experts in large, tertiary centers. Virtual environments for health care delivery and education have been made possible by the same advances in technology that have given us lifelike, computerized video games and military robotic medics" (Predko, 2001). The technology is here to stay and will only be improved. The critical factor will be the ability of health care providers such as the nurse to envision innovative and practical ways to apply the technology to clinical practice and health care management. When it is applied, safety and quality must always be addressed and monitored.

Standards have been developed for most nursing specialties, and telehealth nursing is no exception. The American Academy of Ambulatory Care Nursing (AAACN) has developed some of these standards because "Telehealth nursing has been identified as one of the new and exciting areas of interest and specialty in ambulatory care nursing" (American Academy of Ambulatory Care Nursing, 2001, p. 7). The AAACN recognizes that telehealth nursing is an evolving

BOX 15-1   Key telehealth terms.

Telehealth

The use of telecommunications equipment and communications networks for transferring health care information between participants at different locations. This offers opportunities to provide care when face-to-face interaction is impossible.

Telenursing

A subset of telehealth that allows a nurse to deliver care through a telecommunication system. This may be as simple as just calling a patient on the telephone to more elaborate systems.

Telemedicine

Another subset of telehealth that allows physicians to provide care.

Telepresence

Combines robotics and virtual reality to allow a surgeon to manipulate equipment at a remote site.

Videoconferencing

Provides opportunity for sound and images to be transmitted to a remote site for conferences and consultation with other health care providers or with patients.

Source: Author.

specialty that requires standards. As has been stated by many experts, this area of health care directly affects consumers/patients and the organization's effectiveness. The AAACN definition of telehealth nursing practice describes it as "Nursing practice using the nursing process to provide care for individual patients or defined patient populations through telecommunications media. Telehealth nursing practice occurs in many different health care settings" (American Academy of Ambulatory Care Nursing, 2001, p. 1). Critical criteria for telehealth nursing practice include:

- Using protocols, algorithms, or guidelines to systematically assess and address patient needs.
- Prioritizing the urgency of patient needs.
- Developing a collaborative plan of care with the patient and his/her support systems. The plan of care may include: wellness promotion, prevention education, advice for care counseling, disease state management, and care coordination.
- Evaluating outcomes of practice and care (American Academy of Ambulatory Care Nursing, 2001, p. 2).
- Prioritizing, developing plans of care, and outcome evaluation are typical concerns for nurses, but protocols, algorithms, and guidelines may be new concepts for some nurses. Benefits from using these tools include: consistency, accuracy, quality, completeness, ease, and (some) legal protection. These three tools are often used interchangeably; however, they are somewhat different as can be seen in the following definitions. (See Chapter 9 for more information.)
    - **Protocols** define the ongoing care or management of a broad problem or issue in six areas: (a) assessment/data collection/caller interview process; (b) classification/determination of acuity; (c) nature/type/degree of advice/intervention/direction to the caller; (d) information/education of caller; (e) validation of patient understanding/verbal contracting; and (f) evaluation/follow-up/effectiveness of advice or intervention. A protocol directs the advice/triage/education/ counseling process, assisting in the organization of large amounts of significant information in priority order. It helps show the interrelationship of data, forcing consideration of all possible or likely decision choices and by so doing directs decision making to be based upon data.
    - **Algorithms** are written clinical questions using a branch chain logic (flowchart). An algorithm prescribes what steps to take given particular circumstances or characteristics. Some algorithms also include designated points in the decision-making process where physicians and other caregivers need to discuss with patients or families their preferences

for particular options. Algorithms rely on the nurse's ability to analyze and interpret patient responses to clinical questions.

■ Guidelines are typically a more narrative description of assessment steps that includes education and counseling text to support the nurse during the call (American Academy of Ambulatory Care Nursing, 2001, pp. 22–24).

The nurse who provides telehealth nursing uses these tools to guide clinical decisions. For example, patients who call a nurse telephone advice line that is offered to members of a managed care organization would consult specific protocols, algorithms, or guidelines for questions regarding cardiac, diabetes, or obstetrical concerns. All of these represent standards related to providing care by using technology.

Costs need to be considered for all changes in health care, and the use of technology is no exception. There needs to be careful cost-benefit analysis when decisions are made to use technology. One would assume that **telemedicine** is less costly than more traditional methods of practice if one considers staffing and time required. Whitten and co-authors (2002) conducted a systematic review of telemedicine cost-benefit studies, which included a review of 612 articles about these studies. Only 55, or 9%, of these articles included actual cost-benefit data, and of these articles only 4% met quality criteria. The conclusion from this review, which only covers a small percentage of studies that included cost-benefit aspects, was that no strong evidence existed that telemedicine is a cost-effective means of delivering health care. It is clear that there needs to be more research about this topic. Individual health care providers such as physician offices, clinics, hospitals, home care agencies, and long-term care facilities should all be doing their own cost-benefit analysis before decisions are made about using information technology and telehealth technologies and monitoring cost-benefit factions when these are implemented. It is important to avoid jumping on the bandwagon when a strategy appears new and exciting. It may offer much, but this needs careful analysis.

There are certainly barriers to telehealth that also need to be considered in the cost-benefit analysis. Examples of these barriers include:

■ Reimbursement mechanisms that do not support telehealth. Medicare provides limited reimbursement, but other insurers may not.

■ Lack of communication standards for medical devices causing problems with devices working together and upgrading devices.

■ Lack of affordable or reliable telehealth telecommunication services in some rural and inner city areas.

■ Insufficient broad-based education about home and self-care technologies and their effective utilization hinder acceptance.

■ State regulatory requirements and licensure for health care professionals inhibit cross-border consultative services; this issue has been addressed by some states that have developed multi-state licensure arrangements. Multi-state licensure is a response to this problem (see Chapter 2) (Predko, 2001, p. 79).

Many of these barriers need to be addressed if there is to be effective use of technology. The most critical barrier is a lack of reimbursement or limited reimbursement for these services. The inclusion of this content in nursing education, continuing education, and nursing research focused on this area of practice would help to lower the barriers.

YOUR OPINION COUNTS

Find out what others think about this topic. Post your response and check out other opinions.

Implications for clinical practice

There is some thought that despite the fact that nursing education is trying to prepare new graduates so that they have TIQ, there are still major deficits when it comes to applying IT to nursing practice (Richards, 2001). "Perhaps nurses, traditionally a passive group, are accepting the encroachment of computer technology in patient care with their usual resignation. If this is true, the result may be the integration of technology into nursing practice by individuals other than nurses" (Richards, 2001, p. 8). This would be a devastating result. Nurses need to be upfront, not behind, to ensure that they have a voice in how IT and other technologies are applied to nursing and to health care in general. Health care organizations need nurses who can think ahead, view technologies as opportunities, and can be creative and innovative in their approach to IT. To do this, nurses first need to understand the basics of technology. These new tools and the information that they offer can affect patient care directly. The following are examples of clinical applications of new technology.

- **Automated medication administration:** With increased data indicating that medication errors are an important factor in patient complications and deaths, there is more interest in medication administration methods that might decrease this risk (Institute of Medicine, 1999). "Point-of-service bar coding during medication administration helps caregivers ensure medication safety through automated verification that all of the "five rights" have been met: the right patient, medication, time, dose, and route" (Meadows, 2002, p. 47). Bar coding also offers an opportunity for data collection by providing critical experiential information about medication administration that can be captured in the computer. These data can assist with quality improvement processes, costs and cost effectiveness, and risk management, and help the organization meet insurer and accreditation requirements for these data. A bar code system is expensive; estimates indicate that it will cost the health care industry $1.5 billion to make the changes necessary to implement this type of system (Landro, 2002, July 29). The Institute for Safe Medication Practices (ISMP) has asked the FDA to make bar coding a requirement for all of its products that are available in unit-dose packages, and in 2003, the FDA proposed legislation that would require bar codes (Roark, 2004). The Veteran's Affairs Medical Center in Topeka, Kansas, was able to reduce its medication errors by 86.2% from 1993 to 2001 by using bar coding (Roark, 2004).

  As many drugs are no longer offered in unit-dose packages, health care organizations have had to do their own repackaging so that the unit-dose system can be used, which increases risk for errors (Landro, 2002, July 29). A unit-dose system provides individual prepackaged doses so that the nurse can more easily and safely administer the dose rather than selecting the dose from a multi-dose bottle, and so on. As of 2002, about 10 to 15% of hospitals use patient bedside technology, with nurses scanning a patient's wristband, nurse's identification badge, and the drug to be administered, which then are matched with a computerized list (Landro, 2002, July 29). Checking identification in this way can decrease identification errors that can more easily occur when the nurse just reads the information. To be effective, however, as is true with both identification methods, the nurse must initiate the method correctly. It just does not happen. If a nurse ignores what is expected, the system will not prevent errors.

- **Point-of-care clinical documentation systems:** This application has many positive results for patient care. Particularly important is that nurses document as they provide care, not hours later at the end of the shift. This is possible because electronic documentation methods are used at the bedside or each nurse has direct access to a computer while care is provided. Accuracy can be improved with these methods. No longer do staff need to struggle with interpreting handwriting, which increases the risk of errors. Point-of-care systems may also offer reminders to nurses of tasks that need to be done and help the nurse with planning (Meadows, 2002). Through the use of these documentation system trends, critical data can be obtained. It is important to note that some of these systems can interface directly with patient monitors, such as those used for vital signs, to better improve patient assessment and interventions taken. Communication can be improved as the systems can be used to enhance provider-to-provider communication that is rapid and accurate. These systems are costly; however, the long-term benefits must also be considered: accuracy, decreased errors, decreased time wasted running to get information or to document something critical, less rush at the end of the day to document when nurses are tired and more prone to make errors or may make limited comments just to complete the documentation, and a greater emphasis on bringing the care to the patient (patient-centered care).

- **Clinical data repository:** This type of system "provides longitudinal clinical data storage of patient information fed from all of the other clinical information systems, including patient demographic data" (Meadows, 2002, p. 48). These data can then be used to improve services, in research, and assist with clinical decision making. This type of documentation storage requires less physical storage space, provides more efficient access to historical data, is easier to read, and so on.

Physician order entry: This type of system is often found in health care organizations today. Physicians enter their orders into the computer rather than on a hard copy of the medical record. This has much to offer patient care and nurses. Orders are legible, which helps, as illegibility is a major problem with medical records. Some computer systems alert providers to errors, conflicts such as drug incompatibilities, and allergies. Some systems are "Eliminating errors by addressing the 'golden second'—the point between clinical decision and action" (Meadows, 2002, p. 47). Physicians can be notified when orders need to be reviewed or renewed. This also decreases the need for the nurse to be the "policeman" and remind physicians about orders. How does this help nurses? Time is saved when less time is spent following up on orders. Nurses can feel more confident that the orders are correct. Errors can be decreased—errors made by physicians when orders are incorrect, and nurse errors when orders are followed incorrectly. The medical records become interactive due to these alerts, communicating when something might be wrong or something needs to be done.

- **Electronic medical record:** Documenting in a paperless system has many advantages; for example, decreased time; reduced transcription, storage, copying, and labor costs; improved access for providers; less loss of record material; and improved access for audits (Kerfoot & Simpson, 2002). Data are available when needed with less dependence on memory, which improves clinical decision making. The record is easier to read. Access to the record by staff can occur with more ease. The problem of lost records will be a thing of the past.

- **"Smart" administration pump:** This technology offers a method to administer fluids and medications and at the same time monitor the patient at the bedside for errors (Kerfoot & Simpson, 2002). As time is always important in direct care, it is critical that the equipment maintenance and repair are monitored to ensure safe care.

- **Pharmacy system:** This system provides computerized pharmacy orders, checking, and dispensing, as well as online documentation. (Bar coding may be part of the system.) Online reference systems are also included in this type of system, allowing for application of evidence-based knowledge (Kerfoot & Simpson, 2002).

- **Remote telemetry monitoring:** This technology allows nurses to receive pages or provides a page alarm that notifies the nurse of the patient's identification, heart rate, and a readout of rhythm (Donnelly, 2000). The nurse can then evaluate the patient's condition and take appropriate action.

- **Medical e-mail:** Physicians are using e-mail more and more to communicate with their patients (Hafner, 2002). Advanced practice nurses may also find this to be a useful communication tool. There may, however, be concern that some patients may abuse this communication method, and they may also expect providers to respond quickly. In reality, this concern does not seem to be an actual problem. Some providers are using this method for select patients who send the provider daily monitoring data so that the provider can get a better picture of a problem. Messages need to be clear as misinterpretation or misunderstandings are risks. E-mail does offer a paper trail, documenting what has been told to patients, which can be helpful and decreases communication confusion. E-mail guidelines that have been developed for physicians include the following: (a) inform patient if anyone else will be reading the messages, (b) limit sending group e-mail that lists other recipients, (c) ask patients what type of communication they prefer, and (d) archive the messages (sent and received to patients) (Hafner, 2002). All of these suggestions seem reasonable. Whether or not the system has a Web-based, secure message system is of critical concern, and this should be noted on all messages. Since some people in a family share the same e-mail address, this has a direct implication for confidentiality.

- **Handheld communication systems:** These computer systems can be beneficial to clinical and management staff in all types of health care settings (Austen, 2002). There is more and more software for these systems that allow staff to get information quickly when they need it. Staff can document and search for medical information, search the current *Physician Desk Reference* for drugs or nursing software on drugs, communicate with others, monitor patient information, and make work planning notes. These systems are gradually replacing small note pads and index cards. Some systems have photograph options, which could be used to document visual data. At this time, some of these systems can be expensive, although prices will probably decrease. Most organizations do not provide them for their staff.

■ **Internet prescription:** A patient can now go on the Internet and obtain prescribed drugs. There are great safety and legal risks with this practice as these companies may "operate as if they were outside the scope of traditional state and federal laws and regulations" (Waters, 2002, p. 12). Consumers need to get their drugs through reliable Internet sites.

■ **Home health and IT:** When compared with other health care settings, home health ranks fifth out of 36 in terms of the importance of telehealth in the delivery of care (Dakins, 2002). What is happening in this health care setting? Web-based programs for patient monitoring and interactive video-based programs are expanding. Congestive heart disease, diabetes, and coronary disease are the three conditions that have been focused on when these services have been developed. They are chronic illnesses that if managed well can reduce health care costs. Many personal monitoring devices related to many chronic diseases are either available or in development. Examples of these devices include "a monitor in the bathroom shower that scans for signs of melanoma; a wristwatch-like device that constantly checks pulse, respiration, and temperature; computerized eyeglasses that jog a failing memory with whispered cues; and a 'smart badge' that senses a developing infection and identifies the antibiotic need" (Rickey, 1999-2000, as cited in Predko, 2001, p. 79). There has been an expansion of disease management for chronic illnesses and with this comes the need for greater patient education, self-management, and also monitoring methods. Telehealth offers many options to meet these requirements. Home health also is increasing its use of IT for documentation, with many agencies providing nurses with computers that can be used in the home and on the road. Cellular telephones are clearly a major benefit to home health nurses to keep in touch with patients, home office, and for emergencies.

THINK CRITICALLY

Try this exercise to apply what you have learned about this topic.

Implications for nursing education

Information technology and telehealth certainly have implications for nursing education. If faculty do not make the changes to incorporate more information technology, students will push for it more and more. This whole era is changing the face of learning and education at all levels. Teaching is moving more and more to facilitation of learning. "There is a shift away from traditional pedagogy to the creation of learning partnerships and learning cultures. Pedagogy has to do with optimizing the transmission of information. The children (and young adults) do not want augmented, pre-digested information. They want to learn by doing, where they synthesize their own understanding, usually based on experimentation. Learning, therefore, becomes experimental" (Richards, 2001, p. 7). This movement can be seen in the rapid and solid growth of online courses and degree programs, E-books, increased use of the Web to post course documents, use of e-mail to communicate with students, and video access via university websites. IT also means that there are more and more opportunities for learning to be a continuous, lifelong process, as more and more nurses can easily access it. To attract the Net Generation, schools of nursing will have to turn to these new strategies and adapt their philosophies of learning and teaching, which should focus more on facilitation of learning with faculty in the role of facilitator. This is not only important to attract students into nursing but also to prepare nurses who can function and contribute in a highly technological health care environment. Nurses returning to school for BSN degrees or graduate degrees will have to play catch-up in this new learning environment, and faculty have to be prepared to assist them or lose them. "Baby Boomers lived in a slow-motion world compared to the Net Generation. The children of the digital age expect things to happen fast, because in their world, things do happen fast, including learning" (Richards, 2001, p. 8).

Distance education, or education provided in such a way that the student and instructor are either separated by time or distance, has become an important method for providing continuing education, additional academic degrees, and certification. Benefits of this method, as was discussed in Chapter 13, are flexibility for the student; decreased cost for students such as less travel, parking, and so on; fewer campus buildings needed at schools; increased opportunity to include faculty, such as experts, for short-term teaching; broader mix of students from different geographic areas with different perspectives; opportunity to develop different and innovative teaching strategies; and flexibility for faculty who can travel, teach, and work from home while teaching. Technology can also be used to bring courses to staff within health care organizations and allow organizations with multiple sites to conduct education and training programs without staff travel by using computers, videoconferencing, and other new technology.

Implications for nursing administration

Nurse leaders need to be knowledgeable about IT and its implications for the management of organizations and delivery of health care in all types of settings. The Net Generation wants collaborative workplaces and to feel they are partners with leadership. IT makes this easier and, in fact, a necessity. In the past, information might have been held by management and given out to staff on an as needed basis. Now, staff have greater access of information and can often find a way to obtain this information quickly. The changes in IT alter how people work together and how they communicate. "This technology provides a medium for greater accessibility to shared information and support for rich interpersonal exchange and collaboration across departmental boundaries" (Richards, 2001, p. 11). Nurses now can offer their input quickly in the decision-making process. The following provides some examples of the use of technology and administration.

- **Workforce modeling and prediction:** Kansas City Colleagues for Caring developed a tool that can do workforce modeling and prediction. This type of tool uses data to track workforce demand—both current employment and projected future needs (Mills, Daldrup, & Lacey-Haun, 2002). Tools like this one can be extremely helpful for individual health care organizations and for communities at the local, regional, and state levels. It makes these data more accessible to those who need to make decisions when they need the data. With the growing nursing shortage and need for communities to respond, it is critical to understand the problem, as described by data, and then to use the data most effectively.

- **Pagers to monitor work:** Pagers and headsets to get updates on where patients are in the patient care process are used in some ambulatory care settings such as provider offices, clinics, emergency departments, laboratories, radiology, and other sites where patients wait for care (Tortora, 2001). These methods can inform providers when patients need to be seen, by whom, and so on. This might be viewed as a mechanical approach to care; however, patient wait times can be decreased. Staff can then be more aware of progress or lack of progress through the system so that interventions can be taken.

- **Admission registration:** Computerized admission registration saves staff time and allows for rapid access of information by clinical staff. It also results in more accurate information. Information can also be stored more easily in a computer system.

- **Nurse call systems:** These systems are critical components of a unit's communication system. There are many types of methods, some more complex than others. Clinical units are far past the "yell down the hall" method. Examples of methods are: light signals, buzzers, methods that allow patients to talk directly to nurses, pagers that vibrate, two-way cordless or wireless phones, miniature lapel speaker/microphones, and locator badges with a communication option (McConnell, 2000; Miller, Deets, & Miller, 2001). What makes a good system? First, and foremost, the system must meet the needs of patients, nurses and other unit staff, and secretarial support staff. This is a good example of the importance of including clerical support staff in the decision-making process. A pager method might work well for clinical staff and yet not be effective for the unit clerical support staff who answer the telephones. The system must get the message to the appropriate people as quickly as possible in the most confidential manner with the least amount of interference. It also needs to ensure that emergency situations are communicated quickly and that staff can easily recognize that it is an emergency call and not a routine call. When systems are chosen, the following need to be considered: (a) impact on patients; (b) impact on staff; (c) features; (d) fit with needs; (e) safety; (f) confidentiality; (g) mobility and distance; (h) cost; (i) system integration with present system and requirements; (j) comfort and convenience; (k) environmental factors related to physical or architectural concerns such as noise, physical dimensions, maintenance, and support; and (l) ease of use (McConnell, 2000). Call systems need to (a) save time, (b) improve care, and (c) reduce stress. Efficient call systems can make a very big difference with clinical staff, the management of a service or unit, and patient satisfaction. They can decrease staff fatigue, prevent errors, and get care to patients when they need it.

■ **Voice mail:** Computer-based messaging systems are found in all health care settings today. Staff and consumers/patients encounter them daily. This technology saves time—messages can easily be left when no one answers the telephone. With many calls the message is all that is important, requiring no direct response from the person called. This alone is a plus because it saves time. Voice mail, however, has its critics. It does appear impersonal to many. When a person needs to speak to someone it can be annoying to get the message system, particularly those systems that put the caller on hold or where the caller must key in multiple numbers for various options. Patients can find this difficult when they are ill, have disabilities, and need assistance. Health care organizations need to look carefully at their voice mail call systems and develop technology policy related to their use. The following are examples of some issues that might require policy consideration: "(1) Is it appropriate to turn on voice mail while holding an office meeting? (2) Should an extension be included with a name? (3) Should employees change their greetings if they take a vacation? (4) How many rings should there be before voice mail picks up? (5) What should the time interval be between incoming message and return call?" (Hoban, 1999, p. 56). Improving patient/consumer satisfaction is a key focus of developing guidelines for staff about voice mail usage.

Implications for patient education

E-health is now commonplace in many health care organizations. "The Internet has emerged as a new and important vehicle for accessing health care information. In fact, recent reports in several publications demonstrate that after the physician, the Internet is the second most used source by health consumers. A Harris Poll conducted in 1999 indicated that seventy million of the 97 million Americans who used the Internet in 1999 accessed health advice" (Lin, Truong, Smeltzer, & Williams-Brinkley, 2001, p. 69). This technology is not perfect, and there are concerns about the quality of health material posted on the Web. Much of the information, however, is of good quality and helpful to health care providers and patients/consumers. E-health is "the use of emerging information and communication technology, especially the Internet, to improve or enable health and health care" (Eng, 2001, p. 3). Connectivity is one of the key factors in today's personal and work environment, which includes the health care environment. Consumers and providers expect more and more information to be quickly available, but they also want credible information. "Wireless access to data potentially increases that effectiveness by giving caregivers remote access to clinical data anywhere, anytime through web-enabled telephones, wireless personal digital assistants (PDAs), or E-mails containing clinical alerts that require intervention. The combined effect of mobility and instant alerts enables faster, more accurate decision making, and ultimately better outcomes" (Meadows, 2002, p. 295). What do consumers want? They want to be able to get to their health care information quickly and easily. Many are also interested in communicating with their health care providers via many of the possible technologies (for example, e-mail and voice mail).

Many health care organizations have developed their own websites. A key purpose of these sites is marketing and public relations. Coughlin (2000) notes that these sites serve a purpose;

however, it is often difficult to identify nursing on the sites. Why is it important for nursing to make a clear contribution to these sites? "A web-based presence is a cost-effective way to tell the world who we are and why nursing is special. This is a proactive and innovative approach to improve the professional image of nursing" (Coughlin, 2000, p. 569). For acute care sites the answer is simple. Nurses provide most of the care in hospitals, and consumers should see them featured on these sites. Nursing leadership in health care organizations needs to step up and insist that nurses are featured on the website, and nurses also need to be involved in developing the site, with nurse leaders involved in major decisions related to e-health. Nurse leaders also need to develop their own technological skills and those of the nursing staff to improve TIQ. These websites can also assist with the organization's recruitment and retention (advertising jobs, recognizing expertise, sharing what nurses are contributing); patient education and consumer guidelines; nursing continuing education; linking the nursing staff with resources via the Web; communication of nursing activities such as committees, and so on. Some of this information must be available via pin number or some sort of privacy system, and other parts should be available to the public.

The following are some consumer- or patient-oriented materials that could help nurses in the management of care if they were made available to patients on the organization's website.

- Preoperative instructions
- Patient education guides for common problems (for example, diabetes, cardiac, and so on)
- Postoperative experience
- Admission process
- Discharge process
- Discharge planning
- Family visiting guidelines
- Patient rights
- Intensive care guidelines for family members
- Helping your child with hospitalization
- Hospital diets
- Helping your child cope with a parent/grandparent in the hospital
- Appropriate flowers and plants to send to ensure safety
- Reimbursement issues and procedures
- Talking with your doctor
- Talking with your nurse
- Who is who? Finding your way around our staff
- Patient satisfaction and patient advocacy

These are only a few examples. Any educational content and information also needs to be individualized when patients receive care, and patients would then need to have contact with staff for questions and discussion.

THINK CRITICALLY

Try this exercise to apply what you have learned about this topic.

Implications for nursing research

Informatics has had and will continue to have an effect on nursing research. This effect is felt both in the use of informatics as a tool to facilitate research and as a focus of research—application in the clinical practice and administration. There is a greater need to understand informatics and its implications for the profession. Many health care organizations, with their increasing ability to access technology, will probably increase their research activity. There is greater ability to communicate across organizations and to seek information and consultation. "The information highway has opened the door for a wide exchange of data, information, and knowledge between practitioners and scientists. The capacity for a mega-repository of clinical and research findings will allow for a richer science derived from multiple perspectives. Nurses have the responsibility to initiate practice-based inquiry, participate in clinical nursing research, and use nursing research to enhance patients' well-being and contribute to the body of nursing knowledge" (Appleton, 1998, as cited in Richards, 2001, p. 10).

Technology and managed care

With the rapid growth of information technology, the management and provision of health care have been radically changed. Information is available via many different types of technology today, giving health care providers the opportunity to track patient information across health care settings and virtually anywhere in the world. Recognizing the importance of this technology, in 1999, the American Nurses Association published two monographs, *Competencies for Telehealth Technologies in Nursing* and *Core Principles on Telehealth*. The competencies are found in Box 15-2.

CURRENT ISSUES

Learn about events around the globe that relate to the chapter content.

BOX 15-2 Competencies for use of telehealth technologies in nursing.

The registered nurse:

- Integrates telehealth into nursing practice for client assessment, diagnosis, identification of desired outcomes, plan of care, plan implementation, evaluation, and referrals.
- Establishes a therapeutic relationship, which creates a sense of nursing presence that engages the client.
- Assesses and adjusts communication techniques to maximize the nurse-client relationship.
- Assesses the appropriateness of specific telehealth technologies for individual situations or populations.
- Determines whether client needs can be met with telehealth, using concurrent evaluation, and makes appropriate changes to the management plan.
- Ensures that clients are informed of their choices regarding use of telehealth.
- Demonstrates skills in seeking, using, and providing consultation and participates in interdisciplinary collaboration to meet clients' needs.
- Demonstrates competent knowledge of and skill in specific telehealth technology and relevant telehealth clinical skills.
- Ensures that public and institutional policies related to privacy, confidentiality, informed consent, and information security are employed during telehealth use.
- Uses results of telehealth performance improvement activities to modify practice.
- Documents and integrates into information systems the structure, process, and outcomes of telehealth events.

Source: American Nurses Association. (1999). *Competencies for telehealth technologies in Nursing*. Washington, DC: Author, pp. 7–9. Reprinted with permission.

Managed care organizations (MCOs) are finding that telephone patient advice is an excellent triage method that allows patients to speak directly with a health care professional, who is often a nurse. This method can be used for triage, counseling, disease management, education, self-care support, and appointment and referral services (Greenberg & Schultz, 2002). Questions can be answered, which may prevent the need for an office visit. Patients can also be assessed and referred to the best resource for service. Patient education and guidance can also be provided. Assessment over the phone requires a highly skilled practitioner who can identify critical information that may be communicated in subtle ways. Nurses with their assessment skills and ability to collaborate with physicians are particularly effective. Patient advice systems via telephone require clear documentation policies and guidelines that include content related to who is called, when, for what reason, and required assessment data and interventions. Follow-up is a critical topic as it should be part of the services and the documentation of those services. This form of communication between nurses and patients must take into consideration the importance of trust, establishing a good relationship, and the need to individualize care. The latter is important because many organizations that use patient advice systems follow very specific protocols, algorithms, and guidelines. If, however, this care is not individualized it could have serious consequences. "Cookbook" care must be avoided. The assessment is the key to successful telephone nursing—providing the interventions for needs that should be addressed, which may or may not be found in the guidelines. There are four typical interventions used by nurses in this practice arena: telephone consultation, telephone follow-up, surveillance via telephone, and triage via telephone (Androwich & Haas, 2001; Haas & Androwich, 1999).

The easiest and probably the most common of the four typical interventions used in patient advice systems is using the telephone for patient follow-up. Staff from a day surgery unit call patients before surgery to discuss preoperative requirements and after discharge to determine their status and whether they are following discharge advice. Many health care providers are using the telephone to contact patients and remind them of appointments to decrease the number of patients who do not show up for appointments. Missed appointments are expensive for providers because this time could have been used to see other patients. Health care providers, particularly hospitals, are using the telephone to obtain initial intake information and thus reduce admission time, while at the same time providing the patient with pertinent information. Managed care organizations call patients who have failed to keep appointments or to obtain satisfaction data. The telephone is certainly not new; however, health care providers are now using this technology to their advantage. The use of the telephone for these purposes does take staff time, and this does affect costs; however, it usually is less time than would be required for an in-person encounter— it saves time for the provider and the patient. Staff who make the calls need training, policies, and guidelines related to the purposes of the calls, privacy issues, who to call and what to say, and documentation.

BENCHMARKS

Now let's take a moment to test your knowledge of the concepts you have studied in this section.

Chapter Wrap-Up

Now that you've reached the end of the chapter, you may wish to explore the concepts you've been reading about in greater detail, or test yourself to see how well you've comprehended the material.

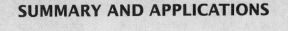

SUMMARY AND APPLICATIONS

- Summary
- Practice Quiz
- Key Terms
- Tying It All Together

- Experiential Exercises
- Case
- Links

REFERENCES

American Academy of Ambulatory Care Nursing, Telehealth Nursing Practice Standards Task Force. (2001). *AAACN telehealth nursing practice administration and practice standards*. Pittman, NJ: Author.

American Nurses Association. (1999). *Competencies for telehealth technologies in nursing*. Washington, DC: Author.

American Nurses Association. (2002) Using innovative technology to enhance patient care delivery. Washington, DC: Author.

Androwich, I., & Haas, S. (2001). Ambulatory care nursing. In J. Dochterman & H. Grace (Eds.), *Current issues in nursing* (6th ed., pp. 150–158). St. Louis: Mosby, Inc.

Appleton, C. (1998). Nursing research: Moving into the clinical setting. *Nursing Management, 29*(6), 43–45.

Austen, I. (August, 22, 2002). For the doctor's touch, help in the hand. *New York Times*, E1, E7.

Coughlin, C. (2000). Where is nursing's presence on the medical center's web site? *Journal of Nursing Administration, 30*(12), 569–570.

Dakins, D. (2002). Home is where the healthcare is. *Telemedicine Today, 9*(2), 18–21.

Donnelly, J. (2000). Integrated communication cascade: Better information, faster response. *Nursing Management, 31*(3), 28–29.

Eng, T. (2001). *The health landscape: A terrain map of emerging information and communication technologies in health and healthcare*. Princeton, NJ: Robert Wood Johnson.

Greenberg, M., & Schultz, C. (2002). Telephone nursing: Client experiences and perceptions. *Nursing Economics, 20*(4), 181–187.

Haas, S., & Androwich, L. (1999). Telephone consultation. In G. Bulechek & J. McCloskey (Eds.), *Nursing interventions: Effective nursing treatments*. Philadelphia: Saunders.

Hafner, K. (2002, June 6). 'Dear doctor' meets 'return to sender.' *New York Times*, E1, E6.

Hoban, L. (1999). Humanizing voice mail in healthcare. *Journal of Nursing Administration, 29*(2), 50–56.

Institute of Medicine. (1999). *Crossing the quality chasm: A new health system for the 21st century*. Washington, DC: National Academy Press.

Kerfoot, K. (2000). TIQ (Technical IQ)—A survival skill for the new millennium. *Nursing Economics, 18*(1), 29–31.

Kerfoot, K., & Simpson, R. (2002). Knowledge-driven care: Powerful medicine. *Reflections on Nursing LEADERSHIP* (third quarter), 22–24, 44.

Kissinger, K., & Borchardt, S. (Eds.). (1996). *Information technology for integrated health systems. Positioning for the future*. New York: John Wiley & Sons, Inc.

Kosko, B. (1999). *Fuzzy future*. New York: Harmony Books.

Landro, L. (2002a, July 29). FDA is urged to hasten efforts to require bar codes on drugs [Electronic Version]. *The Wall Street Journal*.

Landro, L. (2002b, June 10). Health care goes digital [Electronic Version]. *The Wall Street Journal*.

Lin, S., Truong, C., Smeltzer, C., & Williams-Brinkley, R. (2001). Benchmarking. A tool for management decision-making. In J. Dochterman & H. Grace (Eds.), *Current issues in nursing* (6th ed., pp. 69–74). St. Louis: Mosby, Inc.

McConnell, E. (2000). Communication systems make a caring connection. *Nursing Management, 31*(3), 49, 52.

Meadows, G. (2002). The nursing shortage: Can information technology help? *Nursing Economics, 20*(1), 46–48.

Miller, E., Deets, C., & Miller, R. (2001). Nurse call and the work environment: Lessons learned. *Journal of Nursing Care Quality, 15*(3), 7–15.

Mills, N., Daldrup, D., & Lacey-Haun, D. (2002). The future of organizational work: Web-based resource networking. *Journal of Nursing Administration, 29*(12), 6–9.

Predko, J. (2001). Use of distance technology for education, practice, and research. In J. Dochterman & H. Grace (Eds.), *Current issues in nursing* (6th ed., pp. 75–81). St. Louis: Mosby.

Richards, J. (2001). Nursing in a digital age. *Nursing Economics, 19*(1), 6–10, 34.

Rickey, T. (1999-2000, winter). Memory glasses, wristwatch monitors, and smart socks . . . here's to your health. *Rochester Review,* 21–23.

Roark, D. (2004). Bar codes & drug administration. *AJN, 104*(1), 63–66.

Simpson, R., & Keegan, A. (2002). How connected are you? Employing emotional intelligence in a high-tech world. (Nursing informatics). *Nursing Administration Quarterly, 26*(2), 80–87.

Snyder-Halpern, R., & Chervany, N. (2000). A clinical information system strategic planning model for integrated healthcare delivery networks. *Journal of Nursing Administration, 30*(12), 583–591.

Stix, G., & Lacob, M. (1999). *Who gives a gigabyte?* New York: John Wiley & Sons.

Tortora, A. (2001). Bzzzz: Your exam room table is ready. *Business Courier Cincinnati/Northern Kentucky Region, 18*(18), 3, 11.

U.S. Department of Health and Human Services. (1998). *Healthy People 2010.* Washington, DC: Author.

U.S. Human Resources and Services Administration, Office of Advancement for Telehealth (OAT). (1999). http://tlelhealth.hrsa.gov.

Waters, R. (2002). Thinking outside the box helps break through barriers. *Telemedicine Today, 9*(2), 9–17.

Whitten, P., et al. (2002). Systematic review of cost effectiveness studies of telemedicine interventions. *British Medical Journal, 324*(June), 1434–1437.

Wiley, R. (2002). Bioterrorism bill includes funding for telemedicine network expansion. *Telemedicine Today, 9*(2), 8.

ADDITIONAL READINGS

American Nurses Association. (2001a). *Developing telehealth protocols: A blueprint for success.* Washington, DC: American Publishing, Inc.

American Nurses Association. (2001b). *Scope and standards for nursing informatics practice.* Washington, DC: Author.

Andolina, K. M. (2000). The automation of clinical pathways. In M. J. Ball, J. Hannah, S. K. Newbold, & J. V. Douglas (Eds.), *Nursing informatics: Where caring and technology meet.* New York: Springer.

Berendt, M., Schaefer, B., Heglund, M., & Bardin, C. (2001). Telehealth for effective disease state management. *Home Care Provider, 6*(4) 67–72.

Christensen, C., Bohmer, R., & Kenagy, J. (2000). Will disruptive innovations cure health care? *Harvard Business Review,* September–October, 102–110.

Coenen, A., McNeil, B., Bakken, S., Bickford, C., & Warren, J. J. (2001). Toward comparable nursing data: American Nurses Association criteria for data sets, classification systems, and nomenclatures. *Computers in Nursing, 19*(6), 240–246.

Dick, R. S., Steen, E. B., & Detmer, D. E. (Eds.). (1997). *The computer-based patient record: An essential technology for healthcare, revised edition.* Washington, DC: National Academy Press.

Docimo, A., et al. (2000). Using the online and offline change model to improve efficiency for fast-track patients in an emergency department. *Journal of Quality Improvement, 26*(9), 503–514.

Gordon, M., et al. (Eds.). (1999). *Nursing diagnoses: Definitions and classification 2001–2002.* Philadelphia: North American Nursing Diagnosis Association.

Greenberg, M., & Cartwright, J. (2001). Identifying best practices in telehealth nursing: The telehealth survey. *Nursing Economics, 19*(6), 283–285.

Horak, D. (2000). Designing and implementing a computerized tracking system: The experience at one level trauma center emergency department. *Journal of Emergency Nursing, 26*(5), 473–476.

Huber, D., Schumacher, L., & Delaney, C. (1997). Nursing management minimum data set (NMMDS). *Journal of Nursing Administration, 27*(4), 42–48.

Jenkins, T. (1988). New roles for nursing professionals. In M. Ball, K. Hannah, U. Gerdin Jelger, & H. Peterson (Eds.), *Nursing informatics: Where caring and technology meet* (pp. 88–95). New York: Springer.

Johnson, M., Bulechek, G., Dochterman, J., Maas, M., & Moorhead, S. (2001). *Nursing diagnosis, outcomes, interventions: NANDA, NOC, and NIC linkages.* St. Louis, MO: Mosby Year Book.

Johnson, M., Maas, M., & Moorhead, S. (Eds.). (2000). *Nursing outcomes classification (NOC)* (2nd ed.). St. Louis, MO: Mosby Year Book.

Kastens, J. (1998). Integrated care management: Aligning medical call center and nurse triage services. *Nursing Economics, 16*(6), 322–329.

Kohn, L., & Corrigan, J. (1999). *To err is human: Building a safer health system.* Washington, DC: National Academy Press.

Kremsdorf, R. (2002, June 12–14). "Using innovative technology to enhance patient care delivery." Presented at the Proceedings of the American Academy of Nursing Conference on "Using Innovative Technology to Decrease Nursing Demand and Enhance Patient Care Delivery," Washington, DC.

LaDuke, S. (2000). NIC puts nursing into words: A common language empowers nurses to describe, validate, and control their practice. *Nursing Management, 31*(7), 43–44.

Larson-Dahn, M. (2000). Tele-Nurse practice. A practice model for role expansion. *Journal of Nursing Administration, 30*(11), 519–523.

Martin, K., & Scheet, N. (1992). *The Omaha system: Application for community health nursing.* Philadelphia: Saunders.

McCloskey, J., & Bulechek, G. (Eds.). (2000). *Nursing interventions classification (NIC), Iowa interventions project* (3rd ed.). St. Louis, MO: Mosby.

McConnell, E. (1999). Get the buzz on nurse call systems. *Nursing Management, 30*(6), 43.

McCormack, K., & Jones, C. (1998, September 30). Is one taxonomy needed for health care vocabularies and classifications? *Online Journal of Issues in Nursing.* Available: http://www.nursingworld.org/ojin/tpc7/tpc7_2htm.

Nelson, L. (1999). Step-by-step guide to selecting mobile wireless devices. *Nursing Management, 30*(11), 12–13.

Neuhauser, P. (2000). Culture.com. Leading the way to E-nursing. *Journal of Nursing Administration, 30*(12), 580–582.

North American Nursing Diagnosis Association (NANDA). (2001). *Nursing diagnosis: Definitions and classification 2000–2001.* Philadelphia: NANDA.

Russo, H. (2000). The Internet: Building knowledge & offering integrated solutions in health care. *Caring 19*(7), 18–31.

Saba, V. K. (1992). The classification of home health care nursing: Diagnosis and interventions. *Caring Magazine, 11*(3), 50–57.

Sabin, M. (1998). Telephone triage improves demand management effectiveness. *Journal Healthcare Financial Management, 52*(8), 49–51.

Sorrels-Jones, J., & Weaver, D. (1999). Knowledge workers and knowledge-intense organizations. Part 1: A promising framework for nursing and healthcare. *Journal of Nursing Administration, 19*(7/8), 12–18.

Waldo, B. (2000). Redefining the healthcare landscape with the Internet. *Nursing Economics, 18*(2), 99–100.

CHAPTER 16

Health Care Quality Improvement and Safety

CHAPTER OUTLINE

MediaLink
www.prenhall.com/finkelman

The Interactive Exercises for this chapter can be found in the OneKey course at www.prenhall.com/finkelman. Click on Chapter 16 to select from the following activities: Test Your Understanding, Benchmarks, Current Issues, Your Opinion Counts, Think Critically, and Summary and Applications.

What's Ahead

This chapter discusses the critical issues of quality care and safety in the health care delivery system. With the complex system that is changing daily, the task of determining quality of care and the best way to improve care are difficult to accomplish. "The pursuit of excellence in nursing care is a goal that requires objectivity, openness to change, creativity, critical abilities, and support and participation from all levels of nursing staff (Finkelman, 1996, p. ix). Each nurse plays a daily role in ensuring quality care while care is provided but also is responsible for participating in organizational quality improvement (QI) efforts. All health care organizations should have QI programs, which can be found in hospitals, home care, long-term care, and so on. It is important to note that the United States has no comprehensive system to monitor health care, judge improvement, or to determine the best strategies to improve health care. Content in this chapter, however, indicates that this is changing. Since nursing care represents a major component of all health care, nurses should participate in all levels of QI and also address specific nursing issues related to the quality of care.

OBJECTIVES

Before you begin, take a moment to familiarize yourself with the key objectives of this chapter.

- Critique critical issues related to defining quality.
- Define structure, process, and outcomes as they relate to quality.
- Identify two factors that support an increased interest in quality care.
- Summarize the recent activity of the Institute of Medicine and its importance to health care.
- Describe the accreditation offered by the Joint Commission Accreditation of Healthcare Organizations.
- Describe two methods used to measure and ensure quality, safe care.
- Describe a quality report card and its relevance.
- Discuss nurse and physician reaction to the quality of managed care organizations and their effect on health care.

TEST YOUR UNDERSTANDING

Before we begin our exploration of this chapter, take a short "warm-up" test to see what you know about this topic.

YOUR OPINION COUNTS

Find out what others think about this topic. Post your response and check out other opinions.

The Changing View of Quality

Quality is a complex concept, with many factors affecting it. There have recently been some strong influences on the increasing interest in quality, safe care. Assessing and improving care is not a static process. The following discussion includes information about the increased interest in quality of care and the definition of quality care and its critical elements.

Increased interest in quality care

What are factors in the health care delivery environment that indicate there is increased interest in the quality of care? Increased legislation is one indication, which shows a public concern for care. In 2003, bills related to quality care and health care safety were submitted in the U.S. House of Representatives, the Patient Safety Act, H.R. 877, which was originally drafted by the ANA, and in the U.S. Senate, the Patient Safety and Quality Improvement Act, S. 720. These bills demonstrate that there is not an open national debate about the quality of care. The Institute of Medicine (IOM) reports from 1999 to 2003 certainly stimulated some of this legislative activity.

BOX 16-1   Department of Health and Human Services (DHHS).

The government agency that protects the health of the people and offers essential services for those who need assistance providing for themselves. Perhaps the most recognizable programs are Medicare and Medicaid. HHS provides more than 60,000 grants yearly, making it the largest grant-making agency in the federal government. There are 11 operating divisions.

Public Health Service Operating Divisions

- National Institutes of Health

  Supports 35,000 research projects for diseases such as AIDS, cancer, Alzheimer's, diabetes, arthritis, and heart problems.

- Food and Drug Administration

  Assures safety and efficacy of drugs, foods, cosmetics, biological products, and medical devices.

- Centers for Disease Control and Prevention

  Provides disease prevention strategies, monitors and prevents disease outbreaks, and maintains national health statistics. Includes environmental and workplace safety. The director is the administrator of the Agency for Toxic Substance and Disease Registry.

- Indian Health Service

  Provides hospitals, health centers, school health, and village clinics to 1.5 million American Indians and Alaskan natives of 557 recognized tribes.

- Health Resources and Service Administration

  Provides health care to underserved areas that include the poor and the uninsured. Offers supportive services for HIV/AIDS patients through the Ryan White Act.

- Substance Abuse and Mental Health Services Administration

  Supplies substance abuse prevention, treatment, and mental health services. Funds states (federal block grants), towns, and counties to address drug abuse trends, mental health needs, and related public health concerns.

- Agency for Research and Quality

  Conducts and supports research in the areas of quality, cost, access, patient safety, and medical errors.

Human Services Operating Divisions

- Center for Medicare and Medicaid Services (formerly Health Care Financing Administration)

  Administers both programs, provides health insurance for the elderly and disabled. Medicaid provides coverage for adults, children, and nursing home residents with low incomes. Co-administers the State Children's Health Insurance Program (SHIP or SCHIP) with the Health Resources and Services Administration. Acts with the Departments of Labor and Treasury to help small companies get and keep coverage and works against discrimination based on health status for those buying insurance.

- Administration for Children and Families

  Administers statewide welfare programs, child support enforcement systems, and Head Start. Supports child-care, foster care, and adoption assistance, as well as child abuse and domestic violence prevention programs.

- Administration on Aging

  An advocate for the concerns of the elderly. Provides support for Meals on Wheels. Regional and state offices plan, coordinate, and develop community based programs.

- United States Public Health Service Commissioned Corp

  A uniformed service of health professionals who serve in many federal agencies.

Source: U.S. Department of Health & Human Service website, http://dhhs.gov/, What We Do http://dhhs.gov/news/press/2002/pres/profile.html. Retrieved March 1, 2003.

The Department of Health and Human Services (DHHS) plays a major role in health care delivery in the United States and in assessing quality care. Box 16-1 highlights some of the activities of DHHS. The DHHS can get involved in this due to its responsibility to develop rules and regulations for most health care laws and due to its role as the administrator for Medicare and Medicaid.

Another indication of interest in health care quality is not governmental but rather focuses on the purchasers of care in the private sector. The Leapfrog Group, a consortium of Fortune 500 companies and other large private and public health care purchasers of health care benefits, covering more than 34 million people, has developed a clear interest in health care quality (Leapfrog Group, 2003, July 9). The group's mission is to "trigger a giant leap forward in quality, customer service, and affordability of health care of all types by (1) making the American public aware of a small number of highly compelling and easily understood advances in patient safety and (2) specifying a simple set of purchasing principles designed to promote these safety advances, as well as overall customer value" (Leapfrog Group, 2003, July 9). There is no doubt that businesses want value for the money they spend on health care, and employers are the major purchasers of care because they provide health care coverage for their employees.

Health care professional organizations are also involved in the increased interest in health care quality. The Joint Commission on Accreditation of Healthcare Organizations (JCAHO) is directly involved with quality and safety issues and has become more concerned with safety due to the recent IOM reports. It initiated a program that the ANA supports, "Speak Up: Help Prevent Errors in Your Care" (American Nurses Association, 2002). This initiative urges patients to do the following to help prevent health care errors or to "Speak Up."

- **S**peak up if you have questions or concerns, and if you don't understand, ask again. It's your body and you have a right to know.
- **P**ay attention to the care you are receiving. Make sure you're getting the right treatments and medications by the right health care professionals. Don't assume anything.
- **E**ducate yourself about your diagnosis, the medical tests you are undergoing, and your treatment plan.
- **A**sk a trusted family member or friend to be your advocate.
- **K**now what medications you take and why you take them. Medication errors are the most common health care errors.
- **U**se a hospital, clinic, surgery center, or other type of health care organization that has undergone a rigorous on-site evaluation against established state-of-the-art quality and safety standards, such as those provided by JCAHO.
- **P**articipate in all decisions about your treatment. You are the center of the health care team (Joint Commission on Accreditation of Healthcare Organizations, 2003, July 9).

Health care safety and quality are interrelated, and these topics are frequently found in the media—television, newspapers, and other print media. Stories are presented about complications patients experience due to errors, interventions, or inappropriate care. Examples of this type of media can be found at the local, state, and national levels. Consumers hear these stories and worry about the care that they receive, and this increases interest in health care quality.

The most important recent demonstration of increased interest that really has propelled this topic forward was President Clinton's Presidential Advisory Commission on Consumer Protection and Quality in the Health Care Industry, which was established in March, 1997, for a specific time period. This commission addressed many of the concerns about quality care and the need to make changes to improve care. Three nurse leaders served on the 32-member commission. The purpose of the commission was to advise the President about the impact of health care delivery system changes on quality, consumer protection, and the availability of needed services (Wakefield, 1997). The commission consisted of four subcommittees.

1. The first subcommittee's purpose was to develop a Consumer Bill of Rights, Protections, and Responsibilities. Critical issues covered were coverage, choice of practitioners, privacy and confidentiality, disclosure of practitioner qualifications, and external appeals processes. Despite the recommendations from this commission, the United States still does not have a

Consumer Bill of Rights. This is really the only element of this commission's work that has not been successful.

2. The second subcommittee was created to identify performance measurement and quality oversight that would improve the validity and reliability of performance measurement data.
3. The third subcommittee, which was chaired by a nurse, considered the creation of a quality improvement environment and the internal and external barriers and facilitators of quality improvement.
4. The fourth subcommittee focused on the roles of public and private oversight entities, strategies to reach a balance between market-driven quality incentives and regulatory requirements, and the responsibilities of group purchasers to protect quality.

The final report from the commission, *Quality First: Better Health Care for all Americans*, was published in 1999. Box 16-2 describes the commission's recommendations. This commission and its report stimulated the development of the Quality of Health Care in America project initiated by the Institute of Medicine in June, 1998. The purpose of this project is to develop strategies that will improve quality of care over the next 10 years. Box 16-3 highlights the key Institute of Medicine reports that are a part of this project.

As indicated by the number of reports and their content, much work has been done since Clinton's advisory commission in 1997. The following discussion provides an overview of the content of these critical reports related to quality health care.

To err is human. Building a safer health system

The first report, *To Err Is Human. Building a Safer Health System* (Institute of Medicine, 1999), focused on safety within the health care delivery system. Data indicated that there have been and continue to be serious safety problems. Examples include:

■ When data from one study was extrapolated, the result was at least 44,000 Americans die each year as a result of a medication error. Another study indicated the number could be as high as 98,000 (American Hospital Association Statistics, 1999; as cited in Institute of Medicine, 1999).

■ More people die in a given year as a result of medical errors than from motor vehicle accidents (43,458), breast cancer (42,297), or AIDS (16,516) (Centers for Disease Control and Prevention, 1998; as cited in Institute of Medicine, 1999).

■ Health care costs represent over one-half of total national costs, which include lost income, lost household production, disability, and health care costs (Thomas et al., 1999; as cited in Institute of Medicine, 1999).

There are clear problems, and to date the focus has only been on hospital errors. This, however, does not negate the presence of medical errors in home care, long-term care, ambulatory care or primary care areas, and other health care settings. These are settings that require further exploration.

What are some of the outcomes from errors that cause further problems? Cost is certainly a concern, and medication errors can result in a variety of costs. Complications that result from errors may lead to increased health care costs. Opportunity costs occur when repeat diagnostic tests are required or interventions are needed to counteract adverse drug events. Another critical concern is patients' loss of trust in the health care system and its providers. If a patient experiences an error, this has a direct impact on the patient's trust in the health care system; however, the increase in media coverage of health care quality can also have just as serious an impact on patient trust in the system.

Historically, accrediting and licensing organizations have not focused much on the issue of errors, but this has changed (Institute of Medicine, 1999). The decentralized and fragmented health care system certainly has been a factor in contributing to unsafe conditions, and it interferes with improvement. Multiple providers and ineffective communication also are other problems that affect patient safety. Third-party payers (managed care organizations and other insurers) have not been very involved in encouraging providers to improve safety even though they have had some power to do this.

BOX 16-2 The President's Advisory Commission on Consumer Protection and Quality in the Health Care Industry: Recommendations.

Purpose of the health care system must be to continuously reduce the impact and burden of illness, injury, and disability, and to improve the health and functioning of the people of the United States.

Initial Set of National Aims

Reducing the underlying causes of illness, injury, and disability

Expanding research on new treatments and evidence on effectiveness

Ensuring the appropriate use of health care services

Reducing health care errors

Addressing oversupply and undersupply of health care resources

Increasing patients' participation in their care

Measurable objectives need to be specified for each of these aims.

Advancing Quality Measurement and Reporting

A core set of quality measures should be identified for standardized reporting by each sector of the health care industry. There should be a stable and predictable mechanism for reporting. Steps should be taken to ensure that comparative information on health care quality is valid, reliable, comprehensible, and widely available in the public domain.

Creating Public-Private Partnerships

An Advisory Council for Health Care Quality should be created in the public sector to provide ongoing national leadership in promoting and guiding continuous improvement of health care quality. It would track and report on the progress of achieving the national aims for improvement, undertake related quality measurement and reporting, and implement the Consumer Bill of Rights and Responsibilities. A Forum for Health Care Quality Measurement and Reporting should be created in the private sector to improve the effectiveness and efficiency of health care quality measurement and reporting. Widespread public availability of comparative information on quality care needs to be provided.

Encouraging Action by Group Purchasers

Group purchasers, to the extent feasible, should provide their individual members with a choice of plans. State and federal governments should create further opportunities for small employers to participate in large purchasing pools that, to the extent feasible, make a commitment to individual choice of plans. All public and private group purchasers should use quality as a factor in selecting the plans they will offer to their individual members, employees, or beneficiaries. Group purchasers should implement strategies to stimulate ongoing improvements in health care quality.

Strengthening the Hand of Consumers

Widespread and ongoing consumer education should be developed to deliver accurate and reliable information and encourage consumers to consider information on quality when choosing health plans, providers, and treatments. Some consumers will require assistance in making these choices. Further research should be conducted addressing the use of consumer information.

Focusing on Vulnerable Populations

Additional investment should be provided for developing, evaluating, and supporting effective health care delivery models designed to meet the specific needs of vulnerable populations.

Promoting Accountability

The Consumer Bill of Rights and Responsibility should be included in private and public sector contractual and oversight requirements.

Reducing Errors and Increasing Safety in Health Care

Interested parties should work together to develop a health care error reporting system to identify errors and prevent their recurrence.

Fostering Evidence-Based Practice and Innovation

Federal funding for health care research, including basic, clinical, prevention, and health services research, should be increased and the necessary research infrastructure supported. Collaborative arrangements between researchers and private and public sectors should be developed. Research should target those areas where the greatest improvements in health and functional status of population can occur and where gaps in knowledge exist.

(continued)

BOX 16-2 The President's Advisory Commission on Consumer Protection and Quality in the Health Care Industry: Recommendations—*Continued.*

Adapting Organizations for Change

Health care organizations should provide strong leadership to confront quality challenges and pursue aims for improvement. They should commit to reducing errors and increasing safety. Organizations need to develop long-term relationships with all stakeholders.

Engaging the Health Care Workforce

The training of physicians, nurses, and other health care workers must change to meet the demands of a changing health care industry. Minimum standards for education, training, and supervision of unlicensed paraprofessionals should be established. Steps should be taken to improve the diversity and the cultural competence of the health care workforce. Health care workers must be encouraged to identify and report clinical errors and instances of improper or dangerous care. Action must be taken to reduce the unacceptably high rate of injury in the health care workforce. Efforts must be taken to address the serious morale problems that exist among health care workers in many sectors of the industry. Further research should be conducted into how changes in the roles and responsibilities of health care workers are affecting quality.

Investing in Information Systems

Purchasers of health care services should insist that providers and plans be able to produce quantitative evidence of quality as a means of encouraging investment in information systems.

Source: The President's Advisory Commission on Consumer Protection and Quality in the Health Care Industry. (1999). *Quality first: Better health care for all Americans.* Washington, DC: U.S. Government Printing Office.

The report on safety clearly states that there is no one answer to solving this problem. This report defines safety as "freedom from accidental injury" and defines error as "the failure of a planned action to be completed as intended or the use of a wrong plan to achieve an aim" (Institute of Medicine, 1999, p. 3). Errors are directly related to outcomes, which is a significant concern in quality improvement efforts. There are two types of errors: error of planning and error of execution. Errors harm the patient and some that do injure the patient may have been preventable adverse events. An adverse event is "an injury resulting from a medical intervention, or in other words, it is not due to the underlying condition of the patient" (Institute of Medicine, 1999, pp. 3–4). Not all adverse events are due to errors and not all are preventable. Analysis is required to determine the relationship of an error to an adverse event.

Patient safety is a critical component of quality (Institute of Medicine, 1999). The report describes the influence of the environment on quality by identifying three dimensions.

1. Dimension of quality, which includes safe care, practice that is consistent with current medical knowledge, and customization (evidence-based practice).
2. Dimension of the critical factors in the external environment that affect quality improvement efforts, which include regulatory/legislative activities and economic and other incentives.
3. Dimension of "the ability to meet customer-specific values and expectations, permitting the greatest responsiveness to individual values and preferences and maximum personalization or customization of care" (Institute of Medicine, 1999, p. 16).

In 1998, the Institute of Medicine identified three types of quality problems that are used in the measurement of quality.

1. **Misuse:** avoidable complications that prevent patients from receiving full potential benefit of a service
2. **Overuse:** potential for harm from the provision of a service that exceeds the possible benefit
3. **Underuse:** failure to provide a service that would have produced a favorable outcome for the patient (Chassin & Galvin, 1998, p. 1003)

This initiative represents a collaborative effort from a health care professional organization, an accrediting organization, and consumers. Getting the patient involved is a very important strategy; however, the critical next step is listening to the patient. JCAHO also developed a

BOX 16-3 Current reports on health care quality.

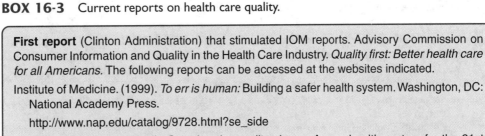

First report (Clinton Administration) that stimulated IOM reports. Advisory Commission on Consumer Information and Quality in the Health Care Industry. *Quality first: Better health care for all Americans.* The following reports can be accessed at the websites indicated.

Institute of Medicine. (1999). *To err is human:* Building a safer health system. Washington, DC: National Academy Press.

http://www.nap.edu/catalog/9728.html?se_side

Institute of Medicine. (2001). *Crossing the quality chasm:* A new health system for the 21st century. Washington, DC: National Academy Press.

http://books.nap.edu/catalog/10027.html?onpi_newsdoc030101

Institute of Medicine. (2001). *Envisioning the national health care quality report.* Washington, DC: National Academy Press.

http://www.nap.edu/catalog/10073.html?se_side

Institute of Medicine. (2002). *Leadership by example: Coordinating government roles in improving health care quality.* Washington, DC: National Academy Press.

http://www.nap.edu/catalog/10537.html?se_side

Institute of Medicine. (2003). *Who will keep the public healthy?* Educating public health professionals for the 21st century. Washington, DC: National Academy Press.

http://www.nap.edu/catalog/10542.html?se_side

Institute of Medicine. (2003). *Health professions education: A bridge to quality.* Washington, DC: National Academy Press.

http://www.nap.edu/catalog/10681.html?se_side

Institute of Medicine. (2003). *Priority areas for national action: Transforming health care quality.* (2003). Washington, DC: National Academy Press.

http://www.nap.edu/catalog/10593.html?onpi_newsdoc010703

Institute of Medicine. *Keeping patients safe: Transforming the work environment of nurses.* Washington, DC: National Academy Press.

http://www.nap.edu/catalog/10851.html

Institute of Medicine. (2003). *Patient safety: Achieving a new standard for care.* Washington, DC: National Academy Press.

http://www.nap.edu/catalog/10863.html

Source: Author.

safety focus, which was implemented in the 2003 accreditation cycle. It focuses on accurate patient identification, effective communication, safe use of high-alert medications, elimination of wrong site surgery, safe use of infusion pumps, and safe use of clinical alarms, all of which are discussed in this IOM report (Kirkpatrick, 2003).

When patient safety is evaluated and addressed, an inevitable issue that arises is worker safety. Patient safety and worker safety are connected. Although worker safety was not a focus of this report, "the committee believes that creating a safe environment for patients will go a long way in addressing issues of worker safety as well" (Institute of Medicine, 1999, p. 20). Worker safety issues are discussed later in this chapter.

The four key messages from this report are: "first, the magnitude of harm that results from medical errors is great; second, errors result largely from systems' failures, not individual failures; third, voluntary and mandatory reporting programs are needed now to improve patient safety; and fourth, the IOM committee and others call on health care systems to focus on error reduction as an important part of their operations and to embrace organizational change needed to reorient error-ridden systems and process" (Maddox, Wakefield, & Bull, 2001, p. 9). Nurses must be involved in developing plans to respond to safety problems on the local, state, and national levels. *To Err Is Human* identified major concerns with patient safety, and its key recommendations are identified in Box 16-4.

BOX 16-4 Institute of Medicine: Patient safety recommendations.

1. Congress should create a Center for Patient Safety within the Agency for Health Care Research and Quality. This center should:
   - Set the national goals for patient safety, track progress in meeting these goals, and issue an annual report to the President and Congress on patient safety.
   - Develop knowledge and understanding of errors in health care by developing a research agenda, funding Centers of Excellence, evaluating methods for identifying and preventing errors, and funding dissemination and communication activities to improve patient safety.
2. A nationwide mandatory reporting system should be established that provides for the collection of standardized information by state governments about adverse events that result in death or serious harm. Reporting should initially be required of hospitals and eventually be required of other institutional and ambulatory care delivery settings. Congress should:
   - Designate the Forum for Health Care Quality Measurement and Reporting as the entity responsible for promulgating and maintaining a core set of reporting standards to be used by states, including a nomenclature and taxonomy for reporting.
   - Require all health care organizations to report standardized information on a defined list of adverse events.
   - Provide funds and technical expertise for state governments to establish or adapt their current error reporting systems to collect the standardized information, analyze it, and conduct follow-up action as needed with health care organizations. Should a state choose not to implement the mandatory reporting systems, the Department of Health and Human Services should be designated as the responsible entity and designate the Center for Patient Safety to: (a) convene states to share information and expertise, and to evaluate alternative approaches taken for implementing reporting programs, identify best practices for implementation, and assess the impact of state programs, and (b) receive and analyze aggregate reports from states to identify persistent safety issues that require more intensive analysis and/or a broader-based response (e.g., designing prototype systems or requesting a response by agencies, manufacturers, or others).
3. The development of voluntary reporting efforts should be encouraged. The Center for Patient Safety should:
   - Describe and disseminate information on external voluntary reporting programs to encourage greater participation in them and track the development of new reporting systems as they form.
   - Convene sponsors and users of external reporting systems to evaluate what works and what does not work well in the programs, and ways to make them more effective.
   - Periodically assess whether additional efforts are needed to address gaps in information to improve patient safety and to encourage health care organizations to participate in voluntary reporting programs.
   - Fund and evaluate pilot projects for reporting systems, both within individual health care organizations and collaborative efforts among health care organizations.
4. Congress should pass legislation to extend peer review protections to data related to patient safety and quality improvement that are collected and analyzed by health care organizations for internal use or shared with others solely for purposes of improving safety and quality.
5. Performance standards and expectations for health care organizations should focus greater attention on patient safety.
   - Regulators and accreditors should require health care organizations to implement meaningful patient safety programs with defined executive responsibility.
   - Public and private purchasers should provide incentives to health care organizations to demonstrate continuous improvement in patient safety.
   - Health professional licensing bodies should (a) implement periodic reexamination and relicensing of doctors, nurses, and other key providers, based on both competence and knowledge of safety practices, and (b) work with certifying and credentialing organizations to develop more effective methods to identify unsafe providers and take action.
   - Professional societies should make a visible commitment to patient safety by establishing a permanent committee dedicated to safety improvement. This committee should (a) develop a curriculum on patient safety and encourage its adoption into training and certification requirements; (b) disseminate information on patient safety to members through special sessions at annual conferences, journal articles and editorials, newsletters, publications, and websites on a regular basis; (c) recognize patient safety considerations in practice guidelines and in standards related to the introduction and diffusion of new technologies, therapies, and drugs; (d) work with the Center for Patient Safety to develop community-based, collaborative initiatives for error reporting and analysis and implementation of patient safety improvements; and (e) collaborate with other professional societies and disciplines in a national summit on the professional's role in patient safety.

BOX 16-4 Institute of Medicine: Patient safety recommendations—*Continued.*

6. The Food and Drug Administration (FDA) should increase attention to the safe use of drugs in both pre- and post-marketing processes through the following actions:
   - Develop and enforce standards for the design of drug packaging and labeling that will maximize safety in use.
   - Require pharmaceutical companies to test (using FDA-approved methods) proposed drug names to identify and remedy potential sound-alike and look-alike confusion with existing drug names.
   - Work with physicians, pharmacists, consumers, and others to establish appropriate responses to problems identified through post-marketing surveillance, especially for concerns that are perceived to require immediate response to protect the safety of patients.
7. Health care organizations and professionals affiliated with them should make continually improved patient safety a declared and serious aim by establishing patient safety programs with defined executive responsibility. Patient safety programs should:
   - Provide strong, clear, and visible attention to safety.
   - Implement non-punitive systems for reporting and analyzing errors within their organizations.
   - Incorporate well-understood safety principles, such as standardizing and simplifying equipment, supplies, and processes.
   - Establish interdisciplinary team training programs for providers that incorporate proven methods of team training, such as simulation.
8. Health care organizations should implement proven medication safety practices.

Source: Institute of Medicine. *To err is human. Building a safer health system.* Washington, DC: National Academy Press, 1999. Reprinted with permission.

Crossing the quality chasm

The second major report from the Committee on the Quality of Health Care in America was *Crossing the Quality Chasm* (Institute of Medicine, 2001a), which focused on developing a new health care system for the 21st century, one that improves care. The first conclusion from the report is that the system is in need of repair, one of fundamental change. As this text has emphasized throughout, the report also emphasizes the impact of the rapid change in the health care system: new medical science, new technology, rapid availability of information, and so on. Health care providers cannot keep up, and "performance of the health care system varies considerably" (Institute of Medicine, 2001a, p. 3). As was noted in *To Err Is Human*, the system is fragmented and poorly organized. It is a system that does not make the best use of its resources. Another conclusion from the report is the impact that the increase of chronic conditions has had on the system. With people living longer, mostly due to the advances in medical science and technology, more are living with chronic conditions. "Chronic conditions, defined as illnesses that last longer than 3 months and are not self-limiting, are now the leading cause of illness, disability, and health problems in this country, and affect almost half of the U.S. population" (Hoffman et al., 1996; as cited in Institute of Medicine, 2001a, p. 27). Many of these patients also have comorbid conditions. They have complicated problems and require collaborative treatment efforts, "involving the definition of clinical problems in terms that both patients and providers understand; joint development of a care plan with goals, targets, and implementations strategies; provision of self-management training and support services; and active, sustained follow-up using visits, telephone calls, e-mail, and Web-based monitoring and decision support programs" (Von Korf et al., 1997; as cited in Institute of Medicine, 2001a, p. 27). The complex, fragmented, and disorganized health care system is ineffective in dealing with these problems. The report supports changes that were identified by Wagner, Austin, and Von Korff (1996):

1. Need for evidence-based, planned care
2. Reorganization of practices to meet the needs of patients who require more time, a broad array of resources, and closer follow-up
3. Systematic attention to patients' need for information and behavioral change
4. Ready access to necessary clinical expertise
5. Supportive information systems

FIGURE 16-1   Six aims for improvement of the health care system.

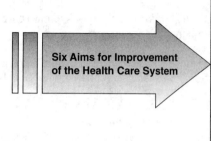
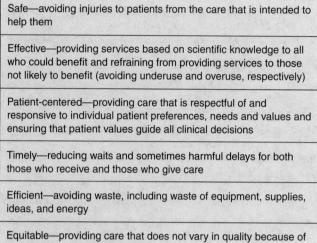

Six Aims for Improvement of the Health Care System

Safe—avoiding injuries to patients from the care that is intended to help them

Effective—providing services based on scientific knowledge to all who could benefit and refraining from providing services to those not likely to benefit (avoiding underuse and overuse, respectively)

Patient-centered—providing care that is respectful of and responsive to individual patient preferences, needs and values and ensuring that patient values guide all clinical decisions

Timely—reducing waits and sometimes harmful delays for both those who receive and those who give care

Efficient—avoiding waste, including waste of equipment, supplies, ideas, and energy

Equitable—providing care that does not vary in quality because of personal characteristics such as gender, ethnicity, geographic

Source: Author and summarized from Institute of Medicine. (2001). *Crossing the quality chasm.* Washington, DC: National Academy Press, pp. 5–6. Reprinted with permission.

This 2001 report identifies quality as a system property. It states that there are six aims for improvement—safe, **effective**, patient-centered, timely, **efficient**, and **equitable**—which are identified in Figure 16-1.

"Health care has safety and quality problems because it relies on outmoded systems of work. Poor designs set the workforce up to fail, regardless of how hard they try. If we want safer, higher-quality care, we will need to have redesigned systems of care, including the use of information technology to support clinical and administrative processes" (Institute of Medicine, 2001a, p. 4). These identified problems are complex and not easily resolved. Some of them have been addressed, such as redesigning, but the results have not always improved care. How should health care providers resolve them and improve? The report's recommendations for an agenda crossing the quality chasm, which are directly related to nursing care, include the following.

■ All health care constituents, including policy makers, purchasers, regulators, health professionals, health care trustees and management, and consumers, commit to a national statement of purpose for the health care systems as a whole and to a shared agenda of six aims for improvement that can raise the quality of care to unprecedented levels. *This is related to the six aims identified by the report and included in earlier chapter content. This will not be easy to accomplish, and it has never been done.*

■ Clinicians, patients, and the health care organizations that support care delivery adopt a new set of principles to guide the redesign of care processes. *Identifying critical concerns will be important. Often clinicians, patients, and health care organizations do not agree.*

■ The DHHS identifies a set of priority conditions to focus initial efforts, provide resources to stimulate innovation, and initiate the change process. *See comments about the report,* Priority Areas for National Action, *later in this section. This report followed the* Crossing the Quality Chasm *report, and it does identify specific conditions.*

■ Health care organizations design and implement more effective organizational support processes to make change in the delivery of care possible. *As has been discussed, change is ever present, and health care organizations and their leaders and staff must learn more effective methods for coping with change to improve.*

■ Purchasers, regulators, health professions, educational institutions, and the DHHS create an environment that fosters and rewards improvement by (a) creating an infrastructure to support evidence-based practice, (b) facilitating the use of information technology (IT), (c) aligning payment incentives, and (d) preparing the workforce to better serve patients in a world of expanding knowledge and rapid change. *There is no doubt that these are key issues, which have been discussed in this text. DHHS has provided some infrastructure to support evidence-based practice through its website, but more support is needed. As was identified in Chapter 15, much has been done to develop information technology. Financial issues and reimbursement are major areas of deep concern. Nursing education as well as other health care professional education must make changes to meet the new demands* (Institute of Medicine, 2001a, p. 5).

Envisioning the national health care quality report

Much has been said about the lack of health care quality. To pursue improvement means that the United States needs methods to determine if care has been improved. The goal of *Envisioning the National Health Care Quality Report* (Institute of Medicine, 2001b) is to develop these methods, which should complement other reports on quality as well as *Healthy People 2010*, which identifies public health objectives (U.S. Department of Health and Human Services, 2000). To be effective there needs to be effective communication and collaboration among the quality efforts. The report recommends that there be a classification matrix of measures, which includes two dimensions: (a) the consumer perspective and (b) components of health care quality. Box 16-5 describes the dimensions and their elements.

"The matrix is a tool to visualize possible combinations of the two dimensions (consumer perspectives and components of health care quality) of the framework and better understand how various aspects of the framework relate to one another" (Institute of Medicine, 2001b, p. 8). In order to develop a national health quality report and analyze data, there needs to be a new health infrastructure with uniform data standards and computerized clinical data systems. The infrastructure has developed to the point that it can be used to meet this goal. How would a national health care quality report affect efforts to improve quality?

- Supply a common understanding of quality and how to measure it that reflects the best current approaches and practices
- Identify aspects of the health care system that improve or impede quality
- Generate data associated with major quality initiatives
- Educate the public, the media, and other audiences about the importance of health care quality and the current level of quality

BOX 16-5   Matrix for the national health care quality report.

Elements for Consumer Dimension
Two dimensions are consumer perspectives of health care needs and components of health care quality

Consumer Perspectives
- Staying healthy
- Getting better
- Living with illness or disability
- Coping with the end of life

Components
- Safety
- Effectiveness
- Patient centeredness
- Timeliness

Source: Author and summarized from Safety Recommendations; Institute of Medicine. (2001). *Crossing the quality chasm.* Washington, DC: National Academy Press, pp. 5–6. Reprinted with permission.

- Identify for policy makers the problem areas in health care quality that most need their attention and action, with the understanding that these priorities may change over time and differ by geographic location
- Provide policy makers, purchasers, health care providers, and others with realistic benchmarks for quality of care in the form of national, regional, and population comparisons
- Make it easier to compare the quality of the U.S. health care system with that of other nations
- Stimulate the refinement of existing measures and the development of new ones
- Stimulate data collection efforts at the state and local levels (mirroring the national effort) to facilitate targeted quality improvements
- Incorporate improved measures as they become available and practicable
- Clarify the many aspects of health care quality and how they affect one another and quality as a whole
- Encourage data collection efforts needed to refine and develop quality measures and, ultimately, stimulate the development of a health information infrastructure to support quality measurement and reporting (Institute of Medicine, 2001b, p. 31)

Leadership by example

This report, requested by Congress, examines the federal government's quality enhancement processes (Institute of Medicine, 2003a). It focuses on six government programs: Medicare, Medicaid, The State Children's Health Insurance Program (SCHIP), The Department of Defense TRICARE and TRICARE for life programs, the Veteran's Administration program, and the Indian Health Services program. A total of about 100 million people are covered by these programs. The report's conclusion is that improvement in this process is particularly needed.

1. There is a lack of consistent performance measurement across and within programs.
2. The usefulness of quality information has been questioned.
3. There is a lack of a conceptual framework to guide the evaluation.
4. There is a lack of computerized clinical data.
5. There is a lack of commitment to guide decisions.
6. There is a lack of a systematic approach for assessing the quality enhancement activities.

Each one of these problems will require substantial changes in the health care delivery system.

The report notes that federal leadership is needed because the federal government is in a unique position to assume a lead role to develop a national health care quality improvement initiative. The federal government is a "regulator; purchaser; health care provider; and sponsor of research, education, and training" (Institute of Medicine, 2001, p. 6). It is the largest purchaser of care, and thus it could have a major impact on many people. It provides direct care to many: military personnel and their families, Native Americans, and veterans. Through these programs the federal government could establish models to improve care. This has already been demonstrated through Medicare and Medicaid. As a regulator, it also can affect many health care providers who are not in the federal system; for example, as has been noted earlier in this text, health care organizations that accept Medicare or Medicaid funds must comply with federal regulations, which impacts all of its patients. It should be noted that regulation is not the best way to make improvement changes because "the regulatory approach is a blunt tool that generally fails to differentiate among grades of quality" (Institute of Medicine, 2001b, p. 7). Regulation should not be relied on as the only approach to the problem. Through sponsorship of research, education, and training, however, the federal government can have a major impact. The report's conclusions recommend that the federal government lead by example and coordinate government roles in improving health care quality. In doing this, the government will have an impact on all parts of the health care delivery system.

Who will keep the public healthy?

This report from the Institute of Medicine addresses the needs for public health in a world that is affected by globalization, rapid travel, scientific and technological advances, and demographic changes. In order to address public health problems, public health professionals need to be prepared to deal with the problems. "A public health professional is a person educated in public health or a related discipline who is employed to improve health through a population focus" (Institute of Medicine, 2003b, p. 4). The eight content areas that are important for today's and future public health professions are: informatics, genomics, communication, cultural competence, community-based participatory research, global health, policy and law, and public health ethics. These areas are in addition to the long held core components of public health: epidemiology, biostatistics, environmental health, health services administration, and social and behavioral science. This report provides an in-depth exploration of the educational needs for improved public health.

Health professions education

In the report *Health Professions Education* (Institute of Medicine, 2003c), the education of health professions is viewed as a bridge to quality care. This discussion does not just focus on education, but rather on the need to have qualified, competent staff in order to improve health care. The report indicates that health professions' education is in need of change to meet the growing demands of the health care system today. "All health professionals should be educated to deliver patient-centered care as members of an interdisciplinary team, emphasizing evidence-based practice, quality improvement approaches, and informatics" (Institute of Medicine, 2003c, p. 3). All of these critical areas have been discussed in this text because they are very relevant to nurses and nursing care.

Priority areas for national action: Transforming health care quality

The IOM report *Crossing the Quality Chasm* (2001a) identifies that the first step the United States needs to take to address quality of care is to conduct a systematic identification of the priority areas for quality improvement in order to make the necessary changes (Institute of Medicine, 2003d). The *Priority Areas for National Action* (Institute of Medicine, 2003d) developed this list by identifying 20 priority areas. The first two areas are to promote care coordination and self-management/health literacy, both of which affect a broad range of groups. The other areas are concerned with the continuum of care across life span, preventive care, inpatient/surgical care, chronic conditions, end-of-life care, and behavioral care. The 20 areas include:

- Care coordination
- Self-management/health literacy
- Asthma—appropriate treatment for persons with mild/moderate persistent asthma
- Cancer screening that is evidence based, with a focus on colorectal and cervical cancer
- Children with special health care needs (who are at increased risk for chronic physical, developmental, and behavioral conditions)
- Diabetes—focus on appropriate management of early disease
- End-of-life with advanced organ system failure—focus on congestive heart failure and chronic obstructive pulmonary disease
- Frailty associated with old age—preventing falls and pressure ulcers, maximizing function, and developing advanced care plans
- Hypertension—focus on appropriate treatment of early disease
- Immunization—children and adult
- Ischemic heart disease—prevention, reduction of recurring events, and optimization of functional capacity
- Major depression—screening and treatment
- Medical management—preventing medication errors and overuse of antibiotics
- Nosocomial infections—prevention and surveillance
- Pain control in advanced cancer
- Pregnancy and childbirth—appropriate prenatal and intrapartum care
- Severe and persistent mental illness—focus on treatment in the public sector
- Stroke—early treatment in the public sector
- Tobacco dependence treatment in adults
- Obesity (emerging area) (Institute of Medicine, 2003d, p. 3)

These areas should be used as a guide by health care providers as they develop their QI programs. It is felt that improving care in these 20 areas will make a major difference on quality of care. Communities can also use this list to develop their community health focus and thus improve the quality of life and care of populations in the community.

Keeping patients safe: Transforming the work environment of nurses

The IOM report *Keeping Patients Safe: Transforming the Work Environment of Nurses* (Institute of Medicine, 2004a) clearly is an important report for nurses in all types of settings. This extensive report addresses critical quality and safety issues with a particular focus on nursing care and nurses and examines these issues from the perspective of the work environment. As the report states, "When we are hospitalized, in a nursing home, or managing a chronic condition in our own homes—at some of our most vulnerable moments—nurses are the health care providers we are most likely to encounter, spend the greatest amount of time with, and be dependent upon for our recovery" (Institute of Medicine, 2004a). From the review of the critical work environment the report then discusses methods for designing the work environment so that nurses may provide safer patient care. The content identifies concerns related to the nursing shortage, health care errors, patient safety risk factors, central role of the nurse in patient safety, and work environment threats to patient safety. Recommendations for resolving these concerns include: patient safety defenses; evidence-based model for safety defenses; reengineering issues; transformational leadership and evidence-based management; maximizing workforce capability through safe staffing levels, need for knowledge and skills and clinical decision making, and interdisciplinary collaboration; workspace design; and building and creating a culture of safety. This report will undoubtedly have a major impact on the practice of nursing, health care delivery, and should affect how nursing is taught.

Patient safety: Achieving a new standard of care

This IOM report expands the work done on safety in earlier reports (Institute of Medicine, 2004b). It emphasizes the need to establish a national health information infrastructure and need for data standards. Why is this important? It is impossible to monitor and then address safety issues without data, and the goal is to have national data as patients receive care from multiple providers. The ultimate goal should be prevention of errors and not resolution of errors after they have occurred. Routine use of electronic health records would give health care providers and patients immediate access to complete patient information as well as tools to guide decision making and help prevent errors (Institute of Medicine, 2004b). In addition, each health care organization needs to develop a patient safety program. Safety is not a topic that has been ignored by health care organizations; however, there is clearly a need for improvement in this area.

THINK CRITICALLY

Try this exercise to apply what you have learned about this topic.

Definition of quality

Can quality of care be defined? This has been a recurring health care question for a long time. The Institute of Medicine (IOM) defines quality as "the degree to which health services for individuals and populations increase the likelihood of desired health outcomes and are consistent with current professional knowledge" (Chassin & Galvin, 1998, p. 1000). There are many definitions that have been suggested; however, we will use this definition in the text. Box 16-6 identifies some examples of specific elements that are considered when quality is assessed.

Reviewing these elements provides some idea about the complexity of the quality of care concept. These elements and others need to be included when staff assess care and plan how to improve care.

BOX 16-6   Examples of quality elements.

- Resource utilization (e.g., use of providers, suppliers, services; length-of-stay; readmission; prevention of need for expensive services)
- Avoids adverse effects
- Improved patient physiological status
- Reduced signs and symptoms of illness
- Improved functional status and well-being
- Accessibility of care
- Appropriateness of care
- Continuity of care
- Effectiveness of care
- Efficacy of care
- Efficiency of care
- Patient perspective issues (e.g., satisfaction data)
- Safety of the care environment
- Timeliness of care
- Risk management (e.g., infection rates, medication errors, patient falls, comorbidities)

Source: Author.

To improve care requires measurement of the status of care delivery, but can quality be measured or are there some aspects that cannot be measured? It is not easy to measure quality, and health care organizations struggle to arrive at the best methods. What are some examples of the difficulty of measuring quality? Measuring the quality of the nurse–patient or the physician–patient relationship quantitatively is not easy as there are many variables involved. Just the issue of personalities and communication methods make it difficult. Another example of care that is difficult to measure is the dying process: "A good death is really an intuitive process by the patient, family, and the caregivers" (Thurber, 1997, p. 179). If knowledge about a specific illness is incomplete, such as with chronic fatigue syndrome, it will be difficult to measure quality care for that particular disorder. More research is required before standards and guidelines can be developed to describe the best treatment for many illnesses. These are just a few examples, but since quality is affected by so many different elements there can be great differences from one experience to another.

Critical quality elements

Typically when quality is discussed three accepted elements of quality are identified.

- **Structure,** the environment in which services are provided
- **Process,** the manner in which services are provided
- **Outcome,** the result of services

These elements usually serve as the framework for the assessment of health care quality, and are related to those identified in Box 16-6. For example, resource utilization is related to structure; improved functional status and well-being is an outcome; and continuity of care is related to process.

Why is quality care so difficult to understand and to monitor? It would seem that patients receive care and get better, or receive care and do not. Care is more complex than this, as many variables make it difficult to measure. Some examples of these variables include:

- **Health care is not a single product.**
  There are many different types of health care (e.g., acute care, home care, primary care, long-term care, medical, surgical, pediatrics, psychiatry, obstetrics, and so on), and patients may

receive care in a number of these settings. In some cases, it is not even clear how to define the product or the service that is received.

■ **Different interventions require different measurements.**

There are many different types of treatment and drugs, and they can be used in a variety of combinations.

■ **Different groups focus on different issues when considering quality.**

Many demographic characteristics affect how one views health and health care and how one responds to health care interventions (e.g., age, gender, ethnic, rural, urban, type of employment, education level, and so on).

■ **Overuse, underuse, and misuse are critical in determining quality.**

Receiving too much care (e.g., medications), not enough care (e.g., not getting follow-up for diagnostic tests), or getting the wrong treatment or no treatment when needed.

■ **Organizations need a culture of quality to improve.**

Organizations that do not want to improve or are not committed—as demonstrated by lack of funding and staff to support efforts—will have great difficulty improving.

■ **Assessment of quality is expensive, and this cost is shifted to purchasers and consumers.**

Health care organizations have to spend money to assess care and plan for improvement. Changes that may need to be made typically affect costs. Staff are required to do this work. The organizations will try to charge more for their services to cover these costs.

■ **Patient satisfaction is a questionable measure of the quality of care.**

It is not clear how patient satisfaction affects quality or even what it means. For example, if a patient describes quality of care by the fact that staff were friendly and yet expected outcomes were not met (Patient is not able to administer self insulin), did the patient receive quality care? The patient may say "yes" while the health care provider would say "no" (Bodenheimer, 1999, p. 489).

If quality of care can be defined (even though it is complex), quality measured, and problems identified, can care be improved? Can improvement be achieved for patients at a cost that society can afford? Honest appraisal of the scientific facts suggests that health care can be improved by closing the wide gaps between prevailing practices and the best known approaches to care and by inventing new forms of care (Berwick & Nolan, 1998). A recommended model for improvement suggested by Berwick and Nolan (1998) focuses on several questions.

1. What is the organization trying to accomplish?
2. How will the organization know whether a change is an improvement?
3. What change can the organization try that it believes will result in improvement?

These questions try to arrive at a description of what the organization considers to be quality care. New nurses soon hear about QI when they begin their first jobs. Organizations typically have staff who work exclusively on QI and often they are nurses. Committees that focus on QI typically include nurses, physicians, social workers, medical records, laboratory staff, and other staff.

Critical health care safety issues

Clearly, there are many safety issues in health care; some relate specifically to patients and others to staff. Some of the critical patient issues are medication administration, use of restraints, violence (as patient violence can lead to injuries for the patient or other patients), nosocomial infections, and wrong patient receiving treatment or patient receiving the wrong treatment. Each one of these is a complex issue. There are standards related to these safety issues (for example, use of restraints) and the critical steps of medication administration (e.g., right patient, right drug, right dose, right time, and right route). Medication administration, as noted in *To Err Is Human* (Institute of Medicine, 1999), can lead to errors. Some of the reasons for errors in this area are: time pressures, fatigue, understaffing, lack of knowledge about the drug and/or the patient, documentation, and systems failure. The American Nurses Association has developed

BOX 16-7 Principles for documentation.

Unique patient identification must be assured within and across paper-based and electronic health care documentation systems.

Documentation systems must assure the security and confidentiality of patient information.

Documentation must be: accurate and consistent; clear, concise, and complete; reflecting patient response and outcomes related to nursing care; received timely and sequential; retrievable on a permanent basis in a nursing-specific manner; able to be audited.

Documentation must meet existing standards such as those promulgated by state and federal regulatory agencies (to include HIPAA as enforced through the Department of Justice (DOJ), the Centers for Medicare and Medicaid Services (CMS), and through accrediting organizations such as the Joint Commission on Accreditation of Healthcare Organizations (JCAHO) and the National Committee for Quality Assurance (NCQA)).

Entries into the medical record (including orders) must be legible, complete, and authenticated and dated by the person responsible for ordering, providing, or evaluating the care provided (JCAHO).

Abbreviations, acronyms, and symbols utilized in documentation must be standardized (JCAHO).

The nurse must be familiar with organizational policies and/or procedures related to documentation.

Several terminologies have been recognized by ANA which specify the domain of nursing and contain terms used in the planning, delivery, and evaluation of the nursing care of the patient or client in diverse settings. An ANA-recognized terminology should be employed in documentation so that data can be aggregated. However, in instances where clinicians are using electronic information systems and structured data linked to a reference terminology, the use of an ANA-recognized terminology at the interface may be unnecessary.

Source: American Nurses Association. (2003). *Principles for documentation.* Washington, DC: Author. Reprinted with permission.

documentation principles, which are described in Box 16-7, to assist nurses in their documentation, a critical factor in ensuring safe care.

"Given that nurses comprise the largest component of the health care workforce and are involved with the provision, management, research, and education related to patient care, safety and error reduction in health care are central concerns for the profession and a responsibility for every nurse" (Maddox, Wakefield, & Bull, 2001, p. 8). How should nurses be involved in the CQI effort? First, nurses need to understand the problem and circumstances related to errors. Contributory factors are important in the analysis of errors or situations when errors could have occurred. These factors can be categorized in the following manner.

- **Institutional:** regulatory context, medicolegal environment
- **Organization and management:** financial resources and constraints, policy standards and goals, safety culture and priorities
- **Work environment:** staffing levels and mix; patterns of workload and shift; design, availability, and maintenance of equipment; administrative and managerial support
- **Team:** verbal and written communication, supervision and willingness to seek help, team leadership
- **Individual staff member:** knowledge and skills, motivation and attitude, physical and mental health
- **Task:** availability and use of protocols, availability and accuracy of test results
- **Patient:** complexity and seriousness of condition, language and communication, personality and social factors (Vincent, 2003, p. 1050; Vincent, Taylor-Adams, & Stanhope, 1998)

It is also important to collect data about possible errors and share this data and its analysis so that prevention strategies can be developed. As the IOM report indicated, it is important for nurses to recognize that the focus should not be on individual nurses who make errors but rather system characteristics that make errors possible.

This culture of blame will not be easy to change. There needs to be new systems of care that prevent errors; for example, computerized drug order entry systems, review of drug orders by pharmacists, greater standardization and simplification, use of written protocols, and other strategies to prevent errors and improve care. Other issues include providing space and time for staff breaks, providing education about care and safety, developing improved information management, including patients and families in care and reduction of errors, and enhancing interdisciplinary teamwork (Maddox, Wakefield, & Bull, 2001).

Nurse staff-to-patient ratios also affect errors (Kovner & Gergen, 1998). The *To Err Is Human* report identified five principles that might be helpful in designing safe health care systems. These include: (a) providing leadership, (b) respecting human limits in the design process, (c) promoting effective team functioning, (d) anticipating the unexpected, and (e) creating a learning environment. These principles apply to nursing and are related to what has been discussed in this text about leadership and management.

For staff, some of the key safety issues are needlesticks, ergonomic safety, violence, latex allergies, and infections, such as what occurred with SARS when so many health professionals in other countries contracted the disease from patients. Violence is found in all settings but is a particular concern in emergency departments, psychiatric/substance abuse services, and in long-term care. Staff need to learn how to protect themselves and others without harming the patient who is violent. Concern also exists about the emotional response that follows after staff experience these incidents. Each one of these safety issues is complex and requires that staff are educated about prevention and that organizations provide support and prevention services as required. The Occupational Safety and Health Administration (OSHA) is the federal agency that is responsible for monitoring safe workplaces.

CURRENT ISSUES

Learn about events around the globe that relate to the chapter content.

BENCHMARKS

Now let's take a moment to test your knowledge of the concepts you have studied in this section.

Quality, Safe Care: Measurement and Improvement
The accreditation process

Accreditation of organizations is important to many different types of organizations. For example, schools of nursing are accredited, meaning they receive some type of official approval that they can offer services, which in the case of schools of nursing are courses toward a nursing degree. Hospitals and other types of health care organizations are also accredited. Evaluation is a fact of life; however, it is not simple and can have major ramifications for a health care organization—costs, staff time and energy, public relations. It may require that the organization institute changes or, in extreme cases, stop providing services. The following discussion offers some information about accreditation in the health care delivery system as a measurement and improvement process.

What is accreditation?

Accreditation is the process by which organizations are evaluated on their quality, based on established minimum standards. Health care facilities have been accredited for a long time, but the process still has its critics. An important criticism is whether or not quality can be defined. "Quality, like obscenity, is difficult to define, but most surveyors (accreditation) assume they know what it is when they see it. Yet there are no absolute and few relative measures of quality that are generally recognized and agreed on by both surveyors and providers. As a result, quality measurement by surveyors is more a matter of faith than science" (Barter, 1988, p. 707). Previous discussion in this chapter identifies a recognized definition for quality of care although there are many other definitions that have been proposed by a number of authorities. Accreditation focuses on quality, and thus a definition is important to the process. Accreditation has undergone many changes in the last 10 years as it has adjusted to the health care environment and to changes in perspectives of the quality care. The most important change has been the increased focus on continuous quality improvement (CQI or QI) or ongoing efforts to improve care, focusing on systems rather than just focusing on health care provider performance and blame. Accreditation is something that all nurses will experience but the level of that experience varies depending upon the nurse's position. Today when hospitals are surveyed all staff are expected to be prepared and participate in the process. The goal is to include more direct care providers rather than just management staff. One can conclude that accreditation is not perfect, has changed over time, now focuses on improvement, and requires understanding and participation from nurses.

Outcomes

As health care providers and organizations have become more experienced in assessing quality, they have turned more to performance-based quality care evaluation, which has been strongly supported by the Joint Commission on Accreditation of Healthcare Organizations (JCAHO). The critical question in assessing the quality of care is did the patient benefit from the care received? If so, how? If not, why? This means that quality care really needs to be defined from the perspective of outcomes, which is supported in the IOM definition of quality (Hansten & Washburn, 1999). Quality really cannot be measured until quality is defined and outcomes are identified. These questions are critical and form the basis of outcomes. It is not uncommon to find "nursing care outcomes" in nursing literature and to hear nurses discussing them. However, this is an incorrect term. Hegyvary (1991) stated that this term should reflect the patient's response to care, not the provider response or the patient's outcome (Rantz, Bostick, & Riggs, 2002). When outcomes are assessed, there are several aspects to include.

- ■ It is necessary to first develop indicators that identify areas of potential problems or improvement of care. This is the content or focus of assessment or evaluation. An **indicator** is a measurable dimension of quality, specifying patient care activities and event occurrences for outcomes that can be monitored. Indicators are criteria in that they are "variables known to be relevant, measurable indicators of the standards of practice" (American Nurses Association, 1991, p. 8).

- ■ Indicators must also include a quantity element or threshold. This preestablished level indicates the need for more intensive assessment, which can emphasize relative rate or trends that need further investigation. For example, an initial, preoperative, and postoperative pain assessment might include (a) localization of pain, (b) type of pain, (c) duration of pain, (d) time of onset, (e) factors associated with pain, and (f) interventions taken and the outcomes, with a threshold of 92%. The threshold indicates when further evaluation needs to be done—if more than 8% of the patient assessments do not meet this indicator, further investigation is required.

- ■ Other indicators focus on sentinel events or events that always require investigation (e.g., suicide attempt, cardiac arrest in labor and delivery, lack of referral to specialist and patient dies).

The components of quality indicators are described in Box 16-8.

Examples of some outcomes are mortality rates, length-of-stay, adverse incidents, complications, readmission rates, patient/family satisfaction, referrals to specialists, patient adherence to the discharge plan or treatment plan, and prevention adherence (e.g., mammogram, Pap smear,

BOX 16-8 Components of quality indicators.

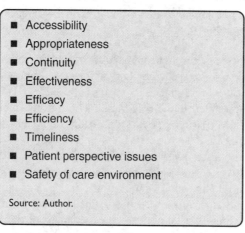

- Accessibility
- Appropriateness
- Continuity
- Effectiveness
- Efficacy
- Efficiency
- Timeliness
- Patient perspective issues
- Safety of care environment

Source: Author.

immunizations). Indicators may also focus on process (actual activities done by health care providers) or structure (facilities, equipment, staff, finances), but the outcome focus (short-term and long-term results, complications, health status and functioning) has become more important.

Joint Commission on Accreditation of Healthcare Organizations

JCAHO has been in existence in some form since 1951. This nonprofit organization accredits more than 17,000 health care organizations, including hospitals, long-term care organizations, home care agencies, clinical laboratories, ambulatory care organizations, behavioral health organizations, and health care networks or managed care organizations. It is the most important accrediting organization in the United States. Its purpose is to improve the quality of care provided to the public by assessing performance based on its standards. The organization establishes minimum standards and benchmarks for health care organizations to use as they improve care. The goals of JCAHO are to:

- Improve the actual delivery of care
- Increase the value and productivity of the accreditation process involving customers and the health care environment as a whole
- Decrease cost and enhance resource allocation
- Promote a continual process of quality of improvement
- Promote high-quality care and patient safety
- Increase the public's confidence in health care organizations
- Customize the survey process
- Promote a collaborative continuous flow of information between health care organizations
- Improve consistency and relevancy of standards and surveyors (Joint Commission on Accreditation of Healthcare Organizations, 2003, July)

Each of these goals is related to nurses and nursing care.

JCAHO standards have been developed, evaluated, and have changed over the years to meet the changing needs of health care delivery. These standards form the framework for JCAHO accreditation. Standards cover the following areas.

1. Nursing
2. Leadership
3. Surveillance
4. Prevention and control of infection
5. Medication management
6. Management of the environment of care
7. Provision of care
8. Treatment and services

9. Ethics, rights, and responsibilities
10. Improving organization performance

The JCAHO survey emphasizes continuous QI throughout the organization. Organizations need to identify and address sentinel events, defined as "an event that had a negative outcome with a patient that people do not want to happen" (Paolucci, 2001, p. 8). A root cause analysis or a systematic review of the event is conducted. The key is to assess the process, not the individual staff who were involved—blame is not the goal but rather prevention of further events. This supports the recommendations from the IOM reports. The QI approach was a major change in the accreditation. Prior to the use of QI standards, accreditation required extensive data collection, and there was a tendency to take a punitive approach. Health care organizations felt that once they met a certain requirement there was nothing else that needed to be done. An analogy would be the student who makes an "A" who then thinks there is nothing else to learn or that there is no risk of the grade going down. Health care organizations did not consistently look for ways to improve but rather just focused on problems. This has now changed as QI has become more acceptable, expected, and continuous.

Related to this effort, JCAHO has developed a core measure initiative so that organizations will focus on what matters. JCAHO defines core measures as "standardized performance measures, with precisely defined data elements, calculation algorithms, and standardized data-collection protocols" (Nolan, 2004, p. 28). These measures should determine if patients are getting the care that they should receive and provide benchmarks. As of 2004, hospitals must select three of the JCAHO core measures, which for 2004 were: community acquired pneumonia (CAP), acute myocardial infarction (AMI), heart failure (HF), and pregnancy and related conditions (including newborn and maternal care). JCAHO has developed specific rules for collecting and reporting data to ensure better comparison of data from one organization to another. Hospitals must develop strategies to improve care for the core areas, and all of these core areas are highly dependent on nursing care. Nurses need to be directly involved in the core measure initiative.

JCAHO surveys the organizations it has accredited every 3 years for routine accreditation. Health care organizations voluntarily request this accreditation; however, for health care organizations that offer medical training programs, provide clinical experiences for nursing students, and receive federal funding, this accreditation is required. It is thus difficult to view accreditation as truly voluntary. Recently, JCAHO began to have random, unannounced surveys. This change was made due to criticism found in the DHHS report *The External Review of Hospital Quality: A Call for Greater Accountability* (Gallagher & Kany, 2000; Gropper, 1999). The concern was expressed that since hospitals had ample time to prepare for scheduled surveys, the hospitals put all their energy into preparation just prior to a survey and were less involved in maintaining standards between surveys. In addition, surveyors will now spend more time on patient units and receive more detailed information about the organization before the actual survey, so that they are better prepared for the survey. Hopefully, these changes in the JCAHO process will result in more effective evaluations of health care organizations that JCAHO accredits.

As is clear from recent IOM reports, the United States has a problem with health care quality and safety despite the long-term presence of accreditation provided by JCAHO. Accreditation has not prevented or solved the problem. A recent Congressional report also indicated that there were criticisms about the JCAHO assessments. It notes that JCAHO is not reliable in assessing Medicare Conditions of Participation. The Medicare conditions of participation are the standards or requirements that organizations providing care to Medicare beneficiaries must meet. Of particular concern is the use of organization self-assessment in the accreditation process ("Stark Urges," 2003). Since JCAHO is planning on moving more toward greater emphasis on organization self-assessment methods, this may be a problem. It is clear that JCAHO accreditation is not the perfect solution to guaranteeing health care quality, but it continues to be used and really is all that is available at this time.

Nurses and JCAHO

All nurses eventually encounter JCAHO—through application of its standards, preparation for surveys, and then participation in surveys. Nurses assume leadership roles in all of these phases. Quality improvement should be continuous with no end. As some areas are improved, organizations then focus on new areas and also revisit areas to determine if improvement continues. Each organization needs to develop plans to ensure that care is assessed and that problems are addressed. The JCAHO survey should not be the focus, although it usually is; rather, the focus should be on continuous improvement. What usually happens is the survey preparation and process become all consuming. Key steps that organizations complete to meet the improvement goal are:

1. Develop a plan (includes units, services, departments, and organization wide)
2. Implement the plan
3. Collect data and analyze the data
4. Develop reports that summarize the data and analysis so that it can be useful in decision making
5. Share data and analysis with staff
6. Develop and implement corrective actions for identified problems
7. Begin again—with more assessment

Nursing staff should be involved in all of these steps. As JCAHO survey time approaches, organizations begin to prepare for the survey. All staff need education about the QI program, JCAHO, and the survey process. Tension usually increases at the time of a survey. Losing accreditation, although this rarely occurs, is extremely serious. The organization may be required to make changes and report these changes by specific deadlines, which may require additional surveys. All of this is costly and affects the organization's public image.

Some health care organizations such as home care agencies are using national evaluation approaches that are not sponsored by JCAHO. Home care agencies use a specific outcome-based approach to quality improvement (QI) called Outcome Assessment Information Set (OASIS), which was developed in the 1990s by the DHHS to provide a "systematic process that would yield consistent data to improve care outcomes" (Mosocco, 2001, p. 205) while focusing on a group of data elements that represents core items of a comprehensive assessment of home care patients. The focus is on whether or not the patient benefited from the care, which should be the focus of care in all types of settings. The OASIS has had its problems. It is complex and takes time to collect the data; however, changes have been made in the system to improve it. The process has two stages.

1. The first is outcome analysis, which includes data collection using the OASIS assessment form, and then processing, editing, and transmitting the data to a central location that collects data from multiple home health agencies. Then each agency receives a risk-adjusted outcomes report, which compares each agency with other agencies providing a quality report card.
2. The second stage is outcome enhancement when each agency that participates in the process selects outcomes for further evaluation—such as identifying problems and strengths, developing best practices, developing a plan of action, implementing and monitoring the plan, and evaluating the effect of these actions in subsequent reports (Mosocco, 2001). Agencies that receive Medicare reimbursement, which constitutes most of them, are required to participate in OASIS.

THINK CRITICALLY

Try this exercise to apply what you have learned about this topic.

Methods used in establishing quality, safe care

Many methods are used in the QI process. Some are used for data collection, while others are used for guidance to improve health care. The methods that are described here include: standards of care, credentialing, utilization review/resource management, clinical guidelines, clinical pathways, benchmarking, evidence-based practice, assessment of access, and risk management. Some of these have been discussed in more detail in earlier chapters so some of this content is review. It is important to remember that quality usually cannot be assessed by using only one method.

Standards of care

Standards of care provide minimum descriptions of accepted actions expected from a health care organization or professional who has specific skill and knowledge levels. They are important in establishing expectations. Standards are developed by professional organizations, legal sources such as nurse practice acts and federal and state laws, regulatory agencies such as accreditation bodies and federal and state agencies, and health care facilities, and are supported by scientific literature and clinical pathways.

Credentialing and licensure

Credentialing is the review process used by a health care organization or insurer to guarantee that a provider or health care professional (e.g., physician, nurse-midwife, nurse practitioner) may practice or provide care to its patients or members. This review typically includes an evaluation of licenses, certification, evidence of malpractice insurance as required, history of involvement in malpractice, and education. Licensure verification is also important to ensure the RNs as well as other clinical staff are licensed to practice.

Utilization review/management

Utilization review/management (UR/UM) is the process of evaluating necessity, appropriateness, and efficiency of health care services for specific patients or patient populations. UM or utilization review has been used in acute care settings for a long time; however, it is also very important to managed care. Nurses are frequently hired as UM staff. They have the clinical skills and knowledge necessary to evaluate patient needs and services to determine the necessity, appropriateness, and timeliness of services.

To reduce costs, it is necessary to assess appropriateness of care and timeliness and influence decisions that are made by providers. "Appropriateness" ties UM to QI. UM is not just looking at numbers such as how many days of treatment. It also focuses on what is appropriate care for the patient's problem. Typically, utilization/resource management or review focuses on length-of-stay or treatment, use of services, complications, readmission rates, number of transfers, number and type of prescriptions, number of referrals to specialists, number of procedures, and so forth. Nurses have the necessary skills for utilization/resource management: clinical knowledge; understanding of health care organizations, nursing process, and communication and collaboration within multidisciplinary teams; and understanding of documentation. This function also requires that the nurse is knowledgeable about managed care, reimbursement, provider options, benefits, and costs. Case managers are also very involved in resource management, and authorization of services is the key task in resource management. How does UM/UR affect nursing care? Two examples, one in a rural hospital and another in a Veteran's Administration (VA) hospital, provide suggestions about the roles that nurses might play and how UM affects care.

■ A rural medical center in Vermont with 188 beds recognized that it had a problem with its length-of-stay that needed to be resolved (Winstead-Fry, Bormolini, & Keech, 1995). The most important decision the hospital made was the first one: to include physicians and nurses in the decision-making process. The hospital leadership did not want to identify who was to blame for the problem, but rather to understand the problem and resolve it. Nursing, as well as the hospital leadership, felt that hospitalization is always the last option, and the goal should be to return the patient to his or her home as soon as possible. The assessment team identified six groups or contributors that might have an impact on a patient's length-of-stay: patients, physicians, family, outside forces, other health care team members, and nurses. Decreased LOS meant that nurses had decreased time for coordination and planning, and yet at the same time, there was an increased need for documentation, patient teaching, and communication. Nursing staff were very important in reaching an understanding of length-of-stay and the effects that a decreased length-of-stay might have on workload and patient care quality. The hospital was using more part-time nursing staff, and part-time staff often have a more difficult time contributing to coordination and planning because they are working sporadically.

After identifying the contributors, the team had to identify methods for resolving the problem. The solutions had to be cost neutral, because the hospital could not afford to increase its expenses to solve the length-of-stay problem. With the help of a physician and a nurse facilitator, the project team identified 10 recommendations, which included use of mobile chart racks to facilitate physician rounds, involvement of nursing in high-level committees, improvement of the beeper system, and education in assertiveness skills for nurses. A major recommendation focused on nursing when the project team recommended that the clinical units use clinical care coordinators. The goal was to improve time management and decision making. Early identification of problems and involvement of family at the time of admission were recognized as very important to the patient's length-of-stay. Nursing leadership strongly supported the entire evaluation process, and this was critical to its success. At the end of the first year, the length-of-stay had decreased. Nursing staff and physicians provided favorable evaluations of the changes, and the clinical care coordinators found their new roles rewarding. This is a good example of nurse–physician collaboration and how it can have a positive impact on health care delivery through utilization and quality.

■ The VA hospital in Milwaukee, Wisconsin, applied the concepts of coordinated care, case management, and continuous quality improvement to improve continuity and coordination between their inpatient units and outpatient programs (Holle, Rick, Sliefert, & Stephens, 1995). This example illustrates the need to begin to assess the articulation of inpatient and outpatient care. The project goals were to:

■ Coordinate inpatient and outpatient care

■ Improve continuity of care

■ Improve communication between inpatient and outpatient staff

■ Reduce duplication of effort between inpatient and outpatient staff

■ Improve efficiency of resource use and improve cost-effectiveness

■ Reduce incidence of unnecessary admissions

■ Reduce incidence of prolonged inpatient stays

■ Facilitate post-discharge follow-up care

■ Enhance patient and significant other involvement in health care planning

■ Improve access to outpatient services

■ Improve patient and staff satisfaction

It was recognized early on in the project that inpatient and outpatient staff knew little about the work that each did or their patient outcomes. Seventeen outpatient clinics and 12 inpatient units were selected for service integration. Transition project teams, each with a project coordinator, implemented the project. The following are the guidelines that were used in the project, which help to understand the issues related to articulating inpatient and outpatient services that can arise when projects such as these are undertaken.

■ Identify patient populations who receive care across the continuum of outpatient and inpatient services, including home care, nursing home care, and referrals to external health care providers.

■ Identify patient self-care and compliance issues (both inpatient and outpatient).

■ Outline discharge planning issues that affect follow-up care.

■ Identify factors that influence quality care (patient outcomes) and length-of-stay.

■ Consider space, staffing, and cross-training issues.

■ Evaluate the roles of registered nurses, licensed practical nurses, nurse assistants, clinical nurse specialists, nurse practitioners, and nurse managers as they affect efficiency and effectiveness of patient care delivery.

■ Identify workload data.

■ Develop/review evaluation methodology to measure overall goals.

■ Review the process of referrals to outpatient services (both medical and nursing referrals).

■ Conduct a literature review of pertinent trends in coordinating/integrating care (Holle et al., 1995).

As changes were made, patient outcomes were tracked and compared. Positive results occurred, including decreasing the length-of-stay, completion of patient education, proper completion of procedures, and treatment follow-through.

These two examples demonstrate the important nursing roles in projects that make major changes to improve care and respond to the demands of the health care environment and the managed care environment.

Clinical guidelines

The use of **clinical guidelines** is a method that focuses on improvement of care. The Agency for Healthcare Research and Quality (AHRQ) is the most prominent agency that develops clinical or practice guidelines. As guidelines identify outcomes and support best practice, they can be useful in determining quality and cost of health care. Professional organizations have also become very active in developing guidelines. How do guidelines enhance the quality of care?

- By identifying possible quality problems arising from underuse, overuse, or incompetent provision of care
- By improving the level of understanding that patients have about their care and thus about the informed consent they might give to have, or forgo, certain treatments
- By enhancing important patient outcomes and incorporating them into patient satisfaction surveys and other instruments designed to assess or improve performance
- By determining priorities for improving or standardizing specific patterns of clinical care (Lohr, 1995, p. 23)

The AHRQ is an important governmental agency that focuses on health care quality issues. Its mission is "to support research designed to improve the outcomes and quality of health care, reduce its costs, address patient safety and medical errors, and broaden access to effective services" (Agency for Healthcare Research and Quality, 2003, July 9). Its goals are to: (a) support improvements in health outcomes, (b) promote patient safety and reduce medication errors, (c) advance the use of information technology for coordinating patient care and conducting quality and outcomes research, and (d) establish an Office of Priority Populations (to ensure that they receive care—low-income groups, minorities, women, children, the elderly, and individuals with special needs). AHRQ has developed quality indicators for inpatient, safety, and prevention. Box 16-9 provides a description of these indicators.

Clinical pathways

Clinical pathways are discussed in more detail in Chapter 9; however, it is important to recognize their use in the assessment of quality and cost of health care. Pathways focus on outcomes and the assessment of their achievement. They provide a benchmarking method for individual patients. The promotion of appropriate use of resources in a timely manner is an important component of each pathway, and this promotes cost-effectiveness. When outcomes are not met, then variances are analyzed to determine causes and actions that need to be taken to prevent further problems. This information also provides data that can be used to improve care for other patients who might have similar problems.

Benchmarking

Benchmarking is a tool that identifies "best practices" (Czarnecki, 1995). (See Chapter 9 for further information on benchmarking.) It is, however, important to note that it is also a tool that links standards of care, guidelines, documentation, quality improvement programs, and clinical pathways. Benchmarking allows organizations to compare their performance both within the organization and with other organizations. It is a process that uses data to improve. It requires that staff use data-driven, decision-making processes and in so doing makes the organization and its staff aware of options. "Benchmarking results in real introspection and the development of a new

BOX 16-9   Agency for Healthcare Research and Quality (AHRQ) Quality Indicators.

The AHRQ Quality Indicators (QIs) are measures of health care quality that make use of readily available hospital inpatient administrative data. Software and a user guide are now available that will help users apply the Quality Indicators to their own data.

Why Were the AHRQ Quality Indicators (QIs) Developed?

Health care decision makers need user-friendly data and tools that will help them:

- Assess the effects of health care program and policy choices.
- Guide future health care policy making.
- Accurately measure outcomes, community access to care, utilization, and costs.

AHRQ has developed an array of health care decision-making and research tools that can be used by program managers, researchers, and others at the federal, state, and local levels. One of these tools is the AHRQ Quality Indicators (QIs), which use hospital administrative data to highlight potential quality concerns, identify areas that need further study and investigation, and track changes over time. They represent a refinement and further development of the Quality Indicators developed in the early 1990s as part of the Healthcare Cost and Utilization Project (HCUP).

What Are the AHRQ QIs?

The AHRQ QIs are a set of quality indicators organized into three "modules," each of which measures quality associated with processes of care that occurred in an outpatient or an inpatient setting. All three modules rely solely on hospital inpatient administrative data:

1. *Prevention QIs*—or ambulatory care sensitive conditions—identify hospital admissions that evidence suggests could have been avoided, at least in part, through high-quality outpatient care.
2. *Inpatient Quality Indicators* reflect quality of care inside hospitals and include:
   - Inpatient mortality for medical conditions.
   - Inpatient mortality for procedures.
   - Utilization of procedures for which there are questions of overuse, underuse, or misuse.
   - Volume of procedures for which there is evidence that a higher volume of procedures is associated with lower mortality.
3. *Patient Safety Indicators* also reflect quality of care inside hospitals, but focus on surgical complications and other iatrogenic events.

What Questions Can the AHRQ QIs Help Users Answer?

Hospitals and hospital systems can use the AHRQ QIs to help answer the following types of questions:

- How does our hospital's cesarean section rate compare to the state or the nation?
- Do other hospitals have similar mortality rates following hip replacement?
- How does the volume of coronary artery bypass graft in my hospital compare with other hospitals?

State data organizations and community health partnerships can use the AHRQ QIs to ask questions that provide initial feedback about clinical areas appropriate for further, more in-depth analysis, such as:

- What can the pediatric AHRQ QIs tell me about the adequacy of pediatric primary care in my community?
- How does the hysterectomy rate in our area compare with the state and national average?

Federal policy makers can use the AHRQ QIs to track health care quality in the United States over time and to assess whether health care quality is improving, for example:

- How does the rate of coronary artery bypass grafts vary over time and across regions of the United States?
- What is the national average for bilateral cardiac catheterization (a procedure that is not generally recommended) and how has this changed over time?

How Can the AHRQ QIs Be Used in Quality Assessment?

Hospitals and other organizations may use the AHRQ QIs without collecting new data by following these steps:

1. Identify the performance measure(s) of particular interest from the list of QIs. For example, a group interested in studying children's health might select the pediatric care indicators.
2. Determine what hospital(s) will be included in the assessment. For example, a local organization examining access to primary care in the community might include data from all local-area hospitals.

BOX 16-9 Agency for Healthcare Research and Quality (AHRQ) Quality Indicators—*Continued*.

3. Acquire the relevant hospital discharge data from individual hospitals, state association or data organization, or state agency that makes discharge data available.
4. Calculate the QI rates, using the AHRQ QI software, hospital discharge data of interest, and other statistical software.
5. Use the calculated rates as a first step in tracking hospital outcomes and primary care access. A hospital might compare rates with existing benchmarks.

   For those QI rates that suggest potential for improvement, develop a plan to study the clinical outcomes and associated processes in more depth.

For complete, current information, see the website http://www.qualityindicators.ahrq.gov/data/hcup/qinext.htm.

Source: Agency for Healthcare Research and Quality. (March 2003). *AHRQ quality indicators*. Rockville, MD. http://www.qualityindicators.ahrq.gov/data/ncup/qinext.htm.

vision for health care—a vision that is built on the detailed redesign of basic processes" (Czarnecki, 1995, p. 2). It begins by identifying the areas of greatest need and those for which there is comparable performance data (Czarnecki, 1996). Time should not be wasted on correcting problems that will not have an impact or for which it is difficult to obtain data.

Evidence-based practice

Evidence-based practice helps to identify and assess high-quality, clinically relevant research that can be applied to clinical practice and is used by nurses and physicians. Evidence-based practice is "a problem solving approach to practice that involves the conscientious use of current best evidence in making decisions about patient care. EBP incorporates a systematic search for and critical appraisal of the most relevant evidence to answer a clinical question along with one's own clinical expertise and patient values and preferences" (Melnyk & Fineout-Overholt, 2005, p. 587). The results are synthesized so that they can be used to improve care. These systematic reviews:

- Estimate the effect of health care interventions.
- Provide generalizable answers, because they are based on a number of studies in different settings and include a variety of participants.
- Identify the individual, clinical, and contextual factors that influence effectiveness.
- Identify uncertainties and gaps in research (Dickson & Entwistle, 1997, p. 3).

Evidence-based practice requires that information is available for specific questions. The research literature is reviewed using explicit scientific methods and includes all relevant research. This valuable information is then available to practitioners and should be helpful in directing their care decisions.

Assessment of access to health care

Access to care is a critical issue in today's health care environment. Assessment of access to determine who is able to access care and who is not is an important measure of the quality of care. Reduced access may result in poorer outcomes of care (Gold, 1998). How easy is it for a patient to receive care? Economic factors, transportation, and availability of appropriate health care providers may make it difficult for the patient to receive care when it is needed. Access has been greatly affected by the diverse health care delivery and financial arrangements that are currently present in the health care environment. There is also an ethical issue interwoven in any discussion of access. Is health care a right? This issue has not been resolved, as there is no state or federal law that says it is a right. The country spends more money on health care than any other service and yet not all citizens receive it. If barriers to coverage and proximity are removed, will the result be equitable access? This is also an unknown.

Access includes more than just initial entry into the health care system; it also includes how services are received within the system and the outcomes of that care. As the health care delivery system has changed, greater strain has been put on safety net providers (for example, free-care clinics, public and teaching hospitals, and other health care facilities that provide care to those with limited funds or insurance coverage). These providers are less able to provide uncompensated care without sustaining major financial hardships. In addition, the strain and overload on the health care delivery system affects the quality of the services provided. Given these facts, the improvement of care will require that these problems are addressed to make care more accessible to all who need care.

Other factors that are important in considering access are convenience, timeliness, handicap provisions, accommodations for language or sight, hours of operation, provider choice, waiting time for urgent and routine care, and timeliness of laboratory tests. Each of these can be used as indicators to determine accessibility of care and thus assist in the evaluation of the quality of care. The Institute of Medicine described access to care as the consumer's ability to access personal health services a person needs when needed to reach the best outcomes (Institute of Medicine, 1993). The major focus today is on accessible primary care, particularly in relation to continuity, time, and provider type. Managed care emphasizes the use of the primary care provider as the gatekeeper or controller of access.

Access for special populations is also a growing concern. These vulnerable populations, such as the mentally ill, homeless, substance abusers, low-income, uninsured, and the disabled (Lurie, 1997), are more vulnerable and often less "attractive" to providers and the community. Efforts have been made to resolve some of these concerns, and some of these efforts have been more successful than others.

Two other special groups that often have problems with access are adolescents and children with special needs. Confidentiality is an issue with adolescents, particularly those who may use mental health, substance abuse, contraceptives, or abortion services. Many teens need to receive services at clinics that have difficulty obtaining funding to maintain their services. This affects adolescent access to needed services. Children with special needs have problems with continuity between the various providers, such as primary and specialty care providers, public health agencies, social service, and the school system (Ireys, Grason, & Guyer, 1998). Access for special populations needs to be addressed whenever changes are made that may limit their access to care. In addition, organized efforts are needed to address present barriers to care for this population.

Risk management

Risk management (RM) focuses on limiting an organization's financial risk associated with the delivery of care, particularly with lawsuits, hopefully before incidents occur. The role of a risk manager in an organization is "to maintain a safe and effective health care environment and prevent or reduce loss to the health care organization" (Pike, Janssen, & Brooks, 2002, p. 3). Strategies that health care organizations use include:

- Purchasing insurance or self-insuring to protect against financial risk
- Identifying exposures, types, where they occur, frequency, and level of risk
- Implementing medicolegal factors to protect against undue risk
- Implementing organizational programs to prevent occurrence of events that might increase financial risk (e.g., incident report system, staff education about risk and documentation, data collection to assist in identifying potential problems)
- Investigating incidents, which might result in a potential lawsuit, as soon as possible after the incident occurs
- Monitoring strategies for prevention of risk

Risk management staff work closely with QI staff as their responsibilities are interrelated. The key source of information is the organization's occurrence or incident reporting system (Pike, Janssen, & Brooks, 2002). Nurses participate in this process by completing the required forms when involved in an incident and following policies and procedures. Most incidents, however, do not result in a lawsuit.

Nurses participate in risk management every day when they ensure patient safety and quality care. Typical areas of high risk include: medication administration, falls, overall patient safety, use of technology and equipment (for example, ensuring that equipment is working correctly before using it in the operating room), assessment and communication of allergies, and any action or intervention that might harm the patient. Health care organizations must also consider the risks to anyone who enters the organization such as visitors, community members, family members, and so on (e.g., a visitor falls in the hallway). Health care organizations and providers also retain legal services to assist them with risk management. Frequently, nurse attorneys are used because they have both the legal and clinical experience to understand the complex problems that arise. These preventive efforts are expensive; however, they are not as expensive as the cost of malpractice suits. Attorneys provide counsel about documentation and actions to be taken if an incident occurs that might put the organization at financial risk. If a nurse is involved in a malpractice suit, the nurse would be covered by the employer's attorney; however, the nurse should also consult an attorney who would just represent the nurse. Malpractice insurance, which every nurse should carry, covers most if not all of the legal expenses.

THINK CRITICALLY

Try this exercise to apply what you have learned about this topic.

Quality report cards

Quality **report cards**, which have become more common in health care, provide specific performance data about an organization at specific intervals. The organization may then compare their data with data from other similar organizations. The goal is to provide information that is helpful to the organization and assists in improving the organization's health care services. Patients and consumers are slowly beginning to find that these report cards might be helpful in assessing health plans, health care providers, and health care organizations such as hospitals to determine the best possible care for them.

Report cards also offer excellent opportunities for health care organizations to examine and compare performance across health care organizations and to develop national, regional, and state averages and benchmarks for specific measures of care and service. Report cards, however, are not perfect. They are costly from the perspective of data collection, analysis, and then sharing the results with others. A report card may indicate improvement in specific areas covered by specific indicators, but there is no assurance that this affects other aspects of care. Interpretation must be done carefully. There is also no guarantee that releasing this information affects quality or consumer's health care choices. Many decisions that consumers make about their health care are not always based on quantitative data, but rather more on what patients think makes them feel better. Patients often seek out information and guidance from family members and friends, who have their own personal views and values that may not be based on facts. In 1996, the Agency for Healthcare Research and Quality conducted a survey in which more than 80% of those surveyed who had seen a report card thought it would be useful to people who were making decisions about health care; however, only one-third had actually used the information (Hochhauser, 1998). To be effective, report cards must be used by consumers and purchasers of care as they make health care decisions. Understanding these new data and finding data may not always be easy, although the Internet is making some report cards more accessible. This will probably increase access over time.

One study examined the relationship between consumers' health plan choices and health plan performance ratings (Chernew & Scanlon, 1998). It included data from a company that had more than 325,000 employees, retirees, and their dependents. The company selected the health plans and fees that were then made available to its employees. All plans were required to offer a standard benefit package; however, the plans differed (e.g., nature of physician network, control over physicians, costs). The plans were required to report data about their performance. The results of this study indicate that employees do not seem to be overly responsive to plan performance measures. In addition, employees may have different values than their employer. For example, employers and some employees may consider long waiting time for appointments as negative, whereas some employees may see this as an indication of physician quality or popularity.

Nursing and quality report cards

What has been the nursing profession's role in the process of describing quality care? One example of how nurses have added to the knowledge of a better understanding of quality care is a 1997 study that reviewed the results of the *American Journal of Nursing* Patient Care Survey of 7,355 nurses (Shindul-Rothschild, Long-Middleton, & Berry, 1997). The purpose of the review was to determine which of the identified 43 variables could be used by nurses to predict the quality of nursing care, and the study was able to obtain an overall prediction rate of 84%. The variables that predicted "good" or "excellent" nursing care were:

1. Registered nurse (RN) staff is not reduced.
2. Nurse executive position is filled.
3. The amount of time that is available to provide nursing care.
4. Nurses are able to uphold their professional standards.
5. Nurses are likely to remain in nursing.
6. There are fewer patient and family complaints, pressure ulcers and skin breakdown, injuries to patients, medication errors, and complications.

Nurses consider these variables to be important in their daily practice. These variables are also connected to structure, process, and outcome, which really form the major perspective of quality at this time. For example, numbers 1, 2, and 5 are connected to structure, numbers 3 and 4 to process, and number 6 to outcomes. These same variables are also similar to the Forces of Magnetism identified in Magnet hospitals, which were discussed in Chapter 6.

In 1994, the ANA initiated an investigation of the impact of workforce restructuring and redesign on the safety and quality of patient care in acute care settings. The purpose of this report was to "explore the nature and strength of the linkages between nursing care and patient outcomes by identifying nursing quality indicators" (Pollard, Mitra, & Mendelson, 1996, p. 1). The result provided a framework for educating nurses, consumers, and policy makers about nursing's contributions within the acute care setting (American Nurses Association, 1996; Moore, Lynn, McMillen, & Evans, 1999; Whitman, Davidson, Rudy, & Wolf, 2001). The project tracked the quality of nursing care provided in acute care settings and considered the current efforts hospitals and health care systems used to track measures of hospital performance with linkages to nursing services (American Nurses Association, 1996). Box 16-10 describes the eight indicators that were selected for inclusion in this quality report card.

This is not a comprehensive list of nursing quality measures, but they represent core indicators for acute care that could be refined or expanded. This was a major step forward for nursing. To ensure quality data, nurses need to develop standardized data reporting processes. As additional measures to assess care are considered, the ANA recommends that two criteria be used to set the priority of measures: (a) the perceived strength of the indicator's relationship to nursing quality (research-based), and (b) the burden associated with data collection (e.g., whether or not the data needs to be aggregated manually). Collaboration with other organizations (e.g., state nursing organizations, state and local governments, the JCAHO, third-party payer, and so on) will result in the development of a more effective report card system for nursing (Oermann & Huber, 1999).

CURRENT ISSUES

Learn about events around the globe that relate to the chapter content.

There continues to be a need to identify objective measures to assess health care provider performance. Managed care has made this even more important as consumers and providers have become more concerned about the quality of care and provider performance as costs are reduced. Identifying nurse-sensitive quality measures was critical in the 1994 ANA report; however, it must be recognized that outcomes measurement in health care is still a relatively new area. There

BOX 16-10   Acute care nursing quality indicators.

Patient-Focused Outcome Indicators
- Mortality rate
- Length-of-stay
- Adverse incidents
- Complications
- Patient/family satisfaction with nursing care
- Patient adherence to discharge plan

Process of Care Indicators
- Nurse satisfaction
- Assessment and implementation of patient care requirements
- Pain management
- Maintenance of skin integrity
- Patient education
- Discharge planning
- Assurance of patient safety
- Responsiveness to unplanned patient care needs

Structure of Care Indicators—Nurse Staffing Patterns
- Ratio of total nursing staff to patients
- Ratio of RNs to total nursing staff
- RN staff qualifications
- Total nursing care hours provided per patient
- Staff continuity
- RN overtime
- Nursing staff injury rate

Source: Author; content summarized from Pollard, P., Mitra, K., & Mendelson, D. of Lewin-VHI, Inc. (1996). *Nursing care report card for acute care*. Washington, DC: American Nurses Association.

is much to learn about it. In general, concern exists that databases and report cards that focus on measuring quality have not included nursing-specific quality indicators.

Three types of indicators were used in the report, which are considered the three critical elements discussed earlier in the chapter: patient-focused outcome, process of care, and structure of care-nurse staffing patterns. Outcome indicators focus on how patients and their conditions are affected by their interaction with nursing staff. Process indicators focus on care delivery. The study identified two types of process indicators: (a) how nurses perceive and discharge their roles or nursing satisfaction, and (b) the nature, amount, and quality of care nurses provide to patients. Structure indicators measure staffing patterns that were expected to affect the quality and quantity of nursing care. Box 16-11 identifies some examples of indicators that apply to each of the three types of indicators.

The conclusions from the 1994 survey identified two major problems. There was a lack of data availability, which interfered with measuring and tracking many of the identified indicators. The second problem was that many of the indicators, particularly patient outcomes indicators, did not have nursing specificity. Since these factors limited the development of a report card, the report explored various approaches that might be taken. One approach was to develop a report card that focused on a core set of nursing quality indicators for which data were available. These included:

- Mix of registered nurses (RNs), licensed practical nurses (LPNs), and unlicensed staff
- Total nursing staff to patients
- RN education

BOX 16-11   Examples of indicators.

Outcome Indicators

- Length-of-stay
- Adverse incidents
- Mortality rates
- Complications
- Patient/family satisfaction
- Patient adherence to treatment plan; to discharge plan

Process Indicators

- Pain management
- Patient education
- Discharge planning
- Nurse satisfaction
- Assurance of patient safety
- Maintenance of skin integrity
- No self harm

Structure Indicators

- Staff continuity
- RN-patient ratio
- RN qualifications
- RN-UAP ratio
- RN overtime
- Staff injury rate
- Staff sick time

Source: Author.

- Nursing staff turnover
- Use of agency nurses (Pollard, Mitra, & Mendelson, 1996, p. 112)

All of these indicators monitor structure outcomes that are directly related to nursing quality, but their relationship with patient outcomes requires further research. A second approach was to collect more data about all outcome indicators that have a strong theoretical or empirical link to nursing. These might eventually be used in a nursing report card. The recommended indicators were:

- Nosocomial infections
- Decubitus ulcers
- Medication errors
- Patient injury rate
- Patient satisfaction (Pollard, Mitra, & Mendelson, 1996, p. 113)

Data needed to be collected on the institutional level and required risk adjustment to provide comparability of data. These data could then be collected on the national, state, or institutional level and on a unit basis within institutions. This type of approach would provide nursing benchmarks to improve nursing care and consequently the quality of care in general. These data have been collected by nurses in many hospitals.

Developing indicators that measure the impact of nursing care on patient outcomes is a natural progression in measuring and ensuring quality health care. The ANA also acknowledges the need for nursing-sensitive indicators across the continuum of care, not just in acute care settings. The ANA has identified 10 nursing-sensitive indicators for use in community-based, non-acute care settings. The development of these indicators is part of the ANA's nationwide Nursing Safety and Quality Initiative, a multiphase effort to investigate the impact of health care restructuring on the safety and quality of patient care and on the nursing profession, which includes the indicators for acute care that were previously discussed. Evidence-based methods were used to identify the acute care indicators and were also used to develop the community-based, non-acute care indicators. The criteria used in identifying the indicators included, but were not limited to: (a) clinical relevance, (b) availability of data, (c) validity and reliability of the indicators, (d) believed relevance of the indicator to nursing practice, and (e) usefulness of data in influencing nursing practice. The 10 indicators approved for pilot testing in long-term care facilities, schools, home care, and other types of community-based organizations included:

1. Pain management
2. Cardiovascular disease prevention
3. Consistency of communication
4. Caregiver activity
5. Staff mix
6. Identification of primary caregiver
7. Client satisfaction
8. Psychosocial interaction
9. Prevention of tobacco use
10. Activities of daily living (ADL)/instrumental activities of daily living (IADL)

These are good examples of community indicators, and when compared with the acute care indicators identified earlier in Box 16-10, they do differ from indicators used to assess acute care.

An example of professional perspectives on the quality of care

Nurses and physicians have been increasingly active in criticizing managed care, particularly its efforts to control clinical decisions. The Kaiser Family Foundation and the Harvard University School of Public Health conducted a survey of nurses and physicians in 1999, which included a national random sample of 1,053 physicians and 768 nurses nationwide (Kaiser Family Foundation & Harvard University School of Public Health, 1999). The survey collected quantitative information from nurses and physicians about their experiences with health plans and their attitudes toward health plans, particularly related to patient care. Respondents were also asked about the consequences of health plan denials of care for their patients. The results from the survey indicated that nurses and physicians were greatly troubled with the changes in health status of their patients caused by managed care. The following is a summary of the survey results.

1. Experiences with health plans
   - Almost nine out of ten physicians (87%) said that their patients experienced some type of denial of coverage for health services by a health plan over the last 2 years.
   - Across all types of services, physicians reported that, in their judgment, between one-third and two-thirds of denials result in "serious" decline in a patient's health status.
   - Almost half of the nurses (48%) also reported that they saw health plan decisions causing a decline in patient health on a relatively frequent basis.
   - Nurses (30%) and physicians (26%) said they exaggerated the severity of a patient's condition often or sometimes to get coverage for them, and physicians reported frequent—and often successful—efforts advocating on behalf of their patients with plans (42%).
   - Among physicians 42% reported that health plans sometimes made efforts to aid them in improving patient care.
   - Over one-third (37%) of physicians said that they dropped participation in a plan over the last 2 years because they were unsatisfied, frustrated, or unhappy (52% said they had not).

- In reflecting on their own experiences in medicine, 58% of the physicians cited administrative issues as a great concern, while 60% of the nurses pointed to inadequate staffing levels.

2. **Attitudes toward health plans**
   - Most nurses and physicians (70% and 79%, respectively) said their views of managed care are shaped a great deal by their experiences as health providers.
   - Both nurses and physicians said that managed care has had a generally negative effect on the health care system, although many also reported positive influences. Particularly noted were increased administrative paperwork (nurses 46%, physicians 95%), decreased time to spend with patients (nurses 85%, physicians 88%), and decreased quality of care (nurses 78%, physicians 73%). The positive effects were the use of practice guidelines and disease management protocols and increased availability of preventive services.
   - Nurses (46%) and physicians (59%) expressed greater concern than the general public (30%) about how plans balance patient care and cost concerns.

3. **Physician experiences and attitudes for different specialties**
   - Physician experiences and attitudes varied considerably by their specialty designation as to the negative impact of managed care on patient care (primary care 66%, specialists 52%).
   - Physician reports also varied based on their relationship with health plans. Physicians who were primarily affiliated with a single HMO (52%) were more likely to report positive views or experiences than those who contracted with a large number of plans (74%).

This survey indicates that much needs to be done to improve care and the relationship between reimbursement organizations, physicians, and nurses. It also indicates that the quality of care is influenced by many factors. Nurses are affected and have valuable opinions about the quality of care and may benefit from collaborating with other health care providers such as physicians who have similar views. A collaborative effort will have a greater impact on changing health care delivery to improve care.

There is no doubt that managed care has stimulated many improvements in health care delivery, but there also have been increasing concerns and complaints about these changes. Some of these concerns are due to the changes that providers have had to make in their practice. When change becomes personal, more complaints will be heard. California has a long history of managed care, and has also been experiencing a backlash against managed care. The governor and state legislature created a task force to examine "the appropriate role of government in guaranteeing the highest standards in quality of care" (Enthoven & Singer, 1998, p. 95). Despite the problems that were identified, such as loss of provider choice and decreasing referrals to specialists, most people in California were satisfied, from 74% to 83%, depending on the type of MCO. The task force investigated the issue of consumer demands for lower costs and unlimited care. Physicians were most concerned with loss of their autonomy and authority and complex contracts that put them in adversarial relationships with third-party payers. Nurses experienced staffing cutbacks and at the same time experienced increased demands for productivity. California nurses played a major role in identifying concerns about the quality of care in their state. California is one example of how a state that has a long managed care history is beginning to assess where it stands on managed care, its impact on quality care, and asking health care professionals for feedback, including nurses.

The future direction: Nursing quality issues

Rantz, Bostick, and Riggs (2002) were commissioned by the ANA to conduct the third review of nursing quality measurement. From 1995 to 2000, they identified 315 nursing studies and 7 discussion/process articles on quality of care. It is notable that compared with the second review, covering 1989 to 1994, there were 180 more studies in the third review. As has been discussed in this chapter, this is another indication of the growing interest in quality of care, and more than just interest but also action to improve. The review included studies related to ambulatory care, community health, home health, hospital-based care, Veteran's Affair medical centers, long-term care, studies across all settings, and quality measurement and nurse-sensitive outcomes. This third review made the following recommendations, which are similar to the recommendations made in the second review.

■ Staff should incorporate the NMDS (Nursing Minimum Data Set) elements into all computerized medical record systems and into federal and state databases as they are revised. Collecting these elements should be reviewed as essential data as regulations are promulgated to enforce legislation written to ensure quality of health care services.

■ Staff should document nursing hours of care per patient, educational preparation of the nurse provider, and the use of assistive personnel in the delivery of care. Each nurse should have a unique provider identifier. Care delivery hours should be included in all large data sets for all settings.

■ A system for determining what constitutes appropriate outcomes for patients in different settings is needed. Data elements for these outcome measures must be included in large data sets for all settings. The system must be sensitive to an individual's potential for self-care or recovery.

■ Continued support for research efforts to identify nurse-sensitive outcomes and the relationship among nursing diagnoses, interventions, outcomes, staffing, and staff mix is essential. Support of standardization so that these elements are included in large data sets is also essential.

■ Nursing care should provide leadership in quality improvement for health care. Nurses have a long and strong history of quality measurement research that can be invaluable to the outcomes of patients and collaboration with other health care providers (Rantz, Bostick, & Riggs, 2003, p. 7).

Data from studies that address how staffing affects patient outcomes have also increased. Chapter 12 discussed nurse staffing in more detail; however, it clearly is relevant to this chapter's content. Needleman et al. (2002) reported, based on their study of 1997 data from 799 hospitals in 11 states, which included both medical and surgical patients, that "a higher proportion of hours of nursing care provided by registered nurses and a greater number of hours of care by registered nurses per day are associated with better care for hospitalized patients" (p. 1715). Another study covering 1998 to 1999 and including 210 hospitals in Pennsylvania revealed similar results (Aiken et al., 2002). The objective of this study was to "determine the association between the patient-nurse ratio and patient mortality, failure-to-rescue (deaths associated with complications) (Clarke & Aiken, 2003) among surgical patients, and factors related to nurse retention. The study indicated that hospitals with the highest patient-to-nurse ratios were at considerable risk (twice as likely) to have nurses who experience burnout and job dissatisfaction, factors that can affect quality and safety in health care delivery. Nurses were shown to be important in preventing death given that staffing levels allowed for effective care—surveillance, early detection, and timely interventions that save lives. The study not only considered patients with the risk of death but also those for whom complications could be prevented. Nursing staffing levels also had an effect on these patients. The conclusion from the study is that nurse staffing levels do affect patient outcomes. The DHHS study that was based on 1997 data also supports the conclusion that there is a strong link between patient outcomes and nurse staffing in hospitals (U.S. Department of Health and Human Services, 2001). The ANA concurs with the need to recognize the importance of staffing levels and effects on patient outcomes (quality and safety), but the ANA was concerned that the IOM report, *To Err Is Human*, did not address this issue ("Health care errors report sparks major debate, 2000"). The latter report, *Keeping Patients Safe: Transforming the Work Environment of Nurses*, discusses this issue (Institute of Medicine, 2004a). The ANA and nurses in general still must do more to educate policy makers, health care leaders, and consumers about this issue. Studies, such as the ones mentioned here, will do much to provide the data that are needed to support greater recognition that improvement of staffing levels and the qualifications of staff can help in major ways to improve the quality and safety of health care, a key concern of health care providers including nurses, consumers, employers, third-party payers, and the government.

BENCHMARKS

Now let's take a moment to test your knowledge of the concepts you have studied in this section.

Chapter Wrap-Up

Now that you've reached the end of the chapter, you may wish to explore the concepts you've been reading about in greater detail, or test yourself to see how well you've comprehended the material.

SUMMARY AND APPLICATIONS

- Summary
- Practice Quiz
- Key Terms
- Tying It All Together

- Experiential Exercises
- Case
- Links

REFERENCES

Agency for Healthcare Research and Quality. Retrieved on July 9, 2003, from http://www/ahrq.gov.

Aiken, L., et al. (2002). Hospital nurse staffing and patient mortality, nurse burnout, and job dissatisfaction. *Journal of Medical Association, 288*(16).

American Hospital Association. (1999). *Hospital statistics.* Chicago, IL.

American Nurses Association. (1991). Task force on nursing practice standards and guidelines: Working paper. *Journal of Nursing Quality Assurance, 5*(3), 1–17.

American Nurses Association. (1996). *Nursing quality indicators.* Washington, DC: American Nurses Publishing.

American Nurses Association. (2002, May/June). ANA supports JCAHO prevention program. *The American Nurse,* 5.

Barter, J. (1988). Accreditation surveys: Nit-picking or quality seeking? *Hospital and Community Psychiatry, 39*(7), 707.

Berwick, D., & Nolan, T. (1998). Physicians as leaders improving health care. *Annals of Internal Medicine, 128*(4), 289–292.

Bodenheimer, T. (1999). The American health care system: The movement for improved quality in health care. *New England Journal of Medicine, 340*(6), 488–492.

Centers for Disease Control and Prevention. (National Center for Health Statistics). (1998). Births and deaths: Preliminary data for 1998. *National Vital Statistics Report, 47*(25), 6.

Chassin, M., & Galvin, R. (1998). The urgent need to improve health care quality. *Journal of the American Medical Association, 280*(2), 1000–1005.

Chernew, M., & Scanlon, D. (1998, Spring). Health plan report cards and insurance choice. *Inquiry, 35,* 9–22.

Clarke, S., & Aiken, L. (2003). Failure to rescue. *American Journal of Nursing, 103*(1), 42–48.

Czarnecki, M. (1995). *Benchmarking strategies for health care management.* Gaithersburg, MD: Aspen Publishers, Inc.

Czarnecki, M. (1996). Benchmarking: A data-oriented look at improving health care performance. *Journal of Nursing Care Quality, 10*(3), 1–6.

Dickson, R., & Entwistle, V. (1997, February). Systematic reviews: Keeping up with research evidence. *Systematic Reviews: Examples for Nursing,* 3.

Enthoven, A., & Singer, S. (1998). The managed care backlash and the task force in California. *Health Affairs, 17*(4), 95–110.

Finkelman, A. (1996). *Quality assurance for psychiatric nursing.* Gaithersburg, MD: Aspen Publishers, Inc.

Gallagher, R., & Kany, K. (2000). Does JCAHO see the truth? *American Journal of Nursing, 100*(4), 74.

Gold, M. (1998). Beyond coverage and supply: Measuring access. *Health Services Research, 33*(3), 625–652, 681–684.

Gropper, E. (1999). Expect truly unannounced surveys (and more) from the Joint Commission. *Nursing Management, 30*(10), 36–38.

Hansten, R., & Washburn, M. (1999). Seven steps to shift from tasks to outcomes. *Nursing Management, 30*(7), 24–27.

Health care errors report sparks major debate. (2000, January–February). ANA calls for closer look at staffing's impact on errors. *The American Nurse,* 8.

Hegyvary, S. (1991). Issues in outcomes research. *Journal of Nursing Quality Assurance, 5*(2), 1–6.

Hochhauser, M. (1998). Why patients have little patience for report cards. *Managed Care, 7*(3), 15–18.

Hoffman, C., Rice, D., & Sung, H. (1996). Persons with chronic conditions. Their prevalence and costs. *JAMA, 276*(18), 1473–1479.

Holle, M., Rick, C., Sliefert, M., & Stephens, K. (1995). Integrating patient care delivery. *Journal of Nursing Administration, 25*(7/8), 32–37.

Institute of Medicine. (1993). *Access to health care in America.* Washington, DC: National Academy Press.

Institute of Medicine (1999). *To err is human: Building a safer health system.* Washington, DC: National Academy Press.

Institute of Medicine. (2001a). *Crossing the quality chasm: A new health system for the 21st century.* Washington, DC: National Academy Press.

Institute of Medicine. (2001b). *Envisioning the national health care quality report.* Washington, DC: National Academy Press.

Institute of Medicine (2003a). *Leadership by example: Coordinating government roles in improving health care quality.* Washington, DC: National Academy Press.

Institute of Medicine (2003b). *Who will keep the public healthy? Educating public health professionals for the 21st century.* Washington, DC: National Academy Press.

Institute of Medicine. (2003c). *Health professions education: A bridge to quality.* Washington, DC: National Academy Press.

Institute of Medicine. (2003d). *Priority areas for national action: Transforming health care quality.* Washington, DC: National Academy Press.

Institute of Medicine. (2004a). *Keeping patients safe: Transforming the work environment of nurses.* Washington, DC: The National Academy Press.

Institute of Medicine, (2004b). *Patient safety: Achieving a new standard for care.* Washington, DC: National Academy Press.

Ireys, H., Grason, H., & Guyer, B. (1998). Assuring quality of care for children with special needs in managed care. *Pediatrics, 98*(2), 178–185.

Joint Commission on Accreditation of Healthcare Organizations. Retrieved on July 6, 2003, from http://www.jcaho.org.

Kaiser Family Foundation & Harvard University School of Public Health. (1999). *Survey of physicians and nurses.* Menlo Park, CA: Kaiser Family Foundation.

Kirkpatrick, C. (2003). Safety first. The JCAHO introduces new patient safety goals. *Nurse Week, 2*(4), 18–20.

Kovner, C., & Gergen, P. (1998). Nurse staffing levels and adverse events following surgery in U.S. hospitals. *Image: Journal of Nursing Scholarship, 30,* 315–321.

Leapfrog Group. Retrieved on July 9, 2003, from http://www.leapfroggroup.org.

Lohr, K. (1995). Guidelines for clinical practice: What they are and why they count. *Journal of Law, Medicine & Ethics, 23,* 49–56.

Lurie, N. (1997). Studying access to care in managed care environments. *Health Services Research, 32*(5), 691–701.

Maddox, P., Wakefield, M., & Bull, J. (2001). Patient safety and the need for professional and educational change. *Nursing Outlook, 49*(1), 8–13.

Melnyx, B., & Fineout-Overholt, E. (2005). *Evidence-based practice in nursing and health care.* Philadelphia: Lippincott Williams & Wilkins.

Moore, K., Lynn, M., McMillen, B., & Evans, S. (1999). Implementation of the ANA report card. *Journal of Nursing Administration, 29*(6), 48–54.

Mosocco, D. (2001). Data management using outcomes-based quality improvement. *Home Care Provider, 6*(12), 205–211.

Needleman, J., et al. (2002). Nurse-staffing levels and the quality of care in hospitals. *New England Journal of Medicine, 346*(22), 1715–1722.

Nolan, E. (2004). Quality at the core of JCAHO initiative. *Nursing Spectrum/Midwestern Edition, 5*(6), 28.

Oermann, M., & Huber, D. (1999). Patient outcomes. A measure of nursing's value. *American Journal of Nursing, 99*(9), 40–47.

Paolucci, M. (2001). The Joint Commission gains an RN perspective. *Nurse Week Great Lakes, 1*(5), 8.

Pike, J., Janssen, R., & Brooks, P. (2002). Role and function of a hospital risk manager. *Journal of Legal Nurse Consultants, 13*(2), 3–13.

Pollard, P., Mitra, K., & Mendelson, D. (1996). *Nursing report card for acute care*. Washington, DC: American Nurses Publishing, Inc.

Rantz, M., Bostick, J., & Riggs, C. (2002). *Nursing quality measurement: A review of nursing studies 1995–2000*. Washington, DC: American Nursing Publishing, Inc.

Shindul-Rothschild, J., Long-Middleton, E., & Berry, D. (1997). Ten keys to quality care. *American Journal of Nursing, 97*(11), 35–43.

Stark Urges DHHS Inspector General to increase oversight of JCAHO. (2003, January 15). Retrieved on July 7, 2003, from http://www.house.gov/stark/documents/108th/jcaholtr.htm.

Thomas, E., et al. (1999). Costs of medical injuries in Utah and Colorado. *Inquiry, 36*, 255–264.

Thurber, C. (1997). Commentary: Quality of managed care: Where is the fit? *American Journal of Medical Quality, 12*(4), 177–182.

U.S. Department of Health and Human Services. (2000). *Healthy people 2010*. Washington, DC: U.S. Government Printing Office.

U.S. Department of Health and Human Services. (2001). *Nurse staffing and patient outcomes in hospitals*. Washington, DC: Author and the Health Resources and Services Research and Quality, Agency for Healthcare Research and Quality, Centers for Medicare and Medicaid Services (formerly Health Care Financing Administration), and the National Institute of Nursing Research.

Vincent, C. (2003). Understanding and responding to adverse events. *New England Journal of Nursing, 348*(11), 1051–1056.

Vincent, C., Taylor-Adams, S., & Stanhope, N. (1998). Framework for analyzing risk and safety in clinical medicine. *British Medical Journal, 316*, 1154–1157.

Von Korf, M., et al. (1997). Collaborative management of chronic illness. *Annals of Internal Medicine, 127*(12), 1097–1102.

Wagner, E., Austin, B., & Von Korff, M. (1996). Organizing care for patients with chronic illness. *Milbank Quarterly, 74*(4), 511–542.

Wakefield, M. (1997). Pioneering new ways to ensure quality health care. *Nursing Economics, 15*(4), 225–227.

Whitman, G., Davidson, L., Rudy, E., & Wolf, G. (2001). Developing a multi-institutional nursing report card. *Journal of Nursing Administration, 31*(2), 78–84.

Winstead-Fry, P., Bormolini, S., & Keech, R. (1995). Clinical care coordination program: A working partnership. *Journal of Nursing Administration, 25*(7/8), 46–51.

ADDITIONAL READINGS

Alford, P., & Allred, C. (1995). Value = Quality + cost. *Journal of Nursing Administration, 25*(9), 64–69.

American Nurses Association. (1995). *Nursing care report card for acute care*. Washington, DC: American Nurses Publishing.

American Nurses Association. (1996). *Nursing quality indicators: Definitions and implications*. Washington, DC: American Nurses Publishing.

American Nurses Association. (1997a). *Implementing nursing's report card: A study of RN staffing, length of stay and patient outcomes*. Washington, DC: American Nurses Publishing.

American Nurses Association. (1997b). *NIDSEC (Nursing Information and Data Set Evaluation Center): Standards and scoring guidelines*. Washington, DC: American Nurses Publishing.

American Nurses Association. (1998a). *Nursing's blueprint for managed care*. Washington, DC: American Nurses Publishing.

American Nurses Association. (1998b). *Standards of clinical nursing practice* (2nd ed.). Washington, DC: American Nurses Publishing.

American Nurses Association. (2002). *Principles for documentation*. Washington, DC: Author.

American Nurses Association. (2003). *Principles for staffing*. Washington, DC: Author.

Averill, C., et al. (1998). ANA standards for nursing data sets in information systems. *Computers in Nursing, 16*(3), 157–161.

Bartscht, K. (1999). Management engineering. In L. Wolper (Ed.), *Health care administration* (pp. 359–388). Gaithersburg, MD: Aspen Publishers, Inc.

Beardsley, D. (1999). *First do no harm: A practical guide to medication safety and JCAHO*. Marblehead, MA: Opus Communication.

Blouin, A., & Brent, N. (2000). Above all, do no harm. Patient and staff safety. *Journal of Nursing Administration, 30*(12), 571–573.

Bower, F., & McCullough, C. (2000). Restraint use in acute care settings. *Journal of Nursing Administration, 30*(12), 592–598.

Burt, S. (1999). What you need to know about latex allergy. *Nursing Management, 39*(8), 18, 20–26.

Classen, D., et al. (1997). Adverse drug events in hospitalized patients: Excess length of stay, extra costs, and attributable mortality. *Journal of the American Medical Association, 277*(2), 307–311.

Create a report card. (2003, May 31). *Measuring the quality of America's health care*. Retrieved July 7, 2003, from http://hprc.ncqa.org/about.asp.

Croke, E., & Mayberry, A. (2001). Physical restraint guidelines and care standard for use in nonpsychiatric acute care setting. *Journal of Legal Nurse Consultants, 12*(1), 3–7.

Dingman, S., Williams, M., Fosbinder, D., & Warnick, M. (1999). Implementing a caring model to improve patient satisfaction. *Journal of Nursing Administration, 29*(12), 30–37.

Ditmyer, S., et al. (1998). Developing a nursing outcomes measurement tool. *Journal of Nursing Administration, 28*(6), 10–16.

Eisenberg, J., Bowman, C., & Foster, N. (2001). Does a healthy health care workplace produce higher-quality care? *Journal of Quality Improvement, 27*(9), 444–457.

Fitzgerald, K. (1997). Clinical benchmarking: Implications for perinatal nursing. *Journal of Perinatal and Neonatal Nursing, 12*(1), 23–30.

Fitzwater, E., & Gates, D. (2002). Testing an intervention to reduce assaults on nursing assistants in nursing homes: A pilot study. *Geriatric Nursing, 23*(1), 18–23.

Frauenheim, E. (2001). Sharper images. Despite needlestick legislation nonsafe sharps still go unchecked. *Nursing Excellence, 1*(2), 6–7.

Freudenheim, M. (2000, February 2). Corrective medicine. New technology helps health care avoid mistakes. *New York Times*, C1, C26.

Grachek, M. (2000). Joint commission accreditation: A framework for coordinating care for older adults. *Geriatric Nursing, 21*(6), 326–327.

Grimaldi, P. (1997). Are managed care members satisfied? *Nursing Management, 28*(6), 12–15.

Gulzar, L. (1999). Access to health care. *Image: Journal of Nursing Scholarship, 31*(1), 13–19.

Hannon, E. (1999). The relation between volume and outcome in health care. *New England Journal of Medicine, 340*(21), 1677–1679.

Heeschen, S. (2000). Making the most of quality indicator information. *Geriatric Nursing, 21*(4), 206–209.

Hellinger, F. (1998). The effect of managed care on quality: A review of recent evidence. *Archives of Internal Medicine, 158*(4), 833–841.

Ignatavicius, D. (2000). Do you help staff rise to the fall-prevention challenge? *Nursing Management, 30*(1), 27–30.

Jech, A. (2001). The next step in preventing med errors. *RN, 64*(4), 46–49.

Jennings, B., et al. (2001). Lessons learned while collecting ANA indicator data. *Journal of Nursing Administration, 31*(3), 121–129.

Joint Commission on Accreditation of Healthcare Organizations. (2005). *2005 accreditation manual for hospitals*. Oakbrook Terrace, IL: Author.

Jones, K., Jennings, B., Moritz, P., & Moss, M. (1997). Policy issues associated with analyzing outcomes of care. *Image, 29*(3), 261–267.

Jones, M. (2001). Medical errors. *Journal of Legal Nurse Consultants, 12*(3), 16–19.

Karch, A., & Karch, F. (2001). Take part in the solution. How to report medication errors. *American Journal of Nursing, 101*(10), 25.

Kovner, C. (2001). The impact of staffing and the organization of work on patient outcomes and health care workers in health care organization. *Journal of Quality Improvement, 27*(9), 458–468.

Lamb, K., et al. (1999). Help the health care team release its hold on restraint. *Nursing Management, 303*(12), 19–23.

Lassen, A., Fosbinder, D., Minton, S., & Robins, M. (1997). Nurse/physician collaborative practice: Improving health care quality while decreasing cost. *Nursing Economics, 15*(2), 87–91.

Longo, D., et al. (1997). Consumer reports in health care: Do they make a difference in patient care? *Journal of American Medical Association, 278*(19), 1579–1590.

Mark, B., Salyer, J., & Wan, T. (2003). Professional nursing practice. Impact on organization and patient outcomes. *Journal of Nursing Administration, 33*(4), 224–234.

McConnell, E. (1999). Infection control: More than a matter of economics. *Nursing Management, 30*(6), 64–65.

McNeil, B. (2001). Shattuck lecture—Hidden barriers to improvement in the quality of care. *New England Journal of Medicine, 345*(22), 1612–1620.

Milstead, J. (2002). Leapfrog group: A prince in disguise or just another frog? *Nursing Administration Quarterly, 26*(4), 16–25.

Nicotra, D., & Ulrich, C. (1996). Process improvement plan for the reduction of nosocomial pneumonia in patients on ventilators. *Journal of Nursing Care Quality, 10*(4), 18–23.

Noetscher, C., & Morreale, G. (2001). Length of stay reduction: Two innovative hospital approaches. *Journal of Nursing Care Quality, 16*(1), 1–14.

Ohldin, A. (2001). Observations from a home-based congestive heart failure intervention. *Home Care Provider, 6*(12), 212–217.

Pear, R. (2000a, January 24). U.S. health officials reject plan to report medical mistakes. *New York Times,* A14.

Pear, R. (2000b, February 22). Clinton to order steps to reduce medical mistakes. *New York Times,* A1, A15.

Perry, J. (2001). Attention all nurses! New legislation puts safer sharps in your hands. *American Journal of Nursing, 101*(9), 24AA, 24CC.

Pew Health Professions Commission. (1995). *Critical challenges: Revitalizing the health professions for the twenty-first century.* San Francisco: Author.

President's Advisory Commission on Consumer Protection and Quality in the Health Care Industry. (1999). *Quality first: Better health care for all Americans.* Washington, DC: U.S. Government Printing Office.

Presley, D., & Robinson, G. (2002). Violence in the emergency department. *Nursing Clinics of North America, 37*(1), 161–169.

Rantz, M. (1995). *Nursing quality measurement: A review of nursing studies.* Washington, DC: American Nurses Association.

Redmond, G., Riggleman, J., Sorrell, J., & Zerull, L. (1999). Creative winds of change: Nurses collaborating for quality outcomes. *Nursing Administration Quarterly, 23*(2), 55–64.

Reed, S. (2000). 106th Congress. Patient protections top legislative agenda. *American Journal of Nursing, 100*(2), 24.

Roark, D. (2004). Bar codes & drug administration. *AJN, 104*(1), 63–66.

Rowell, P. (2001). Lessons learned while collecting ANA indicator data. The American Nurses Association responds. *Journal of Nursing Administration, 31*(3), 130–131.

Rozich, J., & Resar, R. (2002). Using a unit assessment tool to optimize patient flow and staffing in a community hospital. *Journal of Quality Improvement, 28*(1), 31–41.

Shamian, J., Hagen, B., Hu, T., & Fogarty, R. (1994). The relationship between length-of-stay and required nursing care hours. *Journal of Nursing Administration, 24*(7/8), 52–58.

Sims, C. (2003). Increasing clinical satisfaction and financial performance through nurse driven process improvement. *Journal of Nursing Administration, 33*(2), 68–75.

Smith, G., Manderscheid, R., Flynn, L., & Steinwachs, D. (1997). Principles for assessment of patient outcomes in mental health care. *Psychiatric Services, 48*(8), 1033–1036.

Snowden, F. (1998). National benchmarking is on the way. *Inside Care Management, 5*(9), 2–3.

Spath, P. (2000). *Error reduction in hospitals.* San Francisco: Jossey-Bass Publishers.

Stattler, B. (2002). Environmental health in the health care setting. *The American Nurse, 34*(2), 25–40.

Steefel, L. (2002). Nix medication errors the new-fashioned way. *Nursing Spectrum Midwest Region, 3*(6), 26.

Thompson, P. (2000). Patient safety: Pieces of a puzzle. *Journal of Nursing Administration, 30*(11), 508–509.

Trossman, S. (1998). Quality managed care: A nursing perspective. *American Journal of Nursing, 98*(6), 56, 58.

Trossman, S. (2002). New ergonomics 'plan' lacks teeth. *The American Nurse, 34*(3), 9.

Wirt, S. (2003). Latex allergy: When 'protection' becomes the problem. *Journal of Legal Nurse Consultants, 14*(1), 7–9.

DIVERSITY

The profession aims for diversity that reflects the patient population, in order to better meet population needs.

Desired Future Statement (Vision)

Nursing increasingly reflects the population it serves. Our profession derives strength from its ethnic, cultural, social, economic, and gender diversity, thereby enhancing its capacity to respond to the health care needs of a diverse nation. Nursing is a model for other professions in demonstrating the value of diversity.

Five strategies were identified to achieve the vision and one of these was identified as the primary or driving strategy. They are:

Increase health system leadership that reflects and values diversity. (Primary Strategy)

Create diversity and cultural competence through educational programs and standards in the workplace.

Increase diversity of faculty, students, and curricula in all academic and continuing education.

Focus recruitment and retention programs to greatly increase diversity.

Target legislation and funding for diversity initiatives.

Objectives to Support Primary Strategy

Develop recommendations for regulatory, accrediting, and credentialing bodies to address and incorporate diversity issues into regulations, standards, and examinations.

Encourage state/local chapters of national nursing organizations to partner with health care delivery and academic institutions to increase the diversity of their leaders in nursing and other areas.

Mentor diverse undergraduate and graduate nursing students to prepare them for leadership positions.

Create leadership career paths for nurses from diverse backgrounds to prepare them for corporate/foundation boards.

Advance strategies to bring greater diversity to the membership of each nursing organization.

SOURCE: American Nurses Association. (2002). *Nursing's agenda for the future. A call to the nation*. Washington, DC: Author. Reprinted with permission.

Pulling It All Together: The Culture of the Organization

CHAPTER OUTLINE

MediaLink
www.prenhall.com/finkelman

The Interactive Exercises for this chapter can be found in the OneKey course at www.prenhall.com/finkelman. Click on Chapter 17 to select from the following activities: Test Your Understanding, Benchmarks, Current Issues, Your Opinion Counts, Think Critically, and Summary and Applications.

What's Ahead

This chapter focuses on the issue of culture in organizations. This has become an important topic in organizations, especially health care organizations. What is it that makes an organization feel like a comfortable place to work or receive services? How is an organization described? How do individual staff affect an organization's culture? Getting to this part of an organization is not easy.

Even harder is trying to change an organization's culture. This chapter explores some of these issues surrounding diversity in health care. One could wonder why it is placed at the end of the text. The reason: an organization's culture really encompasses all that has been discussed in this text.

OBJECTIVES

Before you begin, take a moment to familiarize yourself with the key objectives of this chapter.

- Define organizational culture.
- Describe how a dissonance culture can affect an organization and patient care.
- Discuss the importance of culture to the organization.
- Compare and contrast staff culture and patient culture.
- Identify the advantages to having a multicultural staff.
- Discuss the implication of a multicultural patient population for the staff and organization.
- Describe a healing organization.
- Explain why safety is an important aspect of organizational culture.
- Identify two strategies that may be used to improve an organization's culture.

TEST YOUR UNDERSTANDING

Before we begin our exploration of this chapter, take a short "warm-up" test to see what you know about this topic.

YOUR OPINION COUNTS

Find out what others think about this topic. Post your response and check out other opinions.

Culture and Climate: Building Cultural Competency

For an organization to build its cultural competency, it must first understand what **organizational culture** is and then assess its present culture. Is it a **consonant** (functional, effective) culture or a **dissonance** (dysfunctional or ineffective) culture? The goal is to be an effective culture. As this process occurs, there are legal issues that also need to be considered related to the organization's culture. Staff, of course, play a key role in culture. This section of the chapter discusses these critical issues.

Definition of organizational culture and climate

In the late 1920s and early 1930s, a study conducted at an electric company focused on employee performance, productivity, and motivation (Milgram, Spector, & Treger, 1999). Why would this study be important to the topic of organizational culture? The results of this study identified a phenomenon which became known as the Hawthorne Effect. During the study environmental factors such as light and noise were altered, and productivity was monitored. Changes in the environment affected productivity. The study also noted that when employees participated in decisions their job satisfaction increased. In the long term these particular experiments have been questioned; however, they did begin the process of increased interest in productivity and job satisfaction factors, which are related to an organization's culture.

This interest in the culture of organizations has grown in all types of businesses including health care. Curtin (2001), a nursing leader, has written about this very important issue. "There is in each institution an implicit, invisible, intrinsic, informal, and yet instantly recognizable *welenschaung* that is best described as 'corporate culture'. Like most important things, it is difficult to define or even describe. It is not 'corporate climate', 'organizational climate', or 'corporate identity'. The corporate culture embodies the organizational values that implicitly and explicitly specify norms, shape attitudes, and guide the behaviors of the members of the organization" (Curtin, 2001, p. 219). Health care organizational culture is more complex than culture found in other businesses as it also includes professional culture due to the presence of health care professionals. Professional culture focuses on highly skilled individuals who are members of a profession and their performance of skilled tasks, whereas bureaucratic culture focuses more on defining "discrete roles carefully and specific role rights and obligations clearly" (Curtin, 2001, p. 220). Health care organizations have struggled to develop their own cultures, blending the typical organizational culture factors with the professional culture factors. The result is often "a dysfunctional production-oriented overlay to their traditional bureaucratic-professional culture" (Curtin, 2001, p. 220). This culture is discussed in this chapter and has been reflected on throughout this text. "Culture is generally defined as a shared system of values, beliefs, traditions, behavior, verbal, and nonverbal patterns of communication that hold a group of people together and distinguish them from other groups" (Salimbene, 1999, p. 26).

Consonant and dissonant cultures

If an organization ignores its culture, this can lead to major problems for the organization. To prevent this, leaders within the organization must recognize the importance of culture to the organization and work toward developing a consonant or an effective organizational culture. This culture includes shared **values**, which are the important concerns and goals shared by most of the people in the organization, and group behavior norms, which are the most common ways of acting within the group in the organization (Jones & Redman, 2000). New people come into the organization and learn about the culture by making a connection between behaviors and their consequences. An adaptive organizational culture is able to meet the challenge of change to become more effective and meet their outcomes. Rigid organizational cultures are not able to do this and become a dissonant or ineffective organizational culture.

Values have a major effect on organizations and provide direction for organizations, which can be demonstrated in staff loyalty and commitment to the organization. "Values encompass the abstract of what is right, worthwhile, or desirable" (Omery, 1989; as cited in McNeese-Smith & Crook, 2003, p. 261). They help when decisions and judgments are made. Do values always mesh? No, they do not, and when they do not, problems often arise. "Lack of congruency between a nurse's personal values and those of the organization decrease satisfaction and effectiveness and may lead to burnout and turnover" (McNeese-Smith & Crook, 2003, p. 260). There is no doubt that there are major problems with burnout and turnover in health care delivery systems today. As these organizations struggle to understand these issues and resolve them, gaining a better understanding of the status of the culture—whether it is dissonant or consonant—may help. It is initially important to identify what is a dysfunctional or dissonant culture. Sovie (1993) identified characteristics of dysfunctional or dissonant hospital cultures. These included:

- Organized to serve the providers and not the patients
- Unclear about individual and department expectations
- Do not regularly measure quality of service
- Lack patient involvement in decision making
- Limited concern about employee satisfaction
- Limited educational/training programs for employees
- Frequent turf battles
- Do not recognize staff accomplishments (As cited in Jones & Redman, 2000, p. 605)

THINK CRITICALLY

Try this exercise to apply what you have learned about this topic.

Characteristics such as these can be used to assess the status of an organization's culture. These characteristics have been discussed in earlier information about leadership and management; these styles are directly related to organizational culture.

Today, health care organizations are experiencing an evolving culture of oppression, which affects organizational culture. One reason this has happened is the limited input that staff nurses have in decisions about nursing practice. Certainly retention and recruitment problems have made this problem worse. Along with these problems, the loss of trust in people and systems has become a critical problem (Aiken et al., 2001). Nurse leaders are needed to resolve this loss of trust. "Trust involves a risk of one person approaching another in the hope of a response. Trust is a central aspect of human existence and within a trusting relationship we care for the lives of others" (Ray, Turkel, & Marino, 2002, p. 1). Making ethical choices is also related to trust. Without trust, there can be no security, no cooperation, no communication, no community, and ultimately no business (Cuilla, 2000). The health care workplace appears to be out of sync—something is missing (Parker & Gadbois, 2000). This missing piece may be the need for more community in the workplace—a place where staff are valued and trust is present. There is also a need to decrease mechanized practice and make practice more human and caring. This is difficult to accomplish when the environment is struggling with staff shortages, stress, rapid change, and organizations that frequently have dissonant cultures.

An effective, creative, and productive workplace

The organization's culture identifies the acceptable attitudes and values within the organization. Formal and informal frameworks define the culture (Milgram, Spector, & Treger, 1999). The formal framework includes the organization's structure, chain of command, and rules and regulations. The informal framework includes use of open-door policies, accessibility of management, dress codes, special events and rituals, and standard manners of speech and behavior. Both frameworks are important and interrelated.

Some health care organizations are more outwardly driven by financial issues, and in other organizations staff interpret that this is the case when it may not actually be true. Both perspectives affect the organization's culture. Why is this the case? Many health care professionals feel a real conflict in their work environment. They want to advocate for the patient and yet they feel extreme stress at work, which makes it difficult to provide the required care. While blaming administration for real and unreal problems, perceptions can become part of an organization's culture, making it an ineffective culture. Organizational caring has been studied within the hospital organizational culture. The theory of bureaucratic caring focuses on the complex nature of the meaning of caring and how health care staff implement caring in their practice (Nyberg, 1991; as cited in Ray, Turkel, & Marino, 2002). Developing an environment of caring must come from leadership so that it is part of the entire organizational environment. "Caring, financial and managerial knowledge, and ethics are integrated by leaders who will create a work environment that encourages autonomy and creativity and where organizational caring is supported by structures and systems devised in the organization" (Ray, Turkel, & Marino, 2002, p. 5; Nyberg, 1991).

Ray, Turkel, and Marino (2002) also investigated the loss of trust, as well as decreased loyalty to employers (hospitals) and the disillusionment of nurses. The study included 46 hospitals, one military hospital, and three civilian not-for-profit health care systems, involving 32 registered nurses and 14 top-level administrators. Data were collected by using semi-structured, 30- to 60-minute participant interviews. The results indicated that the nurses felt administration's decision making centered only on financial issues, which is a common theme heard when nurses discuss organizational culture. Some nurses were concerned about the loss of supplies or running out of supplies, which interfered with their practice. Others noted that administrators made comments about nurses not making the hospital money, but the nurses acknowledged that without nurses there would be no hospital care. The nurses were also concerned about hospitals not covering the cost for people who did not have insurance. They were disillusioned with nursing practice as well as with the impact of the work environment on the nurse-patient relationship. They commented that they were not able to connect with their patients in the best ways possible. Nurses wanted to feel respected and valued as professionals in the organization, but they did not. They felt that improved communication at all levels in the organization was a key strategy for rebuilding trust. Nurses needed to know what was going on when decisions were made. Other nurses complained about the lack of visibility of administrators, which decreased trust. Administrators agreed that visibility was important, but they were too busy with work, which kept them from the clinical areas. Nurses wanted to be seen as equal partners without fear that they would lose their position or be labeled as troublemakers if they made complaints or voiced their opinions about decisions. Participative decision making was critical to autonomy, which would allow the nurses to make more decisions about what they could do and could not do. This was another important way for administration to demonstrate trust in staff. Nurses wanted to feel empowered but instead they felt that they had little voice in decision making. What is really described in the results of this study is the organization's culture. Culture involves key factors that affect how people work together, pleasure or dissatisfaction in work, and so on.

The Competing Values Framework is a method that can be used to define an organization's culture. This framework includes four orientations (Cameron & Quinn, 1994; Jones & Redman, 2000).

1. **Group/clan orientation** in which the organization focuses on concern for people and sensitivity to customers. This type of organization has a friendly work environment that emphasizes loyalty, high cohesion, and tradition. The leader(s) emphasizes teamwork and consensus building.
2. **Developmental/"adhocracy orientation"** is a type of organization in which the focus is on innovation and individual initiative and freedom. This is a dynamic and creative environment with many entrepreneurs. Risk-taking is highly valued.
3. **Irrational/market orientation** focuses on getting the job done with positive results. In this organization the staff is competitive and goal-oriented.
4. **Hierarchy orientation** is a formalized structure organization. The focus here is on procedures and not on people. Efficiency is most important with staff following the rules.

Jones and Redman (2000) have applied these four cultural orientations to two dimensions: (a) flexibility versus control and (b) internal versus external. Considering these two dimensions, how do the four orientations apply? Clan and adhocracy cultural orientations would be placed in the flexibility dimension while market and hierarchy orientations would be placed in the control dimension. Clan and hierarchy orientations also focus on internal processes while adhocracy and market orientations focus on external challenges. Box 17-1 provides a summary of this view of organizational culture.

Strategies have been developed to assist organizations to change their orientation and culture. In today's health care environment, most health care organizations recognize the need to be more flexible and to respond more to both external and internal factors, not just one. These organizations then need to change their orientations to accomplish this effectively. They would want to promote adhocracy and clan values and decrease hierarchy and market values. The study discussed earlier conducted by Ray, Turkel, and Marino (2002) highlighted nurses' concerns about organizations that focus on financial factors over and above other critical issues. This overemphasis on market values suggests this organization would need to change its focus to other goals and emphasize quality. Examples of strategies that might be used to promote group/clan val-

BOX 17-1   One approach to organizational culture: competing values framework.

Flexibility vs.	Control Dimension	Internal vs.	External Dimension
Clan Orientation	Market Orientation	Clan Orientation	Adhocracy Orientation
Adhocracy Orientation	Hierarchy Orientation	Hierarchy Orientation	Market Orientation

Source: Author.

ues would be to survey staff about their needs and ideas, improve team-building skills, and improve employee recognition programs. To promote developmental/adhocracy values, the organization might encourage and reward innovative ideas and develop an effective continuous quality improvement program. To reduce hierarchy values, the organization would need to eliminate ineffective policies and procedures and decrease micromanagement. An organization's culture can be changed, but it takes a planned effort to accomplish this change. The first step should be to assess the culture. A place to begin with the assessment is to consider the many factors within the organization that have an impact on the organizational culture. These factors include:

- Structure and process
- Communication, both formal and informal (e.g., use of memos, e-mail, effect of gossip, accessibility of information, secrecy, how soon do staff know about changes, how effective is its communication, information overload, and so on)
- Acceptance of new members/staff
- Willingness to allow new members to offer suggestions or new ideas
- Management's willingness to include staff in change process
- Morale
- Staff turnovers
- Feedback

The organization's vision, mission statement, and goals reveal important information about the organization and how the organization views itself and its staff; however, these documents may be just more paper to put into binders. The key is to decide if what is written in these documents is actually demonstrated in behavior and communication. Organizations with a consonant culture emphasize the sum of their parts rather than their many separate parts. An organization that is tied up in focusing on its parts and has problems with viewing itself as a whole would have a dissonant culture. It will feel out of sync. From a systems perspective, the organization will not be as effective as it could be. Some aspects of an organization are helpful in describing and understanding the organizational culture. These are the cultural artifacts, which are "the obvious signs and symbols of corporate culture, such as written rules, office layouts, organizational structure, and dress codes" (Dessler, 2002, p. 54). Patterns of behavior can be used to identify traditions, written and verbal comments, and staff behaviors. The values and beliefs are a critical part of the culture. "Stories illustrating important company values are also widely used to reinforce the firm's culture" (Dessler, 2002, p. 55). Managers, team leaders, and preceptors play an important role in clarifying expectations about organization values to the staff, but to do this effectively, they need to understand the culture.

Some key terms are often mentioned when an organization's culture is discussed (Curtin, 2001). Staff, of course, have personal values, and as staff interact and function in their positions within organizations *role-related values* are developed when personal values are shared with others within the culture. *Attitudes* are also important, but what does this mean? Attitudes are formed when staff apply values to real situations. *Institutional values* are critical in understanding organizational structure, and these are developed "over time and reflect shared beliefs about desirable rules of conduct and desirable states of existence" (Curtin, 2001, p. 219). The greater the consistency between the staff values and values of the organization and its managers, the better the organization will function.

THINK CRITICALLY

Try this exercise to apply what you have learned about this topic.

Legal issues

An organization's culture is affected by the people within that organization—its staff, patients, and families that receive the health care services. In today's multicultural society diversity is a critical factor that affects health care organizations. "**Workforce diversity** refers to the mix of people from varied backgrounds in the labor pool" (Shea-Lewis, 2002, p. 6). The critical federal regulations and state labor laws that affect workforce diversity are Title VII of the Civil Rights Act of 1964 and Executive Order 11246, which prohibits employer discrimination on the basis of race, color, religion, sex or national origin, and the American Disability Act of 1990. (See Chapters 10 and 12 for additional information.) It should be noted that since most health care organizations receive reimbursement from Medicare, which is a federal payment system, and Medicaid, which is a joint federal and state reimbursement system, most health care organizations must meet the requirements of these laws and regulations. This means that staff must be prepared with education and training for work in a culturally diverse environment. Diversity within the workforce must also be improved within health care organizations. It is necessary to evaluate the effectiveness of diversity education programs to improve a culturally diverse work setting. "Workforce diversity in health services organizations is of extreme importance. Diversity provides a more comprehensive range of knowledge and abilities. Diversity allows for better decision-making based on different life experiences and perspectives. A diverse workforce can better provide health services to diverse populations" (Shea-Lewis, 2002, p. 6).

Cultural barriers within these organizations for staff and for patients must be assessed and resolved. Language barriers are particularly important (Griffin, 2002). This, of course, includes availability of interpreters when they are needed to assist staff. Family members are not the best choice for interpreters; they are too personally involved, and their culture may affect how and what they translate. For example, in some cultures the husband is the decision maker and the wife simply agrees. In this situation, if the husband is interpreting for his wife (the patient), the husband's attitude would probably limit the wife's participation. Another issue with language is the health care provider needs to be in control of the conversation, and this is difficult to accomplish when staff do not know the language (Griffin, 2002). Patients from different cultures need time to understand what is said and what it means, and they will also process the communication through their own cultural filter. Cultural filters are the way that individuals perceive the world and their experiences. These filters are created and adopted by members of a culture. For example, how a person communicates, verbally, nonverbally, and behaviorally, goes through this filter. If staff are not sensitive and aware of culture and do not have knowledge of other cultures, they may misinterpret words and behaviors. This filter also affects how people define health and illness, whether or not they seek care, from whom they seek care, and their attitudes about the quality of their lives.

Organizational culture must also consider how staff respond to persons with disabilities as employees. Some of this response is dictated by laws. The American Disability Act (ADA) of 1990, which became effective in 1992, has had a major impact on health care workforce issues (Sullivan & Decker, 2001). This law makes it illegal for employers to discriminate against persons with disabilities in employment, and provides for enforcement of equal access to jobs and accommodations. Employers of 15 or more are affected by this law, which certainly includes most health care organizations. How is a disability defined in the law? A disability is (a) a physical or mental impairment that substantially limits one or more of the major life activities of such individuals, (b) a record of such impairment, and (c) being regarded as having such impairment. Examples of disabilities that would apply to the health care workforce include: emotional or mental illness, alcoholism/drug abuse (person would need to be participating in a supervised rehabilitation program), multiple sclerosis, HIV infection/AIDS, cancer, diabetes, heart disease, orthopedic impairments, hearing/vision/speech impairments, communication disorders, and learning disabilities (Sullivan & Decker, 2001). The law does more than prohibit discrimination as it also requires reasonable accommodation, which means that efforts must be made to provide leaves of absence with or without pay, job reassignment, or job restructuring. In addition, the hiring process is affected by this law. A qualified person is a person who can perform the essential job functions, with or without reasonable accommodation. During the process questions about general medical conditions, state of health, specific diseases, or nature/severity of disability cannot be asked. The focus must be on whether or not the person meets essential job functions. It is thus critical that employers clearly define essential job functions, which should be based on the employer's judgment, the job description, and the amount of time spent performing the given function (Guido, 2001). The presence or lack of an atmosphere of acceptance is an important factor in an organization's culture.

The staff and their culture

Health care staff affect an organization's culture and are also affected by the culture. They bring their own personal culture into the organization; in addition, the staff represent several generations, which has a major impact on the organizational culture. Staff and their personal cultures represent a critical component of building cultural competency in an organization.

A *culturally diverse staff*

"Global management recognizes that workers from different cultures exhibit different behaviors" (Milgram, Spector, & Treger, 1999, p. 210). Managers need to understand the impact of cultures on the organization, daily work, and the staff and use cross-cultural management. This requires an open mind and understanding. Acceptance of others who may be different is critical, as is encouragement of staff to share their feelings and reactions. Staff members need to be appreciated for their individual strengths. The focus is on differences, not on right and wrong.

De Ruiter and Saphiere (2001) note that today 20% of physicians are foreign trained. There is also an increase in nurses from other countries who have come to work in the United States due to the nursing shortage. Diversity, however, is not just found in staff who have come from other countries for short periods of employment. There are many staff who have lived here for some time or were born in the United States, but they are members of minority cultures. The multicultural work environment means that nurse leaders must consider its impact on productivity, recruitment, and retention. This requires an awareness of cross-cultural issues. Staff may respond to other staff and patients from cultures different from their own in ways that may be ineffective. This must be addressed in order to build cultural competency.

Seago (2000) investigated "thinking and behavioral styles that are used to measure the concept of organizational culture among registered nurses and unlicensed assistive personnel in acute care hospitals" (p. 278). This study surveyed staff members who worked at least 20 hours per week in selected hospitals. The results indicated that there were differences in how staff members think and behave in these organizations. Why is this so important? Managers whose staff include people of color need to implement management strategies that promote behaviors to improve patient care. Understanding cultural diversity from the perspectives of thinking and behavior may help managers and other staff understand differences in how problems are approached and how staff respond. This study used Cooke and Lafferty's (1987) *Organizational Culture Inventory*. This inventory is based on a definition of organizational culture as "the shared norms and expectations that guide the thinking and behavior by the group members" (Cooke & Rousseau, 1988, p. 246). This is a typical definition of culture. The inventory includes 12 thinking and behavioral styles. These self-reported thinking and behavioral styles are used to measure the ways that group members are expected to think and behave within the organization's culture. This particular inventory is mentioned here as it provides one viewpoint of organizational culture and highlights some important factors and styles. There are three thinking/behavioral factors, and each has specific styles of thinking and behavior.

1. **Constructive factor:** This factor is satisfaction-oriented and includes the following styles. The humanistic or helpful style assumes that people are basically good and that the staff members enjoy teaching and assisting others. The affiliative style is described as warm, accepting, and cooperative. Staff members prefer friendly work relationships. The achievement style focuses on the need to do well, planning, ambitiousness, and enthusiasm. The fourth style is self-actualization, which is the need to meet individual goals, seek growth, and enjoy self-respect.
2. **Passive-defensive factor:** This factor is people-security-oriented and includes the following styles. The approval style focuses on the need to be accepted and trying to please. The second style is conventional, which means staff follow rules and meet expectations. The dependence style also includes following the rules, with an emphasis on the good follower. The avoidance style focuses on self-blame and guilt, and the staff member avoids conflict.
3. **Aggressive-defensive factor:** This factor is task-security-oriented and includes the following styles. The oppositional style focuses on staff resistance to authority. The second style is power, in which staff need to use influence, power, and control. The competitive style

BOX 17-2   Thinking and behavioral factors related to thinking and behavioral styles.

Thinking and Behavioral Factors	Thinking and Behavioral Styles
Constructive Factor	• Humanistic or Helpful Style • Affiliative or Cooperative/Warm Style • Achievement or Enthusiastic/Ambitious Style • Self-Actualization Style
Passive-Defensive Factor	• Approval or Need to Please Style • Conventional or Need to Follow the Rules Style • Avoidance of Conflict or Guilt Style
Aggressive-Defensive Factor	• Oppositional Style • Power Style • Competitive Style • Competence/Perfectionist Style

Source: Author.

includes staff who need to win, and everything is a challenge. The fourth style is competence/perfectionist, when staff need to appear independent and competent and will try harder to reach higher goals to seek perfection (Seago, 2000, p. 279). Box 17-2 highlights the thinking/behavioral factors and their related thinking and behavioral styles. Of these three factors, the constructive factor allows for the the most positive organizational culture.

Seago (2000) applied these thinking and behavioral factors to health care organization redesign. The findings indicate that many organizations are hiring and using more unlicensed assistive personnel (UAP) resulting in a greater staff skill mix, typically with more UAPs than RNs. Therefore, it is important that managers understand how this change in skill mix might change staff culture and behavior. Since in this study UAPs scored much higher on dependence and opposition than RNs, it is important to understand what this might mean to a nurse manager. UAPs may feel that they need to use these thinking and behavior styles (dependence and opposition) to be successful and a "good follower." Typically, this is interpreted as not being threatening or challenging; however, is this really what organizations need in today's health care environment? There is no doubt that teams need good followers to be effective, as was discussed in earlier chapters; however, health care organizations today also need staff, RNs, and other staff who challenge themselves and the organization to do better. The nurse manager and staff nurses need to provide more positive recognition of the UAPs and their work. They need to listen to them more and try to facilitate more decision making within this group, but still provide appropriate recognition of UAP job position limitations as to what they can do. This all needs to become part of the culture of the unit, service/department, and organization. The results of the study also indicate the following.

■ Both groups of staff, RNs and UAPs, want positive interpersonal relationships, are generally accepting and cooperative, need to do well, and enjoy helping and assisting others.

■ Staff members of color, regardless of position, scored higher on the thinking and behavioral styles of approval, avoidance, and competitiveness, whereas UAPs, regardless of race or ethnicity, scored higher on the thinking and behavioral styles of dependence and opposition.

■ Those in this study who were people of color, regardless of the position, gender, or education, scored higher than white people on approval, avoidance, and competitiveness. They tended to want to please more, required more acceptance, and avoided conflict. They also tended to try harder and set high goals for themselves (Seago, 2000, pp. 278, 285).

This study provides information about how changing the skill mix of a unit or workgroup will change the culture of that group. If the goal is to change the culture so that staff work better as a team and feel that they can participate in decision making, the three factors (constructive, passive-defensive, and aggressive-defensive) and their respective styles can make a difference in the success of this effort.

YOUR OPINION COUNTS

Find out what others think about this topic. Post your response and check out other opinions.

Generational issues and their effects on organizational culture

Some authors have discussed the importance of understanding the generation that staff represent and how this influences their different responses to the work environment (Zemke, Raines, & Filipczak, 2000). "Managing diversity here is defined as creating and maintaining an environment in which each person is respected because of his or her differences" (Davis, 2001, p. 161). Nursing now has the unique experience of including four generations working in the same place (Gerke, 2001). This situation can lead to a rich diversity of viewpoints and practice; however, it can also lead to conflict and problems within the organizational culture. Key questions to consider are: (a) What are the four generations? (b) What are their characteristics? (c) What can be done to gain the most for this matrix of generations? The focus of this discussion will be on the last two generations; however, to appreciate these two generations it is necessary to briefly describe the first two generations. Box 17-3 highlights the four generations.

1. The traditional, silent, or mature generation, born from 1930 to 1940. This generation is less apparent due to its age, but it had a major impact on nursing. Many from this generation were nurses in World War II. They can be characterized as hard-working, loyal, valuers of duty, and family focused. Hierarchy was accepted by them as an important characteristic of the organizations in which they worked.
2. Baby Boomers, born from 1943 to 1960. This generation fills most of the nursing positions, both in practice and nursing education. Typically, this group had a choice of only two careers, nursing or teaching (Bertholf & Loveless, 2001). This group will be retiring soon, leading to a greater nursing shortage in both practice and education. This generation works independently, accepts authority, causes few problems, feels that loyalty is an important work value, is less able to cope with new technology, and has been described as workaholics (Bertholf & Loveless, 2001). Gerke (2001) describes this group as preferring consensus leadership, competitive, and more focused on material gain. It is important to recognize that there is variation within the generational group (for example, many in this generation have been the leaders and pushers for greater use of technology in health care). This can be supported by the increased use of computer technology in nursing education and in practice documentation. This would have never happened if some members of the generation had not pushed for it.

Generation X, who were born from 1960 to 1980, and Generation Y, who were born from 1980 to 2000, will be discussed in more detail in this chapter. Why is it important to understand the differences in the last two generations of staff? At this time, they are the major age groups

BOX 17-3   The four key generations in nursing.

1. Traditional Generation	Born 1930–1940
2. Baby Boomers	Born 1943–1960
3. Generation X	Born 1960–1980
4. Generation Y	Born 1980–2000

Source: Author.

that are increasing in nursing and will take on the leadership of the profession as the Baby Boomers retire. It is believed that characteristics of the age groups affect how they work, why they work, and leadership that is required within organizations (American Hospital Association, 2002). Generation X, who are nurses in their 20s and 30s, are different from the Baby Boomer generation (Coupland, 1992; Santos & Cox, 2002). Generation X nurses are described as the "original 'latch key kids' and have grown up mastering information technology and creative thinking" (Bertholf & Loveless, 2001, p. 169). They have grown up during a time of extreme change. Generation X nurses want to be led, not managed. They need to develop self-confidence and empowerment. They want effective, intelligent leaders who mentor staff, and they want to be trusted and respected by their leaders. Nurturing is a key leadership characteristic that is important to Generation X, and it forms the base for their other important characteristics: motivational, receptive, positive, good communicator, team player, good people skills, approachable, and supportive (Wieck, Prydun, & Walsh, 2002). This generation is not made up of joiners, and this will be a problem for professional organizations. They do not value job longevity, which has an impact on loyalty to employers. They also feel strongly about maintaining a balance between work and personal life.

The core values of Generation X staff are diversity, thinking globally, balance, technoliteracy, fun, informality, self-reliance, and pragmatism. The job assets of this generation are: adaptable, technoliterate, independent, intimidated by authority, and creative. How might their values affect their assets? Generation X staff are motivated by organizational messages such as:

- "Do it your way."
- "We've got the newest hardware and software."
- "There aren't a lot of rules here."
- "We're not very corporate."

"Generation Xers are pessimistic and rightfully so given the world they grew up in. They are loyal to themselves and the people with whom they have familial-like relationships. They like to feel that they are part of something bigger. They expect and respond well to things that contribute to their own professional knowledge and competency. Xers are flexible and very comfortable with change. . . . They are technoliterate. . . . Because Generation X often views a job as a stepping stone to the next job, benefits and rewards geared to the present rather than the future are the most valuable in recruitment and retention" (Ulrich, 2001, p. 152). This description of Generation X explains some of the conflict or tension that can be seen between these nurses and Baby Boomer nurses, who are just ahead of them. Baby Boomer nurses are more willing, although not happy about it, to work overtime and are often shocked when younger nurses say they are leaving. This is driven by the fact that more Baby Boomer nurses have a long-term commitment to employers (Santos & Cox, 2002). These are not characteristics found in the generation that is replacing the Baby Boomers.

Generation Y (Nexters), the newest generation entering nursing, demonstrates the core values of optimism, civic duty, confidence, achievement, social ability, morality, street smarts, and diversity. Their important on-the-job assets are: collective action, optimism, tenacity, heroic spirit, multitasking capabilities, and technology savvy. They are interested in technology and feel competent around it. Compared to Generation X, they have more trust in centralized authority (Gerke, 2001). Change is part of their lives, and thus they tolerate it better. Related to this, they are seen as being greater risk-takers and want to be challenged and excited about their work. What organizational messages motivate this generation (Santos & Cox, 2002)?

- "You will be working with bright, creative people."
- "Your boss is in his/her 60s."
- "You and your co-workers can help turn this company around."
- "You can be a hero here."

The first step is to recognize the importance of distinguishing between generations, and the second is develop strategies to improve collaboration and culture. It is clear that these generational groups need to communicate with one another to increase understanding of where each group is coming from and recognize the values that are important to each group. Some strategies that have been recommended to accomplish this include:

- Develop coaching behaviors in preceptors/educators to enable learning by doing and supporting the newer employee in asking "why" questions.
- Design care delivery models to support collaborative practice.
- Utilize participatory management strategies to develop relationships.
- Recognize and accept that all employment is temporary.
- Lighten up.
- Be specific.
- Realize that you have more in common than different.
- Assess the organization for its ability for inclusion.
- Discuss openly how you see your team working with new members (Bertholf & Loveless, 2001, pp. 170–171).

BENCHMARKS

Now let's take a moment to test your knowledge of the concepts you have studied in this section.

Cultural Perceptions of Health and Illness: Need for a Caring, Healing Environment

As organizations and their culture are considered, it is important to recognize that health care delivery organizations are more than just organizations in which people work. This is one part of the culture but not the only part. Whether or not the organizational culture supports an environment in which patients can be cared for is another critical issue. This section discusses factors related to a caring, healing environment.

A diverse patient population

The Institute for the Future (2000) forecasts more diversity for the United States as its population becomes more and more diverse. While the population is still primarily white non-Hispanic (73%), the number of African American, Hispanic, Asian, and Native Americans are increasing because of birth rates and immigration. It is predicted that by 2010 the country's population will be 32% minority ethnic. Absolute numbers will still be small until after 2050 (The Institute for the Future, 2000). The important issue with the diverse population is its regional impact. The regions with the higher concentrations of diverse populations, in order of size, are: the South, the West, Northeast, and Midwest.

There is no doubt that nurses are caring for patients who come from a variety of cultural backgrounds. It is time for nurses to consider how their own cultural backgrounds affect the care they provide and their leadership. What is done with this information? How does it impact the health care delivery system? Why should a nurse leader be concerned? "One of the newest requirements of a nurse leader is to function as a bridge person between people of different cultures" (De Ruiter & Saphiere, 2001). This means that nursing leaders must understand the implications of staff members' personal cultural background, and how this relates to patient cultural background, the cultures in the local community, and of course, the culture of the health care organization.

How do these demographic facts affect the health care delivery system? There will be new demands to provide more culturally appropriate health care. This means more than language competency, which is highly problematic in many areas and for individual health care organizations that must provide interpreters when needed. Where to find this resource and the cost factors are major problems. There are, however, other considerations. These are:

- The effects of lifestyle and cultural differences on health status
- The implications of the diverse genetic endowment of the population
- The impact of patterns of assimilation on health status
- Underdiagnosis and treatment differences among minority groups (The Institute for the Future, 2000, p. 20)

The last issue of differences in health care quality for minority Americans was recently addressed in a report, *Diverse Communities, Common Concerns: Assessing Health Care Quality for Minority Americans* (Collins et al., 2002). It identifies "three factors in ensuring that minority populations receive optimal medical care: effective patient-physician communication, overcoming cultural and linguistic barriers, and access to affordable health insurance" (p. 6). Minority groups are the primary groups that have been affected by uninsurance, underinsurance, and limited access to providers in many communities. Migrant health care is also a critical issue in many areas—and a complex one. The Children's Health Insurance program established by President Clinton to increase the number of children with health insurance coverage has made some impact on these disparity problems, but there have been problems with it, too. The money is there for the coverage; however, many states have struggled with getting families to register for it. One barrier is families who are concerned about sharing information required for registration, such as illegal aliens. Additionally, the process is complex in some states. Language and culture also affect willingness to share information. Fear of government interventions is a concern with some groups. Many states have been successful in addressing some of these critical barriers, and others have been less successful. For this reason, a program that looks like it might help is not as successful as hoped in some regions of the country.

Another aspect of a diverse health care system is education of staff about other cultures. How should this be done to ensure that staff have the needed information and apply it? More of this content is included in nursing education today. This, however, does not get to staff who have practiced for a time and yet still need updates. The Mayo Clinic developed a transcultural patient care website to assist its staff (De Ruiter & Larsen, 2002). This site is available to staff 24–7, whenever the information is needed, and includes information related to the following categories.

- Information about countries, ethnic groups, religious groups, and special populations
- Communicating with the non-English-speaking patient/family
- Cultural assessment guide
- Nutritional assessment tool/resources
- Patient education database
- Departmental information
- Classes on a variety of diversity issues
- Internet transcultural websites

This type of resource would be helpful for any health care organization that has a diverse patient and/or staff population. Obviously, the Mayo Clinic site is for its staff; however, that does not exclude other organizations from developing their own sites.

What is a healing environment?

Curtin (2001) has indicated that "today's hospitals do not have to change their cultures; they have to heal themselves" (p. 219). This is a different perspective of organizational culture. She concludes that the growing emphasis on market-based culture in health care with all of its concern for financial issues and getting a bigger piece of the market has had a serious detrimental effect on the health of health care organizations. She concludes that this value approach needs to be addressed to help hospitals heal. This certainly relates to comments made earlier in this chapter about nurses' concerns about the overemphasis on financial issues. Related to this problem are intrinsic and extrinsic values, which are values that are affected by age, life cycle, and professional status (McNeese-Smith & Crook, 2003). At the same time, some organizations are describing themselves as healing environments. Can this really happen? Can organizations that need to heal themselves be healing environments?

Defining healing environments is not easy. There are a variety of components that are associated with healing environments such as privacy, air quality, noise levels, views, and visual characteristics. As needs among people vary, there is no doubt that the perfect environment for healing cannot be developed, but there has been recognition that efforts should be taken to develop healing environments. "Throughout history health care providers, architects, and psychologists have noted a strong link between the environment and human behavior" (McCullough & Wille, 2001, p. 111). Florence Nightingale commented on the need for healing environments which she associated with fresh air, warmth, cleanliness, quiet, diet, and light (McCullough & Wille, 2001). "Traditionally, physicians and nurses have been the center of action in health care, and patients were expected to adapt to the routines of the facility. Today, patients and families are the central focus of health care, and health care facilities are being designed to address their needs. Regulations, market pressures, and a desire to improve the health care experience foster patient-centered movements" (McCullough & Wille, 2001, p. 110). When health care organizations began to change their focus, they had to confront their weaknesses and try to make difficult changes. Some have been more successful than others.

If one reflects on personal experiences in acute care facilities as well as other types of health care settings, the environment often is not all that conducive to healing—noise interferes with rest and relaxation, lack of cleanliness, difficulty finding one's way around, the lack of warmth as far as color and furnishings, confusion over staff identities, and unresponsive staff. Some organizations, of course, have made successful efforts to improve their environments. One particular example is the California Pacific Medical Center, the Planetree Unit, begun in 1995. This unit was actually created by a health care consumer (McCullough & Wille, 2001). The approach was based on a concept that became known as the Planetree concept, which is based on eight principles of humanistic care, all directed at humanizing, personalizing, and demystifying the health care system for patients and their families. In this type of environment the focus of care is on the whole patient—body, mind, and spirit—with active consumer involvement. In addition, the following also are important.

- The physical environment is vital to the healing process and should be designed to promote healing and learning and encourage patient and family participation.
- A nurturing environment—one that is supportive, friendly, and caring—is an essential component of providing high-quality health care.
- Patients have the right to open and honest communication in warm, caring environments.
- Patients have the right to access information about all aspects of their health, illness, and hospitalization including reading and writing in their medical records.
- All people—patients, families, and professional staff—play unique and vital roles on the health care team.
- Patients have many physical, emotional, intellectual, spiritual, and aesthetic facets and are not isolated units but members of families, communities, and cultures.
- Patients are individuals with rights, responsibilities, and choices regarding their own health and lifestyles.
- Illness can be a time of personal growth for patients. It can also be a time to reevaluate life goals and values, clarify priorities, and discover inner resources (Planetree, 1995).

Some hospitals have been applying the Planetree concept to make necessary changes to improve their healing environments. In reviewing the key strategies that support the Planetree concept, they are clearly strategies that are integral to quality nursing care. They are also highly supportive of a positive culture that not only moves the patient into an important role but also provides a more positive work culture.

The Picker Institute and the Center for Health Care Design conducted research on the patient's perspective of the health care environment, which included over 350,000 interviews. From these interviews, eight dimensions of care valued by patients have been identified.

- Respect for patients' values
- Easy access to care
- Emotional support
- Information and education
- Coordination of care
- Physical comfort
- Involvement of family and friends
- Continuity and transition (Picker Institute, 1999)

These discussions of care are very familiar to nurses.

The Center for Health Design went one step further and identified consumer environmental rights in health care facilities. Environments should:

- Be easy to navigate.
- Offer restricted access to nature through views, gardens, landscaped patios, terraces, courtyards, atria, and natural elements.
- Have an easy-to-control personal environment including lighting, noise and sound reduction, odor elimination, thermal comfort, and privacy.
- Offer the capability to select positive distractions including television, games, videotapes, computers, art, telephone, music, social opportunities, access to nature, and reading material.
- Have activities in spaces conducive to their purpose.
- Make it easy for staff to bring food, medicine, and other supplies related to the care.
- Have access to furniture and equipment that is comfortable and user-friendly.
- Allow maximum opportunities for regular lifestyle activities.
- Have access to a continuous sequence of environments that support one's dignity and the dignity of others.
- Be clean, neat, and orderly.
- Be free from hazards.
- Provide for personal safety and security for personal possessions.
- Inspire trust and confidence.
- Symbolize values appropriate to patients and others.
- Provide for local cultural backgrounds and diversity in the community.
- Be appropriate for the various ages, genders, and physical and cognitive abilities of the people who use it.
- Support interaction with others including care-partners.
- Decrease unnecessary stress for all patients or residents, visitors, and staff.
- Be aesthetically appealing (The Center for Health Design, 2000).

CURRENT ISSUES

Learn about events around the globe that relate to the chapter content.

Safety: A component of organizational culture

Safety is part of an organization's culture, both for staff and for patients, as well as anyone who enters the facility. "**Patient safety culture** is defined as a product of social learning ways of thinking and behaving that are shared and that work to meet the primary objective of patient safety" (Schein, 1999, p. 186). Organizational leaders such as the CEO and the nurse executive are responsible for facilitating the development of a safety culture (Mustard, 2002). The organization's board of directors must also buy into the need for a safe culture as they are the final decision makers and control final budget decisions. Why is it necessary to have the leaders so responsible, and how is safety really connected to the organization's culture?

Safety is related to organizational culture because a critical element of ensuring safety is the identification of errors and improvement areas. If staff do not feel comfortable in reporting errors, which is directly related to organization values, trust, collaboration, communication, and so on, then the organizational culture will have a difficult time addressing patient and staff safety. The goal should be to decrease the shame/blame culture that does exist when errors occur in health care organizations; however, "the shame/blame culture in hospitals can probably never be totally eliminated because 'to err is human' and there will always be the risk of fatal human errors from unthinking and uncaring behavior and the need for minimal punishment or retribution" (Mustard, 2002, p. 113). The important aspect is to try and change this negative culture as much as possible as it affects the willingness of staff to report errors and thus affects safety. The new type of culture that is required is one in which staff can unlearn ineffective practices to improve and reduce safety risks. How does one arrive at this type of culture? It requires: "social capital [results from relationships as peers help one another and support each other], mutual trust and respect, which are essential for this collaborative learning environment" (Mustard, 2002, p. 114). In addition, health care organizations need to increase their awareness of safety risks and how they might reduce or eliminate them. Addressing many of these safety issues such as medical waste, healthy buildings, use of pesticides and cleaners, and purchasing safe products will require political advocacy, collaboration, and networking.

The American Nurses Association (ANA) encourages all nurses to be leaders in advocating for safe health environments (*The American Nurse*, 2001). In supporting this effort, ANA has joined with other organizations such as the Association of Perioperative Nurses, Association of Women's Health Obstetrics and Neonatal Nurses, Infusion Nurses Society, International Council for Nursing, Oncology Nursing Society, American Holistic Nurses' Association, and others by participating in the Health Care Without Harm (HCWH) organization. This is an international coalition of hospitals and health care systems, medical professionals, community groups, health-affected constituencies, labor unions, environmental health organizations, and religious groups who have joined together to focus on the mission of "transforming the health care industry worldwide, without compromising patient safety or care, so that it is ecologically sustainable and no longer a source of harm to public health and the environment" (Health Care Without Harm, 2003). The following are the goals of HCWH.

1. To work with a wide range of constituencies for an ecologically sustainable health care system.
2. To promote policies, practices, and laws that eliminate incineration of medical waste, minimize the amount and toxicity of all waste generated, and promote the use of safer materials and treatment practices.
3. To phase out the use of PVC (polyvinyl chloride) plastics and persistent toxic chemicals in health care and to build momentum for a broader PVC phase-out campaign.
4. To phase out the use of mercury in all aspects of the health care industry.
5. To develop health-based standards for medical waste management and to recognize and implement the public's right to know about chemical use in the health care industry.
6. To develop citing and transportation guidelines that are just and conform to the principles of environmental justice; no communities should be poisoned by medical waste treatment and disposal.
7. To develop an effective collaboration and communication structure among campaign allies.

To accomplish these goals an organization's culture must be open with active staff participation and recognize the importance of a safe working environment. Such an environment suggests the cultures described. They feed on one another.

The physical environment as part of a healing environment

Making health care organizations more appealing spaces is also important. In the last 15 to 20 years, more efforts have been made by hospitals to make their environments more comfortable and soothing (Leighty, 2003). This effort can also be seen in other types of health care settings, too (for example, clinics, M.D. offices, and long-term care facilities). Some evidence exists that these strategies actually have an important impact on patient outcomes and staff. A nurse-friendly environment is one in which the work environment is conducive to safe practice. Examples of these strategies are reducing travel time between work areas, better lighting, connecting areas that relate, and providing space for staff to take breaks. These efforts decrease staff stress, fatigue, and physical burden and thus improve efficiency and nurses' attitudes, which may affect retention and recruitment. When nurses are asked to participate in renovation planning or in new expansions, then the environment typically is a more nurse-friendly environment and more patient-oriented nurses understand what is a healing environment. The staff are the ones who really know what they need to get their work done. Leighty (2003) noted that increased use of private patient rooms (a) decreases requests for transfers, which decreases costs and increases patient satisfaction; (b) increases patient sleep and rest, which affects outcomes and patient satisfaction; (c) along with location of sinks and airflow, decreases nosocomial infections, which affects costs due to complications and outcomes; and (d) can even affect market share because patients want to come to hospitals where they get private rooms. More research needs to be done about environmental factors and how they affect organizational culture. Most would agree that it is much easier to work in a pleasant, attractive environment and that these factors make it easier for patients and families during times of stress, but more information is needed on the effect of these strategies and how they can be improved.

Facilitating diversity and cultural diversity within health care organizations

If an organization has a dysfunctional or dissonant culture, what should be done? Many authorities recommend that this be approached carefully as the problems may not be major ones (Curtin, 2001). "Three key steps related to an assessment and analysis of the culture are: (a) identify and develop an appropriate list of organizational values, (b) measure the degree to which employees and managers share those values, and (c) measure the degree to which they perceive the institution as demonstrating those values" (Curtin, 2001, p. 222).

As organizations assess their cultures and then realize that changes are needed, they will find that increasing participation from all levels of the organization will go a long way in improving the organization and increasing trust among staff and between staff and the organization. Lack of trust can be a major blockage to improving the organization's culture, as was noted earlier in this chapter. "All change in health care organizations is dependent upon trust, the foundation of all constructive human relationships. Trust is solidarity with others; trust is the surrender of our lives to each other in the hope of a response—a bond of caring fostering growth and development" (Logstrup, 1971 p. 18).

How do organizations get a better match between employee values and those of the organization? ". . . we should hire to values, seek diversity, and train to skills. Shared values help create a culture that sends the consistent message and focus. Through shared values and beliefs organizational cultures emerge. Diversity of the team, not simply ethnic diversity but also diversity in thinking, creates a true opportunity for organizational learning to occur. Through this diversity we are able to challenge our own thinking or think out of the box. Through diversity of thinking conflict can emerge and true dialogue can occur. Through this new level of dialogue more creative approaches can emerge and better decisions can be made" (Tornabeni, 2001, p. 7). Tornabeni identifies a key issue. Typically, one thinks of diversity as different cultures; however, it can and should be more than this. Diversity in thinking is also important. McNeese-Smith and Crook (2003) recommend that managers annually discuss and examine employee values in relationship to the organization's values. A good time to do this is at the time of performance evaluations. The goal should be to help staff and support their values as this may help to prevent burnout and loss of staff. This goes along with comments made earlier in this text about the need for leaders to help staff grow and develop, to encourage self-assessment and development of goals, and to recognize the need that to keep staff they must feel a part of the system and the culture.

If an organization concludes after an extensive assessment of its culture that improvement is needed, what should the organization do? Leaders who want to change an organization's culture need to follow these key principles as they develop and implement strategies to improve the organization's culture.

- Involve people in the problems and programs that affect them.
- Do not place blame.
- Clarify battles, objectives, purposes, and tasks.
- Focus on short-term and long-term results.
- Work from a sound information base.
- Use multilevel change strategies.
- Integrate concern for people and achievement of organizational goals.
- Emphasize sustained culture change (Allen & Kraft, 1982; as cited in Jones & Redman, 2000, p. 605).

A key aspect of the organization's culture is how staff and managers view diversity and their level of cultural competency. The basic components of cultural competency in nursing care include:

1. An awareness, sensitivity, and tolerance to differences in culture and language.
2. An ability to refrain from making assumptions (or judgments) about the beliefs, behaviors, needs, and expectations of patients or colleagues of a different cultural background from oneself.
3. An understanding of the role culture plays in forming the health/illness prevention, beliefs, and practices of patience.
4. The ability to recognize the role that one's own culture and background plays in determining one's attitudes and beliefs about such factors as what constitutes acceptable behavior, cleanliness, a happy lifestyle, the roles of family and friends, and so forth.
5. Enough knowledge about the cultures that one serves to avoid breaching the patient's taboos, health care beliefs, or rules of interaction.
6. Enough knowledge about the cultures that one serves to anticipate possible barriers to access or compliance with care.
7. The skill to deliver culturally and linguistically appropriate patient advice and education.
8. The skill to utilize interpreters effectively so that language barriers do not impact the extent or quality of care.
9. The knowledge and flexibility to modify both one's mode of interaction and one's manner of delivering care so that it is culturally and linguistically appropriate to the patient while it meets the hospital's or clinic's standards of quality patient care.
10. Confidence in one's ability to offer quality care to patients of other cultures (Salimbene, 1999, p. 31).

These are helpful guidelines for developing staff/manager competencies. Do they have these competencies? If not, training and education need to be addressed to increase the level of cultural competency. Culture is a sensitive subject so it is important that education programs consider the best learning methods and relevancy of content to the staff and organization. It is important to avoid a paternalistic approach, stereotyping, and biases when this content is presented.

CURRENT ISSUES

Learn about events around the globe that relate to the chapter content.

The recent Institute of Medicine report *Crossing the Quality Chasm* (2001) addresses some key issues related to organizational culture in health care delivery systems. The process of developing this report included the participation from experts in medicine, nursing, safety, pharmacy, and health administration, which resulted in a broad base of viewpoints.

- Care based on *continuous healing relationships:* Patients need a health care system that is responsive to their needs when they need care, and the type of services or entry into services should consider all possible methods, including innovative ones when necessary, such as Internet, telephone, and so on.

- ■ *Customization* based on patient needs and values: Health care delivery must consider the needs that are frequently found in the population; however, it must be flexible enough to address those unexpected needs and consider individual patient choices and preferences.

- ■ The *patient as the source of control:* To be in control patients need information, and health care providers need to be able to accommodate differences.

- ■ *Shared knowledge* and the free flow of information: Patients need access to their health information in an easily accessible manner. The focus should be on sharing information.

- ■ *Evidence-based* decision making: The best possible scientific information needs to be used in providing care.

- ■ *Safety* as a system property: All health care provider settings and providers need to offer a safe environment in which to receive safe and appropriate care.

- ■ The need for *transparency:* Information needs to be shared with patients, which includes information about the provider's performance on safety, evidence-based practice, and patient satisfaction.

- ■ *Anticipation* of needs: Health care providers need to be proactive in relationship to patient needs.

- ■ *Continuous* decrease in waste: Resources should not be wasted, and this includes patient's time.

- ■ *Cooperation* among clinicians: Individual providers and provider organizations need to collaborate to ensure appropriate, timely care and exchange of information (Institute of Medicine, 2001; as cited in Curtin, 2001, p. 218).

Each one of these descriptors is directly related to nursing care, although some have been addressed more effectively than others.

The most effective organizational cultures will be those that have a credible culture. These cultures build and maintain trust, and feature leaders who are role models and who set the culture's tone. Communication is recognized as important and is viewed as being effective. Staff and management are clear about expectations. How does an organization and its leadership go about building a credible culture?

- ■ Reward people who communicate openly and build trust in the workplace; punish those who don't.

- ■ Talk about the values of your organization from the top down and encourage conversation about issues.

- ■ Build your own credibility bank by practicing open communication; if you make a mistake, you will get the benefit of the doubt.

- ■ Encourage questions. Trust thrives on open lines of communication. The people who work for you need to know it's OK to question a decision or priority.

- ■ Don't assume people know what is expected; be clear about the kind of behavior and communication you expect and find acceptable (Bates, 2003, p. 38).

BENCHMARKS

Now let's take a moment to test your knowledge of the concepts you have studied in this section.

Chapter Wrap-Up

Now that you've reached the end of the chapter, you may wish to explore the concepts you've been reading about in greater detail or test yourself to see how well you've comprehended the material.

SUMMARY AND APPLICATIONS

- Summary
- Practice Quiz
- Key Terms
- Tying It All Together

- Experiential Exercises
- Case
- Links

REFERENCES

Aiken, L., et al. (2001). Nurses' report on hospital care in five countries: The ways in which nurses' work is structured have left nurses among the least satisfied workers, and the problem is getting worse. *Health Affairs, 20*(3), 43–53.

Allen, R., & Kraft, C. (1982). *The organizational unconscious*. Upper Saddle River, NJ: Prentice Hall.

American Hospital Association. (2002). *In our hands. How hospital leaders can build a thriving workplace*. Chicago, IL: Author.

The American Nurse. (September/October, 2001). ANA strengthens efforts for a healthier environment. Washington, DC: Author.

American Nurses Association. (1995). *Scope and standards for nurse administrators*. Washington, DC: American Nurses Publishing.

Bates, S. (2003). Creating a credible culture. *Nurse Leader, 1*(1), 37.

Bertholf, L., & Loveless, S. (2001). Baby Boomers and Generation X: Strategies to bridge the gap. *Seminars for Nurse Managers, 9*(3), 169–172.

Cameron, K., & Quinn, R. (1994). *PRISM 5: Changing organizational culture: A competing values workbook*. Ann Arbor, MI: University of Michigan.

The Center for Health Design. (2000). The healthcare consumer's environmental bill of rights. Retrieved from http://www.healthdesign.org.

Collins, K., et al. (2002). *Diverse communities, common concerns: Assessing health care quality for Minority Americans*. (Findings from the Commonwealth Fund 2001 Health Care Quality Survey) New York: The Commonwealth Fund.

Cooke, P., & Rousseau, D. (1988). Behavioral norms and expectations. *Group Organizational Studies, 13*, 245–273.

Cooke, R., & Lafferty, J. (1987). *Organizational culture inventory*. Plymonth, MI: Hanar Synergistics.

Coupland, D. (1992). *Generation X: Tales for an accelerated culture*. New York: St. Martin's Press.

Cuilla, J. (2000). *The working life: The promise and betrayal of modern work*. New York: Times Books/Random House.

Curtin, L. (2001). Healing health care's organizational culture. *Seminars for Nurse Managers, 9*(4), 218–227.

Davis, S. (2001). Diversity and generation X. *Seminars for Nurse Managers, 9*(3), 161–163.

De Ruiter, H., & Larsen, K. (2002). Developing a transcultural patient care web site. *Journal of Transcultural Nursing, 13*(1), 61–67.

De Ruiter, H., & Saphiere, D. (2001). Nurse leaders as cultural bridges. *Journal of Nursing Administration, 31*(9), 418–423.

Dessler, G. (2002). *Management*. Upper Saddle River, NJ: Prentice Hall.

Gerke, M. (2001). Understanding and leading the quad matrix: Four generations in the workplace: The traditional generation, boomers, gen-X, nexters. *Seminars for Nurse Managers, 9*(3), 173–181.

Griffin, C. (2002). Embracing diversity. *NurseWeek Midwest/Great Lakes, 2*(12), 12–13.

Guido, G. (2001). *Legal and ethical issues in nursing* (3rd ed.). Upper Saddle River, NJ: Prentice Hall.

Health Care Without Harm. Retrieved on June 6, 2003, from http://www.hcwh.org.

The Institute for the Future. (2000). *Health and health care 2010: The forecast, the challenge*. San Francisco: Jossey-Bass.

Institute of Medicine. (2001). *Crossing the quality chasm*. Washington, DC: National Academy Press.

Jones, K., & Redman, R. (2000). Organizational culture and work redesign: Experiences in three organizations. *Journal of Nursing Administration, 30*(12), 604–610.

Leighty, J. (2003). Healing by design. *NurseWeek Midwest/Great Lakes, 2*(5), 14–16.

Logstrup, K. (1971). *The ethical demand*. Philadelphia: Fortress Press.

McCullough, C., & Wille, R. (2001). Healing environments. In C. McCullough (Ed.), *Creating responsive solutions to healthcare change* (pp. 109–134). Indianapolis, IN: Center Nursing Press.

McNeese-Smith, D., & Crook, M. (2003). Nursing values and a changing nurse workforce. *Journal of Nursing Administration, 33*(5), 260–283.

Milgram, L., Spector, A., & Treger, M. (1999). *Managing smart.* Houston, TX: Cashman Dudley.

Mustard, L. (2002). The culture of patient safety. *JONA's Healthcare Law, Ethics, and Regulation, 4*(4), 111–115.

Nyberg, J. (1991). Theoretical explorations of health care and economics. *Advances in Nursing Science, 13*(1), 74–84.

Omery, A. (1989). Values, morals, reasoning, and ethics. *Nursing Clinics of North America, 24*(2), 499–507.

Parker, M., & Gadbois, S. (2000). Building community in the healthcare workplace, Part 3. *Journal of Nursing Administration, 30*(10), 466–473.

Picker Institute. (1999). New visions for healthcare: Ideas worth sharing. *Picker Institute Bulletin,* p. 7.

Planetree. Retrieved on June 6, 2003, from http://www.planetree.org.

Planetree. (October, 1995). *Planetree cost-effectiveness: Third annual Planetree conference* (pp. 1–3). Nebraska City, NE: Author.

Ray, M., Turkel, M., & Marino, F. (2002). The transformative process for nursing in workforce redevelopment. *Nursing Administrative Quarterly, 26*(2), 1–14.

Salimbene, S. (1999). Cultural competence: A priority for performance improvement action. *Journal of Nursing Administration, 13*(3), 23–35.

Santos, S., & Cox, K. (2002). Generational tension among nurses. *American Journal of Nursing, 102*(1), 11.

Schein, E. (1999). *The corporate culture survival guide.* San Francisco, CA: Jossey-Bass.

Seago, J. (2000). Registered nurses, unlicensed assistive personnel, and organizational culture in hospitals. *Journal of Nursing Administration, 30*(5), 278–286.

Shea-Lewis, A. (2002). Workforce diversity in health care. *Journal of Nursing Administration, 32*(1), 6–7.

Sovie, M. (1993). Hospital culture: Why create one? *Nursing Economics, 11*(2), 69–90.

Sullivan, E., & Decker, P. (2001). *Effective leadership and management in nursing* (5th ed.). Upper Saddle River, NJ: Prentice Hall.

Tornabeni, J. (2001). The competency game: My take on what it really takes to lead. *Nursing Administration Quarterly, 25*(4), 1–13.

Ulrich, B. (2001). Successfully managing multigenerational workforces. *Seminars for Nurse Managers, 9*(3), 147–153.

Wieck, K., Prydun, M., & Walsh, T. (2002). What the emerging workforce wants in its leaders. *Journal of Nursing Scholarship, 34*(3), 283–288.

Zemke, R., Raines, C., & Filipczak, B. (2000). *Generations at work.* New York: American Management Association.

ADDITIONAL READINGS

American Association of Colleges of Nursing. (January, 2002). *Hallmarks of the professional nursing practice environment.* Washington, DC: Author.

Bodensteiner, L. (2001). Decreasing attrition rates across the generations through values alignment. *Seminars for Nurse Managers, 9*(3), 173–181.

Child, R., Lingle, G., & Watson, P. (2001). Managing diversity in the environment of care. *Seminars for Nurse Managers, 9*(2), 102–110.

Cuilla, J. (2000). *The working life: The promise and betrayal of modern work.* New York: Times Books/Random House.

Doty, E. (2002). Organizing to learn: Recognizing and cultivating learning communities. *Seminars for Nurse Managers, 10*(3), 196–205.

Felgen, J., & Kinnaird, L. (2001). Dynamic dialogue: Application to generational diversity. *Seminars for Nurse Managers, 9*(3), 164–168.

Fields, M., & Zwisler, S. (2001). Guiding across the generations: Rediscovering nursing's promise. *Seminars for Nurse Managers, 9*(3), 154–156.

Frusti, D., Niesen, K., & Campion, J. (2003). Creating a culturally competent organization. *Journal of Nursing Administration, 33*(1), 31–38.

Gantz, N. (2002). Leading and empowering the multicultural work team. *Seminars for Nurse Managers, 10*(3), 164–170.

Jones, J. (2003). Dual or dueling culture and commitment. *Journal of Nursing Administration, 33*(4), 235–242.

Koerner, J. (2001). Weaving an integral culture in a diverse workplace. *Seminars for Nurse Managers, 9*(3), 145–146.

Kohn, L., Carrigan, J., & Donaldson, M. (Eds.). (2000). *To err is human: Building a safer health system.* Washington, DC: National Academy Press.

Laschinger, H., & Wong, C. (1999). Staff nurse empowerment and collective accountability: Effect on perceived productivity and self-rated work effectiveness. *Nursing Economics, 17*(6), 308–316, 351.

OCollins, K. (2002). Diverse communities common concerns: Assessing health care quality for minority Americans. Retrieved on August 8, 2003, from http://www.kaisernetwork.org/health.

Reese, S. (1999). The new wave of gen X workers. *Business and Health, 17*(6), 19–23.

Roberts, S. (1983). Oppressed group behavior: Implications for nursing. *Advances in Nursing Science*, July, 21–30.

Robinson-Walker, C. (2002). Guest editorial: Coaching culture. *Seminars for Nurse Managers, 10*(3), 148–149.

Robinson-Walker, C. (2002). The role of coaching in creating cultures of engagement. *Seminars for Nurse Managers, 10*(3), 150–156.

Schein, E. (1991). *Organizational culture and leadership.* San Francisco, CA: Jossey-Bass.

Wenger, E., & Snyder, W. (2000). Communities of practice: The new organizational frontier. *Harvard Business Review, 78*(1), 139–145.

Weston, M. (2001). Leading into the future: Coaching and mentoring generation X employees. *Seminars for Nurse Managers, 9*(3), 157–160.

INDEX